BMA

D1758836

The Evolution of
Memory Systems

Advance Praise
for *The Evolution of Memory Systems*

Capitalizing on major advances in our understanding of both memory and brain evolution, this book provides the first – and long overdue – account of memory systems placed in an evolutionary context. The result is a captivating and comprehensive survey of two histories, the history of the brain and the history of ideas about memory, which culminates in a new and provocative proposal for the origin of memory. Anyone interested in the brain and behaviour, evolution, or the history of science will find *The Evolution of Memory Systems* a stimulating read.

Morgan Barense, Associate Professor and Canada Research Chair in Cognitive Neuroscience, Department of Psychology, University of Toronto, Canada

The authors convincingly demonstrate that memory systems, and perhaps all neural systems, are best understood in terms of when and why they evolved to meet challenges of the past. Thus, this is a book for those interested in how brains work, and how they differ. This impressive book is like no other in its scope on the successive evolution of memory systems from early vertebrates to present-day humans. I want all my students and co-workers to read it.

Jon H. Kaas, Distinguished Centennial Professor of Psychology, Vanderbilt University, USA

A critical component of defining who we are requires an understanding of our individual past experiences and how they are represented in the brain, as well as how our brain, and in particular memory circuits, evolved in mammals. This book is a tour-de-force on the evolution of memory systems in mammals. It provides a wonderful historical perspective, and an extensive comparative analysis. While the major thrust is to understand human capabilities, particularly circuitry involved in memory, the authors painstakingly review the literature and clearly articulate that these systems did not evolve *de novo* in humans, but that a basic plan was present in our earliest ancestors. This type of discussion is rarely found in a neuroscience community entrenched in studies of single animal models. Kudos to the authors for writing the most comprehensive and interesting text currently available on this topic.

Leah Krubitzer, MacArthur Fellow, Professor of Psychology, Center for Neuroscience, University of California, Davis, USA

Through their combined evolutionary and neuroscience approach the authors beautifully reveal the building blocks of memory systems that combine to produce the complexities of cognition in the human brain.

Trevor W. Robbins CBE, Professor of Cognitive Neuroscience and Experimental Psychology, University of Cambridge, UK

This is an important book for several reasons. First, there is the unique way that the authors formulate their proposals within an evolutionary context, explaining what makes memory special in mammals, in primates, and in humans. Second, their survey of the cognitive neuroscience of memory is guided by an exciting and provocative new taxonomy of memory systems that takes the reader far beyond the hippocampus and medial temporal lobe.

Matthew Rushworth, Professor of Cognitive Neuroscience, Department of Experimental Psychology, University of Oxford, UK

The Evolution of Memory Systems

Ancestors, anatomy, and adaptations

Elisabeth A. Murray

Steven P. Wise

Kim S. Graham

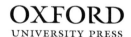
OXFORD
UNIVERSITY PRESS

OXFORD

UNIVERSITY PRESS

Great Clarendon Street, Oxford, OX2 6DP,
United Kingdom

Oxford University Press is a department of the University of Oxford.
It furthers the University's objective of excellence in research, scholarship,
and education by publishing worldwide. Oxford is a registered trade mark of
Oxford University Press in the UK and in certain other countries

© Oxford University Press 2017

The moral rights of the authors have been asserted

First Edition published in 2017

Impression: 1

Published in the United States of America by Oxford University Press
198 Madison Avenue, New York, NY 10016, United States of America

British Library Cataloguing in Publication Data

Data available

Library of Congress Control Number: 2016937962

ISBN 978–0–19–968643–8

Printed and bound by
CPI Group (UK) Ltd, Croydon, CR0 4YY

Oxford University Press makes no representation, express or implied, that the
drug dosages in this book are correct. Readers must therefore always check
the product information and clinical procedures with the most up-to-date
published product information and data sheets provided by the manufacturers
and the most recent codes of conduct and safety regulations. The authors and
the publishers do not accept responsibility or legal liability for any errors in the
text or for the misuse or misapplication of material in this work. Except where
otherwise stated, drug dosages and recommendations are for the non-pregnant
adult who is not breast-feeding

Links to third party websites are provided by Oxford in good faith and
for information only. Oxford disclaims any responsibility for the materials
contained in any third party website referenced in this work.

To our ancestors,
academic and anthropoid alike

Preface

Conception

This book began its life in the back seat of a car, as lives on occasion do. The second author, then a graduate student, accompanied Mort Mishkin and Ted Jones on a quick ride through the campus of Duke University. It was April 1977, and they had to hustle to a symposium somewhere. As the graduate student sat silently in the back seat, Mishkin spoke with building excitement about the famous amnesic patient, H.M. Jones seemed mildly interested, but the graduate student could not have been more enthralled. As an undergraduate he had attended a lecture on H.M., which fertilized a lifelong interest in this seminal clinical case.

During the car ride, Mishkin declared that he had solved a longstanding mystery about H.M. For decades, neuropsychologists had tried and failed to replicate H.M.'s memory impairment in monkeys. In 1977, Mishkin thought he had finally done it by making a lesion that included both the amygdala and the hippocampus. Given what little the graduate student knew about the brain and its evolution, the combination of these two structures seemed odd, but intriguing. At first glance, they did not appear to compose a natural pair. Why, he wondered, would the amygdala and hippocampus hook up in the service of memory, in some sort of exclusive relationship? All the same, a book on the evolution of memory might arouse some interest, he thought, provided that Mishkin's idea stood the test of time. It didn't, but the germ of the book survived in frozen form.

In the interim, the first and third authors studied memory systems intimately, while the second author watched from the back seat, much as he did on that long-ago car ride. Despite undeniable progress in understanding memory systems, no one—even to this day—has successfully placed them in an evolutionary context. Clearly, we would understand memory systems better if we knew when they evolved and the selective pressures that produced them. In 1977, however, and for decades thereafter, brain evolution seemed more mysterious than memory systems would ever be. Slowly, that changed. Neuroscientists now understand brain evolution much better than anyone could have imagined back then. So, after nearly four decades of gestation, it seems like a good time to deliver a book on the evolution of memory systems.

Scope

Although this book considers other species, it emphasizes primates. Not only are all the authors primates, but our proposals depend on the idea that many cortical areas evolved in our order. Readers who view the cortex of other mammals as replicas in miniature or amalgams of primate areas will find our principal thesis unpalatable, to say the least. In Chapter 2 ("New cortical areas")* we summarize some of the evidence supporting our view, but we recognize that many neuroscientists disagree, especially those who study rodents. We respect rodents, but our ancestors diverged from theirs long ago, and primate brains have changed immensely in the meantime. Rodent brains have changed, too.

In addition, some readers might find our neglect of comparative psychology surprising. These studies place the impressive cognitive capacities of our fellow animals beyond doubt, but without generating the kinds of comparisons we need to understand the evolution of memory systems. Instead of comparing the psychology of modern animals, we attempt to understand the adaptations of various ancestors in their time and place.

Likewise, we do not discuss genetic, cellular, or molecular mechanisms. We take it for granted that the central nervous system stores information by adjusting synaptic weights in distributed neural networks. Gene expression, post-translational processing, and protein metabolism—in both presynaptic and postsynaptic components of the relevant neurons—lead to memory formation. If wrong, it hardly matters for our purposes. This book deals with memory at the level of anatomically defined brain systems.

Terminology

Our discussions avoid formal taxonomy, such as *Sus scrofa* for pigs. There is a place for that, but this is not that place. For our purposes, common names will do. We also resort to convenient but slightly erroneous group names from time to time. When we discuss monkeys without further specification, we mean macaques. Other monkeys may complain if they like, but most primate research involves these species. Likewise, we rarely distinguish among the various species of macaques, although we know that they do so with alacrity. By animals and primates, we usually exclude people but sometimes include them, as seems appropriate to the context. Primates are "us" sometimes, at other times "them." When we use a phrase like "monkey neuropsychologist," we trust readers to realize that it refers to research *on* monkeys and not to simian scientists. This is not *Planet of the Apes.*

---

* Throughout the book, references and links to other sections look like this. If no chapter is specified, then the reference is to a section heading within a given chapter.

Acknowledgements

We thank Martin Baum, Charlotte Greene, and Matthias Butler, our editors at Oxford University Press, for their many efforts on behalf of this book. We also thank colleagues who provided comments on selected chapters: Donna Addis, Matthew Apps, Morgan Barense, Mark Baxter, Philip Browning, Tim Bussey, Steve Chang, Paul Cisek, Audrey Duarte, Melissa Duff, Jon Kaas, Leah Krubitzer, Matthew Lambon Ralph, Mark Laubach, Andrew Lawrence, Daeyeol Lee, Lynn Nadel, Dick Passingham, Karalyn Patterson, Charan Ranganath, Peter Rudebeck, Matthew Rushworth, Lisa Saksida, Reza Shadmehr, Matthew Shapiro, Georg Striedter, and Charlie Wilson. Conor Bloomer provided invaluable help with the page proofs. We also express our gratitude to Andrew, Jamie, and Benedict Lawrence. Without their support of this endeavor, one of the authors, and by default the others, might never have finished the book. We also thank Reza Shadmehr for providing the anecdote that begins Chapter 6.

Contents

Abbreviations *xiii*

Glossary *xv*

Epigraph *xix*

Part I **Foundations of memory systems**

1 The history of memory systems *3*

2 The history of the brain *39*

Part II **Architecture of vertebrate memory**

3 The reinforcement memory systems of early animals *85*

4 The navigation memory system of early vertebrates *119*

5 The biased-competition memory system of early mammals *153*

Part III **Primate augmentations**

6 The manual-foraging memory system of early primates *191*

7 The feature memory system of anthropoids *227*

8 The goal memory system of anthropoids *267*

Part IV **Hominin adaptations**

9 The goal and feature memory systems of hominins *305*

10 The social–subjective memory system of hominins *343*

11 The origin of explicit memory in hominins *383*

Part V **Deconstructing and reconstructing memory systems**

12 Deconstructing amnesia *427*

13 Reconstructing memory's past *465*

Epilogue *479*

Index *481*

Abbreviations

A	Amygdala
A1	Primary auditory cortex
AC	Anterior cingulate cortex (area 24)
ADP	Adenosine diphosphate
AgM	Medial agranular (frontal) cortex
AIP	Anterior intraparietal area
ATP	Adenosine triphosphate
BnM	Basal nucleus (of Meynert)
BnST	Bed nucleus of the stria terminalis
CA	*Cornu Ammonis* (Ammon's horn); hippocampal areas
cc	Corpus callosum
CMA(s)	Cingulate motor area(s)
CoA	Cortical nuclei of the amygdala
CR	Conditioned response or conditioned reflex
CS	Conditioned stimulus
DBB	Diagonal band (of Broca)
DC	Dorsal cortex
DMC	Dorsomedial cortex
DREADDs	Designer receptors exclusively activated by designer drugs
DTI	Diffusion tensor imaging
ERh	Entorhinal cortex
ES	Extrastriate visual cortex
FA	Feature ambiguity
FEF	Frontal eye field
fMRI	Functional magnetic resonance imaging
FST	Fundus of the superior temporal sulcus
FDG-PET	Fluoro-deoxyglucose-based positron emission tomography
G	Gustatory cortex
GABA	Gamma-aminobutyric acid, an inhibitory neurotransmitter
GPi	Internal segment of the globus pallidus
GrP	Posterior granular prefrontal area
GrV	Ventral granular prefrontal area
H	Hippocampus
HSVE	*Herpes simplex virus* encephalitis
Ia	Agranular insular cortex
Id	Dysgranular insular cortex
ig	Induseum griseum
IL	Infralimbic cortex
IT	Inferior temporal cortex (excluding PRh)
Lateral PFa	Lateral part of the agranular frontal cortex (OFa and Ia)
LC	Lateral cortex
LIP	Lateral intraparietal area
LOV	Low-order vision
LTD	Long-term depression (of synaptic strength)
LTP	Long-term potentiation (of synaptic strength)
M1	Primary motor cortex
MC	Medial cortex
MIP	Medial intraparietal area
MPTP	Methyl-phenyl-tetrahydropyridine, a neurotoxin that selectively targets dopaminergic cells
MRE	Magnitude of reinforcement extinction effect
MRI	Magnetic resonance imaging
MTL	Medial temporal lobe
MT/MST	Middle temporal area/medial superior temporal area
Oa	Agranular orbitofrontal cortex
PC	Posterior cingulate cortex
PDA	Protostome–deuterostome last common ancestor
PET	Positron emission tomography
PF	Prefrontal cortex
PFc	Caudal prefrontal cortex (area 8, including the frontal eye field)

PFd	Dorsal prefrontal cortex (lateral area 9)
PFdl	Dorsolateral prefrontal cortex (area 46)
PFdm	Dorsomedial prefrontal cortex (medial area 9)
PFo	Granular orbitofrontal cortex (see Table 1.4)
PFp	Polar prefrontal cortex (area 10)
PFvl	Ventrolateral prefrontal cortex (areas 12, 44, 45, and 47)
PH	Parahippocampal cortex
Pir	Piriform cortex
PIT	Pavlovian-to-instrumental transfer
PL	Prelimbic cortex
PM	Premotor cortex (parts of area 6)
PMd	Dorsal premotor cortex
PMv	Ventral premotor cortex
PoRh	Postrhinal cortex
PP	Posterior parietal cortex
PRE	Partial reinforcement extinction effect
PRh	Perirhinal cortex
R–O	Response (action)–outcome association
ROC	Receiver operating characteristic (signal detection)
rs	Rhinal sulcus
RSp	Retrosplenial cortex
rTMS	Repetitive transcranial magnetic stimulation
S	Septal nuclei
S1	Primary somatosensory cortex
S2	Secondary somatosensory cortex
SI	Substantial innominata
S–O	Stimulus–outcome association, Pavlovian memory

S–R	Stimulus–response association, habit
S–R–O	Stimulus–response–outcome association
SEF	Supplementary eye field
SMA	Supplementary motor area
SNc	Substantia nigra pars compacta, a source of dopaminergic cells
SNC	Successive negative contrast effect (case-sensitive abbreviation)
SNr	Substantia nigra pars reticulata
SSA	Supplementary sensory area
SSM	Somatic sensorimotor cortex
ST	Superior temporal cortex
STP	Superior temporal polysensory area
TA	Temporal area A of von Bonin and Bailey
TE/TEa	Rostral parts of the inferior temporal cortex, part of temporal area E of von Bonin and Bailey
TEO	Caudal (occipital) part of the inferior temporal cortex, another part of temporal area E
TMS	Transcranial magnetic stimulation
tt	Tenia tecta
UR	Unconditioned response
US	Unconditioned stimulus
V1	Primary visual cortex, also known as striate cortex (area 17)
V2	Secondary visual cortex
V3	An extrastriate visual area
V4	An extrastriate visual area
VC	Ventral cortex
VIP	Ventral intraparietal area
VP	Ventral pallidum
VTA	Ventral tegmental area, a source of dopaminergic neurons

Glossary

Aegyptopithecus An extinct anthropoid, near the early catarrhines

Agnathans Jawless fishes, specifically hagfish and lamprey, a paraphyletic group

Allocortex A three-layered cortex found in amniotes, including mammals

Amphibians Tetrapods, excluding amniotes; exemplified by frogs, newts, and salamanders, also known as lissamphibians

Amniotes Reptiles, birds, and mammals

Anthropoids Monkeys, apes, and humans

Appendicularians A group of tunicates

Ascidians A group of tunicates

Attribute features Nonmetric features of visual stimuli such as color, shape, visual texture, glossiness, and translucence

Australopiths Extinct hominins

Basal forebrain Ventral telencephalon and diencephalon, including ventral striatum, ventral pallidum, extended amygdala, preoptic areas, and hypothalamus

Carpolestes An extinct plesiadapiform

Catarrhines Old World monkeys, apes, and humans, cf. platyrrhines

Chilecebus An extinct anthropoid, near early platyrrhines

Chordate Notochord-containing deuterostomes

Clade A progenitor species and all of its descendants; an evolutionary lineage

Cladistics An analysis of evolutionary relationships

Cladogram A graphic depiction of evolutionary relationships

Control policy A motor program that specifies the metrics of action

Derived Changed from the ancestral condition

Deuterostomes A clade that includes chordates, tunicates, cephalochordates, echinoderms, and vertebrates

Diffusion tractography A method for tracing fiber fascicles based on imaging the diffusion of water along axonal (white matter) pathways

Episodic memory The explicit memory of events, including the perception of participating in or experiencing the event

Euprimates Primates of modern aspect

Exaptation An evolutionary change that enables future developments

Explicit memory Memories accompanied by a perception of participating or knowing

Gnathostomes Jawed vertebrates, including all modern fishes, amphibians, reptiles, mammals, and birds

Haplorhines Tarsiers and anthropoids

Hippocampal complex Dentate gyrus, cortical fields CA1–CA3, subiculum, fimbria, and fornix

Hominids Chimpanzees, bonobos, gorillas, orangutans, and humans

Hominins Humans and extinct relatives of the same clade, such as australopiths

Hominoids Hominids and gibbons

Homology Trait inherited from a common ancestor

Metric features Measurable features such as durations, distances, temporal order, spatial order, places, sizes, speeds, directions, and number

Orofacial Pertaining to the mouth and/or face, often including the jaws, lips, and tongue

Outgroup A group of species closely related to a clade, but not members of it; *see also*: sister group

Paraphyletic A group of animals with similarities, but not constituting a clade

Parapithecus An extinct anthropoid, near the early anthropoids; also known as *Simonsius*

Panins Chimpanzees and bonobos

Platyrrhines New World monkeys, cf. catarrhines

Plesiadapiform Early primates or close relatives, including *Carpolestes*

Pongids Gorillas, chimpanzees, bonobos, and orangutans

Primitive Resembling the ancestral condition

Problem Behavioral situation in which no previously used process (or similar process) resides in memory to generate a goal

Prosimian Tarsiers and strepsirrhines, a paraphyletic group of primates

Protostome A clade that includes most invertebrate species, such as insects and other arthropods, mollusks, annelids, nematodes, rotifers, and flatworms

Recollection Usually an episodic memory, a form of explicit memory; occasionally a recalled fact, concept, or category (i.e., a semantic memory)

Reptile Amniotes excluding birds and mammals

Semantic memory Explicit memories of facts, accompanied by a perception of knowing; cultural knowledge of concepts, categories, and other generalizations

Sister group The lineage most closely related to the group under consideration

Strepsirrhines Primates excluding haplorhines; includes most prosimians

Subjective memory (1) Belonging to the self; (2) pertaining to or characteristic of one-self; (3) placing emphasis on one's own analyses

Telencephalon Endbrain

Tetrapods Early land animals and their descendants, including amniotes and amphibians

Tunicates A group of deuterostomes

So … apes … descended from men?

Some of us thought so; but it is not exactly that. Apes and men are two separate branches that have evolved from a point in common but in different directions, the former gradually developing to the stage of rational thought, the others stagnating in their animal state. Many orangutans, however, still insist on denying this obvious fact ….

Dr. Zira, *Planet of the Apes* (Pierre Boulle, 1963, pp. 126–7)

Part I

Foundations of memory systems

Two kinds of history influence memory research: the history of ideas about memory and the history of the brain. We introduce these topics in the first two chapters. In Chapter 1 we explain why we wrote the book and provide some background material. In Chapter 2 we present a brief survey of brain evolution.

Chapter 1

The history of memory systems

Overview

Historically, clinical observations and animal research produced a series of conclusions—some right, some wrong—that have shaped our current understanding of memory. Most accounts emphasize a declarative or explicit memory system assigned to four adjacent cortical areas and a habit system attributed to the basal ganglia. The prevailing view of memory systems also segregates memory areas of cortex from perception areas. An evolutionary perspective leads to different ideas in every respect: humans have inherited a diverse assortment of memory systems, each of which evolved in a specific ancestor as it adapted to its time and place; each memory system depends on both the cerebral cortex and the basal ganglia; all cortical areas function in memory; and many contribute to both the memory and perception of their specialized representations.

Memory

What happened to Henry?

In 1953, neurosurgeons removed much of the hippocampus, along with some other brain structures, from Henry Molaison, a patient with severe epilepsy[1]. Soon afterward he became known as H.M., and he had an impact that he would not, and could not, ever know. Although researchers tested H.M.'s memory for more than 50 years[1-6], his principal problem became evident soon after surgery. He had amnesia: in his case, a severe inability to remember newly learned facts and events. He would, for example, forget everything he learned, anything he did, and whoever he met, usually within a few minutes. H.M.'s dramatic impairment inspired generations of psychologists to consider what it means to have—and lose—a memory system. To summarize this book in a single sentence, it explores the evolution of memory systems to better understand the kind of memories that H.M. lost.

Despite its severity, H.M.'s amnesia was of a highly selective kind. He could still learn new motor and perceptual skills, and he could remember most events and facts briefly. He could also remember a lot from his distant past. So as memory researchers attempted to understand H.M.'s amnesia, they focused on what they came to call an anterograde and global impairment in explicit or declarative long-term memory. Unfortunately, these terms do not tell us all that much, and one of them, global, turned out to be misleading (see Chapter 7, "Humans"). In any case, terms that focus on memory impairments tend to neglect intact memories, which they identify only indirectly. The key to understanding H.M.'s amnesia, and that of other such patients, lies as much in their preserved memories as in their impaired ones, and in considering whether terms like anterograde, explicit, and global describe their ailment accurately and adequately.

The term anterograde amnesia emphasizes H.M.'s problem with establishing new memories, and it implies that he retained old ones better. He could remember, for example, where he had lived, as well as famous people from his earlier life. H.M.'s intact memories supported an ability to read, write, and speak, to follow social and moral conventions, and to perform mathematical computations at or near his previous level.

In addition to his relatively preserved retrograde memory, H.M. had a pretty good short-term memory. He could mentally rehearse and manipulate what he had just heard in much the same way as healthy people do, provided that nothing distracted him[7]. In laboratory tests, he attained a nearly perfect memory score for the entire 40-second memory period in one study[8] and remembered a three-digit number for 15 minutes in another[9]. To be clear, H.M. did not have a completely normal short-term memory[8]. As later chapters explain, the pattern of preserved and impaired memories—in H.M. as in other amnesic patients—depends on the kind of representations processed and stored by the missing or damaged areas. But any impairment that H.M. had in short-term memory paled in contrast to his inability to remember new facts and events. He could not have performed more than five decades of memory tests had it been otherwise.

Not only did H.M. have a satisfactory short-term memory, at least for most kinds of information, but he could also establish new long-term memories of many kinds. Accordingly, the literature distinguishes between explicit memory (also called declarative memory), which H.M.'s surgery impaired, and implicit or skill memory (also known as procedural memory, nondeclarative memory, or habits), which remained more-or-less normal. The literature contains many examples of H.M.'s preserved learning of skills. He could, for example, improve at tracing a pattern while viewing his hand in a mirror. He took about 3 days to master this difficult skill, much like healthy people of his age[10]. About 35 years later, H.M. learned how to reach directly to a visual target, despite powerful forces that pushed his hand from the desired trajectory[11]. Practice also improved his perceptual skills, such as reading mirror-image text[1].

Despite his many remaining kinds of memory, H.M.'s amnesia prevented him from living independently. To say merely that H.M. failed to recollect new facts or events does scant justice to the problems that he faced. He could not remember people that entered his life, new places he had been, or events that he had experienced, and so he could not cope with the modern world[1,6]. Milner and her colleagues[3] (p. 217) quoted H.M. as likening his experience to "waking from a dream … every day is alone in itself."

This quotation points to a deeper consequence of H.M.'s amnesia, something difficult to capture with terms like anterograde, explicit, and global. After his surgery, H.M. could not construct a personal narrative of his life experiences. For now we leave it at that, but later, and especially in Chapter 11, we propose that people incorporate representations of themselves into some of their memories and that this capacity results in explicit memory. After his surgery, H.M. could not do that.

What made amnesia monkey business?

From the beginning, memory researchers knew that H.M.'s neurosurgeons had removed several brain structures, including the hippocampus. It therefore seemed reasonable to replicate his amnesia by mimicking that lesion in monkeys and having them perform a memory test[12–14]. We present a history of this effort in Chapter 12 ("The road taken"), but it can be summed up succinctly here: by the 1970s it had failed spectacularly. To the dismay of memory researchers, animals with brain lesions like those in H.M. performed memory tests normally. No one could understand why this experimental approach had failed, but the most popular account invoked vaguely defined "species differences." This notion implied that the memory systems of humans differ from those of monkeys in some crucial—but utterly unspecified—way.

Then, in the mid-1970s, the long run of failures finally ended. Gaffan[15] induced a severe memory impairment in monkeys by cutting the fornix, which conveys axons to and from the hippocampal complex. A few years later, Mishkin[16] observed an impairment on the same kind of memory test that Gaffan had used. Instead of cutting the fornix, Mishkin removed the amygdala and the hippocampus from monkeys, along with some other parts of the brain that received little attention at the time. The reason for the previous failures, according to Mishkin, had nothing to do with species differences. A monkey model of human amnesia merely required making the right kind of lesion in combination with an appropriate memory test.

This book offers a different idea, one that has everything to do with species differences. The psychologists of the 1960s and 1970s failed to replicate H.M.'s amnesia in monkeys because they harbored some outdated ideas about the relationship between humans and monkeys, because memory did not mean to them then what it means to us today, and because they used poorly constrained memory tests, which monkeys can solve in many different ways. In Chapter 12 we explain how these problems, and especially the first one, led some experts astray.

Fortunately, our understanding of these issues has come a long way since the 1970s. First, we now understand the relationships among monkeys, humans, and other animals well enough to avoid the misunderstandings of the past. Evolutionary biology has done away with folk theories that treat monkeys as part of a linear progression from "primitive" animals to modern humans. Although it took a long time to catch on, modern biology can inform our understanding of memory systems in a way that psychologists of the 1970s could scarcely have imagined.

Second, we have a much better idea about what memory means. Computer scientists and information theorists have explained that memory means stored information: nothing more and nothing less. Knowing this, we can understand that H.M.'s amnesia involved selective aspects of memory. As behaviorism gave way to a more cognitive approach to psychology in the 1970s, it became possible to identify different forms of memory in both humans and animals. It has become fashionable to refer to each kind of memory as a system, and much of this book explores what the term *memory system* means. In particular, we ask why memory seems to be organized in systems. Our answer is that new representational systems evolved at certain times and places—in a particular ancestral species—and that they augmented existing representations when they did.

Just as important as what the term memory system means is what it doesn't mean. In this book, if nowhere else in the literature, the term memory system does not imply the lack of additional functions. In a sense, this statement follows from standard logic, and it leads us to use the terms *memory system* and *representational system* interchangeably. In addition to memory, the evidence shows that some representational systems also have perceptual functions (Chapter 7) and others contribute to the control of movements (Chapter 6). Although some experts reject the idea of memory systems altogether[17,18], an evolutionary perspective supports the idea that representational specializations emerged as integrated systems:

- Suites of representational adaptations developed during major evolutionary transitions (see "Homologies"), and the term system recognizes the interdependent adaptive advantages that they provide.

- Evolution commonly produces structures that emerge in response to particular selective pressures, but also perform other functions. To reject the label *memory system* because its neural substrates perform additional functions is like denying that wings function as a mechanical system for flight because animals also use them for social signaling, as many insects and birds do.

- Memory appears to be the function that ties together the several representational systems discussed in this book. Visual areas of cortex, for example, function in both memory and perception (Chapter 7), but they play only an indirect role in controlling action. The premotor areas have a form of memory that guides movements (Chapter 6), but they contribute relatively little to perception.

Third, neuropsychologists now use more sophisticated and rigorous behavioral tests than in the past, in both monkeys and humans. Counterintuitively, some of the most important advances in understanding memory in humans have come from adapting memory tests devised originally for monkey research (see Chapter 7, "The perception–memory dichotomy"). Monkey neuropsychologists now pay more attention to the effect of damage to nearby areas and fiber pathways than in the past. The development of methods for making reversible and selective lesions, which leave nearby axonal pathways relatively intact, has advanced the neuroanatomical rigor of the field immeasurably, and functional brain imaging has added important insights. Likewise, structural brain imaging has dramatically improved the ability of neuropsychologists to assess the extent of brain lesions in neurological and neurosurgical patients, to an extent that would probably have seemed miraculous in the 1970s. Future technological developments promise yet more progress of this kind.

And yet, despite these crucial conceptual and methodological advances, the dominant theory of memory differs little from the one that emerged in the 1970s and 1980s. The situation resembles a living fossil: a species that has remained little changed for millions of years. Ideas about memory systems have not stagnated for quite that long, but an overhaul seems long overdue.

What does the prevailing view say?

Table 1.1 presents the prevailing view of memory systems, the one commonly encountered in textbooks and in most summaries of memory research. Although there is much more to this theory than can be captured in the table, many neuroscientists appear to accept these tenets in particular.

The most common version of the prevailing view holds that the brains of all mammals—including humans and monkeys—have a declarative or explicit memory system, attributed to a conceptual construct called the "medial temporal lobe"[19]. In addition, they have one or a few other memory systems, such as a "habit system" that depends on the basal ganglia[19-21] and various emotional, conditioning, and perceptual priming mechanisms lumped with habits as implicit, nondeclarative, or procedural memories. The prevailing view also holds that other brain areas perform different functions, such as perception, motor control, executive functions, attention, and so forth, but they—for some reason—do not count as memory systems. This book poses a simple question: "Why not?"

Why ask "why not?"

By posing this question, a new view of memory systems emerges, one that makes it natural to ask how representational systems arose in evolution. To understand memory, we need to know not only which brain structures implement each kind of memory, but also when and why they came to do so. And to obtain such knowledge, we need to reconstruct the history of memory systems.

Table 1.1 The prevailing view of memory systems

Memory system	Brain structure
Habits	Basal ganglia
Explicit memory	Medial temporal lobe
Emotional conditioning	Amygdala
Motor conditioning	Cerebellum
Priming	Sensory cortex

The word history sometimes contrasts with prehistory, but the Greek *historia* referred originally to "learning by seeking the truth," and the phrase natural history has long referred to organismal biology. In this vein, we use the word *history* in two senses:

◆ The first deals with evolutionary history. When did the brain areas contributing to a given memory system first emerge? What might have been the selective pressures operating at those times? Few proponents of the prevailing view have asked why the structures that compose memory systems ended up where they are, or where they might have come from. We provide some answers in Chapter 2.

◆ The second deals with intellectual history. How did the prevailing view develop? And how did the focus of memory research settle on a hodgepodge of cortical structures called "the medial temporal lobe"? We address these questions in Chapter 12 ("The road taken").

To reconstruct the history of memory systems, in both senses, we have to ask why the brain and the field of memory research have the history that they have.

Why ask "why?"

As opposed to "how" questions, which evoke answers in terms of anatomy and physiology, "why" questions call for evolutionary answers. Proponents of the prevailing view have rarely addressed evolution and have never done so adequately. When they have tried, they usually relied on outmoded or discredited ideas about evolution. We describe these deficiencies in Chapters 2 ("Outdated concepts" and "Rings and wrongs") and 12 ("The road taken" and "The habit–memory dichotomy"), where we explain how they led the field down the wrong road at times.

The vast majority of writing on memory systems, however, does not suffer from any of these problems because it does not deal with evolution at all. Instead, it simply treats memory systems as if they fell from the sky into the modern world. We know otherwise, of course. The ability to learn from experience is a biological trait. And, like all biological traits, monkeys and humans acquire, store, and retrieve information in ways that reflect their long evolutionary history, much of it common and more recently separate. Accordingly, for reasons that we explain in Chapter 11 ("Conclusions"), we know with certainty that the following two statements are true:

◆ The kinds of memory that H.M. lost did not exist in all of his ancestors.

◆ Yet in some of them it did.

Surely we should want to know more about that. Knowing, even roughly, when, in what kind of animal, or in what ecological circumstances a neural system evolved provides important clues about its most fundamental functions.

We recognize that one can develop a theory of memory systems without reference to evolution. Indeed, many experts say that evolution has little relevance to their research because they study how neuronal systems function or fail in the modern world. One does not need to know how the system reached its current state in order to perform such research.

We also know that some memory researchers believe that the current understanding of brain evolution is so uncertain that it does not merit serious consideration. In the 1970s, when the prevailing view took shape, this opinion had more validity than it does today[22-25]. Obviously, we still do not have all the evidence we want. The same could be said for every research topic, of course, but the problem seems different for evolution. Unlike other aspects of neuroscience, brain evolution deals with events that occurred millions of years ago, when natural selection acted on species that are now extinct. Unlike some structures, such as teeth and bones, brains do not fossilize. Therefore, with the exception of some fossil evidence about brain size and sulci, nearly everything we know about brain evolution comes from comparing modern species. Comparative methods inevitably depend on inference, likelihood, and the principle of parsimony, well short of proof.

On top of that, understanding brain evolution is no easy task. To follow this literature neuroscientists have to wade through a thicket of thorny terms and alien concepts. Consider the following passage:

> Insofar as Gerstang's hypothesis of phylogeny within the chordates is concerned, the finding that appendicularians probably branch more basally than ascidians requires a revision of the presumed ancestral chordate. One solution is just to switch the ancestral chordate from an ascidian to an appendicularian larva. In this case, there need be little change in the notion of a paedomorphic chordate ancestor. Appendicularians would represent a pelagic descendant of the founding deuterostomes, perhaps sister to the enteropneusts. In an alternative evolutionary model, the adult appendicularian ancestor could have given rise to crown appendicularians and to cephalochordates. This scenario obviates any requirement for a paedomorphic origin of the chordate bodyplan.
>
> Valentine[26] (p. 424)

No doubt, evolutionary biologists would struggle with our writings, as we do with theirs. Unfortunately, we need to understand what they have to say, but they can get along perfectly well without reading a word about memory. A partial translation: Gerstang proposed that chordates arose from the larvae of an ancestral species; this might be true, but perhaps not.

Given all this, why not simply ignore evolution? One answer is that by doing so we would forfeit an important source of insight. Take monkeys, for example. No biologist doubts that at some point in evolutionary history monkeys did not exist. Today, there are more than 200 species of monkeys[27]. Chapter 2 explains that certain cortical areas first appeared in a particular ancestor of modern monkeys. The circumstances in which these animals evolved provide some insight into the functions of their new cortical areas. So, in addition to considering cortical function in the usual ways, it might also be valuable to consider the problems and opportunities faced by the animals in which a particular cortical area emerged or elaborated.

We are well aware that the account of memory presented here will need extensive correction and improvement as research progresses. But we hope that our general approach—an attempt to blend structure, function, and evolution—will provide a template for future advances along these lines. We view our book more as a "first word" than a "last word" on the evolution of memory systems.

Why ask anything?

How could we present a "first word" if so much has already been written? Why ask any questions if memory researchers already have the answers? One reason is that previous attempts to discuss the evolution of memory[28] have been dominated by the prevailing view of memory systems. And this is a problem because, as two of us put it previously (Murray and Wise[29], p. 194), the currently dominant theory of memory "is parsimonious, it is attractive, it is extraordinarily popular, and it is wrong." Later chapters spell out the reasons for this conclusion, but four points suffice to introduce the topic:

1. The prevailing view depicts each part of the so-called "medial temporal lobe" as functioning cooperatively in the service of a single kind of memory. The best evidence from monkeys, however, shows otherwise; its different cortical areas perform distinct functions—and sometimes opposing ones[29]. For readers who suspect a straw man argument, we quote one authoritative formulation: "the severity of memory impairment increases as additional components of the medial temporal lobe memory system are damaged" (Zola-Morgan et al.[30], p. 493). We rebut this assertion in Chapter 12 ("The equipotentiality principle").

2. Functional brain imaging studies in humans support the previous point, to such an extent that experts in this field have by-and-large dispensed with this aspect of the prevailing view. We take up this topic in Chapter 7 ("Representational specializations"). Not only do different parts of the so-called "medial temporal lobe" perform different functions[31,32], but the prefrontal cortex and the anterior temporal lobe contribute to memory in ways that the prevailing theory ignores[32–35].

3. A contemporary view of brain organization makes the concept of a "medial temporal lobe memory system," as currently espoused, seem arbitrary and ill-founded: a mere cultural construct rather than a real "thing"[29]. We explain why in Chapter 2 ("Conclusions").

4. The failings of the prevailing view become less surprising in light of the history of the field. Some of its key tenets originated from experiments on monkeys that tested memory on an inappropriate time-scale, lacked proper control procedures, used a poorly constrained behavioral task, and depended upon arbitrarily chosen stimulus material[36]. We examine this literature in Chapters 7 ("The perception–memory dichotomy") and 12 ("The road taken").

We appreciate, however, that it is not enough to criticize the received wisdom on memory systems. According to an old baseball adage, "you can't replace somebody with nobody." In the world of memory science, that maxim doesn't mean very much, and in baseball it doesn't mean a whole lot more. But it makes the point that however frustrating your catcher might be, somebody has to catch. And that's the catch: If we reject the prevailing view, what might replace it? The answer depends on the questions posed.

What should we ask?

We understand memory systems only poorly if we cannot say when they came about and why. Accordingly, we pose three questions in this book:

◆ What representational systems evolved?

◆ When and in what kind of animal did each one develop?

◆ Why did these developments occur, i.e., what adaptive advantages did a particular representational system provide?

As explained earlier (see "Why ask 'why?'"), the last question is especially important[37], and an example from another field illustrates this point. The kidney functions to cleanse the blood of toxins and metabolic waste, to regulate electrolyte levels, and to expel undesirable compounds as urine. To perform this function, the kidney's basic structural unit, the nephron, consists of a knot of capillaries called the glomerulus, aligned with a renal tubule. These structures use passive filtration and selective reabsorption to perform the kidney's functions, which explains a lot about how the kidney works, but not why. The ultimate cause of the kidney's function is its evolutionary history, which led to the kidney being like it is and doing what it does.

Although outdated in its details, and politically incorrect in its language, Homer Smith's *From Fish to Philosopher*[38] addressed both the how and why of kidneys. In 1953, the year of H.M.'s surgery, he wrote about "how our kidneys work, and of how they came to work the way they do—which is the story of the evolution of the vertebrates, of which man is the most notable and intelligent species and the only philosopher" (Smith[38], p. 3). "Superficially," he offered, "it might be said that the function of the kidneys is to make urine; but in a more considered view one can say that the kidneys make the stuff of philosophy itself." If renal physiology has something to say about the origin of philosophy, how much more should we expect from the neuropsychology of memory?

The next three sections provide some answers to our questions: the what, when, and why of memory systems.

What did evolution produce?

We recognize seven memory systems, which we discuss in Chapters 3–10. For convenience, we have given each of these systems a one- or two-word name. Some of these labels refer to the selective pressures that contributed to their emergence, others to the kinds of specialized representations that they have, and still others to functions that they perform. Readers will find ample opportunity to disagree with all of these names, but we emphasize two points about them: (1) none are meant to provide a comprehensive description of the functions that a memory system performs; and (2) a label, in itself, cannot provide a sound basis for rejecting a proposal. These names permit some economy of reference, nothing more, and in most cases it is obvious that they refer to only a part of what a particular memory system does.

We offer answers to the question "What did evolution produce?" chapter by chapter:

◆ *Reinforcement memory* refers to associations among stimuli, responses, and outcomes adjusted by reinforcing feedback (see Chapter 3).

◆ *Navigation memory* depends on a cognitive map that guides foraging and other journeys (see Chapter 4).

◆ *Biased-competition memory* consists of specialized representations that generate a top-down bias on other representations as they compete to control behavior (see Chapter 5).

◆ *Manual-foraging memory* guides choices among valuable items and helps obtain them through visually guided movements (see Chapter 6).

◆ *Feature memory* includes two specific classes of sensory dimensions: attributes and metrics. Attributes include color, shape, visual texture, glossiness, and translucence for vision, along with analogous properties for audition. Metrics include places, numbers, likelihoods, sizes, speeds, order, distances, and durations (see Chapters 7 and 9).

◆ *Goal memory* refers to the objects and places that serve as targets of action, in conjunction with contexts, actions, and behavioral outcomes that become associated with such goals (see Chapters 8 and 9).

◆ *Social–subjective memory* comprises representations of one's self and others that underlie social knowledge and self-reflection (see Chapter 10).

When did memory systems evolve?

These representational systems evolved at different times, in different ancestors, adding to existing systems by a form of accretion:

◆ The reinforcement systems appeared early in the history of animals, as these organisms developed the ability to move and had to make choices about whether, when, and how to do so (see Chapter 3).

◆ The navigation system arose in early vertebrates, along with the telencephalon and brain systems for guiding movements (see Chapter 4).

◆ The biased-competition system evolved in early mammals, which developed the neocortex (see Chapter 5).

◆ The manual-foraging system, which emerged in early primates, was subserved by a suite of new cortical areas that stored memories about how to find, evaluate, reach for, grasp, and manipulate valuable items, along with other movements that draw on similar representations (see Chapter 6).

◆ The goal and feature systems first appeared in anthropoid primates (see Chapters 7 and 8). Later they changed in a key way (see Chapter 9), and some of these developments occurred during human evolution.

◆ The social–subjective system emerged during human evolution (see Chapter 10).

Why did memory systems evolve?

A blend of what, when, and why forms the backbone of this book. The last two sections indicated what representational systems evolved and when. As for why, we suggest the following selective pressures:

◆ The reinforcement systems prepared animals for nutrients and dangers and increased the likelihood of beneficial actions, including those that minimized harm (see Chapter 3).

◆ The navigation system used information from distance receptors, especially those for vision and olfaction, to guide mobile, predatory foraging and to find safe haven based on cognitive maps of the world. Once its specialized representations evolved, they became available for a wide variety of functions well beyond navigation per se (see Chapter 4).

◆ The biased-competition system regulated representations elsewhere in the brain that compete to control behavior. In so doing, its own representations promoted what might be called energy management or energy economics, including high-energy, patient, or urgent foraging strategies when warranted, as well as more flexible switching among the strategies used for obtaining resources (see Chapter 5).

◆ The manual-foraging system exploited the visual developments of early primates by guiding the search for and acquisition of valuable items, as well as by evaluating objects and actions in accord with current biological needs. As with the other memory systems, once its specialized representations emerged they could be adapted to a wide variety of motor functions, including defensive and social behavior (see Chapter 6).

◆ The feature system exploited further developments in primate vision, which occurred in anthropoids and some of their proximate ancestors. This system specialized in representations about the metrics of resources, such as their quantity and distance, as well as qualitative signs of resources, especially at a distance. Among other contributions to fitness, these innovations improved foraging choices (see Chapter 7).

◆ The goal system used sensory information from the feature system to generate goals based on single events and abstract strategies. As a result, anthropoid primates learned faster and made fewer foraging errors than their ancestors: a crucial advantage during shortfalls in resources, especially in the face of severe predation risks (see Chapter 8).

◆ The goal and feature systems later adapted their foraging specializations to general problem-solving and multiple demand cognition, as well as to generalized conceptual and categorical knowledge (see Chapter 9).

◆ The social–subjective system established species-specific representations of one's self and others as an adaptation to the social systems that developed during human evolution. Several far-reaching emergent properties depended on these representations (see Chapters 10 and 11).

Why make it so complicated?

We recognize that these three lists might seem a hodgepodge. Why place so much emphasis on anthropoids? Why give navigation such a fundamental place in the pantheon of brain functions? What does manual foraging have to do with memory systems? What happened to habits and declarative memory? And, above all, why make it so complicated?

Table 1.2 summarizes our proposals and Table 1.3 contrasts them with the prevailing view of memory systems. We know full well that Table 1.2 will not overturn the dominant ideas about memory overnight—or over many nights. Instead, we offer it as a new perspective, one that experts in memory research, investigators in related fields, and students might ponder as they pursue their projects. Although, taken together, our proposals are more complicated than the prevailing view, we hope that they might provide a framework for synthesizing a broad scope of knowledge: concepts that others can consider, correct, and complement in light of their own expertise.

Outdated though it may be, we understand why the prevailing view has retained its popularity for so long: it epitomizes simplicity and parsimony. Not only is it readily remembered, but disputing it demands a detailed discussion. However, a more complicated alternative might thrive if it offers something worthwhile.

Another reason for complexity follows from a fundamental principle of evolution: natural selection produces advantages, not parsimony. Furthermore, it is both a truism and a tautology that evolutionary augmentations arise from an ancestral condition that lacked those traits. Not all such changes increase complexity, of course; simplification and loss of traits often occur as well. But increases in complexity have occurred frequently during evolution, and every descendant species developed from a reasonably successful ancestor. So every evolutionary innovation must be "unnecessary" in some sense because an ancestor got along without it. In Chapters 4–10, we discuss evolutionary changes that

Table 1.2 The evolutionary accretion model

Memory system	Ancestor	Brain structures
Reinforcement	Early animals	Various[a]
Navigation	Early vertebrates	Hippocampal complex
Biased competition	Early mammals	Agranular prefrontal cortex
Manual foraging	Early primates	Posterior parietal, premotor, inferior temporal, and granular prefrontal cortex
Feature	Anthropoids	Posterior parietal, inferior and superior temporal, and perirhinal cortex
Goal	Anthropoids	Granular prefrontal cortex
Social–subjective	Hominins	Granular prefrontal cortex

[a]Basal forebrain, extended basal ganglia, extended amygdala, dopaminergic neurons, cerebellar cortex, deep cerebellar nuclei, and inferior olivary nuclei, among other structures.

Table 1.3 Contrasts between two views of memory

Topic	Prevailing view	Evolutionary accretion model[a]
Functions of cortical areas	Some areas function in memory, others in perception, and still others in "executive" or motor control	All areas function in memory, using specialized representations
Substrate of explicit (declarative) memory	Four cortical areas called "the medial temporal lobe"	Interactions among the navigation, feature, goal, and social–subjective systems[b]
Substrate of implicit (nondeclarative) memory	The basal ganglia as a whole	Cortex–basal ganglia "loops"[c] that have weak links to social–subjective memories[d]
Evolution	Habits and the basal ganglia evolved in "reptiles"; explicit (declarative) memory and the limbic cortex evolved in "primitive" mammals[e]	New, specialized representations emerged as five specific ancestral species adapted to a new way of life, in their time and place

[a] Accretion, in this sense, refers to additions over time.

[b] See Chapter 11 ("Contributing representational systems").

[c] See Plate 1(B).

[d] See Chapter 11 ("Excluded systems").

[e] See Chapter 12 ("The habit–memory dichotomy").

critics will surely view as "unnecessary" or overly complex: lacking parsimony, they will say. If the prevailing view of memory systems explains everything in terms of associations among stimuli, responses, and outcomes[39], why do we need anything more complicated than that? The development, in early vertebrates, of a navigation memory system (see Chapter 4) seems unnecessary from this perspective. So does the idea that early primates developed a new representational system that guides reaching movements with vision (see Chapter 6). Critics will say that invertebrates also navigate and that many animals use vision to guide movements. Of course they do, but new representational systems evolved in early vertebrates and primates anyway because they provided an advantage over the ancestral condition. These advantages provided an increase in fitness in a world of risks and opportunities, not necessarily a qualitatively new capacity. Stated differently, the complexity of our proposals reflects evolution's untidy way of modifying ancestral systems for competitive advantage.

We believe that Table 1.2 agrees better with the available evidence than does the dominant account of memory. But even if it didn't, we would still search for something more than the prevailing view provides. We want to know where our memories come from, and an adequate answer cannot be as simple as "the medial temporal lobe." One reason is that our memories come not only from our brains, but also from our ancestors.

And our mnemonic ancestry goes back a long way. Earlier we mentioned Homer Smith's classic book, *From Fish to Philosopher*[38]. His title recognizes the fact that our ancestry includes not only the first philosophers but also the first vertebrates. Although it is wrong to say that we retain an "inner fish"[40] or a "reptilian brain"[41], it is true that we descended from the first vertebrates, the first land animals (early tetrapods), and the first animals to reproduce on land (early amniotes). Early mammals, early primates, and early hominins also number among our ancestors. Although we are not very fishy, we descend from animals that were; notwithstanding our bipedal habit, we are tetrapods because we descended from the ancestral tetrapods; and although we do not have reptilian parts inside our brains, a common ancestor gave rise to all birds, mammals, and reptiles, including us. When we view ourselves, in full, as vertebrates, tetrapods, amniotes, mammals, primates, and hominins—in addition to philosophers—we can gain the foothold that we need to grasp the evolution of memory systems.

Earlier sections listed the what, when, and why of memory systems separately. It is time to tie the three lists together.

What do we propose?

The epitome of our proposal, which we call the *evolutionary accretion model* of memory, is this: that early vertebrates used one of their innovations, the telencephalon, along with sensory receptors concentrated on their heads, to guide mobile, predatory foraging and defense (see Chapter 2); that the telencephalon included a homologue of the hippocampus, which housed a navigation system that stored and used cognitive maps (see Chapter 4); that, at first, the navigation system functioned mainly in concert with the older reinforcement systems (see Chapter 3), which guided behavior by linking stimuli and actions to biological costs and benefits; that, later, several new representational systems evolved (see Chapters 5–10), each of which reflected the adaptations of a specific ancestor; and that, when the newest one—the social–subjective system (see Chapter 10)—began to interact with older ones, ancestral humans developed the kind of memory that H.M. lost, which involves the perception of knowing facts and participating in events (see Chapter 11).

Where do we go from here?

Stated in a single—albeit very long—sentence, our proposal might seem like a "just so" story. Rudyard Kipling wrote, for example, about how the camel acquired its hump; the ancestral camel simply needed the hump's fat and water to work unceasingly for 3 days, which it had foolishly agreed to do. As the chapters unfold, we hope that readers will appreciate an evidence-based approach, as opposed to presuming how evolution "must have" worked. The evidence is not all that we would like it to be, and it is not what it will some day become. Uncertainties and mysteries abound, but we know enough about evolution in general, and brain evolution in particular, to help us understand memory systems.

To gain this level of understanding, however, requires us to delve into neuroanatomy, neuropsychology, and evolutionary biology. The remainder of this chapter provides some background material on each of these fields in turn.

Anatomy

Terminology

Many discussions in this book assume that readers know about basic neuroanatomy, but we take some liberties with standard terminology. For example, some familiar terms have unfamiliar meanings:

+ Basal ganglia, striatum, and pallidum are used in an extended sense, which includes many telencephalic structures with striatal and pallidal architectures that textbooks typically exclude from the basal ganglia.

+ Neocortex includes all of the cortical areas that evolved in mammals, without reference to subtypes such as proisocortex and periallocortex.

(Two sections—"Basal ganglia" and "Cerebral cortex"—explain our reasons for these choices.)

We also avoid some commonly used terms and invent some new ones. Most experts in memory research consider the hippocampus to be a temporal lobe structure. It does seem to be so in primates, but in Chapter 2 ("Distortions of medial cortex") we explain that as the cerebral cortex expanded in mammals some of its components migrated so much that their ancestral arrangement became difficult to appreciate. Therefore we sometimes describe structures in terms of their ancestral locations rather than their current ones. Referring to the hippocampus as the medial cortex and avoiding the term "medial temporal lobe" has a downside, of course, but we hope that the benefits outweigh the costs.

One novel term involves the poles and axis of the hippocampus. As usual, the septal hippocampus corresponds to the posterior hippocampus in primates and the dorsal hippocampus in rodents. The counterpart is usually called the temporal hippocampus, which corresponds to the anterior hippocampus in primates and the ventral hippocampus in rodents. Because we do not think that the term *temporal* applies properly to any part of the hippocampus, we refer to an "amygdaloid hippocampus" instead, partly because this part of the hippocampus has dense interconnections with the amygdala[42] and partly owing to proximity.

The hippocampus presents some other terminological challenges as well. To simplify matters, we use the term hippocampal complex to refer collectively to the subiculum, the CA1–3 fields, and the dentate gyrus, along with the fimbria and fornix.

In addition, some terms have so many conflicting uses that we simply need to choose one and apply it consistently. In this book, the inferior temporal cortex always excludes the perirhinal cortex, and it includes both the middle and inferior temporal gyri in humans. The anterior cingulate cortex never includes the subgenual, prelimbic, or infralimbic areas.

In general, we use the terms that neuroanatomists use when conversing with each other. Some neuroscientists prefer more formal language: *corpus striatum* rather than striatum, *sulcus principalis* instead of principal sulcus, and so forth. However, neuroanatomists rarely speak in Latin if they can avoid it.

On the other hand, avoiding Latin nomenclature for its own sake would simply confuse everyone. Few readers would benefit if we translated the globus pallidus into the pale sphere, the substantia innominata into unnamed rubbish, or the substantia nigra pars compacta into the dense part of the dark stuff. So we don't. Reading about obscure structures such as the induseum griseum and the tenia tecta might be less than wholly joyful, but we hope that an evolutionary perspective will help readers overcome their agony, if they suffer any.

Brain organization

Figure 1.1(A) presents an overview of vertebrate neuroanatomy, mainly to set the stage for Fig. 1.1(B), which illustrates the motor system. The central nervous system functions to control the body in various ways, with movements being the most conspicuous. Anatomists rarely include neuroendocrine, neurosecretory, and autonomic outputs in the motor system, as Fig. 1.1(B) does, but—like the neuromuscular system—all three of these outputs mediate control of the body by the central nervous system. This abstract statement might seem remote from the topic of memory, but it is relevant because natural selection can only operate on a neural system through motor outputs, however indirectly. Even the most powerful memory system cannot contribute to adaptive success unless it

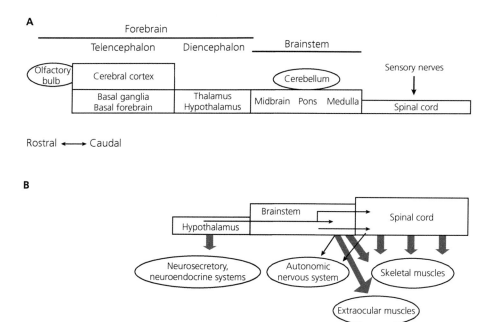

Fig. 1.1 The central nervous system. (A) The major subdivisions of the vertebrate brain and spinal cord. (B) Motor outputs of the central nervous system. From Shadmehr R, Wise SP. *The Computational Neurobiology of Reaching and Pointing*, © 2005, published by The MIT Press.

promotes beneficial behavior. However, for this to be true behavior must be construed in its broadest sense, to include all of the ways in which the central nervous system controls the body.

Basal ganglia

Figure 1.2 illustrates a hierarchical view of telencephalic organization. In traditional anatomy, the telencephalon includes the neocortex, hippocampus, basal ganglia, septal nucleus, amygdala, claustrum, and much more.

Beginning in the 1970s, however, neuroanatomists developed a different view of the telencephalon. Evidence accumulated that many structures in the murky environs of the

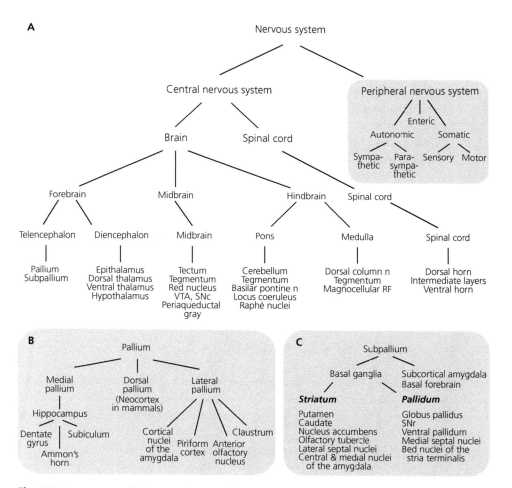

Fig. 1.2 Components of the central nervous system. (A) Hierarchical depiction of the vertebrate nervous system. (B) Components of the pallium. (C) Components of the subpallium, including the basal ganglia. Abbreviations: n, nucleus; RF, reticular formation; SNc, substantia nigra pars compacta; SNr, substantia nigra pars reticulata; VTA, ventral tegmental area.

basal forebrain are actually obscure parts of the basal ganglia. As a result, neuroanatomists began to recognize that telencephalic structures other than the caudate, putamen, and globus pallidus were components of the basal ganglia. Figure 1.2(C) presents a selected list of these structures. Accordingly, when we use the terms striatum, pallidum, and basal ganglia we refer to a much larger collection of telencephalic structures than most textbooks do. In Chapter 2 ("Rings, loops, and memory") we explain why this "hard-core" neuroanatomy has direct relevance to understanding memory systems.

Cerebral cortex

Two fundamental types of cerebral cortex compose the cerebral cortex as a whole. In this book we call them the neocortex and the allocortex. As an approximation, they can be characterized as six-layer and three-layer cortex, respectively.

The word neocortex means new cortex, and in Chapter 2 ("Early amniotes" and "Early mammals") we present evidence that, relative to other kinds of cortex, these areas evolved relatively recently—in early mammals or their immediate ancestors. And when we say "relative to other kinds of cortex," we mean that literally: allocortex means "other cortex."

The literature contains a welter of additional names for varieties of cortex. For reasons that Chapter 2 explains ("Early mammals" and "Rings and wrongs"), we reject the idea that the mammalian cerebral cortex has intermediate types that evolved in successive stages[43]. Instead, we treat all of the areas that evolved in mammals as neocortex. Therefore, as we use the term neocortex it includes juxtallocortex, periallocortex, and proisocortex, which are sometimes classed as transition cortex, as well as many of the areas typically included in the limbic cortex.

In our usage, neocortex means the same thing as isocortex, and it encompasses all varieties, including homotypical, agranular, granular, and dysgranular cortex. Homotypical cortex has a proportionate complement of cortical layers; agranular cortex has no layer 4 or one so sparse as to be difficult to identify; the granular cortex usually means cortex with a hypertrophied layer 4, which is typical of primary sensory areas; and dysgranular cortex has a visible but sparse layer 4. In violation of these definitions, however, we call homotypical and dysgranular regions of the primate prefrontal cortex "granular" because, in a frontal context, any layer 4 attracts attention.

The neocortex of humans and other large primates contains numerous cortical fields, some obvious and well established by a convergence of anatomical, physiological, behavioral, and other data. Others, however, even those repeated in textbooks and brain atlases, result from nothing more than guesswork and precedent. And one can find examples of just about everything in between.

Figure 1.3 shows the terms and subdivisions used in this book, adapted from a cortical map of the macaque monkey brain published by Petrides and Pandya[44]. Figure 1.4 shows the names of sulci and numbers for selected cortical areas. We emphasize macaque monkeys because much of this book depends on data from these species. Figure 1.5 presents a roughly comparable drawing for the human brain.

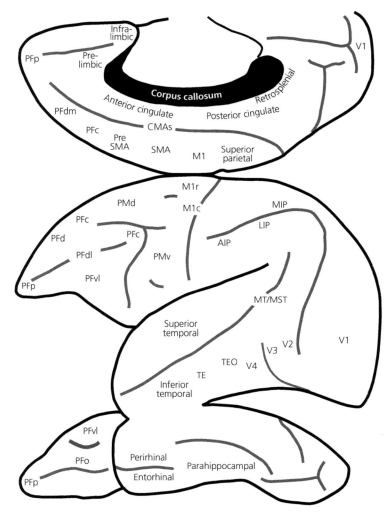

Fig. 1.3 Names for cortical regions in macaque monkeys. Rostral is to the left. From top to bottom: medial view with ventral up; lateral view with dorsal up; ventral view with lateral up. Abbreviations: AIP, anterior intraparietal area; CMA, cingulate motor area; LIP, lateral intraparietal area; M1, primary motor cortex; MIP, medial intraparietal area; MT/MST, middle temporal area/medial superior temporal area; PFc, caudal prefrontal cortex; PFd, dorsal prefrontal cortex; PFdl, dorsolateral prefrontal cortex; PFdm, dorsomedial prefrontal cortex; PFo, granular orbitofrontal cortex (see Table 1.4); PFp, polar prefrontal cortex; PFvl, ventrolateral prefrontal cortex; PMd, dorsal premotor cortex; PMv, ventral premotor cortex; SMA, supplementary motor area; TE, rostral part of the inferior temporal cortex; TEO, caudal (occipital) part of the inferior temporal cortex; V1, primary visual cortex; V2, secondary visual cortex; V3 and V4, extrastriate visual areas. Redrawn from the original by Petrides and Pandya[44]. From Passingham RE, Wise SP. *The Neurobiology of the Prefrontal Cortex*, © 2012, Oxford University Press. Reproduced with permission of OUP.

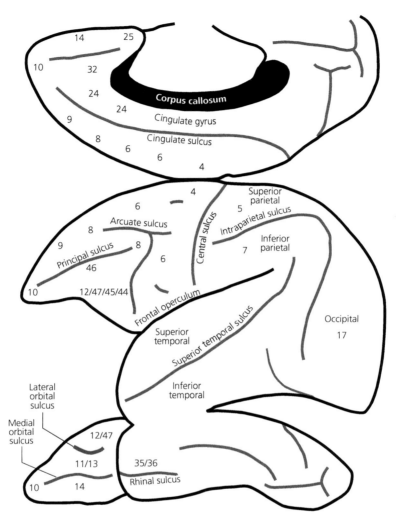

Fig. 1.4 Names for selected regions, sulci, and gyri in macaque monkeys. Numerals indicate cortical areas. Format as in Fig. 1.3. Redrawn from the original by Petrides and Pandya[44]. From Passingham RE, Wise SP. *The Neurobiology of the Prefrontal Cortex*, © 2012, Oxford University Press. Reproduced with permission of OUP.

Of special importance, Fig. 1.3 depicts several prefrontal areas. The brain maps of Walker[45] and Brodmann[46,47] provide the point of departure for their names, but without strict adherence to either. In several figures we have had to resort to abbreviations, including:

- ◆ PFc, the caudal prefrontal cortex (part of area 8), including the frontal eye field;
- ◆ PFd, the dorsal prefrontal cortex (the lateral part of area 9);

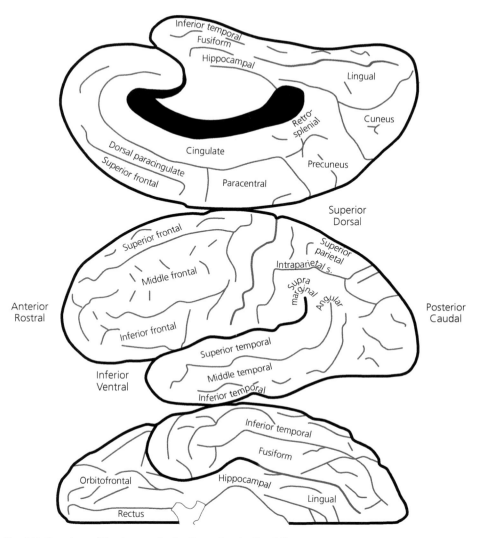

Fig. 1.5 Drawing of the human brain. Format as in Fig. 1.3.

- PFdl, the dorsolateral prefrontal cortex (area 46);
- PFdm, the dorsomedial prefrontal cortex (medial parts of area 9);
- PFo, the granular orbitofrontal cortex (area 11 and granular parts of areas 13 and 14). In our usage, if it is not preceded by the word "granular" the term *orbitofrontal cortex* includes the agranular parts of areas 13 and 14 as well as the agranular insular cortex. We sometimes use the term orbital–insular cortex to emphasize the close relationships among these areas. Although traditional anatomy usually treats the orbitofrontal and insular cortex as distinct entities, a detailed analysis of their architectonics,

Table 1.4 Naming convention for orbital–insular and medial frontal cortex

Overall	General regions		Specific areas	
	Granular cortex	Agranular cortex	Granular cortex	Agranular cortex
Orbitofrontal cortex	PFo	Lateral agranular PF[a]	Area 11, rostral area 13, rostral area 14	Agranular insular cortex, agranular orbitofrontal cortex (caudal area 13, caudal area 14)
Medial prefrontal cortex	PFdm and medial PFp	Medial agranular PF	Medial area 9, medial area 10	Prelimbic cortex (area 32), infralimbic cortex (area 25), anterior cingulate cortex (area 24)

[a] Also known as the agranular orbital–insular cortex.

Abbreviations: PF, prefrontal cortex; PFo, granular orbitofrontal cortex; PFdm, dorsomedial prefrontal cortex; PFp, polar prefrontal cortex.

connections, and topology reveals that the agranular insular areas are integral parts of the orbital neocortex.

◆ PFp, the polar prefrontal cortex (area 10), also known as frontal-pole cortex.

◆ PFvl, the ventrolateral prefrontal cortex (areas 12, 44, 45, and 47).

The term ventromedial prefrontal cortex is different. We avoid this name, for the most part, because it includes both granular and agranular areas of medial frontal cortex, along with some variable extent of orbitofrontal cortex. We do use some general terms, however, such as the medial prefrontal and orbitofrontal cortex, which include both granular and agranular areas. Table 1.4 summarizes our conventions for naming medial and orbital–insular parts of the primate frontal cortex.

Elsewhere in the frontal lobe, the motor cortex consists of the primary motor area (area 4) and the premotor cortex (mainly area 6, but also including parts of area 24). The premotor areas include the supplementary and cingulate motor areas. We never refer to the cingulate motor areas as part of the anterior cingulate cortex, although both come from area 24.

For the parietal lobe, we use a combination of architectonic terms, such as Brodmann's[46,47], along with regional descriptions. There is no particular meaning in these numbers other than that Brodmann named areas as they appeared from top to bottom in a series of horizontal brain sections. For the temporal lobe we sometimes use the terminology of von Bonin and Bailey[48], such as areas TE and TEO. The "T" stands for temporal and the "E" means fifth (after TA, TB, …). The "O" in TEO refers to the more occipital part of area TE. For the occipital lobe, we use physiological names for the most part, such as the primary visual (V1) cortex.

Neuropsychology

Conventions

Much of the book depends on understanding the effects of brain lesions and brain imaging results. In the chapters to come, readers should assume that:

◆ All lesions are bilateral and reasonably symmetrical unless otherwise stated, with the exception of the surgical crossed-disconnection procedure explained later (see "Lesion effects").

◆ Throughout this book, the term *lesion* can refer to any disease or damage that disrupts the function of an area, or to any experimental manipulation that does so, including temporary or permanent disruption of function by pharmacological agents, repetitive transcranial magnetic stimulation (TMS or rTMS), degenerative diseases, surgical ablations, cytotoxins, excitotoxins, or molecular manipulations [as in optogenetics or designer receptors exclusively activated by designer drugs (DREADDs)]. So when we use the term lesion it should not be taken to exclude any of these methods or processes.

◆ Brain imaging refers to functional magnetic resonance imaging, as opposed to structural imaging, unless otherwise stated.

Task names

Memory tests depend on task rules, and tasks have names. In both human and animal neuropsychology the names given to tasks often reflect something about the history of the field or of the task, and they can convey some useful ideas about what kinds of memory they test. They can, however, be misleading. Of course, neuropsychologists claim (and believe) that they take care not to let task names affect their ideas and interpretations too much. But they often do.

For example, tasks called delayed matching-to-sample and delayed nonmatching-to-sample have also been called "recognition memory tasks" or "visual recognition tasks." In these tasks, subjects usually see a sample stimulus, wait for a while after the stimulus goes away, and then try to demonstrate their memory of the sample. Calling this procedure a "recognition memory task" implies to many experts that people can perform the task in only one way, which involves a specific, explicit recollection of the sample stimulus. Unfortunately, subjects can use several different strategies to perform these tasks, some of which involve the use of information about an object's familiarity or about how recently an object has appeared, independent of any specific recollection of the sample. Depending on the details of each memory test, subjects might use any combination of these strategies.

Lesion effects

Regardless of the names given to tasks, the strongest evidence from lesion studies comes from a double dissociation of function. Given two brain structures and two tasks, a lesion of one structure affects the performance of only one task, whereas a lesion of the other structure affects performance only on the other task.

In a form of lesion that comes up repeatedly in this book, investigators selectively lesion a brain structure in one hemisphere and combine this manipulation with a lesion of a different structure in the opposite hemisphere. As a result of such crossed disconnections, the brain as a whole has its normal complement of structures, taking the two hemispheres together. Interactions between the two lesioned areas, however, cannot occur normally, especially within a hemisphere. This type of surgical disconnection tells us that two structures need to interact in order to mediate some aspect of behavior.

In any form, lesions demonstrate that a brain structure plays a necessary role in the normal performance of some task or other behavior, and they show what the remaining parts of the brain can do. With the proviso that changes in functions might occur after permanent lesions, this method provides the strongest form of evidence about the causal contribution of a specific brain structure or pathway to some behavior. In some applications of this method, however, experimenters have inadvertently damaged fiber pathways and cortical areas near the site of the intended lesion. Such unintended—and typically unreported—damage can cause serious misinterpretations of experimental results. For example, in Chapter 12 ("The monkey model") we explain how certain memory functions came to be wrongly attributed to the amygdala. In clinical studies, additional damage often accompanies the largest and most obvious brain lesions, sometimes at distant sites. Unfortunately, these additional lesions are not always evident in structural brain images or in postmortem neuropathology. The difference between temporary and permanent lesions can also be important, as can the difference between surgical ablations of an area and excitotoxic or optogenetic lesions, which largely spare nearby white matter tracts.

Neuropsychologists sometimes limit their analysis to assessing whether a lesion causes an impairment in task performance or not. As a result, they sometimes fail to distinguish between a statistically significant, but mild, impairment and a complete or nearly complete inability to perform or learn some task. When considering a broad range of data, it is easy to make the mistake of treating some brain structure as "necessary" for some task when it makes only a modest contribution to learning or performance. In this book, we try to take into account the magnitude of impairments when interpreting results.

Other methods

In contrast to lesions, which tell us about the structures necessary for a given function, functional brain imaging and neuronal recording studies reveal something about the information processed in a given part of the brain. Each of these methods provides valid information, but only within limits imposed by the measures used:

◆ Brain imaging methods, such as functional magnetic resonance imaging, measure localized changes in metabolism, blood flow, or blood oxygenation. In this book, we call this measure *activation* to distinguish it from the discharge activity of neurons.

◆ Neuronal recordings measure the rates and patterns of action potentials—also known as spiking, discharging, and firing—monitored from individual cells as subjects perform some task. As just mentioned, we use the term *activity* for this measure.

All methods have important limitations, of course. We would understand the brain much better if it were otherwise. Earlier, we mentioned some errors in applying the lesion method, and similar errors have occurred in neurophysiology and brain imaging experiments:

♦ Single-cell recordings show something important about the information that neurons process and encode, but they do not indicate that the cell or its area makes a necessary contribution to a behavior, and they have a very poor ability to rule out hypotheses about the function of a given area. An early paper on the frontal eye field provides an example of this weakness. The authors concluded that this area has nothing to do with initiating eye movements simply because, in their particular experimental conditions, neuronal activity increased only *after* each eye movement had begun[49]. The frontal eye field does sometimes have this property, but only in highly impoverished conditions. In slightly more complex circumstances, many neurons in the frontal eye field increase their activity prior to eye movements[50]. Neurophysiological studies often walk a fine line between oversimplified behaviors that have little relationship to life outside the laboratory and those that are too complex to yield interpretable results.

♦ Functional brain imaging studies have great power, but also many important limitations. First, the measure used in these studies involves synaptic activity within a particular voxel and not, to any large extent, the firing rates of its neurons[51,52]. In areas like the hippocampus and the prefrontal cortex, in particular, increases in this measure might reflect inhibitory influences to an equal or greater extent than excitatory ones. So increases in activation could reflect the suppression of outputs from an area. Or maybe synaptic influences balance and neutralize each other. Second, localization of the measure's source can be problematic. For example, one early brain imaging report attributed emotion-related activation to the amygdala that resulted instead from setting the subject's teeth on edge—and the resulting increase in blood flow that occurred in the nearby masseter muscle[53]. More generally, the vascular architecture of the brain can create signals that reflect venous blood flow far from the activation site, and the signals detected by functional magnetic resonance imaging can be affected by the locations of major arteries or sinuses[54,55].

Any method can lead researchers down the wrong road, of course, but such mistakes represent problems of practice and not deficiencies in principle. Fortunately, many limitations can be addressed by comparing findings and interpretations across methods.

Evolution

This is a book on the evolution of memory systems, not on either evolution or brain evolution. Accordingly, readers need to understand just ten terms and concepts from evolutionary biology in order to follow the proposals presented in this book:

♦ stem group
♦ crown group
♦ clade
♦ sister group

- ◆ paraphyletic group
- ◆ ancestral trait
- ◆ derived trait
- ◆ homology
- ◆ analogy
- ◆ exaptation

Cladistics

A *stem group* lived in the distant past and gave rise to some number of descendant species, living and extinct. Collectively, these descendants are called crown species and compose a *crown group*. Stem and crown species together constitute a *clade*, often illustrated by a cladogram (Figs. 1.6–1.8). These illustrations show the most parsimonious or most likely relationships among various lineages, and they often designate the lineage in which a trait first emerged or vanished.

These days, many cladograms result from molecular phylogenetics, sometimes combined with a large dataset of morphological traits and some combination of parsimony and Bayesian algorithms. Nevertheless, an example using a single trait illustrates the principles underlying cladistics. Figure 1.6 includes a list of animal groups. Those in black type all have a corpus callosum, a massive fiber pathway that connects the two hemispheres. The bottom 3 groups, which lack this trait, appear in gray type.

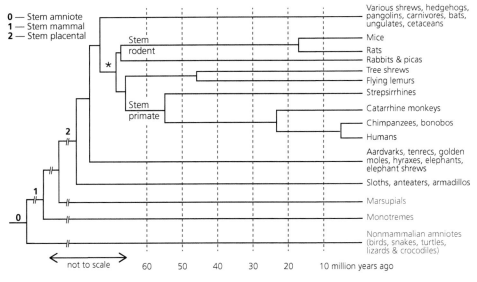

Fig. 1.6 A cladogram of amniotes. The numerals (0, 1, and 2) at the top left correspond to the progenitor species indicated on the cladogram by the same numeral. From 60 million years until the present the divergence times are plotted on an approximately linear scale, shown at the bottom. The asterisk marks the last common ancestor of rodents and primates.

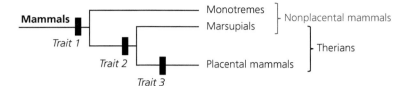

Trait 1 (hair): synapomorphy (shared derived trait) for mammals
but plesiomorphy (ancestral trait) for therians

Trait 2 (live birth): synapomorphy for therians

Trait 3 (placenta): apomorphy (derived trait) for placental mammals

Fig. 1.7 Types of homologies. A simplified cladogram of mammals, with the names of monophyletic groups (clades) in black type and a paraphyletic group in gray type.

Based on the presence or absence of the corpus callosum alone, it seems likely that all of the species listed in black type descend from a common ancestor in which the corpus callosum first emerged. Figure 1.6 marks this ancestral species with the numeral 2.

In addition to having a corpus callosum, all groups in black type nurture their fetuses through a placenta, which gives rise to the name for this group: placental mammals. The more traits that placental mammals share, but other groups do not, the stronger the evidence that placental mammals make up a clade, also known as a monophyletic group.

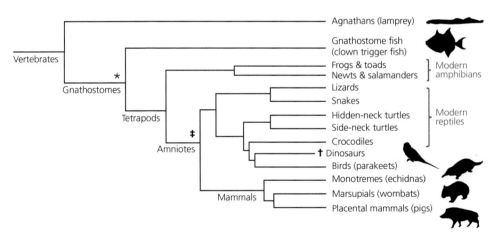

Fig. 1.8 A cladogram of gnathostomes. Some example species are in parentheses to the right. The asterisk marks the last common ancestor of modern fish, amphibians, mammals, reptiles, and birds; the double dagger indicates the last common ancestor of birds and mammals; the dagger indicates an extinct group. Adapted from Fig. 4.1 of Murray EA, Wise SP, Rhodes SEV. What can different brains do with reward? In: *The Neurobiology of Sensation and Reward* (Gottfried JA, ed.), pp 57–92, © 2011, Taylor & Francis. Reproduced with permission. Silhouettes from open source http://phylopic.org/.

This explanation oversimplifies cladistics outrageously, but not in a way that has much relevance to memory systems.

A clade includes all descendants of a progenitor species, and only those species. A *sister group* consists of the species most closely related to that clade. Figure 1.7 presents an example for mammals. Taken together, marsupials and placental mammals all descend from a common ancestor and so represent a clade: therian mammals. The black bar with "Trait 2" beneath it points to one derived trait that therian mammals share, live birth, as opposed to the ancestral condition of laying eggs. Monotremes are the sister group of therian mammals, and they retain the egg-laying habit of stem mammals.

Members of a *paraphyletic group* share a sufficient number of traits to warrant joint consideration but do not constitute a clade. The clades called placental and therian mammals comprise all of the descendants of the progenitor species and only its descendants (Fig. 1.7). The group called nonplacental mammals does not. This paraphyletic group includes some descendants of stem mammals, but not all of them.

Cladistic principles can generate a surprising amount of inferential knowledge. Imagine, for example, the brain of some unknown mammal. If a brain scan reveals a corpus callosum, then we can infer that its mother nourished the creature through her placenta and that it was live born. This example illustrates the power of cladistics, and when we apply these concepts to memory systems we can reap a sizable reward. There are, however, a few pitfalls along the way.

Ancestral and derived traits

As an example of such pitfalls, the terms "primitive" and "advanced" have a long history of abuse. In evolutionary biology they have a very specific meaning: *primitive* means resembling the ancestral condition; *advanced* traits differ from that condition. These terms do not imply any value judgments, although people often read them that way. Primitive anthropoids, for example, did not have the large brains that later anthropoids developed (see Chapter 2, "Anthropoids"), but they count among our heroes all the same. To avoid misunderstandings, however, we mostly refer to *derived traits* and *ancestral traits* and tend to avoid "advanced" and "primitive," except when quoting other sources.

Homologies

Traits passed down to the descendants of a stem species are called homologies, homologues, and homologous. *Homology* is therefore a statement about ancestry, one that does not imply a similar function or any obvious physical resemblance. The inner ear ossicles of mammals, for example, are homologous with components of the ancestral jaw, but they resemble jaws very little and have a dramatically different function. Likewise, the vertebrate jaw derives from gill-support structures, but shares very few traits with them. However, homologues often do have similar functions and frequently resemble each other as well. *Analogy* refers to function, not ancestry, and usually implies a lack of homology. Similarities arise from homology (inheritance from a common ancestor), as well as from convergent and parallel evolution.

Homologies come in two types: traits that emerged in a stem species and those that a stem species inherited from earlier, more distant ancestors. We do not use the specialized terms for these two kinds of homologies, although Fig. 1.7 presents them anyway. Rather than getting bogged down in terminology, Fig. 1.8 illustrates the key points, along with introducing a simple vertebrate cladogram[56]. Earlier, we said that all placental mammals have a corpus callosum. Placental mammals also have jaws, as do all of the groups to the right of the asterisk in Fig. 1.8. The vertebrate jaw, as mentioned earlier, first developed from anterior gill-support structures in a group of animals called stem gnathostomes, and all of their descendants have this trait. So placental mammals have homologues of both the corpus callosum and jaws, but the corpus callosum is an innovation in this clade (a shared derived trait) whereas the jaw is not (a shared ancestral trait, often called a primitive trait). This distinction comes up later, in many forms. In Chapter 6, for example, we emphasize a new memory system and new cortical areas in primates. Along with these innovations, primates also have memory systems and cortical areas that they inherited from more distant ancestors.

Two general principles about homology are important for understanding memory systems:

◆ First, evolutionary innovations often seem to come in suites. For example, jaws evolved in stem gnathostomes along with paired fins and a "free-standing" cerebellum. Stem mammals evolved hair and the new inner ear structure (ossicles) mentioned earlier, along with molars and endothermy (warm-bloodedness). These suites of adaptations appear to have evolved "simultaneously," an illusion that results from the survival of one among many combinations of innovative traits. The various derived traits probably emerged at different times, but a sparse fossil record and the extinction of alternative combinations make it seem as though they arose together. In the following chapters the appearance of several new brain structures in a given ancestor might seem like too much to swallow, but such bursts of innovation are common in evolution.

◆ Second, homologous structures can adopt new functions over time, which means that their functions can differ from each other. The term *exaptation* applies to traits that come to perform different or additional functions after they first evolve. Appendages that began as paired fins later developed into limbs, so fins served as exaptations for limbs and terrestrial locomotion. Likewise, forelimbs served as exaptations for wings and winged flight; and wings served as exaptations for social signaling in certain insects and birds. Several of our proposals on memory systems invoke the concept of exaptation.

We close this chapter by considering three general issues related to homology, which can cause problems in understanding brain evolution.

Independent evolution

Wings commonly serve as a heuristic example of independent evolution. Many kinds of animals have wings, including several kinds of insects, birds, an extinct group of reptiles called pterosaurs, and bats. The wings of all these animals emerged to provide the same fundamental advantage: the use of muscle-generated forces to produce lift for flight (Box 1.1).

Box 1.1 Parallel evolution takes flight

In Chapter 2 ("Early primates" and "Anthropoids") we say, for example, that the inferior temporal cortex, the fovea, and mechanisms for visually guided reaching originated in primates. Given that other large-brained mammals, such as carnivores, have similar areas, retinal specializations, and visually guided reaching, does this mean that these traits "go way back" in evolution, to a common ancestor?

The answer is no. Parallel evolution is ordinary, common, and occasionally necessary, as an example from the fossil record illustrates. As mentioned in the main text, active flight has evolved independently several times: first in insects, later in pterosaurs, then in birds, and most recently in bats. Flight requires wings, of course, but in large animals it also requires a prodigious supply of energy. Vertebrate muscles function optimally at about 37°C. In part to keep their wing muscles warm, especially at takeoff, flying animals maintain their bodies near that temperature, a trait called endothermy. To do so, they need to consume about ten times more energy than cold-blooded (exothermic) animals of comparable size.

Insects have low mass and so can fly without an exorbitant expenditure of energy. Before bats evolved, their earthbound mammalian ancestors had already developed a high-energy life that included endothermy, hairy insulation, and adaptations in diet, metabolism, and dentition. Pterosaurs did not have it so easy because, unlike bats, their ancestors had not developed endothermy. Furthermore, unlike insects, pterosaur wings lifted a lot of mass. The largest of these extinct flying reptiles was three times heavier than the standard 70-kg human[64]. Nevertheless, to initiate and sustain active flight they had to use muscles that functioned best at about 37°C.

So it is hard to imagine how pterosaurs could have evolved if they had not developed some form of endothermy. A large body size helps because it lowers the surface-to-volume ratio and thereby limits heat loss. But without insulation heat loss remains high, and fossil evidence shows that pterosaurs probably developed an insulating fuzz, called pycnofibers, as an adaptation related to endothermy[64]. Perhaps they could not have supported active flight otherwise.

Parallel evolution often reveals itself in the anatomical details of independent adaptations. For example, pterosaurs adapted a different finger to support their wing than did birds and bats. Bats developed wings with the skin surface attached to their fifth digit. The wings of pterosaurs hang from the fourth digit, with the fifth finger vestigial or absent. In birds, the second and third digits are always among the three that provide the scaffolding for wings.

The same principles apply to brain evolution. Similar adaptive pressures often produce comparable solutions. The problems and opportunities faced by all flying vertebrates probably explain the fact that pterosaur brains more closely resemble bird brains than the brains of other reptiles[65]. Pterosaur brains exceed the size expected for a modern reptile of the same body weight, for example. The traditional account for this finding is that flight generated a computational challenge that led to larger brains. The brains of flying reptiles fall just short of the size range for modern birds, however. Perhaps this difference reflects the fact that pterosaurs arose from small-brained reptiles, whereas birds descended from dinosaurs, which had already undergone some brain expansion[64].

Despite their overall similarity in size, the brains of pterosaurs and birds differ in key organizational details. Most notably, the cerebellar flocculus makes up 7.5% of the brain in pterosaurs but less than 2% in birds. This structure plays a key role in stabilizing images on the retina, through ancient reflexes involving vestibular inputs. Its differential expansion in birds and pterosaurs reflects independent adaptations to the requirements of flight.

Dragonflies and bats serve as an example pair of lineages. Insect wings evolved nearly 400 million years ago[57], long before bats or other mammals existed. Furthermore, the last common ancestor of dragonflies and bats had no wings or anything remotely like wings. So dragonfly and bat wings are analogous, not homologous; they evolved through independent evolution. Similarities of this kind often result from developmental constraints or from common selective forces. For example, to produce lift wings must interact with air in ways that constrain their architecture.

To relate this principle to the brain, consider an imaginary animal: Godzilla, a large bipedal lizard, something like *Tyrannosaurus rex*. Earlier (see "Cladistics"), we mentioned that the corpus callosum is an innovation of stem placental mammals. Obviously, Godzilla was not a mammal of any kind, let alone a placental mammal. Suppose that during the evolution of this large animal it developed a corpus callosum as its brain increased in size. Large animals tend to have big brains, so Godzilla probably had a whopper. The existence of a corpus callosum in Godzilla would not change the fact that this trait also originated in stem placental mammals. It would only mean that the corpus callosum evolved independently in "godzilloid amniotes."

Evolutionary changes in the visual system provide examples of this "Godzilla principle" from the real world. When we say, for example, that the fovea evolved in primates, this statement does not imply that primates alone have a fovea. Other vertebrates do, as well. In fact, a fovea evolved several times in vertebrate history. But the existence of a fovea in nonprimate species does not negate the fact that the fovea is a primate innovation. The same goes for other primate traits, such as the granular prefrontal cortex, a large and elaborate inferior temporal cortex, new ways of reaching, feeding, and moving through space, and much else besides (see Chapters 2 and 6). Like Godzilla's corpus callosum, it does not matter for our purposes whether similar traits also evolved in other lineages.

Take the opposite case. What if the corpus callosum regressed in some placental mammal? It never happened, but in principle some mammal could have lost the corpus callosum. This imaginary placental mammal, let's call it the "locavore," would not cease being a placental mammal because it lacked a corpus callosum. Even if the locavore also lost live birth and reverted to laying eggs it would remain a placental mammal by virtue of its ancestry. The same principle applies when we recognize that snakes and whales are tetrapods despite the fact that neither has a leg to stand on.

Independent evolution can obscure the circumstances and ancestors in which a trait arose. In discussions of brain evolution, critics often cite the existence of a trait in one lineage as evidence against the idea that it evolved in another. Too often, these discussions have degenerated into a crusade against unique traits in primates or humans. For example, the observation of language-like vocalizations in a gray parrot has attracted a great deal of attention, although the last common ancestor of birds and humans, marked by a double dagger in Fig. 1.8, surely lacked the vocal behavior of either. In popular science, similarities between human and parrot vocalizations are deemed to disprove the stodgy dogma that language is a uniquely human trait. The key issues, however, concern innovation and ancestry, not similarity or uniqueness.

Independent evolution can also create the illusion that a trait evolved much earlier than it actually did. Of importance for our proposals, the inferior temporal areas of the visual cortex evolved and elaborated independently in primates and in the ungulate–carnivore clade, and so these areas are found in monkeys, humans, cats, and sheep, among other mammalian species. This example is particularly important because in Chapters 6–9 we consider most of the inferior temporal cortex to be a primate innovation. Some authors assume that inferior temporal areas, and especially face recognition areas, are homologous in humans, monkeys, and sheep. This idea leads them to conclude, incorrectly, that the inferior temporal cortex must have originated in some "ancient ancestor"[58]. But the last common ancestor of these species had a very small neocortex, which probably included only one or two visual areas in addition to the primary and secondary visual cortex, areas V1 and V2 (see Chapter 5, "Evolution"). As nocturnal animals, it is safe to assume that whatever inferior temporal areas this ancestral species had, they played little role in visual face recognition. Equally important, stem primates—from which all modern primates have descended—also foraged nocturnally, as dispersed individuals that had infrequent visual interactions (see Chapter 10, "Social factors"). So face recognition and visual signaling could not have contributed very much to their success either. Instead of "ancient ancestry," there is a better explanation. From a common origin, the cerebral cortex enlarged independently in many mammalian lineages, especially those that produced large diurnal animals, as both the primate and the ungulate–carnivore clades did. As brains expanded in these lineages, new inferior temporal areas (almost certainly) arose independently. Face recognition areas in primates are therefore analogous, not homologous, to those in the ungulate–carnivore clade. Convergent and parallel evolution occur very commonly, and undue skepticism about their prevalence has led to many mistaken conclusions about "ancient origins," as in this example.

Homology and nonhomology

Wings exemplify another complication: a trait can be homologous at one biological level, but when considered at a different level the same trait can be analogous and not homologous. This statement seems illogical at first glance: How can a trait be both homologous and not homologous?

Consider the fact that bats and birds both use wings for flying and that their last common ancestor did not. This extinct ancestor lived somewhere around 330 million years ago (double dagger in Fig. 1.8), long before either bats or birds evolved. At one level, then, bat and bird wings are analogous and not homologous; they both provide lift for flight but did not descend from a common ancestor with wings.

Biology can be more complicated than that, however. Both bird wings and bat wings arose from forelimbs, which both birds and bats *did* inherit from a common ancestor. So, as forelimbs, bird wings and bat wings are homologous, although as wings they are analogous and not homologous. Other descendants of stem tetrapods (Fig. 1.8), such as turtles, also have forelimbs, and the forelimbs of all of these animals perform a conserved function: providing force for locomotion. The forelimbs of bats and birds and turtles are therefore homologous, but in bats and birds forelimbs adopted a new function, flight, which evolved independently in these two lineages.

It would be convenient to avoid this complication, but it has direct relevance to understanding memory systems. In many instances, a structure adopts new functions during evolution, yet its ancestry can be traced to something more fundamental. Although the hippocampus is homologous in rodents, humans, and monkeys, in Chapter 11 we propose that it contributes to a new function in humans: explicit memory. This idea might seem implausible to some neuroscientists, but to say that the hippocampus does something qualitatively different in humans, compared with monkeys and rodents, is no more radical than saying that the forelimb does something qualitatively different in bats and birds, compared with turtles. If homology precluded new functions, then no species could ever take flight.

Precursors of the past

One final point: modern species can never have "precursors" of traits in humans (or, for that matter, in any other modern species). The reason is simple; no modern species is the ancestor of any other modern species. Assertions about precursors, like it or not, imply that the trait in question has been inherited little changed from the last common ancestor. This problem undermines assertions about "episodic-like" or "proto-episodic" memory in birds and humans[59,60] (see Box 2.1), "cognitive maps" in honeybees and humans[61], "declarative memory" in rodents and humans[62], and the "precursors of language" in monkeys[63].

The last example is particularly prominent. The idea that the vocalizations of macaque monkeys are precursors of human speech appears commonly in both popular science and prestigious journals. To cite one example, Poremba et al.[63] (p. 448) claimed that "it has often been proposed that the vocal calls of monkeys are precursors of human speech." As a statement about intellectual history, this claim is perfectly true. However, as a statement about evolutionary history it is exceedingly unlikely. Putting aside the question of which monkeys—of the 260 or so species in this diverse paraphyletic group[27]—best represent social signaling in our last common ancestor, the "precursor" view assumes that vocal calls in the lineage leading to macaques have changed little over the millions of years since that ancestor lived. Given the diversity in acoustic signaling among primates, this assumption is almost surely wrong. Instead of viewing monkey calls as "precursors" of speech, it is better to recognize that modern monkeys and humans have vocal communications adapted to their social systems, as our last common ancestor did.

It might seem unlikely that ten terms and concepts suffice for exploring the evolution of memory systems. True enough, they would not get anyone very far in a course on evolutionary biology, but to apply the hard-won accomplishments of contemporary biology to the study of memory systems they can do the job.

References

1. **Corkin, S.** (2013) *Permanent Present Tense* (Basic Books, New York).
2. **Scoville, W.B.** and **Milner, B.** (1957) *J. Neurol. Neurosurg. Psychiatr.* **20**, 11–21.
3. **Milner, B., Corkin, S.,** and **Teuber, H.-L.** (1968) *Neuropsychologia* **6**, 215–234.
4. **Milner, B.** (1972) *Clin. Neurosurg.* **19**, 421–446.
5. **Corkin, S.** (1984) *J. Neurosci.* **2**, 1214–1229.
6. **Corkin, S.** (2002) *Nat. Rev. Neurosci.* **3**, 153–160.
7. **Milner, B.** (2005) *Psychiatr. Clin. North Am.* **28**, 599–611.
8. **Sidman, M., Stoddard, L.T.,** and **Mohr, J.P.** (1968) *Neuropsychologia* **6**, 245–254.
9. **Milner, B.** (1959) *Psychiatr. Res. Rep. Am. Psychiatr. Assoc.* **11**, 43–58.
10. **Milner, B.** (1962) In: *Physiologie de l'Hippocampe*, pp. 257–272 (Centre National de la Recherche Scientifique, Paris).
11. **Shadmehr, R., Brandt, J.,** and **Corkin, S.** (1998) *J. Neurophysiol.* **80**, 1590–1597.
12. **Orbach, J., Milner, B.,** and **Rasmussen, T.** (1960) *Arch. Neurol.* **3**, 230–251.
13. **Correll, R.E.** and **Scoville, W.B.** (1965) *J. Comp. Physiol. Psychol.* **60**, 175–181.
14. **Correll, R.E.** and **Scoville, W.B.** (1967) *Exp. Brain Res.* **4**, 85–96.
15. **Gaffan, D.** (1974) *J. Comp. Physiol. Psychol.* **86**, 1100–1109.
16. **Mishkin, M.** (1978) *Nature* **273**, 297–298.
17. **Gaffan, D.** (2002) *Phil. Trans. R. Soc. B: Biol. Sci.* **357**, 1111–1121.
18. **Saksida, L.M.** and **Bussey, T.J.** (2010) *Neuropsychologia* **48**, 2370–2384.
19. **Squire, L.R., Wixted, J.T.,** and **Clark, R.E.** (2007) *Nat. Rev. Neurosci.* **8**, 872–883.
20. **Fernandez-Ruiz, J., Wang, J., Aigner, T.G.,** and **Mishkin, M.** (2001) *Proc. Natl. Acad. Sci. USA* **98**, 4196–4201.
21. **Broadbent, N.J., Squire, L.R.,** and **Clark, R.E.** (2007) *Learn. Mem.* **14**, 145–151.
22. **Striedter, G.F.** (2005) *Principles of Brain Evolution* (Sinauer, Sunderland, MA).
23. **Kaas, J.H.** (2011) *Brain Behav. Evol.* **78**, 7–21.

24. **Kaas, J.H.** (2012) *Prog. Brain Res.* **195**, 91–102.

25. **Kaas, J.H.** (2013) *Wiley Interdiscip. Rev. Cogn. Sci.* **4**, 33–45.

26. **Valentine, J.W.** (2004) *On the Origin of Phyla* (University of Chicago Press, Chicago).

27. **Mitani, J.C., Call, J., Kappeler, P.M., Palombit, R.A.,** and **Silk, J.B.** (2012) In: *The Evolution of Primate Societies* (eds. Mitani, J.C., Call, J., Kappeler, P.M. et al.), pp. 5–16 (University of Chicago Press, Chicago).

28. **Sherry, D.F.** and **Schacter, D.L.** (1987) *Psychol. Rev.* **94**, 439–454.

29. **Murray, E.A.** and **Wise, S.P.** (2004) *Neurobiol. Learn. Mem.* **82**, 178–198.

30. **Zola-Morgan, S., Squire, L.R.,** and **Ramus, S.J.** (1994) *Hippocampus* **4**, 483–495.

31. **Lee, A.C.H., Buckley, M.J., Gaffan, D., Emery, T.** et al. (2006) *J. Neurosci.* **26**, 5198–5203.

32. **Graham, K.S., Barense, M.D.,** and **Lee, A.C.** (2010) *Neuropsychologia* **48**, 831–853.

33. **Duarte, A., Henson, R.N., Knight, R.T., Emery, T.** et al. (2010) *J. Cogn. Neurosci.* **22**, 1819–1831.

34. **Duarte, A., Henson, R.N.,** and **Graham, K.S.** (2011) *Brain Res.* **1373**, 110–123.

35. **Ranganath, C.** and **Ritchey, M.** (2012) *Nat. Rev. Neurosci.* **13**, 713–726.

36. **Murray, E.A.** and **Wise, S.P.** (2010) *Neuropsychologia* **48**, 2385–2405.

37. **Mayr, E.** (1982) *The Growth of Biological Thought* (Belknap Harvard, Cambridge, MA).

38. **Smith, H.W.** (1953) *From Fish to Philosopher* (Anchor; Doubleday; American Museum of Natural History, Garden City, NY).

39. **Balleine, B.W.** and **O'Doherty, J.P.** (2010) *Neuropsychopharmacol.* **35**, 48–69.

40. **Shubin, N.** (2008) *Your Inner Fish* (Pantheon, New York).

41. **MacLean, P.D.** (1990) *The Triune Brain in Evolution* (Plenum, New York).

42. **Petrovich, G.D., Canteras, N.S.,** and **Swanson, L.W.** (2001) *Brain Res. Rev.* **38**, 247–289.

43. **Sanides, F.** (1970) In: *The Primate Brain* (eds. Noback, C.R. and Montagna, W.), pp. 137–208 (Appleton-Century-Crofts, New York).

44. **Petrides, M.** and **Pandya, D.N.** (2007) *J. Neurosci.* **27**, 11573–11586.

45. **Walker A.E.** (1940) *J. Comp. Neurol.* **73**, 59–86.

46. **Brodmann, K.** (1909) *Vergleichende Lokalisationslehre der Grosshirnrind* (Barth, Leipzig).

47. **Brodmann, K.** (1912) *Ver. Anat. Anz.* **26**, 157–216.

48. **von Bonin, G.** and **Bailey, P.** (1947) *The Neocortex of* Macaca mulatta (University of Illinois Press, Urbana, IL).

49. **Bizzi, E.** and **Schiller, P.H.** (1970) *Exp. Brain Res.* **10**, 150–158.

50. **Goldberg, M.E.** and **Bushnell, M.C.** (1981) *J. Neurophysiol.* **46**, 773–787.

51. **Nielsen, K.J., Logothetis, N.K.,** and **Rainer, G.** (2006) *J. Neurosci.* **26**, 9639–9645.

52. **Logothetis, N.K.** and **Wandell, B.A.** (2004) *Annu. Rev. Physiol.* **66**, 735–769.

53. **Drevets, W.C., Videen, T.Q., MacLeod, A.K., Haller, J.W.** et al. (1992) *Science* **256**, 1696.

54. **Turner, R.** (2002) *NeuroImage* **16**, 1062–1067.

55. **Kim, D.S., Ronen, I., Olman, C., Kim, S.G.** et al. (2004) *NeuroImage* **21**, 876–885.

56. **Murray, E.A., Wise, S.P.,** and **Rhodes, S.E.V.** (2011) In: *The Neurobiology of Sensation and Reward* (ed. Gottfried, J.A.), pp. 57–92 (Taylor & Francis, Boca Raton, FL).

57. **Grimaldi, D.** and **Engel, M.S.** (2005) *Evolution of the Insects* (Cambridge University Press, Cambridge, UK).

58. **Leopold, D.A.** and **Rhodes, G.** (2010) *J. Comp. Psychol.* **124**, 233–251.

59. **Clayton, N.S., Bussey, T.J., Emery, N.J.,** and **Dickinson, A.** (2003) *Trends Cogn. Sci.* **7**, 436–437.

60. **Allen, T.A.** and **Fortin, N.J.** (2013) *Proc. Natl. Acad. Sci. USA* **110 (Suppl. 2)**, 10379–10386.

61. **Collett, T.S.** and **Baron, J.** (1994) *Nature* **368**, 137–140.

62. **Manns, J.R.** and **Eichenbaum, H.** (2006) *Hippocampus* **16**, 795–808.

63. **Poremba, A., Malloy, M., Saunders, R.C., Carson, R.E.** et al. (2004) *Nature* **427**, 448–451.

64. **Witton, M.** (2013) *Pterosaurs: Natural History, Evolution, Anatomy* (Princeton University Press, Princeton, NJ).

65. **Witmer, L.M., Chatterjee, S., Franzosa, J.,** and **Rowe, T.** (2003) *Nature* **425**, 950–953.

Chapter 2

The history of the brain

Overview

The evolution of memory systems depended on new or elaborated brain structures that appeared as specific ancestors adapted to new ways of life. Early vertebrates evolved the telencephalon, including homologues of the hippocampus and basal ganglia. These innovations occurred among a suite of adaptations for mobile, predatory foraging that also included the vertebrate head and sensory organs for olfaction and vision. Early mammals developed the neocortex as they adopted a high-energy life. Later, new parts of the prefrontal, parietal, premotor, and temporal cortex emerged in early primates as they adapted to living in the fine branches of trees. More recently, as anthropoid primates diversified, they increased in size and came to rely on volatile, energy-rich resources distributed over a large home range. Their brains expanded, several new parts of the prefrontal cortex emerged, and their parietal and temporal cortex became more elaborate. Further expansion of these areas occurred during human evolution.

Lunar primates

In 1969 two primates landed on the moon. They used their hindlimbs to walk around for a while; they searched for and chose rocks based on visual features; and they gathered samples with hand tools controlled by visual guidance. Of the 500 million primates who watched them on television, only a few knew that these capacities reflected the evolutionary developments of our earliest primate ancestors. Fewer still knew that they depended on the evolution of memory systems.

The prevailing view recognizes two memory systems: one in the medial temporal lobe for explicit (declarative) memory; the other in the basal ganglia for habits. In this chapter we address two questions about this idea: (1) does the concept of a "medial temporal lobe" make sense in an evolutionary context?; and (2) does the concept of the basal ganglia in the prevailing view agree with comparative neuroanatomy?

To answer these questions, we first need to explore brain evolution, and Figs. 2.1–2.3 foreshadow the main points. Figure 2.1 emphasizes three ideas: (1) the primate cerebral cortex contains a mixture of old and new areas, (2) some of which emerged in early primates, and (3) others of which arose later in primate evolution. Figure 2.2 incorporates the basal ganglia into the picture, in the context of cortex–basal ganglia "loops."

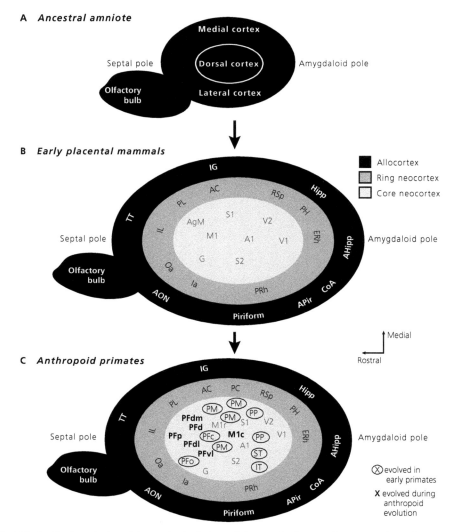

Fig. 2.1 Cortical evolution. Schematic depiction of the cerebral cortex in ancestral amniotes (A), early placental mammals (B), and modern anthropoids (C). In part (C), the areas in bold, black type emerged *de novo* in anthropoids; areas in ovals emerged *de novo* in early primates. For simplicity, we include only a selection of areas and do not distinguish among various posterior parietal, lateral temporal, extrastriate, and premotor areas. Abbreviations: A1, primary auditory cortex; AC, anterior cingulate cortex; AgM, medial agranular cortex, a premotor area; AHipp, amygdalohippocampal transition area; AON, anterior olfactory nucleus; APir, amygdalopiriform transition area; CoA, cortical nuclei of the amygdala; ERh, entorhinal cortex; G, gustatory cortex; Hipp, hippocampal complex; Ia, agranular insular cortex; IG, induseum griseum; IL, infralimbic cortex; IT, inferior temporal cortex; M1, primary motor cortex; M1c, caudal M1; M1r, rostral M1; Oa, agranular orbitofrontal cortex; PC, posterior cingulate cortex; PFc, caudal prefrontal cortex; PFd, dorsal prefrontal cortex; PFdl, dorsolateral prefrontal cortex; PFdm, dorsomedial prefrontal cortex; PFp, polar prefrontal cortex; PFvl, ventrolateral prefrontal cortex; PL, prelimbic cortex; PM, premotor cortex; PP, posterior parietal areas; PRh, perirhinal cortex; RSp, retrosplenial cortex; S1, primary somatosensory cortex; S2, secondary somatosensory cortex; ST, superior temporal cortex; TT, tenia tecta; V1, primary visual cortex; V2, secondary visual cortex.

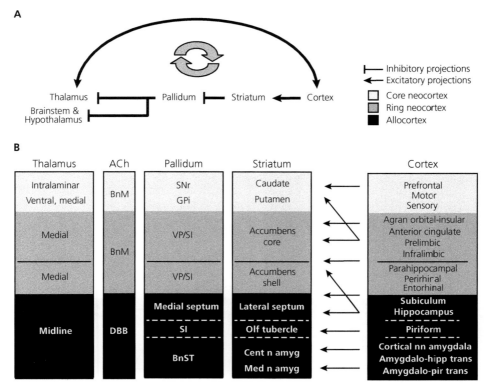

Fig. 2.2 Cortex–basal ganglia "loops." (A) Fundamental "loop" architecture. (B) Selected cortex–basal ganglia modules. The figure omits parts of the amygdala and indirect pathways through the striatum. Abbreviations: ACh, acetylcholine; agran, agranular; Amygdalo-hipp trans, amygdalohippocampal transition area; Amygdalo-pir trans, amygdalopiriform transition area; BnM, basal nucleus (of Meynert); BnST, bed nucleus of the stria terminalis; Cent, central; DBB, diagonal band (of Broca); GPi, internal segment of the globus pallidus; n, nucleus; nn, nuclei; Olf, olfactory; SI, substantia innominata; SNr, substantia nigra pars reticulata; VP, ventral pallidum. Adapted and reprinted from Murray EA, Wise SP. What, if anything, is the medial temporal lobe, and how can the amygdala be part of it if there is no such thing? *Neurobiology of Learning and Memory* 82:178–98, © 2004, with permission from Elsevier.

Figure 2.3 and Plate 1 contrast the prevailing view with the evolutionary accretion model (see Tables 1.2 and 1.3). We return to these figures later in this chapter, but to understand them we first need to sketch a history of the vertebrate brain.

Early vertebrates

To begin the discussion, we need to use eight specialized terms: protostomes, deutero-stomes, chordates, cephalochordates, tunicates (of two types, ascidians and appendicularians), and agnathans. Definitions are given in the Glossary, and Fig. 2.4 places these terms in a phylogenetic perspective.

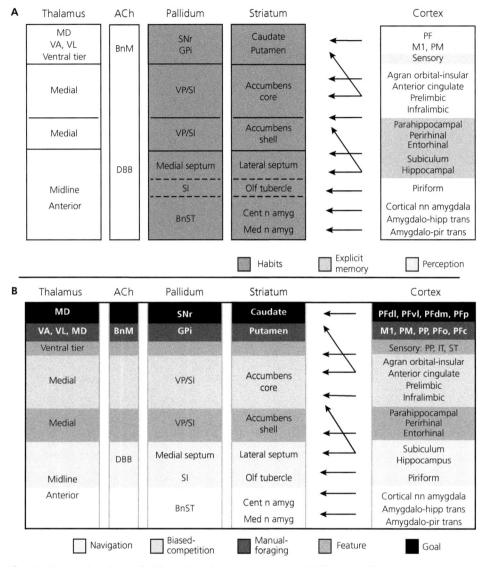

Fig. 2.3 Cortex–basal ganglia "loops" and memory systems. (A) The prevailing view of memory systems. This version applies the "habit system" to the basal ganglia as a whole, in its extended sense. However, most research on habits focuses on the dorsal striatum. (B) An alternative perspective. Format and abbreviations as in Fig. 2.2(B). Additional abbreviations: MD, mediodorsal nucleus; VA, ventroanterior nucleus; VL, ventrolateral nucleus. The unshaded areas remain unclassified according to this scheme, but they contribute to reinforcement learning. Plate 1 presents a color version of this figure and so displays the assignments of cortex–basal ganglia "loops" to representational systems more clearly that the grayscale in this figure. Adapted and reprinted from Murray EA, Wise SP. What, if anything, is the medial temporal lobe, and how can the amygdala be part of it if there is no such thing? *Neurobiology of Learning and Memory* 82:178–98, © 2004, with permission from Elsevier.

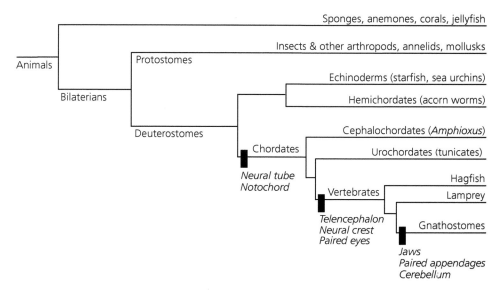

Fig. 2.4 Cladogram of animals. Example groups and species are in parentheses. The traits that evolved *de novo* in a given lineage appear beneath the black bars. Adapted from Figure 4.1 of Murray EA, Wise SP, Rhodes SEV. What can different brains do with reward? In: *The Neurobiology of Sensation and Reward* (Gottfried JA, ed.), pp. 57–92. © 2011, Taylor & Francis. Reproduced with permission.

The origin of vertebrates

Vertebrates evolved more than 500 million years ago from a mobile predator that used its central nervous system to control movement, guided in large part by inputs from visual and olfactory receptors. Vertebrates have existed, therefore, for more than two-thirds of the 750 million years or so since the origin of animals[1,2].

In Chapter 3 ("Evolution") we delve into the origin of animals and the selective factors that produced them. Later animals evolved tubular body plans, with circulatory and digestive systems that permitted dramatic increases in body size and complexity.

Two major groups descended from these early animals: protostomes and deuterostomes (Fig. 2.4). The progenitor of these groups is called the protostome–deuterostome ancestor, often abbreviated as the PDA. Both protostomes and deuterostomes first appear in the fossil record about 530 million years ago[1]. In protostomes (meaning "mouth first"), the first opening of the embryonic tube persists as the mouth and the second becomes the anus. Protostomes are what most people mean by "invertebrates," including insects and other arthropods, mollusks, and various kinds of worms, among others (see Fig. 3.1). In deuterostomes, this sequence is back to front, so to speak, with the second opening forming the mouth.

The PDA probably resembled a worm of some sort. According to the current consensus, nerve nets condensed into concentrated nervous systems independently in protostomes and deuterostomes, although this issue remains unsettled[3,4]. Similarities in the neural expression of developmental regulatory (*Hox*) genes have suggested to some experts that modern brains have descended from a brain in the PDA. Alternatively, these genes may have been co-opted from a role in patterning the anterior body parts of a brainless PDA, prior to the appearance of a central nervous system. In the context of the most likely options for the origins of brains[5], some recent advances in understanding animal evolution[6], and the patterns of gene expression in deuterostomes[7], it seems most likely that a brain evolved independently in protostomes and deuterostomes. Parallel evolution of this kind would explain why protostome brains bear so little resemblance to those of vertebrates.

Among deuterostomes, two kinds of chordates are most closely related to vertebrates: tunicates and cephalochordates (Fig. 2.4). Chordates are named for a rod-like structure, called a notochord, that stiffens their body axis to promote efficient swimming. A notochord also develops in vertebrate embryos, although it typically degenerates.

Cephalochordates include the well-studied creature *Amphioxus*, also known as the lancelet. When biologists first discovered this animal they thought it was some sort of slug. *Amphioxus* turned out to be something very different, but this mistake says quite a lot about it. *Amphioxus* does not closely resemble vertebrates, although it does have something like an eye at its anterior end, along with half a dozen or so neural homologies with vertebrates[8]. Until relatively recently, most evolutionary biologists considered *Amphioxus* to be the closest living relative of modern vertebrates.

A more recent analysis, however, indicates that tunicates are the sister group* of vertebrates[6]. One group of modern tunicates, called ascidians, are immobile (sessile) as adults. These tubular animals attach themselves to a substrate early in life and obtain nutrients by siphoning in suspended particles. Ancestral tunicates might have been more complex than their modern counterparts, but it is hard to imagine these sessile filter feeders as the nearest relatives of vertebrates.

In the late nineteenth century, Gerstang proposed that the immediate ancestors of vertebrates evolved from the mobile larvae of sessile adults[3]. Modern tunicate larvae have some vertebrate traits, such as a notochord and a dorsally situated neural tube (Fig. 2.5B2). Although they do not forage or eat, tunicate larvae do swim, and they continue to do so until they find a suitable substrate. Ascidian tunicates then metamorphose into their sessile form and absorb most of their central nervous system. (An analogous process occurs when scientists take on too many administrative duties.)

Subsequent research has cast some doubt on Gerstang's venerable idea. The stem chordate might have resembled a different kind of tunicate, an appendicularian, rather than an ascidian. Appendicularian tunicates remain mobile throughout their lives and retain their central nervous systems[3]. Figure 2.5(A) depicts a representative appendicularian and its nervous system.

Whatever their precise origins, it is evident that many vertebrate traits arose as adaptations to a mobile life. Like tunicates, all vertebrates have two key chordate traits at

---

* In Chapter 1 ("Cladistics") and in the Glossary we explain the term *sister group*.

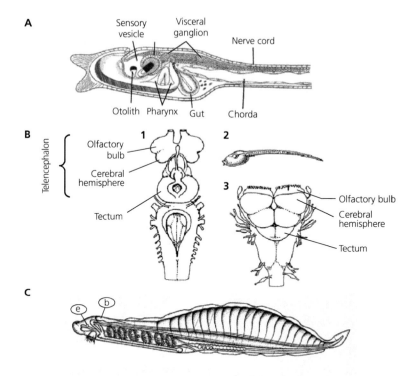

Fig. 2.5 Appendicularians, agnathans, and ancestors. (A) Adult tunicate (an appendicularian). Rostral is to the left. (B) 1: A lamprey brain. Rostral is up. 2: A larval tunicate of a sessile adult (an ascidian). Rostral is to the left. 3: A hagfish brain. Rostral is up. (C) A fossil craniate. Rostral is left. Abbreviations: b, brain; e, eye. (A) Reprinted from Glover JC, Fritsch B. Brains of primitive chordates. In *Encyclopedia of Neuroscience*, © 2009, with permission from Elsevier. (B) From Figure 2.2D, E, and F in Shadmehr R, Wise SP. *The Computational Neurobiology of Reaching and Pointing*, The MIT Press. Originally from Nieuwenhuys R. Deuterostome brains: synopsis and commentary. *Brain Research Bulletin* 57:257–70, © 2002, with permission from Elsevier. (C) From Shu D, Morris SC, Zhang ZF, Liu JN, Han J, Chen L, Zhang XL, Yasui K, Li Y. A new species of yunnanozoan with implications for deuterostome evolution. *Science* 299:1380, © 2003, Reprinted with permission from the American Association for the Advancement of Science.

some point during their development: a dorsal neural tube and a dorsal notochord. They also have a series of bilateral, segmental muscles controlled by a central nervous system.

Fossil evidence supports the idea that a brain had evolved by the time of the earliest vertebrates (Fig. 2.5C). A chordate called *Haikouella* had a clear-cut brain along with paired eyes[9–11], although its relationship to vertebrates remains uncertain[1,12,13]. Other fossils, specifically one named *Haikouichthys*, are unambiguous vertebrates. Specimens from this group, found in rocks about 520 million years old, show evidence of a brain with paired eyes, a notochord, segmented blocks of muscles, and gill-like structures[14]. (Because the brain evolved before bones, many experts prefer the term craniate to vertebrate, but the latter will do for our purposes.) Looking at these fossils more generally, their most obvious structural adaptations supported active swimming[15].

The fossil evidence shows that vision contributed to brain-guided movement from very early in the history of vertebrates, as these animals and their immediate ancestors solved a multitude of problems posed by predatory foraging. Olfactory specializations also developed at this time but did not pre-date vision, as some neuroanatomists have claimed in the past[16]. Together, visual and olfactory receptors provided information from a distance, which these animals undoubtedly used to guide movement.

The origin of the telencephalon

The development of a telencephalon ranks among the most significant of derived vertebrate traits[17]. All modern vertebrates have a telencephalon, including those that diverged from the others longest ago: agnathan fish. Agnathan means "jawless," and these animals not only lack jaws but also paired fins. The modern agnathans, lamprey and hagfish, both have elongated bodies, but fossil agnathans show a broad variety of body shapes[1]. Like all other vertebrates, the agnathan telencephalon includes the olfactory bulbs (Fig. 2.5B1, B3). Figures 1.8 and 2.4 place hagfish and lamprey in a broader evolutionary perspective.

No other animals have a telencephalon. Protostome brains, including insect brains, have nothing resembling a telencephalon and probably have few, if any, homologues of vertebrate brain structures. Among deuterostomes, cephalochordates (*Amphioxus*) also lack a telencephalon, although they might have homologues of the hindbrain and spinal cord, and perhaps part of the diencephalon as well[8,18,19]. Because all vertebrates have an identifiable telencephalon, but no other chordates or protostomes do, we can infer that the telencephalon evolved in the stem vertebrates or their immediate ancestors.

Given the importance of the telencephalon, we would of course like to know what composed the original version. Of most relevance to memory systems, comparative neuroanatomy indicates that it included homologues of both the cerebral cortex and basal ganglia:

- Homologues of the cerebral cortex sometimes go by the term *pallium*, not to be confused with the pallidum (a part of the basal ganglia). In mammals, the pallium comprises the olfactory bulbs, claustrum, and cerebral cortex, including the hippocampus and piriform cortex. The latter two structures probably have homologues in all vertebrates[20–24] (see "Homologies").

- Homologues of the basal ganglia exist in agnathans, specifically lamprey[25]. Because of the broad distribution of homologues of the basal ganglia among vertebrates[22,24,26–33], we can infer that stem vertebrates evolved the basal ganglia, along with their characteristic dopaminergic inputs[34,35].

The vertebrate telencephalon includes several additional structures, such as the amygdala, septal nuclei, and basal forebrain. As explained later (see "Rings and loops"), many of these structures are parts of the basal ganglia or, most enigmatically of all, of the claustrum. The claustrum, like the cortex, derives from the pallium. Because no one knows much about its function, however, we do not discuss it further, except to say that parts of the amygdala have been included in the claustrum, specifically the basal and lateral nuclei[36].

Additional vertebrate traits

Along with the telencephalon, stem vertebrates evolved a complex suite of additional traits. For instance, stem vertebrates evolved a set of sensory organs on their heads, including bilateral eyes. These structures arise from embryonic placodes, thickenings of the ecto-dermal tissue that mature into olfactory, vestibular, and visual organs. Other derived traits arise from neural crest cells, which produce the autonomic nervous system, sensory neu-rons, myelinating cells, skeletal tissue in the head, head muscles, and other cranial struc-tures. In addition, the neural crest and placodes produce such vertebrate innovations as smooth muscle, endocrine glands, and the cartilage that supports feeding and respiration. Two semicircular canals and the lateral-line system sense gravitational forces as well as movements of the body and head. In essence, the innovations of stem vertebrates include the telencephalon, most of the head, several sensory organs, and a respiratory apparatus.

Stem vertebrates also evolved cardiovascular, digestive, renal, and motor sys-tems[37], including a new kind of muscle resulting from the fusion of many myoblasts[38]. Consequently, vertebrate muscles consist of large cells with many nuclei, a property that provides advantages in terms of length and force. Additional innovations include brain-stem mechanisms for controlling eye movements and respiration. Eye movements, for example, probably evolved to hold the eye stable relative to the external world, at least for brief periods[39]. According to this idea, the oculomotor system originated as an adapta-tion for limiting the blurring of visual images during movement. Finally, stem vertebrates developed the anterior pituitary gland, which responds to hypothalamic secretions by producing hormones that regulate growth, metabolism, and reproduction.

Summary

The telencephalon originated in early vertebrates, along with new embryonic tissues that produced the head and its sensory organs, including paired eyes. These animals used information detected at a distance, in large part provided by vision and olfaction, to guide foraging and self-defense. The telencephalon exerted control over the body through its connections with the motor system, broadly construed to include neuroendocrine, neu-rosecretory, and autonomic outputs, as well as skeletal and eye muscles (see Chapter 1, "Brain organization" and Fig. 1.1B). Through interactions with the hypothalamus, the telencephalon of early vertebrates regulated metabolism and maintained homeostasis. Through interactions with the hypothalamus, brainstem, and spinal cord, it also con-trolled reproductive, ingestive, exploratory, and defensive behaviors mediated by skeletal muscles[40]. Of most relevance to memory systems, the telencephalon that emerged in early vertebrates included homologues of both the hippocampus and basal ganglia.

With their newly derived traits, early vertebrates established the fundamental way of life that their descendants have followed ever since. The telencephalon acquired, processed, and stored information about the animal's place in a world of chemicals and objects; it assessed the biological value of objects and places; and, crucially, it made choices about what actions to make or to withhold. Our earliest vertebrate ancestors needed to conserve energy, avoid risk, and yet exploit opportunities for consuming nutritious items. In crude anthropomorphic terms, they were lazy and easily frightened, yet greedy. This combination worked, but they clearly have a lot to answer for.

Early amniotes

This section, like the one on early vertebrates, relies on some specialized terms: in this case gnathostome, tetrapod, and amniote (see Fig. 1.8).

After vertebrates became established, jawed fishes evolved from jawless ancestors. Called gnathostomes (meaning "gnawing mouth"), these animals also developed paired appendages (fins) and a cerebellum. Descendants of the early gnathostomes included the stem tetrapods, which evolved about 370–450 million years ago, as well as the stem amniotes, which appeared about 320–360 million years ago[41,42]:

- ◆ Crown tetrapods[†] include frogs, toads, newts, and salamanders, collectively amphibians (also known as lissamphibians), along with all amniotes (see Fig. 1.8).
- ◆ Crown amniotes include turtles, snakes, lizards, and crocodiles, collectively reptiles, along with all mammals and birds (Box 2.1).

Tetrapods first entered the terrestrial niche, and developments in egg architecture allowed amniotes to live a fully terrestrial life.

The section on early vertebrates mentioned the pallium, a part of the telencephalon. In amniotes, part of the pallium adopted the architecture that characterizes this structure in mammals and reptiles: It became the cerebral cortex.

Cerebral cortex

The neocortex so dominates the appearance of the human brain that other parts of the cerebral cortex recede from the mind's eye. Yet neocortex is only one type of cerebral cortex; the other is allocortex, which includes the hippocampus. Despite this fact, neuroscientists—even experts on the hippocampus—sometimes mistakenly refer to "the hippocampus *and* the cerebral cortex," as if the former was not part of the latter. But it is.

Allocortex and neocortex have a great deal in common. In both, pyramidal cells collect in parallel sheets, with one long dendrite, called the apical dendrite, extending towards the surface of the cortex. Basal dendrites are oriented roughly parallel with the surface, and dendritic spines cover both apical and basal dendrites. Pyramidal cells send excitatory, glutamatergic outputs to subcortical structures and to other parts of the cortex.

....

[†] In Chapter 1 ("Cladistics") and in the Glossary we explain the term *crown group*.

Box 2.1 What about birds?

Readers might wonder why we give such short shrift to birds. The simplest reason is that we want to focus on human memory, and no bird is or ever was an ancestor of humans. Evolutionary biologists have long recognized that birds and mammals evolved from two lineages that diverged early in the history of amniotes, and the brains of both lineages have changed dramatically in the interim (Fig. 2.6A).

Without doubt, birds have impressive cognitive capabilities. The popular description of corvids as "avian primates," however, conveys an unfortunate impression. This laudably anti-chauvinistic sentiment downplays the importance of convergent evolution in cognition, despite its undisputed prevalence in other traits, such as endothermy.

One recent discussion, for example, claims that episodic memory in humans and birds depends on neural structures and circuits inherited from a common ancestor, concluding that "protoepisodic memory systems exist across amniotes and, possibly, all vertebrates" (Allen and Fortin[163], p. 10379). This conclusion relies on the proposition that human episodic memory is homologous to the "what–where–when" memories observed in birds, an oversimplified view that denies both independent evolution and diversity. We address this issue in Chapter 11 ("Episodic-like memory"), but for now we stress a general rule: To search for "precursors" or "proto-functions" by comparing two modern species depends on faulty assumptions (see Chapter 1, "Precursors of the past"). Parallel and convergent evolution occur quite commonly, in part because independently evolving lineages often confront similar problems and opportunities.

For the sake of discussion, however, assume that homologues of the hippocampus subserve "what–where–when" memories in all mammals and birds. Even so, this would not mean that their last common ancestor had episodic memory or that precursors of episodic memory "exist across amniotes" (Allen and Fortin[163], p. 10379). If homologies conveyed that implication, then monkeys would be able to fly. Birds and monkeys have a homologous structure, the forelimb, which supports locomotion. But monkeys cannot fly, except in *The Wizard of Oz*. Likewise, birds and humans have a homologue of the hippocampus, but that doesn't mean that the bird hippocampus does what the human hippocampus does. Indeed, in Chapter 11 we advance a specific proposal to the contrary. Just as a bird's wings are not precursors of human forelimbs, the representations housed in the bird hippocampus are not precursors of those in the human hippocampus.

The concepts of "avian primates" and precursors of episodic memory in birds would be harmless except for two implications that they convey, perhaps inadvertently: Primates have no cognitive capacities that other animals lack, and, even if they do, episodic memory is not among them. Diversity denial of this sort underpins the prevailing view of memory systems, as we explain in Chapter 12 ("The road taken"). To understand the evolution of memory, however, we need to embrace both diversity and primate innovations.

Allocortex has three layers, an outer molecular layer (layer 1) and two layers of output cells. Inputs to allocortex terminate mainly in layer 1 and outputs arise from the pyramidal cells of layers 2 and 3. So neuroanatomists often refer to allocortex as three-layer cortex.

The neocortex has a different and more complicated structure, and it is usually thicker. Although neuroanatomists often refer to neocortex as six-layer cortex, it comes in many variants, with different numbers of layers. To a first approximation, inputs from the thalamus terminate in layers 1, 3, and 4 (for areas that have layer 4); interconnections among cortical areas arise mostly from layers 2 and 3 (with some from layer 5); outputs to most subcortical structures come from layer 5; and projections to the thalamus originate from layer 6.

Because a six-layer neocortex is present in all modern mammals and absent from other amniotes, we can infer that it is an innovation of early mammals or their immediate ancestors.

Homologies

Figure 2.6(A) illustrates some homologies in the vertebrate pallium[43]. Because the telencephalon increases in complexity during development, its simpler embryonic states sometimes reveal homologies that are obscured by later development. Figure 2.6(A) emphasizes two of them:

1. The dorsomedial telencephalon includes a structure called the medial pallium in amphibians and birds, the medial cortex in reptiles, and the hippocampus in mammals.
2. The ventrolateral telencephalon includes a structure called the lateral pallium in amphibians and birds, the lateral cortex in reptiles, and the piriform cortex in mammals. Because it receives direct input from the olfactory bulb through the lateral olfactory tract, a homologue of the piriform cortex has been identified in all vertebrates, including modern agnathans[22].

The entire cerebral cortex has an allocortical architecture in most modern reptiles[27,44], and so it seems likely that the pallium adopted this trait in stem amniotes. Figure 2.7(A) illustrates the cerebral cortex of a lizard, demonstrating its three-layer structure. Taken together, the small-cell (parvocellular) and large-cell (magnocellular) parts of the medial cortex compose the hippocampal homologue (Fig. 2.7A). Figure 2.6(B, C) illustrates its axonal connections in lizards and mammals, respectively[44]. One recent analysis, which also took birds into account, suggests that the parvocellular part corresponds to the hippocampus proper (the CA fields) and the magnocellular part corresponds to the subiculum, with the dentate gyrus being either greatly expanded or evolved *de novo* in mammals[44].

In addition to its three-layer structure, the dendritic architecture of neurons in the reptilian medial cortex supports the proposed homology[27,44]. Like the mammalian hippocampus, the medial cortex of modern reptiles contains an extraordinary amount of heavy metals, mainly zinc, as demonstrated by the Timms stain. Other similarities include the distribution of axon terminals from other cortical areas, which concentrate

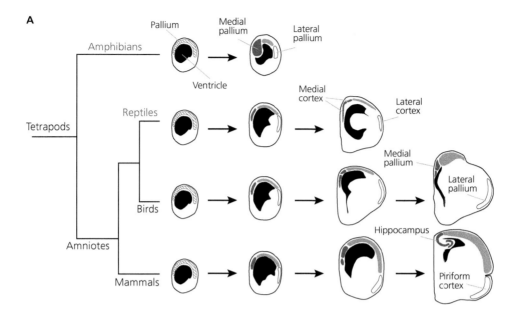

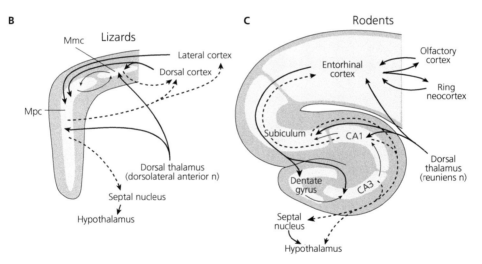

Fig. 2.6 Evolution and development. (A) The evolution of developmental sequences in the cerebral cortex and pallium, in one hemisphere. Medial is to the left, dorsal is up. The key homologues have consistent shading in all drawings. Paraphyletic groups in gray type. (B, C) Connections of the hippocampus homologue in representative reptiles and rodents. Abbreviations: CA1 and CA3, cortical fields in the hippocampus; Mmc, medial cortex, large cell (magnocellular) part; Mpc, medial cortex, small cell (parvocellular) part; n, nucleus. (A) Adapted from Striedter GF. *Principles of Brain Evolution*. Sunderland, MA: Sinauer, © 2005, (B), (C) From Striedter GF. Evolution of the hippocampus in reptiles and birds. *Journal of Comparative Neurology*, 524: 496–517. © 2016, John Wiley & Sons. Reproduced with permission.

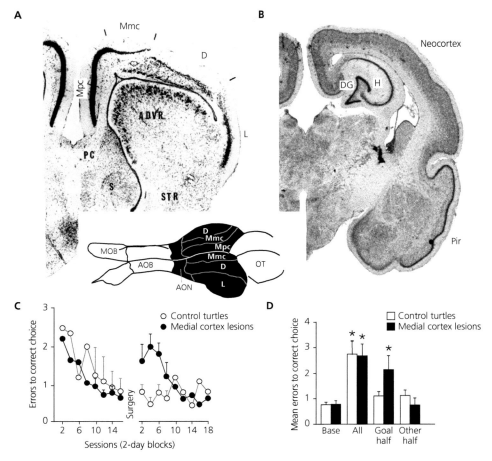

Fig. 2.7 Reptilian cortex. (A) Representative frontal section through a lizard brain. For the brain section, dorsal is up and medial is to the left. For the inset, rostral is to the left. (B) Representative frontal section through a marsupial brain. Format as in (A). Abbreviations: ADVR, anterior dorsal ventricular ridge; AOB, accessory olfactory bulb; AON, anterior olfactory nucleus; D, dorsal cortex; DG, dentate gyrus; H, hippocampus; L, lateral cortex; Mmc, medial cortex, large cell (magnocellular) part; Mpc, medial cortex, small cell (parvocellular) part; MOB, main olfactory bulb; PC, pallial commissure; OT, optic tectum (homologue of the superior colliculus); Pir, piriform cortex; S, septal nuclei; STR, striatum. (C) Effect of medial cortex lesions on a baited version of the Morris water maze in turtles. Error bars: standard error. Only selected variance data are illustrated. (D) Effect of concealing extramaze cues. Conditions: Base, baseline, post-criterion training; All, all extramaze cues concealed; Goal half, extramaze cues concealed in the half of the testing room that contained the goal (food); Other half, extramaze cues concealed in the half of the room without the goal. Asterisks show statistically significant differences from baseline. (A, inset) From Ulinski PS. The cerebral cortex of reptiles. In *Cerebral Cortex: Comparative Structure and Evolution Of Cerebral Cortex*, Part I, eds. EG Jones, A Peters, pp. 139–215, © 1990, With permission of Springer. (B) Reproduced from the Wisconsin Brain Collection (http://www.brainmuseum.org/), supported by the US National Science Foundation and the National Institutes of Health. (C), (D) Redrawn from López JC, Vargas JP, Gómez Y, Salas C. Spatial and non-spatial learning in turtles: The role of medial cortex. *Behavioural Brain Research* 143:109–20, © 2003, with permission from Elsevier.

near cell bodies in layer 2, and terminals from the thalamus, which go to the outer part of layer 1. Both the reptilian medial cortex and the mammalian hippocampus have reciprocal connections with the thalamus and outputs to the septal nuclei[27] (Fig. 2.6B, C).

Behavioral evidence also supports these homologies. In one experiment, lizards searched for a warm rock in a circular field that also contained three additional rocks at room temperature[45]. Unlike mammals and birds, lizards need to absorb energy from their external environment in order to move effectively; so they search for warm rocks. This task parallels the hippocampus-dependent Morris water maze, in which rodents search for a submerged platform in a water tank. Lizards with lesions of the medial cortex learned the task more slowly and took longer to find the heated rock than did control lizards. Lesions of the dorsal cortex had a similar effect, perhaps because they blocked visual inputs to the medial cortex. Despite the similarity between the rodent and lizard versions of the task, probe trials revealed an important difference. The lizards used cues within the testing field rather than distant (extramaze) cues, whereas rodents depend on extramaze cues to perform the Morris water-maze task (see Chapter 4, "The cognitive map through history"). This difference probably reflects the fact that the lizards navigated to a visible goal in this experiment whereas in the water-maze task rodents cannot see their goal and instead must navigate via extramaze cues.

In another experiment, also a version of the Morris water maze, turtles searched for a submerged platform that had been baited with food—out of four platforms[46]. As long as the location of the food remained constant, the turtles learned to swim to its location. Like rodents in such tasks (see Chapter 4, "The cognitive map through history"), the turtles used extramaze cues to guide navigation. After lesions of the medial cortex, the turtles had a performance impairment that persisted through several days of testing (Fig. 2.7C). Although they eventually recovered their ability to find the food, the turtles with medial cortex lesions used a different strategy from control turtles. Turtles in the lesion group used the extramaze cues only in half of the room, the half that contained the food (Fig. 2.7D). Striedter[44] suggests that the lesioned turtles lost their ability to guide foraging via a series of landmarks and locations (discussed in Chapter 4 in terms of a cognitive map). After the lesion, the turtles seem to have instead resorted to snapshot memory, which involves matching current and remembered visual inputs, in this case for the part of the room with food.

In addition to connectional and embryological evidence, the expression of developmental regulatory genes supports the proposed homologies. Figure 2.8(B) and Plate 2(B) illustrate different patterns of gene expression by the level of gray shading or by color, respectively. The studies that led to these drawings show that the hippocampal (medial) cortex of developing mice expresses the same pattern of developmental regulatory genes as does the medial pallium in developing chicks[47-49]. This evidence points to inheritance from a common ancestor that lived early in the history of amniotes (double dagger in Fig. 1.8). Likewise, the piriform (lateral) cortex of developing mice expresses the same pattern of developmental regulatory genes as the lateral pallium in developing chicks[47-49].

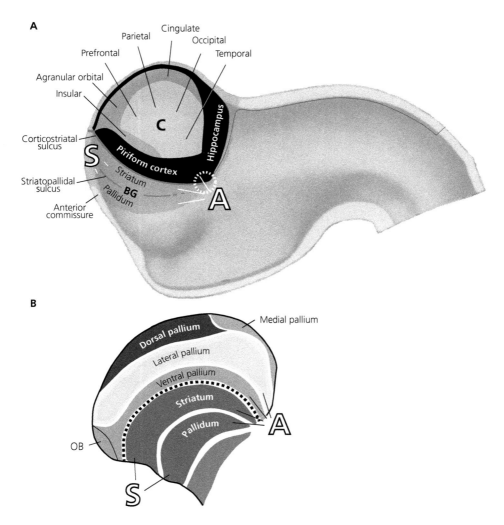

Fig. 2.8 Cortical origins. (A) Location of cortical areas in the embryonic human brain. Rostral is to the left. The dashed white circle shows the region that becomes the frontotemporal junction, which includes the piriform cortex as it makes a transition with the cortical nuclei of the amygdala. The large S and A indicate the general regions that give rise to the septal nuclei and the amygdala, respectively. (B) A schematic of telencephalic regions expressing diagnostic patterns of developmental regulatory genes in mice and chicks. Abbreviations: A, amygdala; BG, basal ganglia; C, neocortex; OB, olfactory bulb; S, septal nuclei. Plate 2 presents a color version of this figure. (A) Reprinted from Swanson LW. Cerebral hemisphere regulation of motivated behavior. *Brain Research* 886:113-64, © 2000, with permission from Elsevier. (B) Modified from Puelles L, Kuwana E, Puelles E, Bulfone A, Shimamura K, Keleher J, Smiga S, Rubenstein JL. Pallial and subpallial derivatives in the embryonic chick and mouse telencephalon, traced by the expression of the genes dlx-2, Emx-1, Nkx-2.1, Pax-6, and Tbr-1. *Journal of Comparative Neurology* 424:409–38, © 2000, John Wiley & Sons, with permission.

[Note that both the piriform cortex and lateral pallium have two subdivisions, called lateral and ventral in Fig. 2.8(B) and Plate 2(B).]

Outdated concepts

Having mentioned modern reptiles, we need to address some outdated ideas about brain evolution[50]. MacLean proposed that humans and other mammals have a "reptilian brain," which he identified with the basal ganglia, to go along with a "primitive mammalian brain" (roughly, the limbic system) and an "advanced mammalian brain." This idea struck a romantic chord with the public, one that has resonated in cult films (*Mon Oncle d'Amerique*), popular science (*The Dragons of Eden*), and, with no restraint whatsoever, on the Internet. In Chapter 5 ("Walnut brains and nutty ideas") we relate an example from popular science.

Few experts take MacLean's ideas seriously, however, and for good reason. Many of the structures that MacLean identified as mammalian "advances," such as the hippocampus and other components of the limbic system, originated much earlier. Mammals do not have "reptilian" structures inside their heads, although they do share homologues of many brain structures with other amniotes, including the basal ganglia.

The term limbic system, which comes from the Latin word for border or rim, also deserves a comment. This concept has heuristic value because, to an approximation, the limbic system consists of structures directly connected to the hypothalamus[40]. This property, however, says little about brain evolution.

Summary

The cerebrum of stem amniotes included the medial cortex and lateral cortex, homologues of the mammalian hippocampus and piriform cortex, respectively. These areas have a three-layer allocortical structure, which differs from mammalian six-layer neocortex. Some experts have objected to the term neocortex, noting the idea that it developed from the amniote dorsal cortex and so was not entirely new. The derived architecture of the neocortex, however, warrants its designation as "new cortex." Nevertheless, the reptilian dorsal cortex does have a homologue of the primary visual cortex of mammals. This part of the reptilian allocortex receives retinal inputs relayed via the thalamus, just as the primary visual cortex does in mammals[51].

Early mammals

The comparative evidence shows that the neocortex emerged during the evolution of mammals, and its initial composition can be inferred by identifying homologous areas in a diverse selection of crown mammals[52,53]. This reconstruction includes at least two visual areas, the primary visual cortex (V1) and a secondary visual area (V2), along with one or two others[54]. It also includes the perirhinal cortex, which is a multimodal sensory area, as well as sensory areas for audition and somatic sensation, including a primary auditory (A1) and primary somatosensory (S1) cortex (Fig. 2.9). In addition, this reconstructed

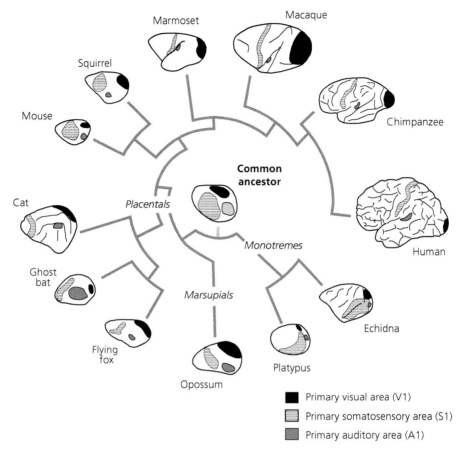

Fig. 2.9 Cortical cladogram. Primary visual, somatosensory, and auditory areas in a selection of mammals, and the inferred common ancestor. Brains are drawn at different scales. (Figure 5.1 illustrates the cortex of the common ancestor in a different way.) Adapted from Krubitzer LA, Seelke AM. Cortical evolution in mammals: the bane and beauty of phenotypic variability. *Proceedings of the National Academy of Sciences U.S.A.* 109 Suppl. 1:10647–54, © 2012, National Academy of Sciences, with permission.

brain has an agranular insular area, which in modern mammals receives relatively direct olfactory, gustatory, and visceral inputs. The areas mentioned so far contribute to sensory processing, but stem mammals also evolved neocortical areas with more enigmatic functions, such as the retrosplenial, cingulate, prelimbic, infralimbic, and agranular orbitofrontal cortex. Figure 2.1(B) illustrates a selection of these areas on a schematic representation of the cerebral cortex. Later, in Chapter 5 ("Evolution"), we illustrate them in a more conventional way (see Fig. 5.1A).

Because this is a book on memory systems, not evolution, we do not dwell here on the many additional innovations of mammals. Most experts estimate that the first true mammals appeared about 210–220 million years ago, in a major evolutionary transition from a specific group of amniotes. This transition involved a multitude of "experiments" with various combinations of derived traits, only some of which involved the brain. The stem mammals adapted to a high-energy, nocturnal foraging niche. To cite just a few of the innovative traits that emerged with early mammals, they evolved a new kind of tooth (the molar), a new kind of ear (and high-frequency audition), a new mode of temperature control (involving hair, endothermy, and instinctive behaviors that conserved heat), and a new mode of nurturing offspring that led to the name "mammal." Molars, for example, are so strongly and uniquely characteristic of mammals that some extinct species are known only by the chance discovery of a single fossilized tooth.

Rings

Figure 2.1 presents a figurative overview of the cerebral cortex. In the amniote ancestors of mammals, allocortex made up the entire cerebral cortex (Fig. 2.1A). In mammals, allocortical areas form a ring around the neocortex (Fig. 2.1B, C). In addition to the piriform (lateral) cortex and the hippocampus (medial cortex), this ring includes several small, obscure allocortical areas, such as the cortical nuclei of the amygdala, the induseum griseum, and the tenia tecta. In addition, the allocortex includes several small areas often called transition areas, such as one between the amygdala and the piriform cortex (the amygdalopiriform transition area) and another between the hippocampus and the amygdala (the amygdalohippocampal transition area). Little is known about the function of these structures, but their layout contributes to the ring structure of the cerebral cortex when viewed as a whole.

Figure 2.1(B) (light gray) depicts some of the sensory and motor areas of the neocortex in early placental mammals. Between these areas and the allocortex lie several additional cortical areas, collectively called "transition areas" (dark gray) by some neuroanatomists. This sense of "transition" differs from its meaning in the previous paragraph, which referred to transitions between one allocortical area and another. Accordingly, we have invented a novel term for the areas adjacent to the allocortex: ring neocortex. The contrasting term, core neocortex, refers to areas that do not border the allocortex.

Memory researchers might have a particular interest in how the parahippocampal and entorhinal cortex fit into this scheme. Their complex lamination clearly excludes them from allocortex. We group both with the ring neocortex, although the primate parahippocampal cortex might be included with the core areas instead. We class the presubiculum and subiculum as allocortex because they lack the laminar complexity of neocortex, but leave parasubiculum and prosubiculum unclassified because their properties seem genuinely intermediate between allocortex and neocortex.

Rings and wrongs

Although the idea of an allocortical ring around the neocortex is nothing new—it can be tracked from page to page in any decent brain atlas—it is controversial because of an association with ideas about cortical evolution advanced by Sanides[55]. He classified components of the ring neocortex as periallocortex, juxtallocortex, proisocortex, and so forth. For example, he called cortex with a pale band between superficial and deep layers periallocortex (or juxtallocortex) and cortex without this band, but also without a layer 4, proisocortex. Sanides suggested that these "transition" areas evolved prior to other parts of the neocortex, which implies that there was a stage during mammalian evolution in which the cortex consisted only of ring ("transition") neocortex and allocortex, with no additional (core) areas. Although this idea remains popular[56–60], no comparative evidence supports it. That does not mean that the idea of cortical rings is a waste of time, just that it is wrong in the way that Sanides and others have applied it.

Furthermore, Sanides advanced an imaginative scheme in which a group of medial cortical areas evolved from the hippocampus, whereas a group of lateral areas arose from the piriform cortex. He claimed that he could spot these medial and lateral "trends" by examining the architecture of cortical areas. Without a strong comparative underpinning, however, these "trends" say nothing about cortical evolution.

Some of Sanides' suggestions do find support in comparative neuroanatomy, however. He said that the hippocampus and piriform cortex correspond to the ancestral medial and lateral cortex, respectively, and that these areas evolved before the neocortex. As explained earlier (see "Early amniotes"), comparative evidence supports these ideas.

Unfortunately, most of Sanides' suggestions about cortical evolution are either demonstrably wrong or entirely speculative, often leaving no way to evaluate their validity. In the former category, Sanides imagined that primary sensory areas, such as the primary visual (V1) cortex, the primary somatosensory (S1) cortex, and the primary auditory (A1) cortex, appeared relatively recently in evolution and were the newest of neocortical areas. The comparative evidence contradicts this idea conclusively. The primary sensory areas were among the earliest neocortical areas to appear during mammalian evolution[52,53], as established by the homologies illustrated in Fig. 2.9. We return to this point in Chapter 5 ("Evolution").

Among the problems with Sanides' approach is the fact that homologues can change during evolution and usually do. So what Sanides saw as evidence for the recent appearance of primary sensory areas probably reflects their long history of accrued modifications. Applying his line of reasoning to the human hand instead of the cortex, one could speculate about the evolutionary history of the fingers based on their relative lengths. Sanides' evolutionary doctrine about the "advanced" and "transition" cortex has no more merit than the supposition that the middle finger evolved most recently because it is longest. (Because fingers fossilize we know that nothing of the sort occurred.)

Some evolutionary sequences are probably lost to history. This can happen because many novel combinations of traits develop during major evolutionary transitions but only one set prevails. Many "experiments" in mammalian architecture became extinct, and so no one can study their brains. Short of some *Jurassic Park*-like resurrection, no one ever will. The fact is that no modern mammals have ring neocortex but lack core neocortex. If there ever was a stage like that, it must have happened early in the transition to true mammals. We will probably never know. Regardless, the comparative evidence shows that the neocortex, ring and core combined, is an innovation of stem mammals.

Embryonic rings

So far, we have considered the ring structure of the cerebral cortex from an evolutionary perspective. The same principle emerges from studying embryological development. Figure 2.8(A) and Plate 2(A) depict an embryonic human brain with the nascent cortex and basal ganglia in the upper left[40]. In this simplified form, the overall organization of the telencephalon is clearer than in newborns and adults. Allocortical areas, specifically the piriform cortex and the hippocampus, reside at the boundary of cortex with subcortex. As such, they compose parts of the outermost cortical ring. Likewise, the insular, orbitofrontal, and cingulate areas that make up the ring neocortex lie "outside" the core neocortical areas of the prefrontal, parietal, temporal, and occipital cortex, but "inside" the allocortex. Figure 2.8(A) and Plate 2(A) do not depict the entire ring structure, however, because some details are too small and difficult to discern in early embryos. Small, obscure cortical areas complete the allocortical ring, as explained earlier. Although cells migrate among telencephalic structures and the overall architecture becomes highly distorted as the brain grows, the fundamental pattern remains evident.

Rings and loops

According to Swanson[40], an archetypal telencephalic architecture encompasses the entire cerebral cortex and basal ganglia, the latter being construed in its extended sense (see Chapter 1, "Basal ganglia"). Figure 2.2(A) illustrates this architecture, called a "loop" because of its recurrent nature[61,62]. According to this idea, the telencephalon regulates behavior through the "loop" pathways of the basal ganglia, which selectively disinhibit motor outputs via a sequential pair of inhibitory projections (Fig. 2.2A), with side branches of the loops providing indirect influences via the subthalamic nucleus (not illustrated).

Swanson's conclusions depend mainly on evidence from cell morphology, axonal connections, neurotransmitters, and embryological origins[36,40,63]. In his view, certain telencephalic structures, which textbooks label as parts of the amygdala or as septal nuclei, are components of the striatum instead of being separate "things." These reclassified structures include the central and medial nuclei of the amygdala, the anterior amygdaloid area, and the lateral septal nucleus (see Fig. 1.2C). Each of these nuclei has GABAergic neurons resembling the medium spiny neurons that characterize the traditional striatum, and they project to other GABAergic cells in much the same way that the striatum projects to the globus pallidus in primates. Like the traditional striatum, these unconventional striatal structures receive glutamatergic, excitatory inputs from the thalamus and cortex. Figure 2.2(B) illustrates some of these cortex–basal ganglia "loops," including several that include unconventional parts of the striatum.

The same conclusions can be derived from a study of the embryonic telencephalon. The region between the corticostriatal and striatopallidal sulci that gives rise to the traditional striatum also produces parts of the amygdala and the lateral septal nucleus. As illustrated in Fig. 2.8(A) and Plate 2(A), the septal nucleus (S) comes from the rostral part of this embryonic territory and the striatal amygdala (A) comes from its caudal part.

The study of developmental regulatory genes provides independent support for these ideas. As mentioned earlier, Fig. 2.8(B) and Plate 2(B) illustrate the pattern of gene expression in mice and chicks[47,48]. The lateral septal nuclei and the striatal amygdala express some of the same diagnostic genes during development as the traditional striatum does. These findings, together with embryological and connectional data, support two related ideas: (1) the lateral septal nucleus is the most rostral part of the striatum and (2) the striatal components of the amygdala are the most caudal parts.

The organization of the pallidum reflects the same principles. In the late twentieth century, neuroanatomists began to recognize an extended amygdala that includes basal forebrain structures such as the bed nucleus of the stria terminalis. These extended aspects of the amygdala can be viewed as parts of the pallidum, albeit complicated ones. So the amygdala, in this capacious sense, includes the caudal parts of both the pallidum and striatum, along with the caudal limit of the lateral cortex [labelled "A" in Fig. 2.8(A, B) and Plate 2(A, B)]. Likewise, the medial septal nucleus corresponds to the rostral limit of the pallidum (labelled "S").

Figure 2.2(B) summarizes the relationship between cortical rings and cortex–basal ganglia "loops" by using the same shading convention as in Fig. 2.1(C). Most research has focused on cortex–basal ganglia "loops" that include the neocortex. In contrast, "loops" that include the hippocampus or piriform cortex have received much less attention. Yet these allocortical areas project to a part of the striatum, engage a part of the pallidum, and have reciprocal connections with the thalamus. Each "loop" also receives cholinergic inputs from the basal forebrain.

Regulatory rings

Areas in the allocortical ring project to the hypothalamus and its motor systems, both directly and via their cortex–basal ganglia "loops." As explained in Chapter 1 ("Brain organization," Fig. 1.1B), the motor system in its broadest sense includes neuroendocrine, neurosecretory, and autonomic outputs along with the traditionally recognized motor outputs that control skeletal and eye muscles. The hypothalamus contributes to all of these functions[40] and thereby influences many aspects of behavior, such as instinctive responses to chemosensory and hormonal inputs, procreation, avoidance of harm, and the quest for nutrients, fluids, and warmth. It therefore seems likely that the ancestral telencephalon controlled motor outputs mainly via an influence over the hypothalamus.

Rings, loops, and memory

Ideas about rings and "loops" have a direct relevance to understanding memory. The dominant theory of memory systems holds that sensory areas of neocortex subserve perception, the basal ganglia corresponds to a "habit system," and something called the "medial temporal lobe" underlies explicit memory (Fig. 2.3A and Plate 1A). In Chapters 7 ("The perception–memory dichotomy") and 12 we challenge this doctrine from a standard neuroscience perspective, but Fig. 2.3 and Plate 1 illustrate some conceptual issues that have received less attention. Specifically, it makes little sense to discuss the function of the so-called "medial temporal lobe" as something apart from the function of the basal ganglia. The hippocampus, for instance, has its territories in the striatum and pallidum just as neocortical areas have theirs. The idea that the "basal ganglia" subserves habits and not "memories" seems incoherent in this context. As we say in Chapter 12 ("The road not taken"), denying that the basal ganglia contributes to explicit memory—despite the fact that some cortex–basal ganglia "loops" include the "medial temporal lobe" areas that supposedly subserve explicit memory—"provides ample signs that something is amiss in world of memory research."

In this context, Fig. 2.3(B) and Plate 1(B) present an alternative perspective, one that relates the cortex–basal ganglia "loops" of Fig. 2.2(B) to the representational systems emphasized in the evolutionary accretion model of memory (see Table 1.2). These illustrations are not meant to imply that the basal ganglia has precisely the same function as the cortical components of a given "loop," but because they function together they need to be considered together in any theory of memory systems.

Summary

The neocortex—including both the ring and core neocortex (Fig. 2.1B)—first appeared in stem mammals, which adapted to a high-energy nocturnal niche. The ring neocortex borders allocortical areas, such as the hippocampus and piriform cortex, which mammals inherited from more distant ancestors (Fig. 2.1A). Like allocortical areas, the ring neocortex has a relatively direct influence on hypothalamic functions, which the core neocortex lacks. Two additional points about cortical evolution are especially important for understanding memory:

◆ There is no comparative evidence for the idea that the neocortex evolved in an ordered sequence beginning with the ring neocortex and ending with the core neocortex. Likewise, there is no evidence for "evolutionary trends" of the sort promoted by Sanides.

◆ All cortical areas participate in cortex–basal ganglia "loops," including allocortical areas such as the hippocampus (Fig. 2.2B). The prevailing view of memory systems, which ignores this fundamental architecture, therefore depends on outmoded ideas about telencephalic organization (Fig. 2.3A).

Early primates

Our discussion of primate evolution requires several specialized terms: strepsirrhine, haplorhine, anthropoid, catarrhine, platyrrhine, plesiadapiform, and euprimate. Strepsirrhines include lemurs, lorises, and bushbabies. Haplorhines consist of tarsiers and anthropoid primates, which split into platyrrhines (New World monkeys) and catarrhines. The latter group includes all Old World monkeys, apes, and humans. Together, the tarsiers and strepsirrhines are often called prosimians, a paraphyletic group[‡] of small primates with a nocturnal foraging habit. Plesiadapiforms are allied to stem primates and

---

[‡] In Chapter 1 ("Cladistics") and in the Glossary we explain the term *paraphyletic group*.

contrast with primates "of modern aspect," also known as euprimates. Figure 2.10 shows how these lineages relate to each other.

Primates evolved about 60 million years ago or perhaps a little earlier. Aside from cortical organization, their major innovations include grasping hands and feet, which had nails rather than claws, frontally directed eyes, and a leaping–grasping form of locomotion[64,65]. These and other innovations developed as early primates adapted to a new way of life, one that involved living and foraging in the fine branches of trees and shrubs. These branches have flowers, nectar, seeds, fruits, and nuts, along with young, tender, nutritious leaves. To understand how the cerebral cortex changed in early primates, we need to appreciate the selective pressures that these animals experienced in the fine-branch niche.

A fossil species named *Carpolestes* is instructive in this regard[66]. It dates to about 55 million years ago (see Fig. 6.1A), and Fig. 2.10 illustrates one idea about its relationship to modern primates. *Carpolestes* lacked the frontally directed eyes and leaping adaptations

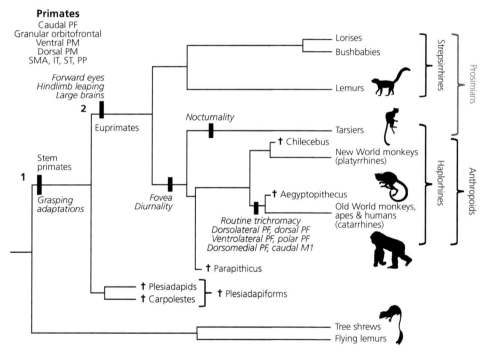

Fig. 2.10 Cladogram of primates. A dagger (†) denotes extinct species. The innovative traits of selected lineages appear above or below the black rectangles. Clades (monophyletic groups) in black; paraphyletic groups in gray. Numerals 1 and 2: two common ancestors of primates. Abbreviations: IT, inferior temporal cortex; PF, prefrontal cortex; PM, premotor cortex; PP, posterior parietal cortex; SMA, supplementary motor area; ST, superior temporal cortex. From Figure 2.5 in Passingham RE, Wise SP. *The Neurobiology of the Prefrontal Cortex*, © 2012, Oxford University Press. Reproduced with permission of OUP, with the addition of silhouettes from open source http://phylopic.org/.

that characterize euprimates, but it had a specialized grasping ability[67]. Grasping adaptations provide obvious advantages for visually guided locomotion[68] and visually mediated foraging[69,70]. The characteristics of *Carpolestes*[66], a plesiadapiform primate, suggest that grasping specializations arose first, in stem primates, followed by the development of frontally directed eyes and hindlimb-dominated leaping in stem euprimates. Together, this suite of adaptations contributed to foraging among flimsy branches[70–72]. Along with their new grasping and leaping ability, early euprimates evolved novel ways of seeing, reaching, and feeding.

Visual and behavioral adaptations in early primates

Early primates foraged in dim light[65], and, like other mammals, lacked either a fovea or trichromatic (full-color) vision. Accordingly, primates probably used their derived visual traits for enhanced stereopsis, depth perception, and light summation in a large binocular field[73–78]. Frontally oriented eyes might also have permitted one eye to have a clear line of sight when the other was blocked[79] and increased the ability to see things in front of and beneath the snout[75]. The visual system in primates is so impressive they have often been called "visual animals," despite the fact that visually guided behavior appeared very early in vertebrate history.

Primates also evolved a unique way of moving[80]. They shifted to hindlimb-dominated locomotion and used less force to move than their ancestors did[72]. These adaptations probably decreased oscillations that attract predators, and they freed the forelimbs and hands for other functions. Among these specializations, grasping hands provided advantages for stability and steering, as well as for manipulating items[72]. Early euprimates probably developed a feeding habit that involved bringing food to the mouth with one hand while stabilizing the body with the other hand, as many modern strepsirrhines do[81] (see Fig. 6.1A). This feeding technique not only involves grasping food items and bringing them to the mouth, but also grasping nonfood items, such as thin branches, and bending them in order to gnaw off valuable items.

In addition, primates developed a new cortical mechanism for reaching toward, grasping, and manipulating items in the fine-branch niche, based on a stereoscopic frame of reference. In Chapter 6 ("Parietal–premotor networks"), we describe this mechanism in some detail.

New cortical areas

The adaptations of early primates depended, in part, on new parts of the premotor, posterior parietal, and temporal cortex. The size of the neocortex expanded relative to body mass, and the amount of cortex increased as a fraction of the brain[82]. We defer a discussion of the areas just listed to Chapter 6 and concentrate here on another innovation of early primates: the granular prefrontal cortex.

A paper by Preuss and Goldman-Rakic[83] established the key points. They described the frontal cortex of a strepsirrhine (prosimian), the bushbaby *Galago*. In an architectonic analysis, Preuss and Goldman-Rakic identified a homotypical and moderately myelinated area in the bushbaby frontal cortex, which they called the posterior granular cortex. As explained in Chapter 1 ("Cerebral cortex"), homotypical areas have a clearly visible layer 4 and are called "granular cortex" in the frontal lobe. Taking connections as well as architectonics into account, Preuss and Goldman-Rakic concluded that the posterior granular cortex in bushbabies is homologous with area 8 in macaque monkeys and humans, which includes the frontal eye fields. In support of this conclusion, low-level electrical stimulation evokes eye movements from this area in bushbabies[84], as it does from area 8 in macaque monkeys[85]. Preuss and Goldman-Rakic[83] also concluded that bushbabies and macaques have homologous granular areas in their orbitofrontal cortex. These findings indicate that strepsirrhines have homologues of two granular prefrontal areas seen in monkeys and humans—the caudal prefrontal cortex and the granular orbitofrontal cortex—and a more recent report has confirmed these conclusions[86].

Rodents lack any granular frontal areas, and bushbabies appear to lack additional granular areas that are observed in the prefrontal cortex of anthropoids. These anthropoid areas have very light myelination, in contrast to the moderate myelination observed in the caudal and granular orbitofrontal cortex. The lightly myelinated prefrontal areas include the ventrolateral, dorsal, dorsolateral, and dorsomedial prefrontal cortex, and probably the polar prefrontal cortex as well (see Fig. 1.3). Figure 2.11 illustrates the relevant homologies among humans, macaque monkeys, and rats.

These conclusions remain controversial because some neuroscientists consider the rodent frontal cortex to be homologous with the granular prefrontal cortex in primates. Proponents of this opinion cite connections of the rodent frontal cortex with the mediodorsal nucleus of the thalamus, dopaminergic inputs to this part of cortex, and the effects of lesions of this area on tasks thought to measure spatial memory. None of these claims holds up, however, as explained in detail elsewhere[82,87,88]. Briefly, both mediodorsal nucleus and dopaminergic neurons project outside the prefrontal cortex of primates; and frontal cortex lesions cause mild and temporary impairments on "spatial memory tasks" in rodents that bear only scant resemblance to the severe and permanent impairments caused by lesions of the prefrontal cortex in monkeys. The idea that primates developed new granular prefrontal areas—but inherited the agranular prefrontal areas[76,89]—finds additional support in four lines of evidence:

1. The agranular prefrontal cortex borders the allocortex in rodents and primates; the granular prefrontal cortex does not.

2. Electrical stimulation evokes autonomic outputs from the agranular prefrontal cortex in rodents and primates; stimulation of the granular prefrontal cortex does not[90-96].

3. The agranular prefrontal cortex projects to and near the ventral striatum in rodents and primates; the granular prefrontal cortex does not and instead projects mainly to the caudate nucleus, part of the dorsal striatum[97-102].

4. The agranular prefrontal cortex receives relatively direct gustatory, olfactory, and visceral inputs in rodents and primates; the granular prefrontal cortex does not and instead receives these inputs indirectly via the agranular prefrontal cortex[103].

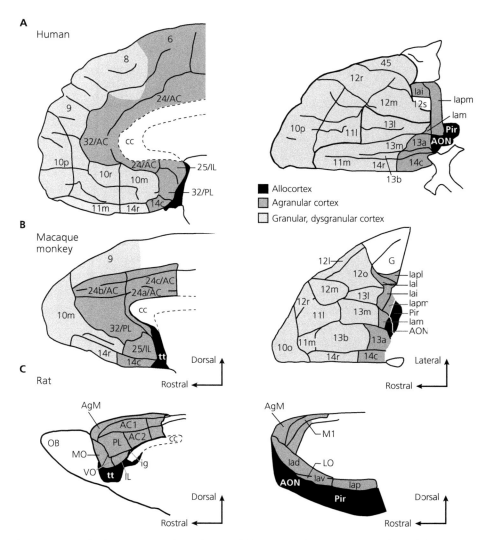

Fig. 2.11 Homologies among prefrontal areas. (A) Humans. (B) Macaque monkeys. (C) Rats. In (A)–(C), the left column shows a medial view of the rostral part of a cerebral hemisphere. Rostral is to the left, dorsal is up. In (A) and (B), the right column shows a ventral view of the rostral part of a cerebral hemisphere. Rostral is to the left, lateral is up. In (C), the right column shows a lateral view. Rostral is to the left, dorsal is up. The drawings have different scales. Abbreviations: AC, anterior cingulate cortex; AgM, medial agranular motor area; AON, anterior olfactory nucleus; cc, corpus callosum; G, gustatory cortex; Ia, agranular insular cortex; ig, induseum griseum; IL, infralimbic cortex; LO, lateral orbitofrontal cortex; MO, medial orbitofrontal cortex; OB, olfactory bulb; Pir, piriform cortex; PL, prelimbic cortex; tt, tenia tecta; VO, ventral orbitofrontal cortex. Subdivision of areas: a and b, arbitrary designations (as in 13a and 24b) or agranular (as in Ia); c, caudal; d, dorsal; i, inferior; l, lateral; m, medial; o, orbital; p, posterior (as in Iapl) or polar (as in 10p); r, rostral; v, ventral. From Figure 2.1 in Passingham RE, Wise SP. *The Neurobiology of the Prefrontal Cortex*, © 2012, Oxford University Press. Reproduced with permission of OUP.

Taken together, the comparative evidence indicates that the agranular prefrontal cortex evolved in early mammals, some parts of the granular prefrontal cortex emerged in early primates, and additional parts of the granular prefrontal cortex appeared later, in anthropoids.

For readers skeptical about these conclusions, Wise[82] and Passingham and Wise[88] present a more comprehensive discussion, along with a consideration of two competing ideas: that small-brained mammals have a replica in miniature of primate brains and that cortical areas in small-brained mammals contain amalgams of several primate areas. These concepts have little to recommend them and, in broad perspective, echo debates from early in the history of biology about preformation (akin to the amalgam theory) versus epigenesis. The amalgam theory, for example, holds that a few, small frontal areas in rodents have all of the traits that the expansive primate prefrontal cortex has, despite the fact that rodents lack any of the primate innovations discussed earlier in this chapter. Proponents of this idea often assemble lists of similarities between rodent and primate prefrontal cortex, but this approach has little probative value. New areas probably emerge through replications, insertions, and differentiation of cortical areas[104], and so nearby areas share many traits, but such similarities provide no support for cortical amalgams[88]. Taken to its logical conclusion, the amalgam theory implies that the neocortex of early mammals had all of the specialized representations seen in the cortex of every descendant species, including the Doppler-shift representations found in the auditory cortex of echolocating bats and the foveal motion detectors observed in the middle temporal cortex of anthropoid primates. None of this makes any sense for the progenitor of mammals, which did not hunt insects with echolocation and did not track moving objects with foveal vision. It would be an odd world indeed in which donkeys and monkeys, rats and cats, and the progenitor of all mammals had the same specialized representations as echolocating bats.

Distortions of medial cortex

With the expansion of the neocortex in primates, other parts of the cerebral cortex underwent considerable distortion. As a result, the hippocampus has traditionally been viewed as a component of the temporal lobe in primates, as emphasized in the prevailing view of memory systems. (The name temporal comes from the location of the temporal plate, a part of the primate brain case that underlies the temple.)

Figure 2.12 depicts how the hippocampus became part of the temporal lobe in primates. In the ancestral condition (Fig. 2.12A), the hippocampal homologue was the medial cortex (M), as explained earlier in this chapter (see "Homologies"). Figure 2.12(B) (left) shows what the brain of an imaginary transitional species might have looked like, with drawings from left to right suggesting how the hippocampus migrated into its current location in primates while maintaining the ancestral topological relationship with the septal nuclei and amygdala. Despite the distortions caused by cortical expansion, the hippocampus of primates remains—as it has been since the advent of stem amniotes—medial cortex (Figs. 2.6 and 2.7). Genuine temporal cortex consists of neocortical areas that have evolved much more recently.

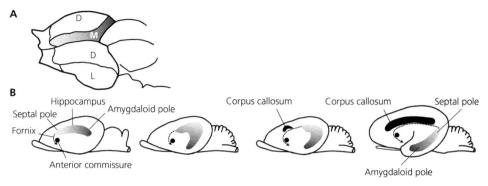

Fig. 2.12 Hippocampal migration. (A) The homologue of the hippocampus in an amniote, using a snake brain to represent the amniote ancestor of mammals. The septal pole is shaded in light gray and the amygdaloid pole is in dark gray. Rostral is to the left. (B) Figurative sequence illustrating how the hippocampus migrated from its ancestral orientation and position (left) to its current disposition in primates (right), as the cerebral cortex expanded. Medial view. Rostral is to the left, dorsal is up. Abbreviations: D, dorsal cortex; M, medial cortex; L, lateral cortex. From Murray EA, Wise SP. Why is there a special issue on perirhinal cortex in a journal called *Hippocampus*? The perirhinal cortex in historical perspective. *Hippocampus* 22:1941–51, © 2012, reproduced with permission from John Wiley & Sons. Adapted from a drawing by Graham RB. *Physiological Psychology*, Wadsworth Publishing © 1990.

Summary

As early primates adapted to a nocturnal life confined to the fine branches of trees, they developed new mechanisms for visually guided locomotion and grasping, their brains expanded, and several new cortical areas appeared, including the first granular prefrontal areas. In Chapter 6 we develop an idea first advanced by Preuss[77] about how these areas support foraging in the fine-branch niche.

Anthropoids

Earlier (see "New cortical areas"), we explained that several new granular prefrontal areas evolved in anthropoid primates (Figs. 2.1C, 2.10, and 2.11). To appreciate the selective pressures involved, we need to explore anthropoid adaptations more generally.

Visual and behavioral adaptations in anthropoids

Both comparative analysis and fossil evidence indicate that early anthropoids foraged diurnally. For example, their fossils have relatively small eye sockets, an indication of a diurnal habit[64]. Furthermore, most modern anthropoids are diurnal, in contrast to most strepsirrhines[105]. Daylight foraging entails a substantial increase in the risk of predation compared with the nocturnal foraging of early primates.

The fovea evolved only once in primates, in early haplorhines, which were the ancestors of both tarsiers and anthropoids[106] (Fig. 2.10). As a result, tarsiers and anthropoids have the high-acuity vision provided by a fovea, but other primates do not. (Foveas have, however, evolved independently in several other vertebrates[106].) Along with the fovea, anthropoids extended some of the derived visual traits of early primates. Early anthropoid eyes are more frontally directed than in early primates, which increases the binocular visual field for stereopsis. Forward-facing eyes correlate positively with the size of the visual cortex, the brain as a whole[73], and the pathway conveying high-acuity signals from the retina to the thalamus[75].

Later, after the tarsier–anthropoid split, some anthropoids evolved trichromatic (full-color) vision (Fig. 2.10). Many mammals, along with most other primates, have only two kinds of photoreceptive pigments (cone opsins), but catarrhines developed a third pigment, resulting in a form of trichromatic vision called *routine*. Some platyrrhine (New World) monkeys developed a different kind of trichromacy[107], which depends on polymorphisms of opsin genes. Instead of developing a new gene, these monkeys achieve trichromacy via two versions of an existing gene. Stem tarsiers might also have had opsin polymorphisms[108]. In addition, New World howler monkeys and some strepsirrhines have evolved routine trichromacy convergently with catarrhines[108].

These visual developments promoted the ability to distinguish potential foods and feeding sites, especially distant ones. As a result, anthropoids spend much of their time looking around and acting on what they see. Red-tail monkeys, for example, spend 20% of their waking life looking around, compared with 5% spent on social contact[109].

As anthropoids diversified, they became larger. Early anthropoids, which appeared not long after the origin of euprimates, weighed only 100–300 mg[64,65]. Anthropoids did not reach the 1–5 kg range until about 34 million years ago, after the divergence of platyrrhines and catarrhines. Thus the development of larger bodies occurred in parallel in New World and Old World primates[107], which has a bearing on changes in the neocortex that we discuss later.

As anthropoids became larger, they moved through the large-branch niche as arboreal quadrupeds[64,110], a form of locomotion still used by many modern anthropoids[72]. Moving from branch to branch with four limbs requires a great deal of energy, especially with changes in elevation[111]. Some later anthropoids, including macaque monkeys, conserved energy by becoming terrestrial quadrupeds.

To meet their high energy needs, anthropoids began to forage over a much larger home range than their ancestors did[112]. They mainly ate ripe fruits and tender leaves[107], although they probably supplemented this diet with insects, flowers, roots, bark, seeds, nuts, and tree gums, as do modern anthropoids. Insects, although prevalent, have relatively low biomass[113] and serve mainly to provide particular vitamins and amino acids. Predation risks and the heat stress associated with tropical daytime conditions probably limited their foraging to periods around dusk and dawn. Because of this limitation and their inability to digest most of the plant matter in the tropics, anthropoids became dependent on the high-energy products of angiosperm trees, especially fruits. They therefore had to overcome the frequent and unpredictable food shortages associated with this resource. In addition, they faced competition with other diurnal foragers, such as fruit-eating birds, other members of their social group, and other primate species. This competition surely escalated during shortfalls in favored nutrients.

Predation risk, time constraints, and competition interacted with the fact that each tree species has its own pattern of fruiting, which varies during the year, from year to year, and from region to region within an anthropoid's home range[114]. Modern monkeys such as mangabeys, for example, have home ranges with tens of thousands of trees, of which only 4% or fewer have fruit at any time[114,115]. Some trees bear fruit only once every 2 or 3 years. A given species might produce fruit in 5% of its trees in one part of an anthropoid's home range, 50% in another, or none at all[116]. Field observations have revealed several features of anthropoid foraging in modern species that probably apply to their ancestors as well:

- Anthropoid monkeys learn about the value of different trees, including the quantities of fruit that they produce[115].
- They learn to visit trees more frequently based on their experience with high-quality fruits in those trees[114].
- Anthropoids change their foraging strategies during shortfalls in preferred foods[113,117], foraging for longer periods of time or changing their diet to fallback foods.
- They make use of sensory signs indicating the location of foods and other resources. Sounds made by competitors, for example, provide one source of such signs[114].
- Anthropoids predict the timing of food production based on when a tree last fruited[118].
- They react to resources seen in one tree of a given species by visiting other trees of the same kind[119].
- They adjust their predictions based on weather, returning to a previously productive tree more often in hot weather when ripening occurs rapidly[114].

Because of their energy-intensive foraging, the unreliability of angiosperm "produce," competition, and predation, anthropoids have a lot to learn. To thrive, they need to avoid poor foraging choices, especially those that run the risk of predation.

Changes in brain size

As anthropoids became larger animals, their brains expanded relative to body mass. Figure 2.13(B) shows that this expansion exceeded the amount accounted for by changes in body size alone, a disproportionate brain enlargement called an *upward grade shift*. A similar grade shift occurred during the transition to euprimates[82], so larger brains— like forward-facing eyes—represent an instance of anthropoids exaggerating a trait that emerged in early primates.

Figure 2.13(A), from Radinsky's pioneering work, illustrates a fossil endocast for the cortex of one extinct anthropoid, *Aegyptopithecus*, an early catarrhine[110]. Such casts conform to the inside of a fossil skull to demonstrate the pattern of sulci and gyri. Radinsky's results show that the frontal lobes expanded more recently than did other parts of the anthropoid cortex[120,121]. *Aegyptopithecus* had a central sulcus (Fig. 2.13A, bottom) but less frontal cortex than seen in modern monkeys (Fig. 2.13A, top). Radinsky's work also leads to the conclusion that the visual areas of cortex began expanding early in primate evolution, and that by the time of *Aegyptopithecus* (about 33 million years ago) these

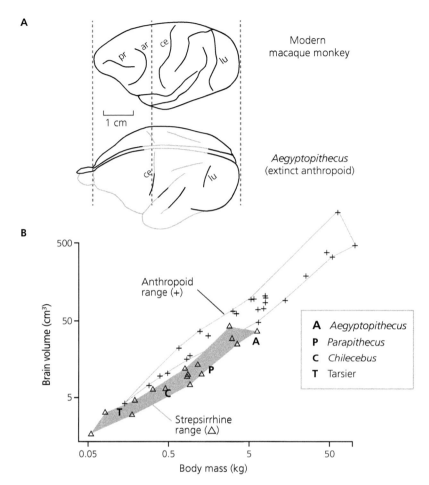

Fig. 2.13 Grade shift in brain size. (A) Top: macaque brain. Bottom: fossil endocast of an extinct early catarrhine, *Aegyptopithecus*. Rostral is to the left, dorsal is up. The light gray lines estimate the locations of sulci and brain boundaries absent from the fossil specimen. The dashed vertical lines give reference locations for the two drawings. (B) Plot of brain versus body size in selected primates. Abbreviations: ar, arcuate sulcus; ce, central sulcus; lu, lunate sulcus; pr, principal sulcus. (A) Redrawn from Radinsky L (1979) The fossil record of primate brain evolution. In: *49th James Arthur Lecture on the Evolution of the Human Brain*, pp. 1–27. New York: American Museum of Natural History. (B) Modified from Passingham RE, Wise SP. *The Neurobiology of the Prefrontal Cortex*, © 2012, Oxford University Press. Reproduced with permission of OUP.

areas had reached their modern size, or nearly so. Because *Aegyptopithecus* lived after the platyrrhine–catarrhine divergence, these findings imply that much of the frontal expansion occurred independently in New and Old World primates[82].

The advantages provided by the larger visual cortex of *Aegyptopithecus* probably involved perceptual learning in central, foveal vision. As we discuss in Chapter 7, the inferior temporal cortex represents visual attributes such as color, which depend on the fovea. Monkeys, like humans, rely on perceptual learning to become "experts" in particular discriminations, among similar shades of red, for example[122]. Brain imaging evidence from the inferior temporal cortex of humans has provided support for a contribution to perceptual learning[123]. Likewise, in monkeys, lesions of the inferior temporal cortex have impaired the ability to distinguish similar hues[124]. Lesions of this area have also disrupted central vision, mediated by the fovea, with much less effect on stimulus arrays that encompassed a larger part of the visual field[125].

Despite its enlarged visual cortex, the *Aegyptopithecus* brain (point A in Fig. 2.13B) falls within the size range of modern strepsirrhines. Two additional fossil anthropoids, *Parapithecus*[126] and *Chilecebus*[127], likewise fall within the prosimian range (points P and C in Fig. 2.13B). The former was an early anthropoid, perhaps prior to the platyrrhine–catarrhine split; the latter was an early platyrrhine. The same conclusion applies to another extinct platyrrhine, *Homunculus*[128], and to modern tarsiers (point T in Fig. 2.13B).

The fact that an early platyrrhine and an early catarrhine both had brains within the prosimian range suggests that the upward grade shift in brain size occurred after the platyrrhine–catarrhine split. As explained earlier, so did an expansion of the frontal lobe and an increase in body size. These conclusions imply that the selective pressures operating early in anthropoid evolution, which led to visual adaptations and an enlarged visual cortex, differed from the factors that subsequently promoted an increase in body size, an upward grade shift in brain size, and expansion of the frontal cortex. Independent brain expansion in New and Old World anthropoids also suggests that new parts of granular prefrontal cortex might have evolved in parallel, at least in part.

Not all anthropoid brain expansion involved the prefrontal and temporal visual cortex. The size and number of areas in the posterior parietal and somatosensory cortex also increased[78], developments that we take up in Chapter 6 ("Evolution").

Brain changes and foraging

The brain expansion that characterizes derived anthropoids, which occurred after the platyrrhine–catarrhine divergence about 34 million years ago, might have come in response to a period of climatic cooling that occurred around 35 million years ago. This cooling regime resulted in widespread shortfalls of resources in the tropics, and, as a result, anthropoids needed to diversify their feeding habits to exploit alternative (fallback) resources. According to Dominy[129], leaf eating intensified at this time, and trichromacy might have evolved in catarrhines to provide them with an advantage in identifying young, tender, nutritious leaves, which often are redder than older, tougher leaves.

In a monograph on the prefrontal cortex, Passingham and Wise[88] propose that the new prefrontal areas of anthropoids helped them overcome periodic shortfalls in preferred, high-energy foods—in part by generating foraging goals in a new way. As a result of this innovation, anthropoids learned faster and with fewer errors, a trait that has obvious importance for a large foraging animal facing predation threats, not to mention heat stress and competition. We return to this topic in Chapter 8 ("Augmentation of older memory systems").

In addition, a new, caudal part of the primary motor cortex evolved in anthropoids. In contrast to the rostral primary motor cortex, neurons in the caudal primary motor cortex project directly (monosynaptically) to spinal motor neurons[130]. This trait contrasts with the corticospinal projection in other mammals. Rodents, for example, have few, if any, direct, monosynaptic projections from their primary motor cortex to spinal motor neurons[131], like the rostral primary motor cortex of anthropoids. According to Kaas[132], the caudal primary motor cortex evolved in anthropoids, and independent work shows that humans also have rostral and caudal divisions of the primary motor cortex[133]. In addition to giving rise to monosynaptic corticospinal projections, this area receives inputs from highly sensitive cutaneous receptors[134,135], with an emphasis on inputs from the hand. Peripheral sensory receptors, such as Meissner corpuscles, signal small amounts of skin stretching, and these cutaneous inputs probably play a role in guiding the manipulation of objects. In large part, they do so by providing feedback concerning skin deformation, which primates use to judge the compliance of ripe fruits such as figs (some species of which do not change color as they ripen). In support of this idea, anthropoids that eat the most fruit have the highest density of Meissner corpuscles on their hands, and especially on their fingertips[136].

Summary

As anthropoids became larger they foraged (in daylight) over a greater home range, required more energy, and faced enhanced predation risks that punished unproductive foraging choices. Their cortex expanded and several new granular prefrontal areas appeared, along with elaborations of the posterior parietal, somatosensory, motor, and temporal cortex. Passingham and Wise[88] propose that the new prefrontal areas generate goals based on metric and attribute representations provided by the posterior parietal and temporal cortex, respectively. By representing new kinds of contexts, speeding up goal-related learning, and applying abstract strategies to unfamiliar foraging problems, anthropoids could forage more safely than their ancestors could. We return to these topics in Chapters 7 and 8.

Hominins

The ape–human lineage diverged from other catarrhines about 24–30 million years ago[137] and hominins diverged from the chimpanzee–bonobo (panin) lineage around 5–7 million years ago. The hominin–panin split occurred in tropical Africa during a period of global cooling and drying that led to decreased forestation and an increase in grassy areas. Many ape species died out at this time, but hominins adapted by spending more time foraging at ground level, which favored bipedal over quadrupedal locomotion[138]. At first, hominins retained considerable tree-climbing capacity, adapting to life on the ground but also foraging, avoiding predators, and sleeping in trees[139]. We discuss hominin evolution in more detail in Chapter 11 ("Evolution"), so here we focus on selected issues involving cortical organization.

Overall brain expansion

Early on, the most dramatic difference between the panin and hominin lineages involved bipedalism, but changes in brain size followed. Early hominins were "remarkably apelike in the small size of their brains" (Klein[138], p. 274). Later, one phase of brain expansion occurred about 2.5 million years ago, another about 1.6 to 1.8 million years ago, and the hominin brain reached its modern shape and size around 200,000 to 600,000 years ago[140,141]. We revisit hominin brain expansion in Chapters 9 ("Evolution"), 10 ("Social factors"), and 11 ("Evolution"), so here we highlight just two topics: regional brain expansion and the possible appearance of new areas.

Regional expansion

The literature on regional brain evolution includes an ongoing debate, which we address in Chapter 10 ("Regional expansion"). Here we bypass that debate by focusing on four studies:

- Because light myelination characterizes the new and elaborated anthropoid areas in prefrontal, posterior parietal, and inferior temporal cortex (see "New cortical areas"), structural brain imaging can reveal their extent[142]. Plate 2(C) shows that these lightly myelinated areas (blue) have expanded dramatically in chimpanzees and humans, in absolute terms, compared with a representative Old World monkey.

- Another approach involves fitting the contours of a chimpanzee brain onto the map of a human brain, using the central sulcus, the posterior part of the lateral sulcus, and visual cortex as reference points[143]. To make this fit work, the prefrontal, posterior parietal, and temporal areas have to be increased in size.

- A similar analysis uses well-established homologies as reference areas, and it leads to much the same conclusion (Plate 3C)[144].

- Finally, we emphasize a recent analysis by Passingham and Smaers[145]. Their investigation shows that the volume of prefrontal gray matter in humans exceeds the amount predicted for nonpongid anthropoids—a paraphyletic group illustrated in Fig. 2.14(C). Basically, nonpongid anthropoids correspond to modern monkeys and gibbons. The remainder of Fig. 2.14 shows that when the estimated volume of the prefrontal cortex is compared with that of two reference regions—the motor and premotor cortex combined (Fig. 2.14A) and the primary visual (striate) cortex (Fig. 2.14B)—the size of prefrontal cortex in humans is many times the predicted value (Fig. 2.14D). This analysis suggests that the granular prefrontal cortex of both hominins and panins expanded relative to the primary visual cortex, but more so in hominins (Fig. 2.14D). Figure 9.1 presents similar data for the temporal and posterior parietal cortex.

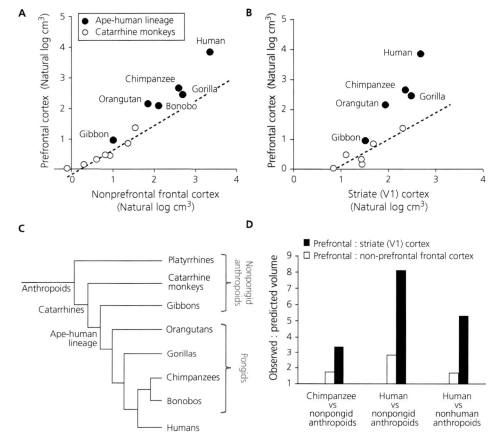

Fig. 2.14 Expansion of the prefrontal cortex. (A) The volume of granular prefrontal cortex plotted against the volume of the remainder of the frontal lobe. (B) The volume of granular prefrontal cortex plotted against the volume of striate (V1) cortex. (C) Cladogram of anthropoids. Paraphyletic groups in gray. (D) Ratio of observed granular prefrontal cortex volume for chimpanzees and humans to that predicted by the group indicated. The comparison in (D) includes platyrrhines, whereas the plots in (A, B) include only catarrhines. Data in (A, B, D) from from Passingham and Smaers[145].

Possible new areas

According to Kaas[53] (p. 42), macaque monkeys have approximately 130 neocortical areas, whereas humans have "as many as 150–200 or more." This conclusion implies that human brains have at least 20 cortical areas that Old World monkeys do not have, and some analyses of the posterior parietal[146,147] and anterior temporal cortex[148] support this idea. But the evidence remains equivocal because the identification of functionally distinct cortical fields depends on methods that differ for each species.

The polar prefrontal cortex (area 10) serves as an example of the problems involved. One architectonic analysis suggested that gibbons lack a lateral part of the polar prefrontal cortex, which both chimpanzees and humans have[149], and a recent architectonic analysis in humans confirmed a distinction between medial and lateral components of the polar prefrontal cortex[150]. A demonstration of subdivisions does not, however, indicate that one of them emerged during ape or hominin evolution.

A series of studies have examined whether new prefrontal areas appeared after the split between the ape–human lineage and other anthropoids. The investigators used both diffusion tractography and functional brain imaging to compare the brains of humans and anesthetized macaque monkeys[151–153]. They first identified clusters of voxels in the prefrontal cortex that have similar connections, and then compared these clusters with correlated activations called coupling. According to this analysis, a region often called the lateral frontal-pole cortex in humans has coupling like the anterior part of the dorsolateral prefrontal cortex in monkeys[152]. In both species, the area in question has connections with a caudal part of the inferior parietal cortex, which the frontal-pole cortex of monkeys lacks[154–156]. These results suggest that at least part of the area commonly labeled lateral frontal-pole cortex in humans corresponds instead to an anterior part of the dorsolateral prefrontal cortex.

The same investigations indicate that the medial[151], ventrolateral[152], and orbital[153] prefrontal cortex consist mainly of areas that seem to be homologous in monkeys and humans, with few human areas "unaccounted for" in monkeys. These homologies include a medial frontal-pole region that, in humans, becomes activated in theory of mind and social-evaluation tasks (see Chapter 10, "Medial frontal cortex", and Plate 5A). Although these studies did not identify a large number of new frontal areas, they did point to a small ventrolateral part of the frontal-pole cortex that might be unique to humans. This area becomes activated in relation to multitasking, the valuation of foregone outcomes, counterfactual propositions, and prediction errors[157–159] (see Plate 5B).

The idea that humans might not have a large number of new areas does not mean, however, that no changes have occurred in the human brain. For example, the temporal cortex has more widespread connections with Broca's area in humans than does the homologous area in chimpanzees[160]. Similarly, whereas the whole extent of the caudal ventrolateral prefrontal cortex has significant coupling with the superior temporal cortex in humans, a more restricted part has this property in monkeys[152]. The latter finding parallels one for a rostral part of the dorsolateral prefrontal cortex[151]. In monkeys, this area shows coupling with most of the superior temporal cortex, but in humans the middle parts of the superior temporal cortex lack coupling, which probably reflects the expansion and reorganization of auditory areas involved in language[144]. In the same vein, diffusion tractography shows that the superior longitudinal fascicle (see Fig. 12.1) differs in chimpanzees, humans, and Old World monkeys; connections between the inferior parietal cortex and the frontal cortex extend further rostrally in humans than in other anthropoids[161].

Summary

Cortical areas that emerged or elaborated in anthropoids—the granular prefrontal, inferior temporal, and posterior parietal cortex—expanded after the ape–human lineage split from other anthropoids (Figs. 2.14 and 9.1, Plates 2C and 3C), as did the brain and cerebral cortex as a whole. Notwithstanding this expansion, the number of new areas in hominins might be smaller than is sometimes assumed.

Conclusions

Brain evolution has direct relevance for theories of human memory, and especially for the prevailing view of memory systems:

◆ Homologues of both the basal ganglia and the hippocampus evolved in our most distant vertebrate ancestors as they adapted to a life of mobile, predatory foraging. The "loop" architecture that links the cerebral cortex and basal ganglia also emerged at this time (Fig. 2.2). Therefore there is no basis for the assumption that the basal ganglia "antedates" other memory-related structures, as some proponents of the prevailing view of memory have assumed (see Chapter 12, "The habit–memory dichotomy"). Mishkin et al.[162] (p. 74), for example, stated that in searching for the neural substrate of habits: "The striatal complex or basal ganglia is an obvious candidate from an evolutionary standpoint in that it antedates both the cerebral cortex and the limbic system in phylogenesis." Earlier (see "Outdated concepts") we traced the source of this misconception.

◆ The cerebral cortex emerged in early amniotes as allocortex. The medial cortex of early amniotes evolved into the mammalian hippocampus; the lateral cortex became the piriform cortex (see "Homologies").

◆ The neocortex evolved in early mammals, including both the core and ring areas (Figs. 2.1B and 5.1A). No evidence supports the popular idea that the ring neocortex, often called either "transition" or limbic cortex, evolved before the core neocortex (see "Rings and wrongs").

◆ Many new cortical areas evolved in early primates, including the first granular prefrontal areas (Figs. 2.1C and 2.10). In Chapter 6 we propose that—along with several premotor and posterior parietal areas, most of the inferior temporal cortex, and other visual and auditory areas—these prefrontal areas supported foraging in the fine branches of angiosperm trees.

◆ Additional parts of the granular prefrontal cortex evolved in anthropoids, and both temporal and posterior parietal regions became more elaborate as well (see Figs. 2.1C, 2.10, 6.1, and 6.3). These ancestral species came to rely on volatile resources and foraged in daylight over a large home range in the face of serious predation risks. Together, these factors produced a strong selective pressure for minimizing foraging errors.

◆ The evolution of hominins and apes saw the expansion of lightly myelinated parts of the granular prefrontal, posterior parietal, and inferior temporal cortex (see Plates 2C and 3C). We expand on this point in Chapters 9 ("Evolution"), 10 ("Regional expansion"), and 11 ("Evolution").

These conclusions place us in a position to answer the two questions posed at the beginning of this chapter:

1. Does the concept of a "medial temporal lobe" make sense in an evolutionary context?
2. Does the concept of the basal ganglia in the prevailing view agree with comparative neuroanatomy?

The answer to both questions is "no." First, the concept of a "medial temporal lobe," as a unified functional entity, makes little sense from a comparative perspective. It mixes allocortex and neocortex, which have very different evolutionary histories and emerged in response to different selective pressures; it includes a few parts of the ring neocortex, but excludes most of the others; and it treats the hippocampus as part of the temporal cortex, which it is not. The hippocampus remains, as it has been since the advent of amniotes, medial cortex. The concept of a "medial temporal lobe" results from the expansion of the primate neocortex and the distortions that this caused among older cortical areas. As the cortex expanded, the hippocampus migrated toward the primate temporal lobe (see "Distortions of medial cortex") and became situated near fiber tracts that connect the temporal and frontal cortex. In Chapter 11 ("Disconnection") we explain how this happenstance has hampered theories of human memory.

Second, according to the prevailing view of memory systems, the basal ganglia subserves habits. The "basal ganglia" that this idea refers to, however, consists only of the parts most conspicuous in mammals—the nuclei identified as the basal ganglia in traditional anatomy textbooks. Neuroanatomists now recognize additional parts of the basal ganglia and appreciate that all cortical areas—allocortex and neocortex included—function in concert with the basal ganglia. Some cortex–basal ganglia "loops" evolved early in the history of vertebrates (black shading in Fig. 2.2B); others evolved more recently, as new cortical areas emerged in stem mammals, early primates, and anthropoids (gray shading in Fig. 2.2B). Theories that treat either the basal ganglia or the "medial temporal lobe" in isolation from their cortex–basal ganglia "loops" (Fig. 2.3A, Plate 1A) fail to recognize the fundamental architecture of the telencephalon. The prevailing view of memory systems wrongly considers the "medial temporal lobe" as something apart from the function of basal ganglia and often views the basal ganglia in a way that neglects many cortex–basal ganglia "loops."

A common simile disparages advances toward some distant and controversial goal as "like the progress monkeys make toward the moon by climbing a tree." As monkeys ascend a typical tree, they get about 40 meters closer to the moon; the final 400 million meters, however, call for a different approach. Memory research seems like that sometimes. So we take comfort from the fact that primates actually did reach the moon and that they began that long journey by climbing trees. Early primates adapted to a life confined to trees; anthropoids developed into arboreal quadrupeds that moved from tree to tree; and early hominins continued to climb trees even as they adapted to life at ground level[139]. Primates landed on the moon just a few million years later: next to nothing on the time-scale of vertebrate evolution. In Chapters 3–11 we explore some of the evolutionary developments that made it possible.

References

1. Erwin, D.H. and Valentine, J.W. (2013) *The Cambrian Explosion: The Construction of Animal Diversity* (Roberts, Greenwood Village, CO).
2. Vermeij, G.J. (1996) *Science* **274**, 525–526.
3. Valentine, J.W. (2004) *On the Origin of Phyla* (University of Chicago Press, Chicago, IL).
4. Grimaldi, D. and Engel, M.S. (2005) *Evolution of the Insects* (Cambridge University Press, Cambridge, UK).
5. Schmidt-Rhaesa, A. (2007) *The Evolution of Organ Systems* (Oxford University Press, Oxford).
6. Dunn, C.W., Hejnol, A., Matus, D.Q., Pang, K. et al. (2008) *Nature* **452**, 745–749.
7. Lowe, C.J., Wu, M., Salic, A., Evans, L. et al. (2003) *Cell* **113**, 853–865.
8. Lacalli, T.C. (2008) *Brain Res. Bull.* **75**, 319–323.
9. Chen, J.-Y., Huang, D.-Y., and Li, C.-W. (1999) *Nature* **402**, 518–522.
10. Shu, D.G., Morris, S.C., Han, J., Zhang, Z.F. et al. (2003) *Nature* **421**, 526–529.
11. Mallatt, J., Chen, J., and Holland, N.D. (2003) *Science* **300**, 1372.
12. Shu, D. and Morris, S.C. (2003) *Science* **300**, 1372.
13. Shu, D., Morris, S.C., Zhang, Z.F., Liu, J.N. et al. (2003) *Science* **299**, 1380.
14. Swalla, B.J. and Smith, A.B. (2008) *Phil. Trans. R. Soc. B: Biol. Sci.* **363**, 1557–1568.
15. Carroll, R.L. (1988) *Vertebrate Paleontology and Evolution* (Freeman, New York).
16. Herrick, C.J. (1948) *The Brain of the Tiger Salamander* (University of Chicago Press, Chicago, IL).
17. Nieuwenhuys, R. (2002) *Brain Res. Bull.* **57**, 257–270.
18. Lacalli, T.C. and Holland, L.Z. (1998) *Phil. Trans. R. Soc. B: Biol. Sci.* **353**, 1943–1967.
19. Wada, H. and Satoh, N. (2001) *Curr. Opin. Neurobiol.* **11**, 16–21.
20. Wicht, H. and Northcutt, R.G. (1992) *Brain Behav. Evol.* **40**, 25–64.
21. Wicht, H. and Northcutt, R.G. (1998) *J. Comp. Neurol.* **395**, 245–260.
22. Northcutt, R.G. (1996) *Brain Behav. Evol.* **48**, 237–247.
23. Northcutt, R.G. (2001) *Brain Res. Bull.* **55**, 663–674.
24. Striedter, G.F. (2005) *Principles of Brain Evolution* (Sinauer, Sunderland, MA).
25. Stephenson-Jones, M., Ericsson, J., Robertson, B., and Grillner, S. (2012) *J. Comp. Neurol.* **520**, 2957–2973.
26. Neary, T.J. (1990) In: *Cerebral Cortex: Comparative Structure and Evolution of Cerebral Cortex, Part I* (eds. Jones, E.G. and Peters, A.), pp. 107–138 (Plenum, New York).
27. Ulinski, P.S. (1990) In: *Cerebral Cortex: Comparative Structure and Evolution of Cerebral Cortex, Part I* (eds. Jones, E.G. and Peters, A.), pp. 139–215 (Plenum, New York).
28. Northcutt, R.G. (2008) *Brain Res. Bull.* **75**, 191–205.
29. Smeets, W.J.A.J., Marín, O., and González, A. (2000) *J. Anat.* **196**, 501–517.
30. Wullimann, M.F. and Mueller, T. (2002) *Brain Res. Gene Expr. Patterns* **1**, 187–192.
31. Wullimann, M.F. and Rink, E. (2002) *Brain Res. Bull.* **57**, 363–370.
32. Medina, L., Brox, A., Legaz, I., Garcia-Lopez, M. et al. (2005) *Brain Res. Bull.* **66**, 297–302.
33. Moreno, N. and González, A. (2007) *J. Anat.* **211**, 151–163.

34. Robertson, B., Huerta-Ocampo, I., Ericsson, J., Stephenson-Jones, M. et al. (2012) *PLoS One* **7**, e35642.

35. Thompson, R.H., Menard, A., Pombal, M., and Grillner, S. (2008) *Eur. J. Neurosci.* **27**, 1452–1460.

36. Swanson, L.W. and Petrovich, G.D. (1998) *Trends Neurosci.* **21**, 323–331.

37. Janvier, P. (1996) *Early Vertebrates* (Oxford University Press, Oxford).

38. Carroll, R.L. (1997) *Patterns and Processes of Vertebrate Evolution* (Cambridge University Press, Cambridge, UK).

39. Walls, G.L. (1962) *Vision Res.* **2**, 69–80.

40. Swanson, L.W. (2000) *Brain Res.* **886**, 113–164.

41. Clack, J.A. (2002) *Gaining Ground: The Origin and Evolution of Tetrapods* (Indiana University Press, Bloomington, IN).

42. Hedges, S.B. (2001) In: *Major Events in Early Vertebrate Evolution: Paleontology, Phylogeny, Genetics and Development* (ed. Ahlberg, P.E.), pp. 119–134 (Taylor & Francis, London).

43. Striedter, G.F. (1997) *Brain Behav. Evol.* **49**, 179–213.

44. Striedter, G.F. (2016) *J. Comp. Neurol.* **524**, 496–517.

45. Day, L.B., Crews, D., and Wilczynski, W. (2001) *Behav. Brain Res.* **118**, 27–42.

46. López, J.C., Vargas, J.P., Gómez, Y., and Salas, C. (2003) *Behav. Brain Res.* **143**, 109–120.

47. Puelles, L., Kuwana, E., Puelles, E., Bulfone, A. et al. (2000) *J. Comp. Neurol.* **424**, 409–438.

48. Puelles, L. (2001) *Phil. Trans. R. Soc. B: Biol. Sci.* **356**, 1583–1598.

49. Brox, A., Ferreiro, B., Puelles, L., and Medina, L. (2002) *Brain Res. Bull.* **57**, 381–384.

50. MacLean, P.D. (1985) *Psychol. Med.* **15**, 219–221.

51. Hall, J.A., Foster, R.E., Ebner, F.F., and Hall, W.C. (1977) *Brain Res.* **130**, 197–216.

52. Kaas, J.H. (2011) *Brain Behav. Evol.* **78**, 7–21.

53. Kaas, J.H. (2013) *Wiley Interdisc. Rev. Cogn. Sci.* **4**, 33–45.

54. Lyon, D.C. (2007) In: *The Evolution of Nervous Systems* (eds. Krubitzer, L. and Kaas, J.H.), pp. 267–306 (Elsevier, New York).

55. Sanides, F. (1970) In: *The Primate Brain* (eds. Noback, C.R. and Montagna, W.), pp. 137–208 (Appleton-Century-Crofts, New York).

56. Barbas, H. and Pandya, D.N. (1989) *J. Comp. Neurol.* **286**, 353–375.

57. Mesulam, M.M. (1990) *Ann. Neurol.* **28**, 597–613.

58. Cummings, J.L. (1993) *Arch. Neurol.* **50**, 873–880.

59. Goldberg, G. (1985) *Behav. Brain Sci.* **8**, 567–616.

60. Ridley, R.M., Durnford, L.J., Baker, J.A., and Baker, H.F. (1993) *Brain Res.* **628**, 56–64.

61. DeLong, M.R. and Georgopoulos, A.P. (1981) In: *Handbook of Physiology* (eds. Brookhart, J.M., Mountcastle, V.B. and Brooks, V.B.), pp. 1017–1061 (American Physiological Society, Bethesda, MD).

62. Alexander, G.E., DeLong, M.R., and Strick, P.L. (1986) *Annu. Rev. Neurosci.* **9**, 357–381.

63. Petrovich, G.D., Canteras, N.S., and Swanson, L.W. (2001) *Brain Res. Rev.* **38**, 247–289.

64. Fleagle, J.G. (1999) *Primate Adaptation and Evolution* (Academic Press, San Diego, CA).

65. Rose, K.D. (2006) *The Beginnings of the Age of Mammals* (Johns Hopkins Press, Baltimore, MD).

66. Bloch, J.I. and Boyer, D.M. (2002) *Science* **298**, 1606–1610.

67. Sussman, R.W. (1991) *Am. J. Primatol.* **23**, 209–233.

68. Martin, R.D. (1990) *Primate Origins and Evolution: A Phylogenetic Reconstruction* (Princeton University Press, Princeton, NJ).

69. Cartmill, M. (1972) In: *Functional and Evolutionary Biology of Primates* (ed. Tuttle, R.), pp. 97–122 (Aldine-Atherton, Chicago, IL).

70. **Cartmill, M.** (1974) *Science* **184**, 436–443.

71. **Cartmill, M.** (1992) *Evol. Anthropol.* **1**, 105–111.

72. **Schmitt, D.** (2010) In: *Primate Neuroethology* (eds. Platt, M.L. and Ghazanfar, A.A.), pp. 31–63 (Oxford University Press, New York).

73. **Barton, R.A.** (1998) *Proc. R. Soc. B: Biol. Sci.* **265**, 1933–1937.

74. **Allman, J.** (2000) *Evovling Brains* (Freeman, New York).

75. **Barton, R.A.** (2004) *Proc. Natl. Acad. Sci. USA* **101**, 10113–10115.

76. **Preuss, T.M.** (2007) In: *Evolution of Nervous Systems* (eds. Kaas, J.H. and Preuss, T.M.), pp. 2–34 (Elsevier, New York).

77. **Preuss, T.M.** (2007) In: *Primate Origins: Adaptations and Evolution* (eds. Ravosa, M.J. and Dagasto, M.), pp. 625–675 (Springer, New York).

78. **Kaas, J.H.** (2012) *Prog. Brain Res.* **195**, 91–102.

79. **Changizi, M.A.** (2009) *The Visual Revolution* (Benbella, Dallas, TX).

80. **Larson, S.G.** (1998) In: *Primate Locomotion: Recent Advances* (eds. Strasser, E., Fleagle, J.G., Rosenberger, A.L. and McHenry, H.M.), pp. 157–173 (Plenum, New York).

81. **MacNeilage, P.F., Studdert-Kennedy, M.G.,** and **Lindblom, B.** (1987) *Behav. Brain Sci.* **10**, 247–303.

82. **Wise, S.P.** (2016). In: *Evolution of Nervous Systems*, 2nd edn (eds. Krubitzer, L.A. and Kaas, J.H.) (Elsevier, Amsterdam) (in press).

83. **Preuss, T.M.** and **Goldman-Rakic, P.S.** (1991) *J. Comp. Neurol.* **310**, 429–474.

84. **Wu, C.W.H., Bichot, N.P.,** and **Kaas, J.H.** (2000) *J. Comp. Neurol.* **423**, 140–177.

85. **Bruce, C.J.** (1985) *J. Neurophysiol.* **54**, 714–734.

86. **Wong, P.** and **Kaas, J.H.** (2010) *Anat. Rec.* **293**, 1033–1069.

87. **Wise, S.P.** (2008) *Trends Neurosci.* **31**, 599–608.

88. **Passingham, R.E.** and **Wise, S.P.** (2012) *The Neurobiology of the Prefrontal Cortex* (Oxford University Press, Oxford).

89. **Preuss, T.M.** (1995) *J. Cogn. Neurosci.* **7**, 1–24.

90. **Bailey, P.** and **Sweet, W.H.** (1940) *J. Neurophysiol.* **3**, 276–281.

91. **Delgado, J.R.** and **Livingston, R.B.** (1948) *J. Neurophysiol.* **11**, 39–55.

92. **Kaada, B.R., Pribram, K.H.,** and **Epstein, J.A.** (1949) *J. Neurophysiol.* **12**, 347–356.

93. **Smith, W.K.** (1945) *J. Neurophysiol.* **8**, 242–255.

94. **Smith, W.K.** (1938) *J. Neurophysiol.* **1**, 55–68.

95. **Wall, P.D.** and **Davis, G.D.** (1951) *J. Neurophysiol.* **14**, 507–517.

96. **Ward, A.A.** (1948) *J. Neurophysiol.* **11**, 13–23.

97. **Ferry, A.T., Öngür, D., An, X.H.,** and **Price, J.L.** (2000) *J. Comp. Neurol.* **425**, 447–470.

98. **Brog, J.S., Salyapongse, A., Deutch, A.Y.,** and **Zahm, D.S.** (1993) *J. Comp. Neurol.* **338**, 255–278.

99. **Haber, S.N., Kunishio, K., Mizobuchi, M.,** and **Lynd-Balta, E.** (1995) *J. Neurosci.* **15**, 4851–4867.

100. **Haber, S.N., Kim, K.S., Mailly, P.,** and **Calzavara, R.** (2006) *J. Neurosci.* **26**, 8368–8376.

101. **Berendse, H.W., Galis-de Graaf, Y.,** and **Groenewegen, H.J.** (1992) *J. Comp. Neurol.* **316**, 314–347.

102. **Freedman, L.J., Insel, T.R.,** and **Smith, Y.** (2000) *J. Comp. Neurol.* **421**, 172–188.

103. **Carmichael, S.T.** and **Price, J.L.** (1996) *J. Comp. Neurol.* **371**, 179–207.

104. **Krubitzer, L.** and **Kaas, J.** (2005) *Curr. Opin. Neurobiol.* **15**, 444–453.

105. **Heesy, C.P.** and **Ross, C.F.** (2004) In: *Anthropoid Origins: New Visions* (eds. Ross, C.F. and Kay, R.F.), pp. 665–698 (Academic/Plenum, New York).

106. **Ross, C.F.** (2004) In: *Anthropoid Origins: New Visions* (eds. Ross, C.F. and Kay, R.F.), pp. 477–537 (Academic/Plenum, New York).

107. Williams, B.A., Kay, R.F., and Kirk, E.C. (2010) *Proc. Natl. Acad. Sci. USA* **107**, 4797–4804.

108. Melin, A.D., Matsushita, Y., Moritz, G.L., Dominy, N.J. et al. (2013) *Proc. Biol. Sci.* **280**, 20130189.

109. Struhsaker, T.T. (1980) *African J. Ecol.* **18**, 33–51.

110. Kay, R.F., Williams, B.A., Ross, C.F., Takai, M., and Shigehara, N. (2004) In: *Anthropoid Origins: New Visions* (eds. Ross, C.F. and Kay, R.F.), pp. 91–135 (Academic/Plenum, New York).

111. Janson, C.H. (1988) *Behaviour* **105**, 53–76.

112. Martin, R.D. (1981) *Nature* **293**, 60.

113. Oates, J.F. (1987) In: *Primate Societies* (eds. Smuts, B., Cheney, D.L., Seyfarth, R.M. *et al.*), pp. 197–209 (University of Chicago Press, Chicago, IL).

114. Janmaat, K.R.L., Byrne, R.W., and Zuberbühler, K. (2006) *Animal Behav.* **72**, 797–807.

115. Zuberbühler, K. and Janmaat, K.R.L. (2010) In: *Primate Neuroetholgy* (eds. Platt, M.L. and Ghazanfar, A.A.), pp. 64–83 (Oxford University Press, Oxford).

116. Chapman, C.A., Chapman, L.J., Struhsaker, T.T., Zanne, A.E. et al. (2004) *J. Trop. Ecol.* **21**, 1–14.

117. Kavanagh, M. (1978) *Folia Primatol. (Basel)* **30**, 30–63.

118. Milton, K. (1988) In: *Machiavelian Intelligence: Social Expertise and the Evolution of Intellect in Monkeys, Apes and Humans* (eds. Byrne, R.W. and Whiten, A.), pp. 285–305 (Clarendon, Oxford).

119. Menzel, C.R. (1991) *Animal Behav.* **41**, 397–402.

120. Radinsky, L. (1975) *Am. Sci.* **63**, 656–663.

121. Radinsky, L. (1979) In: *49th James Arthur Lecture on the Evolution of the Human Brain*, pp. 1–27 (American Museum of Natural History, New York).

122. Gaffan, D. (1996) *Cogn. Brain Res.* **5**, 69–80.

123. Mundy, M.E., Downing, P.E., Dwyer, D.M., Honey, R.C. et al. (2013) *J. Neurosci.* **33**, 10490–10502.

124. Buckley, M.J., Gaffan, D., and Murray, E.A. (1997) *J. Neurophysiol.* **77**, 587–598.

125. Horel, J.A. (1994) *Behav. Brain Res.* **65**, 157–164.

126. Bush, E.C., Simons, E.L., and Allman, J.M. (2004) *Anat. Rec. A Discov. Mol. Cell Evol. Biol.* **281**, 1083–1087.

127. Sears, K.E., Finarelli, J.A., Flynn, J.J., and Wyss, A. (2008) *Am. Mus. Novit.* **3617**, 1–29.

128. Kay, R.F., Kirk, R.C., Malinzak, M., and Colbert, M.W. (2006) *J. Vert. Paleontol.* **26**, 83A–84A.

129. Dominy, N.J. (2004) *Integr. Comp. Biol.* **44**, 295–303.

130. Rathelot, J.A. and Strick, P.L. (2009) *Proc. Natl. Acad. Sci. USA* **106**, 918–923.

131. Wise, S.P. and Donoghue, J.P. (1986) In: *Cerebral Cortex* (eds. Peters, A. and Jones, E.G.), pp. 243–270 (Plenum, New York).

132. Kaas, J.H. (2004) *Anat. Rec. A Discov. Mol. Cell Evol. Biol.* **281**, 1148–1156.

133. Geyer, S., Ledberg, A., Schleicher, A., Kinomura, S. et al. (1996) *Nature* **382**, 805–807.

134. Tanji, J. and Wise, S.P. (1981) *J. Neurophysiol.* **45**, 467–481.

135. Strick, P.L. and Preston, J.B. (1982) *J. Neurophysiol.* **48**, 150–159.

136. Hoffmann, J.N., Montag, A.G., and Dominy, N.J. (2004) *Anat. Rec. A Discov. Mol. Cell Evol. Biol.* **281**, 1138–1147.

137. Zalmout, I.S., Sanders, W.J., Maclatchy, L.M., Gunnell, G.F. et al. (2010) *Nature* **466**, 360–364.

138. Klein, R.G. (2009) *The Human Career.* (University of Chicago Press, Chicago, IL).

139. Kraft, T.S., Venkataraman, V.V., and Dominy, N.J. (2014) *J. Hum. Evol.* **71**, 105–118.

140. Bookstein, F., Schafer, K., Prossinger, H., Seidler, H. et al. (1999) *Anat. Rec.* **257**, 217–224.

141. Conroy, G.C., Weber, G.W., Seidler, H., Recheis, W. et al. (2000) *Am. J. Phys. Anthropol.* **113**, 111–118.

142. Glasser, M.F., Goyal, M.S., Preuss, T.M., Raichle, M.E. et al. (2014) *NeuroImage* **93P2**, 165–175.

143. Avants, B.B., Schoenemann, P.T., and Gee, J.C. (2006) *Med. Image Anal.* **10**, 397–412.

144. Van Essen, D.C. and Dierker, D.L. (2007) *Neuron* **56**, 209–225.

145. Passingham, R.E. and Smaers, J.B. (2014) *Brain Behav. Evol.* **84**, 156–166.

146. Scheperjans, F., Palomero-Gallagher, N., Grefkes, C., Schleicher, A. et al. (2005) *NeuroImage* **28**, 362–379.

147. Caspers, S., Geyer, S., Schleicher, A., Mohlberg, H. et al. (2006) *NeuroImage* **33**, 430–448.

148. Pascual, B., Masdeu, J.C., Hollenbeck, M., Makris, N. et al. (2015) *Cereb. Cortex* **25**, 680–702.

149. Semendeferi, K., Armstrong, E., Schleicher, A., Zilles, K. et al. (2001) *Am. J. Phys. Anthropol.* **114**, 224–241.

150. Bludau, S., Eickhoff, S.B., Mohlberg, H., Caspers, S. et al. (2014) *NeuroImage* **93P2**, 260–275.

151. Sallet, J., Mars, R.B., Noonan, M.P., Neubert, F.-X. et al. (2013) *J. Neurosci.* **33**, 12255–12274.

152. Neubert, F.-X., Mars, R.B., Thomas, A., Sallet, J. et al. (2014) *Neuron* **81**, 700–713.

153. Neubert, F.-X., Mars, R.B., Sallet, J., and Rushworth, M.F. (2015) *Proc. Natl. Acad. Sci. USA* **112**, E2695–2704.

154. Jones, E.G. and Powell, T.P.S. (1970) *Brain* **93**, 793–820.

155. Markov, N.T., Ercsey-Ravasz, M.M., Ribeiro-Gomes, A.R., Lamy, C. et al. (2014) *Cereb. Cortex* **24**, 17–36.

156. Petrides, M. and Pandya, D.N. (2007) *J. Neurosci.* **27**, 11573–11586.

157. Koechlin, E., Basso, G., Pietrini, P., Panzer, S. et al. (1999) *Nature* **399**, 148–151.

158. Boorman, E.D., Behrens, T.E.J., Woolrich, M.W., and Rushworth, M.F. (2009) *Neuron* **62**, 733–743.

159. Boorman, E.D., Behrens, T.E., and Rushworth, M.F. (2011) *PLoS Biol.* **9**, e1001093.

160. Rilling, J.K., Glasser, M.F., Preuss, T.M., Ma, X. et al. (2008) *Nat. Neurosci.* **11**, 426–428.

161. Hecht, E.E., Gutman, D.A., Bradley, B.A., Preuss, T.M. et al. (2015) *NeuroImage* **108**, 124–137.

162. Mishkin, M., Malamut, B., and Bachevalier, J. (1984) In: *Neurobiology of Learning and Memory* (eds. Lynch, G., McGaugh, J. and Weinberger, N.M.), pp. 65–77 (Guilford, New York).

163. Allen, T.A. and Fortin, N.J. (2013) *Proc. Natl. Acad. Sci. USA* **110 (Suppl. 2)**, 10379–10386.

Part II

Architecture of vertebrate memory

Modern memory reflects both inheritance and innovation. In the next three chapters we discuss the ancestral condition of early primates. In Chapter 3 we explain that early animals developed a diverse assortment of reinforcement learning mechanisms. In Chapter 4 we explore an innovation of early vertebrates: a representational system that initially served navigation. Then, in Chapter 5, we discuss a memory system that emerged in early mammals.

The reinforcement memory systems of early animals

Overview

Reinforcement learning evolved early in the history of animals. As a result, animals can remember which actions in which circumstances produced benefits or avoided costs. They can also remember which stimuli and locations were associated with costs or benefits. As new representational systems evolved in vertebrates, the older forms persisted in modified form as our most remote mnemonic ancestry. In vertebrates, a variety of unrelated brain structures subserve reinforcement learning: some involving the cerebellum, others depending on telencephalic structures. Reinforcement learning also occurs in invertebrates, which lack homologues of any of these structures; and both brainless animals and insect ganglia can acquire memories through reinforcement learning. These findings show that reinforcement learning is not the product of a coherent system or neurophysiological "mechanism." Instead, diverse forms of reinforcement learning evolved independently in several lineages: linked by little more than surface similarities.

Pavlovian pronouncement

While you are studying, observing, experimenting, do not remain content with the surface of things ... but try to penetrate to the mystery of their origin.

Ivan Pavlov[1] (p. 572)

Creatures of habit, we strive to adopt easy and safe behaviors that pay off in a big way. In recognition of these facts, a radical form of behaviorism once dominated the field of psychology. Proponents of this now abandoned philosophy believed that humans, along with all other animals, simply take in sensations that become linked to "responses." A few universal learning mechanisms, they hoped, would suffice to "explain" all behavior in pigeons, pigs, and people. Alternative ideas, they liked to say, amount to nothing more than "hand-waving," barely worthy of serious scientific consideration, if at all. Eventually, this radical form of behaviorism died out, but many problems might have been avoided had its proponents heeded the counsel of their progenitor, Pavlov. He suggested that they put aside surface similarities and focus instead on origins.

True enough, many kinds of learning and memory look similar on the surface, and experts can use a common terminology to describe a broad range of experimental results. So it seems to some experts as though memory mechanisms have changed little during evolution, except in their details. But maybe, just maybe, millions of years of vertebrate evolution have produced new forms of memory in addition to new vertebrate species, new parts of the vertebrate body, and new brain structures. We think that this is exactly what happened.

Nevertheless, universal learning laws that apply to all animals have enduring appeal, and to understand why concepts such as reward and reinforcement, stimulus–response–outcome contingencies, and associated formalisms seem to "explain" so much, we need to understand when reinforcement learning evolved, how it changed over time, and how it influenced the representational systems that evolved later.

Evolution

In Chapter 2 ("The origin of vertebrates") we described animal evolution in broad strokes. Animals first evolved about 750 million years ago and diversified dramatically about 200 million years after that. Evolutionary developments in the first animals, relative to the multicellular eukaryotes most closely related to them, included a more diverse array of differentiated cell types and a developmental mechanism to produce them. The word animal derives from the Latin for having breath, but the first breath was a long way off when animals first emerged.

The earliest animals had a sponge-like or sheet-like (planar) architecture. They lived their lives in water and fed on bacteria and other small items in their immediate vicinity. As their descendants became larger, they could forage from progressively larger volumes of water. This increased foraging range provided early animals with the nutrition necessary for a larger size, and some of these organisms adapted to moving along the seafloor. Prominent among these organisms were animals with bilateral symmetry, which often had some kind of skeletal support. By about 525 million years ago, all or nearly all of the major modern animal groups had emerged: a diversification in animal architectures called the Cambrian explosion[2]. Their descendants became larger and more complex, fueled by yet larger foraging ranges. To support their larger mass, these animals foraged on plants, fungi, and bacteria, and eventually on each other.

Not all animals move, but early in the history of animals the ability to do so came to characterize this clade. A multicellular aggregation has a specific advantage over single-celled organisms when it comes to movement. It requires a certain mass, achievable only by grouping cells, for an individual organism to gain sufficient momentum to overcome the viscosity of water[2]. A mobile life has obvious advantages, but it has many drawbacks as well. At the most fundamental level, an organism can damage itself by moving. Even with safeguards against such damage, active foraging entails significant costs of two additional kinds: energy consumption and an increased risk of harm, including predation. Had the benefits of a mobile life not outweighed these costs, anemones might rule the world. (Perhaps, although there is no way of knowing for sure, they would do a better job than its current rulers.) To obtain the benefits of mobility, animals have to choose among movements, their timing, and occasions for withholding them. Early in the history of animals, neural systems developed that improved these choices.

Pavlovian conditioning

Pavlovian conditioning can involve as few as two stimuli: a "neutral" one and one that produces an innate reflex response. When these two stimuli occur in rapid succession, new reflexes emerge in response to the originally "neutral" stimulus. We place neutral in quotation marks because, as we explain later (see "Why Pavlovian conditioning happens"), these stimuli are often less neutral than it seems on the surface.

Pavlovian terminology

The term conditioned stimulus (CS) refers to the originally "neutral" stimulus; an unconditioned stimulus (US) produces an innate reflex, called an unconditioned response (UR), and the new behavior is called a conditioned response or conditioned reflex (CR).

The term "outcome" comes into play as well. A beneficial resource or a harmful stimulus corresponds to the outcome (O) of a sensory event (S). Because these outcomes generate reflex responses, they are also unconditioned stimuli. In this sense, a stimulus–outcome (S–O) association corresponds to a CS–US association.

What happens in Pavlovian conditioning

A textbook example of Pavlovian conditioning, described by Pavlov himself, involves the pairing of a sound with food. A bell rings and food appears after a fixed delay. With repeated presentations the sound elicits a conditioned response, which ranges from significant salivation to downright drooling. It took a while, but investigators finally determined that, for the most part, CS–US associations underlie Pavlovian memories. The details can be found in psychology textbooks.

Pavlovian memories come in many varieties. Some involve detrimental outcomes, called aversive, whereas others involve beneficial outcomes, called appetitive. Animals show at least five categories of Pavlovian learning for appetitive outcomes:

1. *Pavlovian approach* refers to the tendency of animals to move towards a conditioned stimulus, also known as sign tracking. This behavior brings the animal closer to objects associated with a valuable resource. In addition, animals sometimes perform biting, chewing, or licking movements in response to conditioned stimuli. Like many Pavlovian behaviors, these responses prepare animals for the consumption of resources.

2. Pavlovian conditioning can also involve behaviors directed toward a predicted unconditioned stimulus, sometimes known as goal tracking.

3. Pavlovian conditioning includes physiological responses, such as reflexes that anticipate the ingestion of food[3]: secretion of gastric acid; pancreatic enzymes such as insu-
lin; and ghrelin, a hormone that regulates energy economics[4,5]. Not only does the direct
sight or smell of food trigger these reflexes, but so does the expectation of food.

4. Like the third category, Pavlovian conditioning produces a variety of autonomic
responses, including increases or decreases in blood pressure, heart rate, skin conduc-
tance, and pupil diameter.

5. Conditioned orienting cuts across the other categories. Some stimuli—typically novel
ones and those with abrupt onsets—trigger orienting or startle responses, which can
include movements directed toward the stimulus, autonomic responses, and vigi-
lance behaviors[6]. For example, rats presented with a bright flashing light rear on their
hind legs and show other behaviors directed toward the light, as well as autonomic
responses[7,8]. When the light is paired with food, these orienting responses do not
habituate as they otherwise would, which appears to reflect Pavlovian learning[7].

Some of these behaviors, such as Pavlovian approach, depend on the nucleus accumbens, part of the basal ganglia[9]. Consistent with this finding, dopamine release in the
nucleus accumbens correlates with Pavlovian approach behavior (sign tracking) but not
approach to the location of food (goal tracking)[10]. The activity of midbrain dopaminergic neurons, likewise, closely tracks certain Pavlovian approach behaviors in monkeys
(Box 3.1). Categories 3–5 depend, in part, on the amygdala[11].

These examples involve appetitive stimuli, but Pavlovian conditioning also occurs for
aversive stimuli. In a typical example, a visual or auditory stimulus precedes a brief puff of
air to the cornea, which elicits an unconditioned response: an eyeblink or, for animals that
have one, the extension of a membrane to cover the eye (the nictitating membrane). With
repetition, the conditioned stimulus comes to elicit an eyeblink or nictitating-membrane
response. Conditioned responses to aversive stimuli include orienting (category 5), autonomic and physiological reflexes (categories 3 and 4), and movements in relation to the
conditioned or unconditioned stimuli (categories 1 and 2). Defensive reflexes include
avoidance, withdrawal, escape, and freezing.

Certain stimuli elicit defensive and other aversive responses in naive animals, and thus
can serve as unconditioned stimuli of particular biological importance. For example, cat
odor appears to be innately aversive to rodents[12], as are certain chemicals in the urine of
predators[13,14]. A particular defensive behavior depends on the type of danger signal: contact with predators, predator odor, or injurious stimuli, for example. It also depends on
the physical capacities of each species for combat or escape. These observations have led
to the idea that animals have species-specific defensive responses: a set of innate behaviors that evolved to deal with specific threats, as opposed to relying solely on a general-
purpose learning mechanism for the avoidance of harm[15,16].

Two misunderstandings commonly accompany discussions of Pavlovian conditioning.
First, the names applied to conditioned responses can suggest more about the subjective
experience of animals than they should; second, classifications of these memories can
imply fewer and less diverse mechanisms than actually exist.

Box 3.1 Blocking and dopaminergic cell activity

A classic experiment by Kamin[128] showed that conditioned stimuli block new learning. In his procedure some rats experienced noise–foot-shock pairings, but others did not. Next, all the rats experienced a compound stimulus of noise plus light, after which the same foot shock occurred. Rats without the noise–shock memories learned the light–shock association in the usual way, but those with noise–shock memories did not. Somehow, the fact that the noise predicted the shock prevented the rats from learning a light–shock association. This phenomenon is known as the Kamin blocking effect or, more simply, blocking.

In monkeys, the activity of midbrain dopaminergic neurons directly reflects the blocking effect[129]. The key experiment began by conditioning a stimulus–outcome pairing for one visual stimulus, stimulus A, but not for another visual stimulus, B. Stimulus A (but not stimulus B) therefore predicted the availability of fruit juice that the monkeys could lick from a spout. After the monkeys had learned this association, two compound stimuli, AC and BD, were constructed. The monkeys then experienced a training regimen that paired both compound stimuli with the fruit juice. The fact that stimulus A accurately predicted the outcome prevented the monkeys from learning the association between stimulus C and the juice, but they had no problem learning the association between stimulus D and the juice. Accordingly, after stimulus D, alone, the monkeys showed a Pavlovian licking response, but after the presentation of stimulus C, alone, they did not.

During this experiment, about half of the dopaminergic neurons responded more to stimulus D than to stimulus C, and others responded only to stimulus D, despite the fact that both stimuli had equal reward histories. No cells responded more to stimulus C. These results support the idea that dopaminergic cells emit a teaching signal that permitted stimulus D to serve as a conditioned stimulus. Stimulus C, however, could not be associated with the juice outcome because of the Kamin blocking effect.

Fear conditioning exemplifies the first point. These Pavlovian memories involve a set of defensive responses that emerge when an initially "neutral" stimulus predicts an aversive unconditioned stimulus, such as electric shock. After several pairings of a light or a tone with a shock to their feet, for example, rodents freeze upon presentation of the light or tone: a defensive response. Despite the term *fear conditioning*, the fact that animals learn to make defensive responses does not imply that they experience the emotion that humans call fear[17,18], a point that becomes important in Chapter 11 ("Choices based on predicted outcomes" and "Conditioned responses").

On the second point, a classification like *conditioned response* seems to imply a common neural mechanism, which contradicts well-established facts about Pavlovian learning. As already mentioned, some forms of Pavlovian conditioning depend on the amygdala and basal ganglia, both of which are telencephalic structures. Others, however, depend on the cerebellum, a brainstem structure:

◆ Cerebellar-dependent conditioned responses tend to involve defensive or protective responses made by particular body parts, as exemplified by eyeblink conditioning and withdrawal reflexes, and they usually exhibit precise timing.

◆ Amygdala- and basal ganglia-dependent[19] responses can be either defensive, as in the case of fear conditioning, or appetitive; and they usually involve biologically important stimuli, such as signs of predators, food, or conspecifics. In addition, they often involve coordinated autonomic or physiological reflexes, along with movements of the whole body, as exemplified by Pavlovian approach or escape behaviors. Such actions have less precise timing than for cerebellum-dependent conditioning.

Even restricting the discussion to amygdala-dependent Pavlovian memories, a classification such as *conditioned defensive response* can imply a single, unified mechanism where none exists. The conditioned responses to three classes of aversive stimuli—predators, social threats, and painful stimuli—all depend on outputs from the amygdala, for example, but they involve different nuclei and different output pathways. Predation and social threats produce conditioned responses via outputs from the medial nucleus of the amygdala that reach the midbrain only indirectly. Conditioned pain responses, however, involve outputs from the central nucleus of the amygdala that reach the midbrain directly[20].

Why Pavlovian conditioning happens

In order to discuss why Pavlovian conditioning occurs we need to take into account the advantages that it provides and the selective factors that favored its development. In general terms, the prediction of an unconditioned stimulus enables a reflex response to begin sooner, which can increase its effectiveness. When a dog learns that a bell signals the imminent availability of food, it benefits from a longer period of salivation before the food arrives. Likewise, when a visual cue consistently precedes a foot shock or an air puff to the eye, a learned defensive reflex occurs earlier than if the animal awaits the aversive (and potentially damaging) stimulus before responding to it.

Pavlovian associations also link stimuli and locations to a subjective value, defined in terms of biological costs or benefits. (The term subjective refers to the value of an outcome to an animal—given its current state—as opposed to an objective value such as calories for food or volts for shocks.) Ongoing Pavlovian conditioning can adapt an animal's behavior to the subjective value of outcomes currently associated with particular stimuli and locations as they change over time.

Although we have characterized conditioned stimuli as initially "neutral," we put that word in quotation marks because they can be far from neutral. Stimuli in an animal's natural habitat have many sensory features, and a potential conditioned stimulus might share some of these features with an unconditioned stimulus, although not enough to reach the threshold for a response. As a result, learning occurs faster for some conditioned stimuli than for others. Indeed, some experts believe that learning about not-so-neutral stimuli, rather than genuinely neutral ones, provides the principal adaptive advantage of Pavlovian learning[21]. Laboratory experiments that use impoverished stimuli, such as simple tones and shapes, have little prospect of revealing this advantage.

Taste aversion learning illustrates a lack of neutrality for certain classes of conditioned stimuli. Animals quickly learn to avoid foods or fluids that have preceded nausea or malaise in the past, and this learning occurs much faster for gustatory stimuli than for auditory or visual ones[22]. The adaptive advantage of this bias is obvious: Materials entering the body can cause harm in a way that visual or auditory stimuli rarely can. Taste aversion learning probably depends on strengthening existing links between gustatory inputs and aversive responses, pushing them from just below to just above threshold. As a result, animals can learn the association between a taste and a bad outcome very quickly, often after just one ill-fated gastronomic experience. (As a result of one such bad outcome, one of the authors has not had a single sip of Scotch whisky for more than 40 years.)

Another example comes from studies of conditioned snake fear in monkeys. In these experiments, naive monkeys acquired robust defensive responses to fake snakes when they were used as conditioned stimuli, in part by observing other monkeys reacting that way[23–25]. Defensive responses to wooden blocks developed much more slowly, if at all. Although some experts have concluded that defensive responses to snake-like stimuli depend entirely on learning[26], naive monkeys have been observed to display mild responses to fake snakes without any conditioning[27]. A fake snake thus serves as a weak (and often insufficient) unconditioned stimulus. As a result, it can be a much more effective conditioned stimulus than a wooden block could ever be. Conditioned stimuli that share features with unconditioned stimuli can, accordingly, provide a significant advantage in Pavlovian learning, thus preparing animals for outcomes to come.

Evolution of Pavlovian conditioning

Chapter 2 emphasized the history of deuterostomes (see Fig. 2.4). We are all descendants of the stem deuterostome, but to understand the evolution of Pavlovian conditioning we need to pay more attention to protostomes. To this end, Fig. 3.1(A) shows the branching times of their major groups[2].

The literature on reinforcement learning in "invertebrates" almost always involves protostomes, although one important paper describes Pavlovian conditioning in sea anemones (asterisk in Fig. 3.1A). Pavlovian conditioning has been observed in flatworms (*Planaria*), gastropod mollusks (sea slugs and garden slugs), cephalopod mollusks (octopuses and cuttlefish), roundworms (nematodes), annelids (segmented worms), and various arthropods (insects and crustaceans).

In a common experimental design, animals develop a conditioned response to the presentation of a light paired with an electric shock. For example, garden slugs and snails, both terrestrial mollusks, have displayed standard and second-order Pavlovian conditioning. In the latter, a conditioned stimulus reinforces new learning instead of a primary reinforcer doing so. Garden slugs and snails also showed blocking and extinction[28–31].

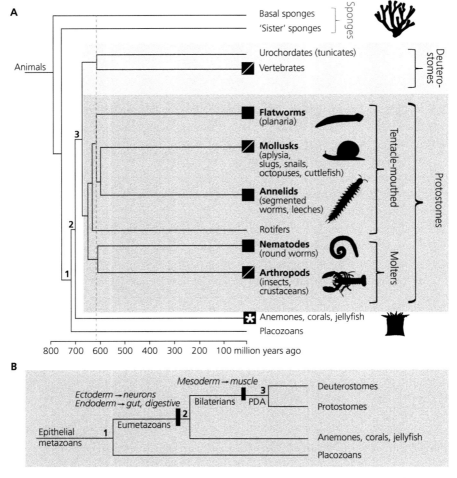

Fig. 3.1 Protostomes and early animals. (A) A time-based cladogram (chronogram) of animals based on molecular methods. Divergence times estimated from molecular data often precede those based on fossils. Black squares (right) designate groups that exhibit Pavlovian conditioning; those showing instrumental conditioning have a white diagonal line within the square. The white asterisk notes the special case of anemones. The vertical dashed line shows when vertebrates diverged from other chordates. Numbered stem species (1–3) match in (A) and (B). (B) Early speciation events in animal history. The derived traits noted above black rectangles refer to the germ layers that give rise to neurons, gut and digestive tissues, and muscles. PDA, protostome–deuterostome common ancestor. (A) Adapted from Erwin and Valentine[2].

Blocking refers to an inability to learn about stimuli that accompany a previously established conditioned stimulus (Box 3.1); extinction involves the masking of conditioned reflexes when the previously reliable outcome fails to occur. Nematodes (roundworms) exhibited both appetitive and aversive learning, and they could also learn to distinguish safe from toxic food items[32].

Some protostomes have been studied extensively. Insects and other arthropods, for example, have exhibited robust forms of Pavlovian conditioning in several studies. Honeybees, for which there is an especially rich Pavlovian-learning literature, have displayed many of the same conditioning properties seen in mammals and birds. For example, experiments in bees have demonstrated extinction, context conditioning, and latent inhibition, among other features of conditioning in mammals[33]. We explained extinction earlier. In context conditioning, a background stimulus sets the occasion for a particular S–O association. Without this occasion-setter, the conditioned response fails to occur or does so less reliably[34]. Latent inhibition refers to the fact that when a neutral stimulus repeatedly appears, but no outcome follows, it becomes difficult to use that stimulus for Pavlovian conditioning. Papini[33], in his Table 8.3, has assembled a "partial list" of two dozen learning traits shared by honeybees and vertebrates, with the promise of more elsewhere.

The diverse distribution of animals that store Pavlovian memories allows us to consider whether they inherited this trait from a common ancestor. Figure 3.1(A) designates the modern groups showing this form of learning by placing a black square at the right end of the line. We have made no effort to make this illustration comprehensive, and there is no need to do so. The evidence cited here suffices to show that Pavlovian memories have a wide distribution among modern protostomes. Their distribution in vertebrates has similar breadth among crown groups[35].

The study of sea anemones is particularly important because these animals are members of a group called radiates or Cnidaria (asterisk in Fig. 3.1A), which branched off before the split between protostomes and deuterostomes. As a result of this early divergence, the cnidarian nervous system differs utterly from that of both protostomes and deuterostomes. The nervous system of anemones consists of sensory cells at the surface of the epithelium— the layer of tissue that covers and protects an animal—and ganglionic neurons deeper in the epithelium. Some of the sensory cells function as photon transducers. Both sensory cells and ganglionic neurons have processes that connect into networks that synapse on each other and on muscle cells. Although neurons and their processes can concentrate to a limited extent in tissue folds, these animals lack the centralized nervous system that characterizes both protostomes and deuterostomes. Even though anemones lack a central nervous system, they can respond to stimuli and move around from time to time.

Haralson et al.[36] demonstrated Pavlovian conditioning in sea anemones. In their experiment, a light served as the conditioned stimulus and shock was the unconditioned stimulus. During training, anemones learned to fold their oral disk and tentacles in response to the light, as well as to emit an electrical response. The demonstration of associative learning requires ruling out interpretations of the results in terms of arousal, sensitization, or pseudoconditioning (a form of sensitization that results from repeated presentation of an unconditioned stimulus). By doing so, Haralson et al.[36] showed that genuine Pavlovian learning occurs in anemones. Because these animals lack a brain or any other kind of centralized nervous system, this finding supports the idea that Pavlovian learning is a general property of neural networks.

Viewed generally, the comparative literature suggests that Pavlovian learning either emerged in the ancestral species denoted by the numeral 2 in Fig. 3.1 (eumetazoans) or did so repeatedly in nervous systems of various kinds. The broad distribution of Pavlovian learning in protostomes and deuterostomes indicates that if this trait evolved independently in both clades—a distinct possibility—it did so early in both, by the time that vertebrates first appeared (indicated by the dashed vertical line in Fig. 3.1A) or shortly thereafter.

The comparative evidence also indicates that Pavlovian memories can be established by diverse kinds of neural systems: epithelial structures in brainless animals (anemones); peripheral ganglia detached from a central nervous system of insects (Box 3.2); the cerebellum; and telencephalic structures such as the amygdala and basal ganglia. Taken together, these findings demonstrate that Pavlovian conditioning does not result from a single neurophysiological "mechanism," notwithstanding surface similarities and common formalisms. The simple fact that Pavlovian conditioning occurs in both "invertebrates" and vertebrates provides sufficient support for this conclusion on its own. These groups have brains that resemble each other very little and probably evolved in parallel (see Chapter 2, "The origin of vertebrates"). Accordingly, even before addressing instrumental conditioning, we can conclude that the concept of a reinforcement learning system is little more than a trash-can category, much like the term "invertebrate" itself. Both terms—"invertebrate" and reinforcement learning—refer to leftovers.

Box 3.2 Brainless conditioning

Pavlovian conditioning occurs in a naturally brainless species, sea anemones, but it is also possible to study protostomes that have had their brains removed. An experiment by Horridge[130] demonstrated response–outcome conditioning in decapitated cockroaches and locusts. Subsequent studies showed that either the ventral nerve cord[131,132] or an isolated peripheral ganglion[133] suffices to acquire and retain these memories.

In a representative experiment, fine wires were inserted into two legs from different animals. One of the legs touched a saline solution when it was sufficiently extended, a response that completed an electrical circuit and produced the unconditioned stimulus: shock. A yoked leg received shock simultaneously. The two legs differed in that the yoked leg had a random joint angle at the time of the shock, whereas the master leg always had a joint angle large enough for its "foot" to touch the saline. Flexion of the leg reduced the joint's angle and terminated the shock. After one leg had been conditioned, both legs were then tested independently. The master leg flexed sufficiently to avoid shock significantly more frequently than the yoked leg did, demonstrating a response–outcome (R–O) memory.

Instrumental conditioning

Pavlovian memories reflect outcomes associated with stimuli, but animals can also learn about outcomes that follow their actions. The terms for these behaviors, operant and instrumental conditioning, reflect this relationship. An animal operates on the world; its actions are instrumental in producing an outcome. Pavlovian approach behavior resembles instrumental responding in a general way, but it differs in that the outcome does not depend on anything the animal does.

Instrumental terminology

In the laboratory, the reinforcing feedback used for instrumental conditioning usually consists of appetitive outcomes, called rewards, although aversive feedback can also condition behavior. Primary reinforcers satisfy biological needs, such as nutritional ones, or have the potential to cause harm. Secondary reinforcers (also called conditioned reinforcers) can condition behavior because of their association with primary reinforcers.

The specialized literature often refers to actions as "responses," even in the absence of any obvious triggering event. Accordingly, "R" stands for both responses to stimuli and other actions. Because this literature often uses the terms goal and outcome interchangeably, it labels behaviors guided by predicted outcomes as goal-directed responding. In this book, however, we recognize other kinds of goals, such as the objects and places that serve as targets for reaching movements in primates. As a result, we refer to outcome-directed behavior where others use goal-directed.

In addition to action–outcome (R–O) associations, stimulus–response (S–R) associations form during instrumental conditioning. Behaviors predominantly guided by these associations, without reference to predicted outcomes, are called habits. This is the meaning of habit used in learning theory, a conceptual framework that seeks to establish universal laws of learning. In cognitive psychology, however, this term has a different meaning. Insensitivity to a competing task demonstrates a habit, not insensitivity to predicted outcomes. Furthermore, in biology the word habit has yet another meaning, one that refers to genetically determined traits. Many rodents, for example, have a fossorial habit, which means that they live underground. Even trees have habits, such as growing tall. In this book, we use the term habit in all three ways, depending on the context. For the remainder of this chapter, however, we limit ourselves to the learning-theory meaning.

What happens in instrumental conditioning

Instrumental conditioning establishes or strengthens associations between actions and outcomes, based on reinforcing feedback. If reinforcement follows an action in the presence of a particular stimulus, that stimulus comes to modulate R–O associations, which results in associations among stimuli, actions, and outcomes (S–R–O associations). Positive and negative reinforcement change the likelihood of repeating a behavior in the future.

Abundant research distinguishes habits from outcome-directed behavior. In theory, animals learn both S–R and S–R–O associations in parallel, but eventually they can compete, cooperate, or operate in nested hierarchies. Habits, as mentioned earlier, involve behaviors guided by S–R associations, with little or no sensitivity to predicted outcomes. Early in learning, however, animals are highly sensitive to the value of a predicted outcome. Only after extensive training does an animal's behavior become insensitive to outcomes.

As Pearce[37] has pointed out, the distinction between habits and outcome-directed behavior dates back more than a century. This old idea has taken on new significance, however, as a crucial (and widely misunderstood) underpinning of the prevailing view of memory systems, as we explain in Chapter 12 ("The habit–memory dichotomy").

Specific experimental procedures can distinguish habits from outcome-directed behavior, including the one that we emphasize here: reinforcer devaluation. In a common experimental design, rats first learned that a cue predicted food delivery, and so the presentation of that cue came to elicit movements toward a food cup[38]. Then the subjective value of the food was reduced experimentally. Several methods can devalue foods and other resources, but two have become common. One involves taste aversion learning, as mentioned earlier: pairing food ingestion with hypodermic injections of a toxin that produces malaise or nausea. In another, animals consume a given food to satiety. Regardless of the method used, when the rats saw a conditioned stimulus after food devaluation, they approached the food cup less frequently or more slowly. This observation demonstrates that the rat's behavior depended on the current subjective value of the outcome. Although this particular example involved Pavlovian conditioning, reinforcer devaluation affects both Pavlovian and instrumental behaviors because both depend on the subjective value of predicted outcomes.

Experiments on rodents and monkeys show that the amygdala plays a necessary role in reinforcer devaluation, and thus in outcome-directed behavior. In one experiment, monkeys learned that the choice of one object produced a particular kind of food (outcome), whereas the choice of a second object produced a different kind of food. After learning about a large number of objects and their associated foods, the monkeys then faced a choice between two objects, one associated with one kind of food and the other associated with a different food. Control monkeys tended to choose the object associated with their preferred food. In the next phase of the experiment, the monkeys ate one of the two foods until sated, which devalued that food. Afterward, the monkeys tended to avoid objects associated with the devalued food and chose the other class of objects instead, a phenomenon called the *devaluation effect*. Lesions of the amygdala diminished the devaluation effect or eliminated it entirely[39,40]. We return to this topic in Chapter 6 ("Orbitofrontal–amygdala interactions") in the context of primate innovations.

In another experiment, injections of an inhibitory neurotransmitter temporarily inactivated the amygdala prior to the selective satiation procedure. Because the inactivation lasts for a long time, this procedure ensured that neurons in the amygdala were inactive as the subject consumed one of the foods to satiety, as well as during the choice phase of the experiment. This inactivation procedure caused a result similar to that of permanent amygdala lesions; it blocked the devaluation effect. Inactivation of the amygdala that was limited to the choice phase, in contrast, had no effect; the monkeys shifted their choices as usual[41]. These findings show that after the satiety-induced devaluation has occurred in these experiments, the amygdala no longer plays an essential role in using altered food value to choose among objects. The updated value of the predicted outcome, therefore, must be stored somewhere outside the amygdala. Nevertheless, the amygdala plays a necessary role in updating these valuations, and for this reason we treat it as a component of the reinforcement system.

Outcomes and predicted outcomes have both general and specific aspects. In rodents, the central nucleus of the amygdala mediates the valuation of the general properties of the outcomes, such as their positive or negative valence, whereas the basolateral nuclei of the amygdala do so for the specific sensory features of outcomes, such as their taste or smell[42]. The basolateral amygdala makes this contribution for both Pavlovian and instrumental learning and across different methods for devaluing an outcome[38].

In many circumstances, Pavlovian and instrumental conditioning work together. In the case of food, for example, the sight of food acts as a conditioned stimulus eliciting Pavlovian approach behavior. The same stimulus prompts an instrumental response based on a predicted outcome, which leads to the same behavior. In this example, S–O and R–O associations cooperate.

In another form of cooperation, when a conditioned stimulus and an instrumentally conditioned action predict the same outcome, animals act as though they have more motivation to perform the action, a phenomenon called Pavlovian-to-instrumental transfer (PIT). Somehow, the combination of the two outcome predictions increases the likelihood or speed of an instrumental response[43]. We mentioned earlier that the central nucleus of the amygdala mediates general outcome valuations, and the basolateral amygdala does so for specific outcome features. The contribution of the striatum to PIT also reflects this distinction, specifically for two parts of the ventral striatum: the core and shell of the nucleus accumbens. For central nucleus-dependent tasks, lesions of the core impaired PIT[44], but for basolateral-dependent tasks lesions of the shell did so[45,46]. Accordingly, interactions between the amygdala and the basal ganglia appear to underlie this form of cooperativity between Pavlovian and instrumental conditioning.

Sometimes, however, Pavlovian and instrumental conditioning mediate conflicting behaviors. An entertaining example of such conflict, sometimes termed "misbehavior," comes from an anecdote about pigs trained to drop a token into a slot to earn food[47]. Although the pigs readily learned the instrumental response (the authors of this report noted the cooperative and ravenous nature of pigs) some pigs held on to the token and rooted around with it rather than dropping it into the slot. Apparently, the Pavlovian response of approaching and manipulating the token conflicted with the instrumental response necessary to obtain food rewards. When the Pavlovian behavior "wins" such a contest, it seems like "misbehavior" to people trying to train the pigs to do something else, and the same goes for other species as well[48].

A report by Hershberger[49] provides a classic example of conflicting Pavlovian and instrumental behaviors. In his experiment, a chick first ate from a visually distinctive bowl and developed a Pavlovian approach behavior toward it. With the aid of mirrors, the bowl later seemed to move away from the chick as the animal approached it. In contrast, if the chick moved away from the bowl the mirrors made it seem as if the bowl was chasing the chick. Extensive instrumental conditioning failed to suppress the Pavlovian approach behavior in this condition, and so the chick continued to run toward the bowl even as it moved farther away. Perhaps the contrived testing situation accounts for this result; after all, chickens do not naturally feed on mobile foods. The standard explanation, however, is that the chicks cannot overcome the competition from Pavlovian approach behavior.

Why instrumental conditioning happens

To summarize "What happens in instrumental conditioning," when a beneficial outcome follows an action, that action becomes more likely in the future. When an action occurs in a specific sensory context and results in a reward, an animal becomes more likely to act in the same way when it next encounters that context or something sufficiently like it (stimulus generalization). According to animal learning theory this occurs through two so-called "mechanisms": habits and outcome-directed behavior[50–55].

Some advantages of instrumental memories seem obvious, and the two "mechanisms" appear to play complementary roles. Habits work well in conditions of low resource volatility, and do so for two main reasons: (1) speed and (2) the fact that a given choice occurs consistently[51,53], thus avoiding the computationally intensive mechanisms that take feedback into account[51,56]. Too much reliance on habits, however, would forego the benefits of more flexible choices. At higher computational cost[57], outcome-directed behaviors can cope with a moderate degree of resource volatility. (In Chapter 8, "Augmentation of older memory systems," we discuss yet higher levels of resource volatility.) When resource distributions change, foraging choices change accordingly. Compared with habits, behavioral consistency decreases and choices come to reflect an average over several outcomes, with a bias toward more recent ones[58–60]. The existence of outcome-directed behaviors, therefore, affects the balance between exploiting reliable resources and exploring alternatives[56,61–65]. Perhaps more importantly, outcome-directed behaviors also enable choices based on current biological needs, as exemplified by selective satiation on a particular kind of food (the devaluation effect)[39,40].

Combined with Pavlovian learning and phenomena such as habituation and sensitization, habits and outcome-directed behavior seem to explain nearly everything worth explaining about behavior, at least according to some experts[53,66]. Reinforcement systems do indeed provide animals with powerful and fairly general learning capacities, which can cope with moderate levels of resource volatility and enable them to exploit reasonably reliable resources. But these phylogenetically ancient learning "mechanisms" hardly explain everything about animal behavior, a point we expand upon later (see "Conclusions").

In part, exaggerations about the importance of instrumental and Pavlovian conditioning stem from the impoverished conditions of the laboratory, which also obscure one of the adaptive advantages that instrumental conditioning provides. Laboratory experiments often involve only a few stimuli, each of which has only one or two relevant features. Actions are limited to simple choices, such as bar presses, nose pokes, or escape from one place to one other place. However, in ecologically realistic situations the sensory stimuli that guide choices have a large number of sensory features[67]. So, too, do the outcomes that result from those choices, such as foods and fluids. Actions in the wild are typically much more complex than bar presses or nose pokes. Accordingly, it is impossible to devote equal computational resources to all of the available sensory information, all aspects of predicted outcomes, and every possible action: a problem called information overload.

Several mechanisms have evolved to mitigate this problem. Reinforcement learning mechanisms do so by regulating the associability of stimuli, as we explain later (see "Stimulus associability"). However, there are other ways that animals deal with information overload. One involves special-purpose mechanisms such as imprinting and taste aversion[22,68,69]. In primates, however, a new representational system mitigates information overload through top-down biased competition[70], a process mediated by the prefrontal cortex (see Chapter 8, "Augmentation of the biased-competition system"). Although learning theorists often refer to both stimulus associability and top-down biased competition by the word "attention," these two mechanisms differ utterly: in their neural substrates, in their most significant properties, and in their evolutionary history, as we explain later (see "Attention versus surprise"). Their surface similarities simply reflect the common problem that both evolved to address: at different times, in different lineages, and in different ecological conditions.

Evolution of instrumental conditioning

Protostomes

Mollusks, such as the well-studied sea slug (or sea hare) *Aplysia*, are among the protostomes that show instrumental conditioning[29,71–73]. *Aplysia*'s feeding behavior, specifically the biting movements that occur during feeding, can be instrumentally conditioned. In one experiment, the investigators replaced primary reinforcement (food ingestion) by stimulating the esophageal nerve, which they timed to follow biting movements (in the absence of food)[73]. After this training, the conditioned sea slugs made more biting movements than members of a control group did. Neural recordings from the buccal ganglion, which generates the motor signals used for ingestion, confirmed the existence of outputs induced by instrumental learning. In an *in vitro* experiment involving a neuron that participates in feeding behavior, the investigators could mimic reinforcement by applying dopamine to this neuron, and this procedure also induced biting-related outputs[74–76].

Pond snails also show instrumental conditioning. These animals absorb oxygen in two different ways: through their skin when under water and via a respiratory orifice, called a pneumostome, when they are at the surface of a pond. Under hypoxic aquatic conditions, these animals approach the surface of the pond and open their pneumostome to bring in oxygenated air. In one experiment, external contact with the pneumostome, using a wooden probe, caused it to close. With repeated stimulation of this kind, the snails ceased to open their pneumostome. Control procedures showed that this type of avoidance learning did not result from either hypoxia or nonassociative mechanisms[77]. These observations demonstrated instrumental conditioning because the snails learned the association between an action (opening their pneumostome) and an aversive outcome (a tactile thwack). In this case, because the stimulus was aversive, the snails learned to withhold the behavior.

In addition to mollusks like sea slugs and snails, insects and other arthropods form instrumental memories. Green crabs, for example, can learn to press one of two available levers, typically via claw extension, to earn food. In one experiment[78], pressing one lever always produced food whereas pressing another lever never did so. The crabs learned to press the food-producing lever at a significantly higher rate than the alternative lever. When the association between the levers and food was reversed, the crabs switched their choice after just two 20-minute sessions. Crabs also dramatically reduced their frequency of lever pressing in extinction sessions.

Among the insects, honeybees show both second-order conditioning and many of the phenomena that characterize instrumental behavior in mammals[33]. An experiment on fruit flies, for example, demonstrated heat-box learning, an avoidance behavior in which movement into one half of a box led to a reduction of the temperature within the whole box. After about 20 minutes of training, the flies moved to the side of the box that decreased the heat level (remaining there about 90% of the time), and these memories persisted for up to 2 hours[79]. Certain mutations of a particular gene, called *ignorant*, affect Pavlovian conditioning in these flies, and others affect instrumental conditioning[79].

Although these examples merely scratch the surface of the relevant literature, they suffice to show that both the major groups of protostomes exhibit instrumental conditioning. Figure 3.1(A) identifies these two protostome groups with brackets to the right. A diagonal white line through a black square indicates the lineages in which instrumental conditioning has been demonstrated.

Nonmammalian vertebrates

We mention here only a few examples of instrumental conditioning in nonmammalian vertebrates because we expect that most readers already assume that such learning occurs among all vertebrates. One experiment exploited the innate tendency of crested newts to snap at small dark objects[80]. Newts saw two visual stimuli pasted on the outside of their tank: a small black circle at one place and a small black triangle somewhere else. Snapping at the correct stimulus earned the newts a piece of worm, and the newts learned to snap correctly. In other work on amphibians, toads have been instrumentally conditioned to cross a runway to obtain water, to make a particular choice in a T-maze, and to later reverse that choice[81].

Work in teleost fish has provided extensive evidence for instrumental learning, for both positive and negative reinforcement. In one experiment, goldfish were placed in a tube and trained to discriminate between a red and green light. In the presence of a red light any movement that broke an invisible beam led to the provision of oxygenated water, a primary reinforcer, for 15 seconds[82]. For a green light, withholding movement for 20 seconds produced oxygenated water. The goldfish learned to make the instrumental response more frequently for the red light than for the green light.

In another experiment, goldfish swam between two small end-tanks separated by a 1-cm wide barrier containing shallow water[83]. Four groups of goldfish were subject to different experimental treatments. Two groups could escape shock in one end-tank by crossing the shallow barrier to the other end-tank; the other two groups couldn't do anything to prevent being shocked. One of the two groups in each category saw an overhead light that predicted shock. After this training, the fish that could both see a predictive visual cue and terminate the shock crossed the barrier most often; the groups that couldn't terminate the shock did so least often.

Another experimental design distinguished Pavlovian from instrumental conditioning by training mormyrid fish and employing a yoking procedure[84]. The master fish could discharge their electric organs to turn off a warning light and avoid electric shock. Yoked fish received the same presentations of light and shock as the master group, but their actions did not affect the frequency or intensity of the shocks. Under these conditions, master fish learned to discharge their electric organs and thus avoid shocks; yoked fish did so less frequently. Because the Pavlovian S–O (light–shock) relationship did not differ between the two groups these results demonstrate instrumental learning. Goldfish have also learned an instrumental avoidance task[85], in which master fish had to cross a barrier to postpone a shock. The barrier-crossing rates of master fish exceeded those of yoked fish, and this behavior was correlated with the response–shock interval.

The literature on instrumental behavior in birds involves a lot of key pecking—often in response to sensory cues—for little more than chicken feed. In one example, pigeons performed instrumentally conditioned pecking responses in total darkness. Darkness eliminated all visual stimuli, and so this manipulation served to rule out an account of the pigeon's behavior in terms of Pavlovian (S–O) memories[86].

Mammals

Among vertebrates, the partial reinforcement extinction (PRE) effect, the magnitude of reinforcement extinction (MRE) effect, latent inhibition, and the successive negative contrast (SNC) effect appear to be limited to mammals[33]. Although honeybees also show latent inhibition and the PRE effect, its rarity among nonmammalian vertebrates suggests that these traits arose independently in mammals and bees[33]:

◆ The PRE effect consists of greater resistance to extinction after partial reinforcement training than after continuous reinforcement training. In the former, the outcome occurs only on some trials; in the latter, it occurs on every trial. However, the PRE effect could be equally well described as a continuous reinforcement effect: a speeding of extinction after continuous reinforcement training.

- ◆ The MRE effect closely resembles the PRE effect, but the key feedback variable consists of the amount of reinforcement rather than its likelihood.

- ◆ The SNC effect involves the rejection of an appetitive outcome after a downshift in its quantity or quality. Experimental subjects respond less than a control group that has only experienced the smaller or less palatable outcomes.

The PRE effect can be demonstrated in maze tasks in which rats need to choose the correct arm of a maze to obtain food, for example. But this can also be done more simply by measuring the time needed for rats to reach the end of a single runway to obtain food. In an experiment involving extinction training, rats slowed down on the trials after they failed to find food, but they slowed down more after continuous reinforcement (Fig. 3.2, unfilled circles) than after partial reinforcement (filled circles)[87]. Extinction in the laboratory corresponds to resource depletion in natural habitats, so these rats gradually learned that the end of the runway was "depleted." As a result, their subjective valuation of the foraging site decreased and they slowed down, but less so (at first) for partial reinforcement schedules.

Like the PRE effect, the SNC effect can be demonstrated by measuring how fast rats run for resources. In one experiment, normal rats decreased their running speed after experiencing a downshift in reward magnitude, with an overshoot in this reduction compared with animals that had never experienced "better times" in the "good old days"[88].

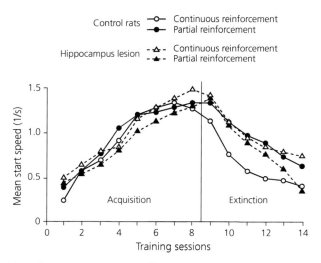

Fig. 3.2 The partial reinforcement extinction effect. The plot shows the speed of rats as they began running down a track toward the previous location of food, as a function of test sessions. It contrasts the effects of continuous reinforcement (unfilled symbols) and partial reinforcement (black symbols), as well as the effect of hippocampus lesions (dashed lines) compared with control rats (solid lines). Adapted from Rawlins JN, Feldon J, Gray JA. The effects of hippocampectomy and of fimbria section upon the partial reinforcement extinction effect in rats. *Experimental Brain Research* 38:273–83, © 1980, with permission of Springer.

The PRE, MRE, and SNC effects, common among mammals but rare or absent in other vertebrates[33], have something in common; they demonstrate greater flexibility in the face of diminishing resources. Mammals have much higher energy requirements than other vertebrates (birds excluded), largely due to the demands of endothermy (see Box 1.1). The reinforcement systems in mammals shift foraging choices relatively rapidly when a resource diminishes or depletes:

◆ The PRE effect results in a faster shift when a consistent resource depletes (continuous reinforcement) compared with an inconsistent one (partial reinforcement).

◆ The MRE effect results in a faster shift after a larger resource depletes compared with a smaller one.

◆ The SNC effect results in a larger shift after a resource diminishes compared with a constant resource at that diminished level.

As we explain in Chapter 4, the hippocampal complex stores many of the memories that guide foraging behaviors. Accordingly, Fig. 3.2 (triangles, dashed lines) shows the results of an experiment in which lesions of the hippocampus blocked the PRE effect in rats[87,89]. Similar results were obtained for lesions of the septal nuclei[90] and of the fimbria and fornix[87], the fiber tracts that connect the hippocampal complex to other parts of the brain. Recall from Chapter 2 that the septal nuclei correspond to the striatal parts of cortex–basal ganglia "loops" involving the hippocampus. In a related experiment, lesions of the hippocampal complex also blocked the SNC effect. Unlike control rats, lesioned rats did not decrease their running speed after downshifts in the magnitude of reward or increase it following an upshift[88] (Fig. 3.3C, D), and comparable results have been reported for maze learning. These findings suggest that, compared with other vertebrates (Fig. 3.3A, B), the reinforcement systems in mammals show enhanced flexibility in the face of depleted or depleting resources[33]. We revisit this topic in Chapter 5 ("Conclusions") in the context of new cortical areas that evolved in early mammals.

Mechanisms

Obviously, we have neither the intention nor the capacity to present a primer on reinforcement learning and its mechanisms. A voluminous literature and many textbooks deal with these topics. Instead, we concentrate on one well-worked example in order to establish the predicate for later chapters.

Comparator functions

According to current models of reinforcement learning, such as the temporal difference model, midbrain dopaminergic cells function as comparators for rewards, contrasting the outcomes that actually occur with those that are predicted[91–95]. Dopaminergic cells usually discharge at a steady rate, but they respond with increased activity for larger than expected or unexpected rewards and with decreased activity for smaller than expected or omitted rewards. In addition, they increase their activity in response to stimuli that predict rewards, based on learned S–O associations[91].

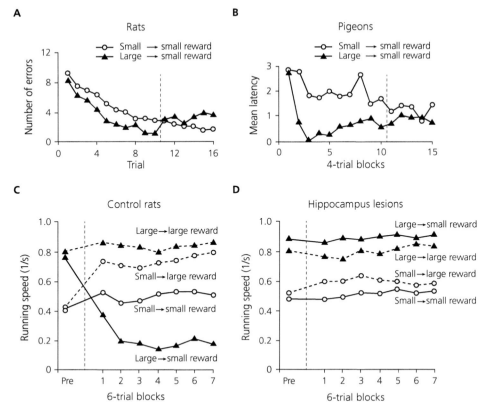

Fig. 3.3 The successive negative contrast effect. (A) Effect of downshifting reward versus consistent reward at the lower level. Note the overshoot of the black triangles after the shift in reward level (dashed vertical line). (B) Lack of the successive negative contrast effect in pigeons, as indicated by the lack of overshoot of the black triangles. (C) Successive negative contrast effect on track running in rats. Dashed lines indicate groups receiving large rewards in the final phase of the experiment; solid lines indicate groups receiving small rewards at that time. (D) Effect of hippocampus lesions on successive negative contrast effects in rats. Note that in (A) the abscissa is "trials" whereas in (B–D) it is "blocks of trials." (A, B) Redrawn from Papini MR. *Comparative Psychology: Evolution and Development of Behavior*, © 2008, Psychology Press, with permission. (C, D) Redrawn from Franchina JJ, Brown TS. Reward magnitude shift effects in rats with hippocampal lesions. *Journal of Comparative and Physiological Psychology* 76:365–70, © 1971, American Psychological Association, with permission.

These models usually share several key assumptions:

◆ Rewards function as reinforcing feedback to strengthen associations that are active in their presence.

◆ Pavlovian and instrumental memories result from strengthening of S–O and R–O (alternatively, action–outcome) associations, respectively.

- Increases in the activity of dopaminergic cells reinforce behaviors and decreases lead to extinction.

- Dopaminergic cells reside in the substantia nigra pars compacta (SNc) and ventral tegmental area (VTA), and they function as comparators that compute a reward-prediction error signal, which serves as a teaching signal for appetitive forms of conditioning[96,97].

- Because some midbrain dopaminergic neurons respond to positively valued stimuli with an increase in activity, as they do for unpredicted rewards, any stimulus can become a secondary reinforcer, which accounts for second-order conditioning.

Not all conditioning relies upon rewards or dopamine, however. As explained earlier (see "What happens in Pavlovian conditioning"), many forms of Pavlovian conditioning depend on cerebellar mechanisms. In these kinds of conditioning, neurons in the inferior olivary nuclei serve as comparators, rather than dopaminergic cells in the SNc or VTA.

To understand the evolution of memory systems, we need to appreciate the comparator mechanisms in some detail. By understanding cerebellar conditioning at the cellular and synaptic level it should become clear that the descriptions and formalisms used in the literature on learning theory reflect surface similarities, not "mechanisms" in the neurophysiological sense. The reason is that the same terms, descriptions, and concepts apply to a variety of neural mechanisms that implement reinforcement learning. The mechanisms that depend on telencephalic structures, such as the amygdala and striatum, are well known, as is the role of their dopaminergic inputs. But another, independent mechanism involves the brainstem, including the cerebellum.

In an extensively studied example of Pavlovian learning, called eyeblink conditioning, an auditory tone serves as the conditioned stimulus and an air puff to the eye provides the unconditioned stimulus. Sensory inputs to trigeminal nuclei, reticular-formation intermediaries, and motor outputs from the facial nucleus produce the unconditioned response, namely eyelid closure (Fig. 3.4B, shaded area).

In eyeblink conditioning, the basilar pontine nuclei relay information about both the conditioned and unconditioned stimuli to the cerebellum. In both cases, mossy fibers convey this information, and they influence both Purkinje cells in the cerebellar cortex and cells in the deep cerebellar nuclei (Fig. 3.4B, upper left). In the cerebellar cortex, mossy-fiber inputs exert their influence via granule cells, which send their parallel fibers to Purkinje cells (Fig. 3.4A).

Cerebellar memories generate a particular kind of prediction: An unconditioned stimulus will occur at a specific time after a conditioned stimulus. This prediction takes the form of an inhibitory signal from the deep cerebellar nuclei to the inferior olivary nuclei. The same signal goes to central pattern generators in the brainstem to generate a conditioned response (Fig. 3.4B, lower left). Inferior olivary neurons not only receive the inhibitory prediction signal just mentioned, but also an excitatory input from the trigeminal nuclei that reflects the unconditioned stimulus (Fig. 3.4B, C), and they project to Purkinje cells via climbing fibers, which provide a teaching signal analogous to dopaminergic projections (Fig. 3.4A, B).

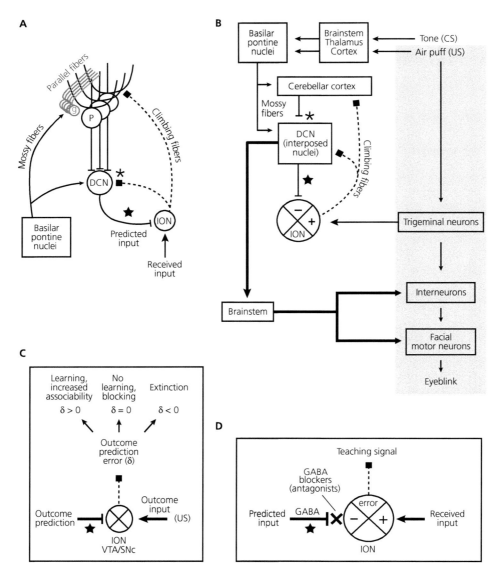

Fig. 3.4 Cerebellar circuits for Pavlovian learning. (A) Cerebellar architecture. Lines that end in arrowheads provide excitatory inputs; lines that end in flat bars provide inhibitory inputs; lines that end in squares modulate synaptic weights. The stars and asterisks are referred to in the text. (B) Neural circuits underlying Pavlovian eyeblink conditioning. Shading: circuit for the unconditioned response. (C) Comparator mechanisms and types of error signals. δ indicates a difference measure. (D) Pharmacological blockers applied to the comparator. Abbreviations: CS, conditioned stimulus; DCN, deep cerebellar nuclei; g, granule cells; GABA, gamma-aminobutyric acid; ION, inferior olivary nuclei; P, Purkinje cells; SNc, substantia nigra pars compacta; US, unconditioned stimulus; VTA, ventral tegmental area. (A)–(D) From Shadmehr R, Wise SP. *The Computational Neurobiology of Reaching and Pointing*, © 2005, published by The MIT Press.

Like dopaminergic cells, most of the time inferior olivary neurons discharge at a steady rate (approximately once per second). This level of climbing-fiber activity suffices to maintain synaptic weights between parallel fibers and Purkinje cells (Fig. 3.4A). When climbing-fiber activity increases, synapses between parallel fibers and Purkinje cells weaken through postsynaptic long-term depression (LTD); when climbing-fiber activity decreases, these synapses strengthen through presynaptic long-term potentiation (LTP).

On the first trial of the conditioning procedure, a tone—which will become the conditioned stimulus—does not predict the air puff or anything else. But when an air puff, the unconditioned stimulus, occurs at a fixed interval after the tone, excitatory inputs to the inferior olivary neurons increase their activity three- to eight-fold at that time. An increase in inferior olivary activity also means an increase in climbing-fiber activity, which weakens selected parallel fiber–Purkinje cell synapses. This decrease in synaptic weight renders Purkinje cells less responsive to future inputs from the parallel fibers, and thus to future inputs from the tone. So when the tone occurs on subsequent trials, the selected parallel fibers excite Purkinje cells less effectively, at some delay, which means that these Purkinje cells will inhibit neurons in the deep cerebellar nuclei less (asterisk in Fig. 3.4A, B). This decrease in the activity of Purkinje cells releases neurons in the deep cerebellar nuclei from inhibition at a specific delay from the onset of the tone. After a number of paired tone–air-puff trials, this release becomes large enough to generate a conditioned eyeblink.

Once the cerebellum has established this Pavlovian memory, the tone accurately predicts the air puff in time and intensity, and so inferior olivary neurons no longer increase their discharge rate in response to the air puff. The inhibitory prediction signal from the cerebellum to the inferior olivary nucleus (star in Fig. 3.4A–D) has come to precisely balance excitatory sensory inputs signaling the air puff. In this circumstance, the comparator produces no prediction-error signal, and so climbing-fiber activity remains constant. As a result, the cerebellum cannot learn about additional stimuli that accompany the tone, a phenomenon known as the Kamin blocking effect (Box 3.1).

An experiment involving the Kamin blocking effect illuminates the comparator's function. When the prediction signal from the cerebellum could not reach the inferior olivary comparator because of a pharmacological blockade (Fig. 3.4D), the air puff could once again generate a teaching signal[98]. Inhibition from the deep cerebellar nuclei no longer balanced the excitatory sensory input, and so the puff again became unpredicted, as far as the comparator could tell. As a result, the cerebellum learned about a new conditioned stimulus, a phenomenon called unblocking. In this sense, synaptic blockers block blocking.

Studies of extinction lead to a similar conclusion. Extinction occurs when the air puff no longer follows the tone. Because the excitatory sensory input from the air puff does not occur, the sensory signal reflecting the unconditioned stimulus no longer balances the inhibitory (predictive) input from the cerebellum. As a result, inferior olivary cells become inactive when the unconditioned stimulus should occur. The associated decrease in climbing-fiber activity causes parallel-fiber synapses on Purkinje cells to strengthen via LTP, which negates the previously established LTD. Afterward, when the tone occurs again, Purkinje cells generate a stronger output and more effectively suppress activity in the deep cerebellar nuclei. After several extinction trials, the cerebellum stops generating both the prediction signal and the conditioned reflex.

Like the experiment on the blocking effect, pharmacological blockade of the prediction signal (star in Fig. 3.4B, D) prevented a decrease in climbing-fiber activity[99]. No air-puff signal reached the comparator because that unconditioned stimulus did not occur, but no prediction signal reached it either because of the pharmacological blockade. Because the activity of inferior olivary cells remained constant, the eyeblink persisted despite the absence of the air puff.

The cerebellar mechanisms for Pavlovian learning establish two key points. First, memories involving inferior olivary and dopaminergic comparators resemble each other closely, yet depend on completely different parts of the brain. Therefore any description of conditioning, blocking, extinction, and so forth as a "mechanism" depends on a computational analogy, not on a structure–function relationship that is subject to natural selection. Second, dopaminergic mechanisms are not alone in mediating learning. The brain implements its learning algorithms with other plasticity mechanisms, such as LTP and LTD in the cerebellar cortex, which change synaptic weights according to principles similar to those for dopamine-mediated plasticity.

Signals involving comparator functions, such as prediction and prediction-error signals, occur in many structures, including the granular[100] and agranular prefrontal cortex, amygdala, and ventral striatum[101,102]. But the ancestral comparators, as such, appear to correspond to dopaminergic cells in the midbrain and inferior olivary cells in the brainstem. Related signals elsewhere in the brain appear to reflect the comparator's outputs or inputs, and outputs in the form of prediction errors have widespread effects on memory[103–105]. In addition to the ancestral comparators, Seo and Lee[100] suggest that new comparators evolved more recently, in the granular prefrontal cortex of primates.

Stimulus associability

Although they did not understand the neural mechanisms just described, psychologists noticed one of their consequences long ago. They realized that changes occur in stimulus associability during various forms of conditioning. Learning theorists sometimes refer to these phenomena as "attention for learning," but this concept should not be confused with the concept of attention as used in cognitive psychology. We explain the difference later (see "Attention versus surprise").

Associative learning models link a learning rate parameter to stimulus associability: the greater the associability, the faster the learning. Models differ in whether they stress the conditioned or unconditioned stimulus as contributing most to changes in associability, with the classic Rescorla–Wagner model[106] emphasizing the former and the Pearce–Hall model[107] the latter. The general principle is the same in both cases: Predictions and prediction errors affect stimulus associability, which in turn affects the rate of learning.

Accurate predictions decrease associability, as explained earlier (see "Comparator functions"). When a conditioned stimulus precisely predicts an unconditioned stimulus, the comparator produces a null output ($\delta = 0$ in Fig. 3.4C). As a result, no teaching signal occurs. Not only does new learning about the conditioned stimulus become difficult, but so does learning about other stimuli that accompany the conditioned stimulus (the Kamin blocking effect, see Box 3.1).

In this context, prediction errors can increase associability. For example, violating the expectancy of the unconditioned stimulus restores its associability after learning, a phenomenon sometimes called surprise. Surprise, in this sense, represents an unsigned error signal. Earlier (see "Comparator functions"), we explained the neural mechanism of this phenomenon. When sensory events do not match predictions, a prediction-error signal promotes new learning, including extinction learning, depending on the sign of the error signal (δ in Fig. 3.4C).

In studying these phenomena, experimental psychologists have found: (1) a degree of independence in the mechanisms for increases and decreases in associability; (2) that positive and negative prediction errors engage different brain systems; (3) that changes in associability affect both conditioned[106] and unconditioned[107] stimuli; and (4) that the direct effects of prediction errors, as mediated by comparators, affect learning differently from indirect influences mediated by structures connected to the comparators[66,108,109].

An extensive literature implicates the central nucleus of the amygdala in surprise-induced enhancements of associability[110], for both stimuli and outcomes[111] and conditioned and unconditioned stimuli[112]. In accord with these findings, neurophysiological studies have described central nucleus neurons that signaled reward-prediction errors after omissions or downshifts in reward ($\delta < 0$ in Fig. 3.4C)[113]. Activity modulations of these neurons correlated with central nucleus-dependent measures of surprise, although selectively in that they did not reflect unexpected rewards or the effects of devaluation.

The effects of outcome omissions rely on the amygdala and the substantia innominata[110,114]. As explained in Chapter 2 ("Rings and loops"), the substantia innominata is part of the ventral basal ganglia and, among other characteristics, it contains cholinergic cells that project elsewhere in the brain. In one experiment, inactivation of the substantia innominata eliminated surprise effects, but not as the surprises occurred during training, only later when the inactivation occurred during subsequent test sessions[115]. Taken together, these results indicate that the amygdala plays a necessary role in registering selected aspects of surprise or in establishing a new level of stimulus associability; in contrast, the substantia innominata functions in the expression of increased associability.

Additional experiments have shown that cholinergic projections from the substantia innominata to the neocortex contribute to surprise-induced enhancements in associability[116]. Furthermore, interactions between the pars compacta of the substantia nigra and the central nucleus of the amygdala are essential[117,118]. Like the central nucleus per se, substantia nigra–central nucleus interactions play a critical role in registering surprise and establishing a higher level of stimulus associability, but not in later expression. Perhaps the central nucleus conveys a prediction signal to dopaminergic neurons in the substantia nigra, which in turn send a prediction-error signal back to the central nucleus[66].

The basolateral nuclei of the amygdala also play a role in regulating stimulus associability. Neurophysiological studies have revealed increases in neuronal activity in these nuclei after changes in reward quantity, whether the change was an increase or decrease in reward[102]. This change in activity correlated with faster orienting to predictive cues, and inactivation of the basolateral amygdala slowed learning in response to changes in outcomes. Neurons in the basolateral amygdala thus appear to provide an unsigned error signal (surprise) ($\delta \neq 0$ in Fig. 3.4C or $|\delta|$). This part of the amygdala plays an especially important role when multiple outcomes occur, which supports its specialization, mentioned earlier, for predicting specific sensory aspects of outcomes[119]. Likewise, a specialization of the central nucleus for outcome omissions agrees with its role in predicting general aspects of outcomes.

Attention versus surprise

Some learning theorists equate surprise in conditioning experiments with "attention." Despite their surface similarity, these two concepts—surprise and attention—differ dramatically, as illustrated in Fig. 3.5. In conditioning-related surprise, accurate predictions

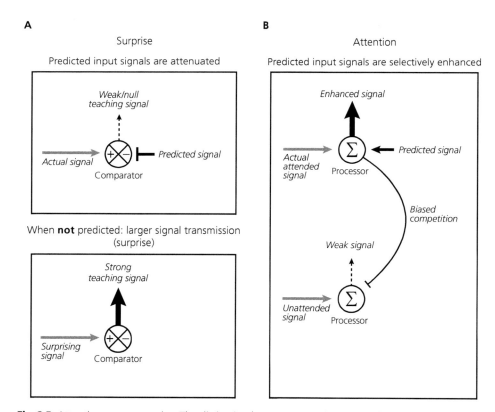

Fig. 3.5 Attention versus surprise. The distinction between attention, as used in cognitive psychology, and surprise, as used in conditioning experiments. Comparator format as in Fig. 3.4(C).

nullify the expected sensory signal. In attention, accurate predictions enhance sensory signals, and as a result of this enhancement attended stimuli and features gain a competitive advantage over unattended ones[70]. Surprise depends on phylogenetically ancient mechanisms, which are common to most if not all vertebrates, whereas attention depends on the granular prefrontal cortex, which evolved in primates (see Chapter 2, "Early primates" and "Anthropoids").

The practice of using the same term, attention, to apply to such different neural mechanisms can cause considerable confusion. It fosters the impression that nothing important has changed during vertebrate (or mammalian) evolution: All species have "attention" and experience surprise. The learning-theory concept of acquired distinctiveness takes notice of this problem, but does little to resolve it or place these traits in a phylogenetic perspective. The problem stems from divorcing the study of memory systems from the ecological conditions in which they evolved. Conditioning-related surprise provides a partial solution to the problem of information overload, which early animals and ancestral vertebrates experienced in their times and places. Later, other ancestors—in other times and places—faced different aspects of information overload, and they mitigated this problem in additional ways (see Chapter 8, "Augmentation of the biased-competition system").

Cost–benefit comparison

The study of dopamine function has cleaved into two schools: one for motor control, the other for reinforcement learning. Perhaps the effects of dopamine on different time-scales can reconcile these two traditions[92], but we think that a simple cost–benefit analysis does so more simply.

Parkinson's disease, which results from the degeneration of dopaminergic neurons, causes patients to make movements that are both abnormally short, called hypometric in the specialist literature, and abnormally slow, called bradykinetic[120]. Likewise, in an experiment on monkeys, inactivation of the internal segment of the globus pallidus caused hypometric and bradykinetic movements[121]. A simple explanation accounts for both observations, assuming that greater costs correspond to lesser benefits and vice versa. Expressed in terms of comparator functions in healthy individuals (Fig. 3.4C), when a movement is faster or larger than optimal, which corresponds to a higher cost, dopaminergic cells decrease their level of activity, as they do for smaller than expected benefits (including omitted rewards). This teaching signal contributes to the extinction of inefficient movements: slowing and shortening them to an optimal level. Parkinson's disease causes a decrease in dopamine release, of course, which makes normal movements seem too costly, and so the motor system slows and shortens them, resulting in bradykinetic and hypometric movements.

Viewed from this perspective, the dopaminergic teaching signal minimizes costs and maximizes benefits—for both energy expenditure and reinforcement. This idea encompasses both the dorsal and ventral basal ganglia and reconciles the motor-control and learning-theory perspectives on dopamine and the basal ganglia. The ventral basal ganglia and their cortex–basal ganglia "loops" (see Fig. 2.2B) optimize primary reinforcement, such as foods and fluids, whereas the dorsal basal ganglia and their cortex–basal ganglia "loops" optimize energy expenditure. A key aspect of striatal function involves the prediction of feedback of either kind, a topic taken up in Chapters 6 ("Autopilot control") and 12 ("If not habits, what?").

Evolution of dopamine mechanisms

Protostomes lack homologues of the basal ganglia, midbrain, and brainstem, but, as explained earlier (see "Evolution of Pavlovian conditioning"), they appear to use analogous conditioning mechanisms, including a contribution from dopaminergic cells. Although it has been suggested that protostomes use different learning algorithms from vertebrates, at least some of them, honeybees for example, learn and strengthen associations in much the same way as vertebrates, including through second-order conditioning[94,122,123]. The mechanisms differ to an extent, however, with octopamine playing a role in protostomes along with dopamine.

The dopamine system evolved relatively early in vertebrate history, pre-dating the split between gnathostomes and other vertebrates such as lamprey (Fig. 2.4). These jawless fish have dopaminergic neurons in their diencephalon, which are probably homologous to the midbrain dopaminergic system in gnathostomes[124,125]. Behavioral pharmacology supports this conclusion. A neurotoxin that produces Parkinson's disease in humans and monkeys, MPTP, does so by killing dopaminergic neurons. Applied to lamprey, it causes similar symptoms, such as bradykinesia[126].

Conclusions

Reinforcement memory evolved early in the history of animals to support fairly general-purpose learning about biological costs and benefits. Collectively, these memories provided advantages over special-purpose reflexes, which adapt through sensitization and habituation. Various reinforcement systems interact to balance computational costs with the ability to adapt to fluctuating resources and changing biological needs.

The contributions of the amygdala exemplify how reinforcement memories contribute to fitness. In Chapter 2 we explained that the amygdala corresponds to the caudal part of the telencephalon, and it enhances fitness in a variety of ways: conditioned orienting; conditioned defensive responses; surprise-mediated changes in stimulus associability; regulating movements for feeding, escape, and procreation; and updating valuations. Its strong link to emotion is unsurprising in this context.

Although reinforcement learning appeared early in animal evolution, the persistence of these traits puts them in a position to influence all the representational systems that evolved later. Three conceptual problems have resulted from this fact: radical behaviorism, diversity denial, and the assumption that surface similarities and formalisms reflect "mechanisms."

Behaviorism

Although behaviorism is "all but dead" as a philosophical matter (Bunge[127], p. 31), its influence persists in contemporary neuroscience, often in cryptic form. As mentioned earlier (see "Pavlovian pronouncement"), the radical version of behaviorism has receded into the background and now rarely generates very much controversy. Some recent writings, inspired in part by animal learning theory, come pretty close though. We quote one version verbatim (Balleine and O'Doherty[53], p. 48):

> Recent behavioral studies in both humans and rodents have found evidence that performance in decision-making tasks depends on two different learning processes; one encoding the relationship between actions and their consequences and a second involving the formation of stimulus–response associations. These learning processes are thought to govern goal-directed and habitual actions, respectively.

As an introduction to two kinds of learning and memory, among many other kinds, this statement is perfectly reasonable. As a comprehensive description of human decision-making, however, it omits a great deal. Experts in learning theory often nod to the existence of something beyond reflexes, Pavlovian conditioning, habits, and outcome-directed behavior, but their approach provides little prospect of accounting for traits such as mental trial and error, scenario construction, constructive episodic simulation, mental imagery, or inferential, logical, relational, metaphorical, and analogical reasoning, not to mention a theory of mind, self-awareness, and self-reflection. By excluding so much, learning theorists can claim to explain a lot—a lot of what they choose to study, that is—but doing so excludes the derived traits that characterize human cognition. We return to these topics in Chapters 9–11.

Diversity denial

Laboratory research has concentrated on very few species. If we are correct, then primates have representational systems that rodents (and other mammals) do not have. In much of the memory literature, however, differences among species are often denied, ignored, or dismissed as the consequence of motor or sensory factors. One of the consequences of such diversity denial is an excessive emphasis on behaviors that all animals can perform, such as the ubiquitous, if dreary, discrimination and matching tasks.

Surface similarities as "mechanisms"

Learning theorists describe the diverse forms of conditioning in a common terminology, with similar formalisms. The fact that some forms of Pavlovian learning depend on the cerebellum, whereas others rely on the amygdala or basal ganglia, demonstrates that they do not correspond to a single neural "mechanism" or "system," at least as these terms are used in neurophysiology. Although the centralized nervous systems of vertebrates and protostomes support Pavlovian learning, so do the neural nets of sea anemones and isolated insect ganglia. Instrumental conditioning, likewise, can occur in diverse kinds of nervous systems. In the epigraph of this chapter, we quoted Pavlov's warning to researchers against remaining "content with the surface of things." The terminology and formalisms used in the learning-theory literature probably reflect analogous neural computations, but they mask the diversity among animal species and obscure evolutionary innovations.

Proposal

For every chapter in Parts II–IV (Chapters 3–11) a proposal appears as a single italicized paragraph. This chapter is unusual in that its proposal comes near the end:

> *Reinforcement learning evolved, piecemeal, among several species of early animals, including the ancestors of vertebrates. Rather than corresponding to a learning "mechanism" that "explains" all animal behavior, reinforcement learning reflects the remnants of our most remote mnemonic ancestry. Subsequent evolutionary developments augmented these ancient mechanisms with innovative and specialized representational systems, each of which provided advantages to particular ancestral species.*

As we explained in Chapter 1 ("Evolution"), the term *paraphyletic* refers to species left over after removing a clade. Likewise, this chapter discusses what remains after removing more recently evolved representational systems, developments that we explore in Chapters 4–10.

References

1. Pavlov, I.P. (1936) *Nature* **137**, 572.
2. Erwin, D.H. and **Valentine, J.W.** (2013) *The Cambrian Explosion: The Construction of Animal Diversity* (Roberts, Greenwood Village, CO).
3. Begg, D.P. and **Woods, S.C.** (2013) *Nat. Rev. Endocrinol.* **9**, 584–597.
4. Woods, S.C. (1991) *Psychol. Rev.* **98**, 488–505.
5. Drazen, D.L., Vahl, T.P., D'Alessio, D.A., Seeley, R.J. et al. (2006) *Endocrinology* **147**, 23–30.
6. Bradley, M.M. (2009) *Psychophysiology* **46**, 1–11.
7. Holland, P.C. (1977) *J. Exp. Psychol. Anim. Behav. Process.* **3**, 77–104.
8. Hunt, P.S. and **Campbell, B.A.** (1997) *Behav. Neurosci.* **111**, 494–502.
9. Parkinson, J.A., Dalley, J.W., Cardinal, R.N., Bamford, A. et al. (2002) *Behav. Brain Res.* **137**, 149–163.
10. Flagel, S.B., Cameron, C.M., Pickup, K.N., Watson, S.J. et al. (2011) *Neuroscience* **196**, 80–96.
11. Braesicke, K., Parkinson, J.A., Reekie, Y., Man, M.S. et al. (2005) *Eur. J. Neurosci.* **21**, 1733–1740.
12. Vazdarjanova, A., Cahill, L., and **McGaugh, J.L.** (2001) *Eur. J. Neurosci.* **14**, 709–718.
13. Fendt, M. (2006) *J. Chem. Ecol.* **32**, 2617–2627.
14. Ferrero, D.M., Lemon, J.K., Fluegge, D., Pashkovski, S.L. *et al.* (2011) *Proc. Natl. Acad. Sci. USA* **108**, 11235–11240.
15. Bolles, R.C. (1970) *Psychol. Rev.* **71**, 32–48.
16. Fanselow, M.S. (1994) *Psychon. Bull. Rev.* **1**, 429–438.
17. LeDoux, J.E. (2013) *Trends Cogn. Sci.* **17**, 155–156.
18. Dunsmoor, J.E. and **Murphy, G.L.** (2015) *Trends Cogn. Sci.* **19**, 73–77.

19. Everitt, B.J., **Cardinal, R.N.**, Parkinson, J.A., and **Robbins**, T.W. (2003) *Ann. NY Acad. Sci.* **985**, 233–250.

20. Gross, C.T. and **Canteras, N.S.** (2012) *Nat. Rev. Neurosci.* **13**, 651–658.

21. Domjan, M. (2005) *Annu. Rev. Psychol.* **56**, 179–206.

22. Garcia, J., Lasiter, P.S., **Bermudez-Rattoni, F.**, and **Deems, D.A.** (1985) *Ann. NY Acad. Sci.* **443**, 8–21.

23. Mineka, S., Davidson, M., **Cook, M.**, and **Keir, R.** (1984) *J. Abnorm. Psychol.* **93**, 355–372.

24. Cook, M. and **Mineka, S.** (1989) *J. Abnorm. Psychol.* **98**, 448–459.

25. Mineka, S. and **Cook, M.** (1993) *J. Exp. Psychol. Gen.* **122**, 23–38.

26. Fichtel, C. (2012) In: *The Evolution of Primate Societies* (eds. Mitani, J.C., Call, J., Kappeler, P.M. et al.), pp. 169–194 (University of Chicago Press, Chicago, IL).

27. Nelson, E.E., Shelton, S.E., and **Kalin, N.H.** (2003) *Emotion* **3**, 3–11.

28. Sahley, C., Gelperin, A., and **Rudy, J.W.** (1981) *Proc. Natl. Acad. Sci. USA* **78**, 640–642.

29. Carew, T.J. and **Sahley, C.L.** (1986) *Annu. Rev. Neurosci.* **9**, 435–487.

30. Samarova, E.I. and **Balaban, P.M.** (2007) *Neurosci. Behav. Physiol.* **37**, 773–777.

31. Samarova, E.I. and **Balaban, P.M.** (2009) *Front. Cell. Neurosci.* **3**, 8.

32. Zhang, Y., Lu, H., and **Bargmann, C.I.** (2005) *Nature* **438**, 179–184.

33. Papini, M.R. (2008) *Comparative Psychology: Evolution and Development of Behavior* (Psychology Press, New York).

34. Holland, P.C. (1992) *Psychol. Anim. Learn. Motiv.* **28**, 69–125.

35. Macphail, E.M. (1982) *Brain and Intelligence in Vertebrates* (Clarendon Press, Oxford).

36. Haralson, J.V., Groff, C.I., and **Haralson, S.J.** (1975) *Physiol. Behav.* **15**, 455–460.

37. Pearce, J.M. (1997) *Animal Learning and Cognition: An Introduction* (Psychology Press, New York).

38. Johnson, A.W., Gallagher, M., and **Holland, P.C.** (2009) *J. Neurosci.* **29**, 696–704.

39. Malkova, L., Gaffan, D., and **Murray, E.A.** (1997) *J. Neurosci.* **17**, 6011–6020.

40. Izquierdo, A. and **Murray, E.A.** (2007) *J. Neurosci.* **27**, 1054–1062.

41. Wellman, L.L., Gale, K., and **Malkova, L.** (2005) *J. Neurosci.* **25**, 4577–4586.

42. Balleine, B.W. and **Killcross, S.** (2006) *Trends Neurosci.* **29**, 272–279.

43. Bouton, M.E. (2006) *Learning and Behavior: A Contemporary Synthesis* (Sinauer, Sunderland, MA).

44. Hall, J., Parkinson, J.A., **Connor, T.M.**, Dickinson, A. et al. (2001) *Eur. J. Neurosci.* **13**, 1984–1992.

45. Corbit, L.H., Muir, J.L., and **Balleine, B.W.** (2001) *J. Neurosci.* **21**, 3251–3260.

46. Corbit, L.H. and **Balleine, B.W.** (2011) *J. Neurosci.* **31**, 11786–11794.

47. Breland, K. and **Breland, M.** (1961) *Am. Psychol.* **16**, 681–684.

48. Boakes, R.A., Poli, M., **Lockwood, M.J.**, and **Goodall, G.** (1978) *J. Exp. Anal. Behav.* **29**, 115–134.

49. Hershberger, W.A. (1986) *Anim. Learn. Behav.* **14**, 443–451.

50. Malmgren, R.D., Stouffer, D.B., **Campanharo, A.S.**, and **Amaral, L.A.** (2009) *Science* **325**, 1696–1700.

51. Rangel, A., Camerer, C., and **Montague, P.R.** (2008) *Nat. Rev. Neurosci.* **9**, 545–556.

52. Sugrue, L.P., Corrado, G.S., and **Newsome, W.T.** (2005) *Nat. Rev. Neurosci.* **6**, 363–375.

53. Balleine, B.W. and **O'Doherty, J.P.** (2010) *Neuropsychopharmacol.* **35**, 48–69.

54. Dickenson, A. (1994) In: *Animal Learning and Cognition* (ed. Mackintosh, N.J.), pp. 45–79 (Academic Press, New York).

55. Dickenson, A. and **Balleine, B.W.** (1994) *Anim. Learn. Behav.* **22**, 1–18.

56. Daw, N.D., Niv, Y., and **Dayan, P.** (2005) *Nat. Neurosci.* **8**, 1704–1711.

57. Shenhav, A., Botvinick, M.M., and **Cohen, J.D.** (2013) *Neuron* **79**, 217–240.

58. **Herrnstein, R.J.** (1961) *J. Exp. Anal. Behav.* **4**, 267–272.

59. **Herrnstein, R.J.** (1974) *J. Exp. Anal. Behav.* **21**, 159–164.

60. **Sakai, Y.** and **Fukai, T.** (2008) *PLoS One* **3**, e3795.

61. **Daw, N.D.**, O'Doherty, J.P., Dayan, P., **Seymour, B.** et al. (2006) *Nature* **441**, 876–879.

62. **Dayan, P.** (2012) *Curr. Opin. Neurobiol.* **22**, 1068–1074.

63. **Frank, M.J.**, Doll, B.B., Oas-Terpstra, J., and **Moreno, F.** (2009) *Nat. Neurosci.* **12**, 1062–1068.

64. **Lau, B.** and **Glimcher, P.W.** (2005) *J. Exp. Anal. Behav.* **84**, 555–579.

65. **Rutledge, R.B.**, Lazzaro, S.C., Lau, B., **Myers, C.E.** et al. (2009) *J. Neurosci.* **29**, 15104–15114.

66. **Holland, P.C.** and **Maddux, J.-M.** (2010) In: *Attention and Learning* (eds. Mitchell, C.J. and LePelley, M.E.), pp. 305–349 (Oxford University Press, Oxford).

67. **Levy, D.J.** and **Glimcher, P.W.** (2012) *Curr. Opin. Neurobiol.* **22**, 1027–1038.

68. **Rozin, P.** and **Kalat, J.W.** (1971) *Psychol. Rev.* **78**, 459–486.

69. **Bateson, P.P.** (1969) *Adv. Sci.* **25**, 279–288.

70. **Desimone, R.** and **Duncan, J.** (1995) *Annu. Rev. Neurosci.* **18**, 193–222.

71. **Carew, T.J.**, Walters, E.T., and **Kandel, E.R.** (1981) *Science* **211**, 501–504.

72. **Brembs, B.** and **Heisenberg, M.** (2000) *Learn. Mem.* **7**, 104–115.

73. **Brembs, B.**, Lorenzetti, F.D., Reyes, F.D., **Baxter, D.A.** et al. (2002) *Science* **296**, 1706–1709.

74. **Nargeot, R.**, Baxter, D.A., and **Byrne, J.H.** (1997) *J. Neurosci.* **17**, 8093–8105.

75. **Nargeot, R.**, Baxter, D.A., and **Byrne, J.H.** (1999) *J. Neurosci.* **19**, 2261–2272.

76. **Nargeot, R.**, Baxter, D.A., Patterson, G.W., and **Byrne, J.H.** (1999) *J. Neurophysiol.* **81**, 1983–1987.

77. **Lukowiak, K.**, Ringseis, E., Spencer, G., **Wildering, W.** et al. (1996) *J. Exp. Biol.* **199**, 683–691.

78. **Abramson, C.I.** and **Feinman, R.D.** (1990) *Physiol. Behav.* **48**, 267–272.

79. **Putz, G.** and **Heisenberg, M.** (2002) *Learn. Mem.* **9**, 349–359.

80. **Hershkowitz, M.** and **Samuel, D.** (1973) *Anim. Behav.* **21**, 83–85.

81. **Schmajuk, N.A.**, Segura, E.T., and **Reboreda, J.C.** (1980) *Behav. Neur. Biol.* **28**, 392–397.

82. **Van Sommers, P.** (1962) *Science* **137**, 678–679.

83. **Scobie, S.R.** and **Fallon, D.** (1974) *J. Comp. Physiol. Psychol.* **86**, 858–866.

84. **Mandriota, F.J.**, Thompson, R.L., and **Bennett, M.V.** (1968) *Anim. Behav.* **16**, 448–455.

85. **Behrend, E.R.** and **Bitterman, M.E.** (1963) *J. Exp. Anal. Behav.* **6**, 47–52.

86. **Rudolph, R.L.** and **Van, H.R.** (1977) *J. Exp. Anal. Behav.* **27**, 327–330.

87. **Rawlins, J.N.**, Feldon, J., and **Gray, J.A.** (1980) *Exp. Brain Res.* **38**, 273–283.

88. **Franchina, J.J.** and **Brown, T.S.** (1971) *J. Comp. Physiol. Psychol.* **76**, 365–370.

89. **Jarrard, L.E.**, Feldon, J., Rawlins, J.N., **Sinden, J.D.** et al. (1986) *Exp. Brain. Res.* **61**, 519–530.

90. **Henke, P.G.** (1974) *J. Comp. Physiol. Psychol.* **86**, 760–767.

91. **Schultz, W.** (2006) *Annu. Rev. Psychol.* **57**, 87–115.

92. **Schultz, W.** (2007) *Annu. Rev. Neurosci.* **30**, 259–288.

93. **Steinmetz, J.E.** (2000) *Behav. Brain Res.* **110**, 13–24.

94. **Suri, R.E.** and **Schultz, W.** (2001) *Neur. Comput.* **13**, 841–862.

95. **Sutton, R.S.** and **Barto, A.G.** (1998) *Reinforcement Learning* (MIT Press, Cambridge, MA).

96. **O'Doherty, J.P.**, Dayan, P., Friston, K., **Critchley, H.** et al. (2003) *Neuron* **38**, 329–337.

97. **Fiorillo, C.D.**, Tobler, P.N., and **Schultz, W.** (2003) *Science* **299**, 1898–1902.

98. **Kim, J.J.**, Krupa, D.J., and **Thompson, R.F.** (1998) *Science* **279**, 570–573.

99. **Medina, J.F.**, Nores, W.L., and **Mauk, M.D.** (2002) *Nature* **416**, 330–333.

100. Seo, H. and Lee, D. (2009) *J. Neurosci.* **29**, 3627–3641.

101. Roesch, M.R., Calu, D.J., Esber, G.R., and Schoenbaum, G. (2010) *J. Neurophysiol.* **104**, 587–595.

102. Roesch, M.R., Esber, G.R., Li, J., Daw, N.D. et al. (2012) *Eur. J. Neurosci.* **35**, 1190–1200.

103. Chen, J., Cook, P.A., and Wagner, A.D. (2015) *J. Neurophysiol.* **114**, 1227–1238.

104. Kim, G., Lewis-Peacock, J.A., Norman, K.A., and Turk-Browne, N.B. (2014) *Proc. Natl. Acad. Sci. USA* **111**, 8997–9002.

105. Henson, R.N. and Gagnepain, P. (2010) *Hippocampus* **20**, 1315–1326.

106. Rescorla, R.A. and Wagner, A.R. (1972) In: *Classical Conditioning: Current Research and Theory* (eds. Black, A.H. and Prokasy, W.F.), pp. 64–99 (Appleton-Century-Crofts, New York).

107. Pearce, J.M. and Hall, G. (1980) *Psychol. Rev.* **87**, 532–552.

108. Tobler, P.N., Dickinson, A., and Schultz, W. (2003) *J. Neurosci.* **23**, 10402–10410.

109. Schultz, W. and Dickinson, A. (2000) *Annu. Rev. Neurosci.* **23**, 473–500.

110. Holland, P.C. and Gallagher, M. (1993) *Behav. Neurosci.* **107**, 235–245.

111. Holland, P.C. and Gallagher, M. (1993) *Behav. Neurosci.* **107**, 246–253.

112. Holland, P.C. and Kenmuir, C. (2005) *J. Exp. Psychol. Anim. Behav. Process.* **31**, 155–171.

113. Calu, D.J., Roesch, M.R., Haney, R.Z., Holland, P.C. et al. (2010) *Neuron* **68**, 991–1001.

114. Chiba, A.A., Bucci, D.J., Holland, P.C., and Gallagher, M. (1995) *J. Neurosci.* **15**, 7315–7322.

115. Holland, P.C. and Gallagher, M. (2006) *J. Neurosci.* **26**, 3791–3797.

116. Bucci, D.J., Holland, P.C., and Gallagher, M. (1998) *J. Neurosci.* **18**, 8038–8046.

117. Lee, H.J., Youn, J.M., O, M.J., Gallagher, M. et al. (2006) *J. Neurosci.* **26**, 6077–6081.

118. Lee, H.J., Youn, J.M., Gallagher, M., and Holland, P.C. (2008) *Eur. J. Neurosci.* **27**, 3043–3049.

119. Chang, S.E., McDannald, M.A., Wheeler, D.S., and Holland, P.C. (2012) *Behav. Neurosci.* **126**, 279–289.

120. Mazzoni, P., Hristova, A., and Krakauer, J.W. (2007) *J. Neurosci.* **27**, 7105–7116.

121. Desmurget, M. and Turner, R.S. (2008) *J. Neurophysiol.* **99**, 1057–1076.

122. Abramson, I., Giray, T., Mixson, T.A., Nolf, S.L. et al. (2009) *J. Insect Sci.* **10**, 1–17.

123. Hussaini, S.A., Komischke, B., Menzel, R., and Lachnit, H. (2007) *Learn. Mem.* **14**, 678–683.

124. Northcutt, R.G. (1996) *Brain Behav. Evol.* **48**, 237–247.

125. Smeets, W.J.A.J., Marín, O., and González, A. (2000) *J. Anat.* **196**, 501–517.

126. Thompson, R.H., Menard, A., Pombal, M., and Grillner, S. (2008) *Eur. J. Neurosci.* **27**, 1452–1460.

127. Bunge, M. (2003) *Philosophical Dictionary* (Prometheus, New York).

128. Kamin, L.J. (1969) In: *Punishment and Aversive Behavior* (eds. Campbell, B.A. and Church, R.M.), pp. 279–296 (Appleton-Century-Crofts, New York).

129. Waelti, P., Dickinson, A., and Schultz, W. (2001) *Nature* **412**, 43–48.

130. Horridge, G.A. (1962) *Nature* **193**, 697–698.

131. Horridge, G.A. (1962) *Proc. R. Soc. Lond. B: Biol. Sci.* **157**, 33–52.

132. Eisenstein, E.M. and Carlson, A.D. (1994) *Physiol. Behav.* **56**, 687–691.

133. Eisenstein, E.M., Carlson, A.D., and Harris, J.T. (1997) *Integr. Physiol. Behav. Sci.* **32**, 265–271.

Chapter 4

The navigation memory system of early vertebrates

Overview

The navigation system evolved in early vertebrates, along with the telencephalon, as an adaptation for mobile foraging—guided primarily by vision and olfaction. Throughout vertebrate history, part of the telencephalon—the hippocampus homologue—has stored memories collectively called a "cognitive map": neural representations of foraging fields and protected places, including objects, odors, and locations, as well as the sequences in which they are encountered during a journey. Cognitive maps allowed early vertebrates to navigate to places outside their immediate sensory range and to use novel routes to reach their goals. At first, the navigation memory system stored the specialized representations needed for foraging excursions and for finding safe haven, and the hippocampal complex of rodents, monkeys, and humans continues to perform these conserved functions. Once it evolved, its representations adapted to support a wide range of derived functions.

Mappa mundi

> There are several … sources of enjoyment in a long voyage …. The map of the world ceases to be a blank; it becomes a picture full of the most varied and animated figures.
>
> Charles Darwin[1] (*Voyage of the Beagle*, p. 555)

What the voyage of the *Beagle* did for Darwin, their foraging journeys did for early vertebrates. They populated a map of the world.

The life of early vertebrates is not, we realize, a topic that one typically finds in the memory literature. To be sure, some experts have embraced the idea that specialized aspects of learning and memory have evolved in different species[2,3], and mainstream memory researchers have considered evolution from time to time[4-6]. But the predominant theories of memory make little use of these ideas. Why would they if memories result solely from reinforcement learning mechanisms that all animals share?

One reason is that stem vertebrates developed some "unnecessary" complexities in response to the selective pressures of their time and place. Among these violations of parsimony, our ancient ancestors developed a neural apparatus that represented maps of their world[7,8].

To suit our overall scheme, we have invented a new name for these specialized representations: the navigation memory system. There is danger in this name, of course. Some readers might take it to imply that this neural system functions exclusively in either navigation or memory, but we do not intend anything of the sort. To say, for example, that Darwin devised a theory of evolution does not imply that he never did anything else. Likewise, to say that a representational system functions in navigation memory does not imply that it never does anything else. Our label emphasizes ancestral selective pressures, not comprehensive functions.

Evolution

Stem vertebrates emerged as mobile predators that used energetic swimming movements to obtain nutrients and avoid harm (see Chapter 2, "Early vertebrates"). Among their derived traits was the telencephalon, which included a structure called the medial pallium. In Chapter 2 we explained that the medial pallium is homologous with both the medial cortex of amniotes and the hippocampus of mammals (see Figs. 2.6 and 2.7). Unlike the lateral pallium and its characteristic olfactory inputs, no single sensory system dominates the inputs of the medial pallium, although projections from olfactory and visual areas of the pallium, as well as from the hypothalamus, probably played an important role from the start.

We could devote this chapter to experiments on fishes[9,10], birds[4,11–13], and other non-mammalian species. In Chapter 2 ("Homologies"), for example, we cited evidence that the medial cortex guides navigation in lizards[14] and turtles[15] (see Fig. 2.7C). In Fig. 4.1(A), all of the lineages with a black square to the right have at least one species in which a lesion of the hippocampus or its homologue impairs navigation. Figure 4.1(B, C) illustrates the effect that lesions of the hippocampus homologue caused in goldfish, which we revisit later (see "Conclusions"). Navigational functions could, in principle, have arisen in the hippocampus homologue convergently[16], but at first glance Fig. 4.1(A) suggests that it performs a conserved navigational function. Like other conserved traits, some lineages can lose them. In cetaceans, the hippocampus has regressed dramatically[17], presumably because other brain mechanisms have superseded its functions.

Notwithstanding comparative data from goldfish, turtles, lizards, and birds, the fact remains that most knowledge about hippocampus homologues comes from studies of mammals. As a conceptual matter, our proposal situates the navigation memory system in a distant vertebrate ancestor. As a practical matter, however, the remainder of this chapter focuses on species that emerged long afterwards. In essence, we highlight some selected results from rodents, monkeys, and humans to place the hippocampus in an evolutionary framework. Accordingly, this chapter concentrates on conserved functions, and we defer to later chapters—especially Chapters 7, 10, and 11—a consideration of derived traits, some of which depend on cortical areas that emerged at various times during primate evolution.

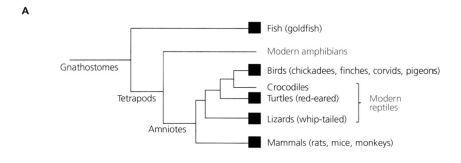

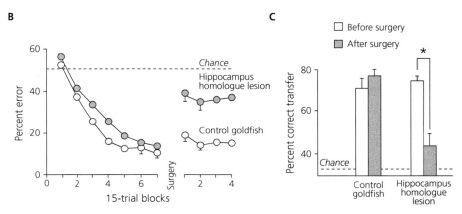

Fig. 4.1 Navigation in vertebrates. (A) Cladogram of gnathostomes, showing the lineages in which lesions of the hippocampus or its homologues cause impairments in navigation (squares). In the format of Fig. 3.1. (B) Maze learning in goldfish before and after lesions of the hippocampus homologue. Error bars: standard error. (C) Transfer test consisting of a novel starting location. (B, C) Redrawn and adapted from Rodríguez F, López JC, Vargas JP, Gómez Y, Broglio C, Salas C. Conservation of spatial memory function in the pallial forebrain of reptiles and ray-finned fishes. *Journal of Neuroscience* 22:2894–903, © 2002, Society for Neuroscience.

Proposal

The navigation memory system evolved de novo in early vertebrates, and from the start it housed specialized representations for mobile foraging and active defense. At first, these map-like representations depended on a homologue of the hippocampus called the medial pallium. Although it developed in response to selective pressures involving navigation, the hippocampus homologue came to perform additional functions that depend on its specialized representations. These functions support choices based on order, recency, scenes, sequences, and contexts, as well as both spatial and temporal relations among stimuli.

Navigation memory in rodents

Although many memory researchers take for granted the idea that our brains create a representation of the world, this has not always been the case. To explain why, we begin this section with a brief history of research on the concept of cognitive maps.

The cognitive map through history

Throughout most of the twentieth century, behaviorism dominated psychology[18], especially in the United States. According to this philosophy, stimulus–response learning accounts for behavior, and influential figures such as Hull, Thorndike, and Skinner showed that it could indeed explain a lot of what animals do.

A challenge to behaviorism came from psychologists who surmised that animals did not always learn in the simplest possible way[19]. Tolman[7,20], for example, wrote extensively on the shortcomings of one set of "laws" governing all learning and memory. This debate continued through the middle part of the twentieth century. In the 1940s, it seemed to come down to a question about navigation. Did navigation rely on learned responses to stimuli or on cognitive maps? The response-learning theory, championed by the behaviorists, held that animals navigate by making a series of learned responses to sensory stimuli.

Although behaviorists dominated psychology in the mid-twentieth century, the alternatives did not disappear entirely. The cognitive map theory held that animals learn spatial layouts in addition to responses. Tolman[7] recounted an experiment performed by one of his students[21], which he took to demonstrate a map-like memory in rats. The key observation involved the ability of rats to generate novel paths to a spatial goal. These experiments began with rats being trained in an apparatus something like a modern T-maze (Fig. 4.2A). From their starting point (numeral 1 in Fig. 4.2A), the rats could see the maze along with various objects and landmarks in the room, such as lights, doors, tables, fans, and wall hangings, collectively called extramaze, distal, or distant cues. In the training phase of the experiment, the rats learned to turn toward one side of the maze to find food. In the testing phase, the rats were placed at the opposite side of the room (numeral 2 in Fig. 4.2B), and the straight path from their starting point only extended for a short distance, unlike in the original training phase (Fig. 4.2A). In Fig. 4.2(B) we use black rectangles to illustrate the available runways. Most of the rats chose paths that led them into the side of the room that had contained food during their original training (Fig. 4.2C, D), although this choice required them to turn in a different direction relative to their own bodies. According to Tolman, rats remember locations in a map-like manner and navigate on the basis of these memories.

In a modern version of these experiments, two groups of rats—a "response" group and a place group—learned to run through a plus-maze (Fig. 4.3A, B). The arm opposite the rat's starting location was blocked, which effectively converted a plus-maze into a T-maze. Rats in the place group acquired food if they ran into a particular arm of the maze, regardless of their starting point; rats in the "response" group got food by making a particular turn at the junction: left or right. Most rats found it easier to learn about places than responses, which is the tendency that Tolman took as evidence for his cognitive map theory.

Research in animal navigation made a dramatic advance with the discovery of place cells in the rat hippocampus[22]. The existence of cells encoding places seemed, at first, to vindicate Tolman's ideas about cognitive maps. In the original description, place cells

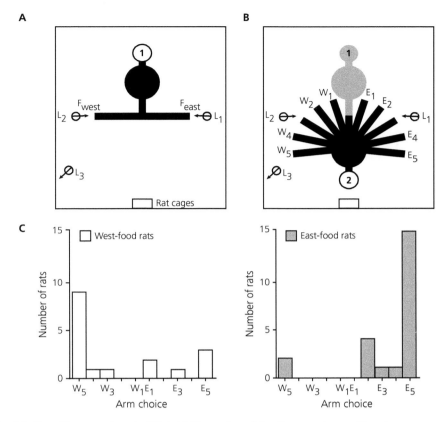

Fig. 4.2 Cognitive maps in rats. (A) A 1940s version of the T-maze, along with extramaze cues. Half of the rats found food in the west side of the room (F_{west}), the other half found it in the east side (F_{east}). During training, rats began at location 1, ran across a circular table, scampered through a chute, and then chose one of the two arms of a maze, east or west. L_1–L_3 show the locations of three lamps and the directions in which they pointed (arrows). (B) During testing, rats began at a different place in the same room, location 2, and they encountered a different maze. The gray shading shows where the now-absent origin location (1), table, and chute had been during the training trials. (C) Left: West-food rats predominantly chose arms to the west (W_1–W_5). Right: East-food rats predominantly chose arms to the east (E_1–E_5). Only a few rats turned in the same direction, relative to their bodies, as in the original training. Adapted from Tolman EC. Cognitive maps in rats and men. *Psychological Review* 55:189–208, © 1948, American Psychological Association.

appeared to signal that a rat occupied a particular location, regardless of the animal's orientation or how it got there. That is, place cells seemed to encode places independent of "responses" or actions: a map-like property. Later studies showed that many (although not all) place cells changed the way they signaled location depending on an animal's actions (or lack thereof)[23]. Place cells have also been shown to encode stimuli, such as objects and odors, in addition to locations. However, at the time of their discovery the apparent independence of place cells from stimuli and "responses" seemed to support the

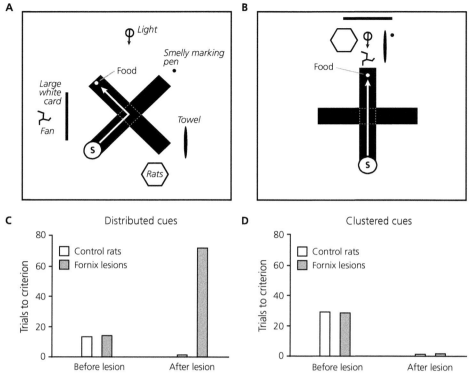

Fig. 4.3 Effect of fornix lesions on navigation using clustered or distributed extramaze cues. (A) In the distributed-cue condition, extramaze cues included an odorous marking pen and two fellow rats, at various places, but none especially near the food (small white circle). The arrow indicates the orientation of a lamp. S marks the starting location. (B) In the clustered-cue condition, all extramaze cues, including the rat cage (hexagon), were located near the food. (C) Trials-to-criterion and the effect of fornix lesions on navigation based on distributed cues. (D) Trials-to-criterion and the effect of fornix lesions on navigation based on clustered cues. From O'Keefe J, Conway DH. On the trail of the hippocampal engram. *Physiological Psychology* 8:229–38, © 1980, with permission of Springer.

cognitive map theory. In a landmark synthesis, O'Keefe and Nadel[8] linked the existence of place cells with evidence that the hippocampus plays an important role in navigation. The hippocampus, they proposed, subserves Tolman's cognitive maps.

An early experiment provided some insight into how rats use these maps. Initially, rats received various types of training on a plus maze[24]. As in Tolman's work, the subjects used extramaze cues for orientation. In this case, however, the investigators manipulated the locations of these cues. In the *distributed condition*, cues were scattered around the outside of the maze (Fig. 4.3A); in the *clustered condition*, all the cues were placed near the arm of the maze containing food (Fig. 4.3B). In both conditions, the rats began at different starting points from trial to trial, and the food-bearing arm remained constant. After the rats had mastered this task, the fornix was lesioned in half of the animals in each group. Two main findings emerged from these procedures. First, intact rats found it easier to learn with distributed cues compared with cues that clustered near the goal. Figure 4.3(C, D) illustrates this finding by the height of the before-lesion bars: The more trials rats took to reach a performance criterion, in this case 90% correct choices, the harder it was for them to perform the task. Second, fornix lesions impaired the performance of rats that relied on distributed cues (Fig. 4.3C) but not those that used clustered cues (Fig. 4.3D). This result showed that when the rats relied on distributed cues, as they do in natural foraging, fornix lesions disrupted their performance. When all the extramaze cues clustered near the food, something that rarely (if ever) occurs in their natural habitat, the rats navigated in some other, fornix-independent way.

These results—and especially the effect of fornix lesions (Fig. 4.3C)—provided support for the idea that the hippocampus plays a conserved navigational function in rats, a conclusion that gained additional weight from studies using the radial-arm maze[25-30]. The cognitive map theory of hippocampal function holds that navigation relies on the specialized representations of stimuli that are encountered at various times and places along a journey to a goal. Results from the distributed-cue condition, which stressed this form of navigation, supported this idea.

As the history of this field unfolded, researchers extended the cognitive map theory from foraging to harm avoidance. In the Morris water maze, for example, rats needed to swim to a submerged, invisible platform in a circular pool of opaque water. Over repeated trials they learned the location of this platform, and lesions of the hippocampus caused a severe impairment on this task[31].

Considering experiments of the 1940s to the 1980s together, the purely behavioral work—as exemplified by Fig. 4.2 and the before-lesion data in Fig. 4.3—strengthened the idea that rats navigate according to cognitive maps. According to this theory, such maps allow animals to navigate to places outside their immediate sensory world without having to rely exclusively on reinforced responses to stimuli. The after-lesion data in Fig. 4.3(C) supported the idea that the hippocampus subserves cognitive maps[8].

These results did not convince all experts, however. According to one school of animal behavior, animals navigate solely according to a combination of stimulus–response, stimulus–stimulus, and stimulus–outcome memories[32,33]. In one formulation, the basal ganglia, hippocampus, and amygdala, respectively, specialize in these three kinds of associations[34]. From this perspective, what seems like evidence for cognitive maps merely reflects conditioned place–outcome memories combined with some stimulus–stimulus complexities.

The impasse

Thus, by the mid-1980s, the field had arrived at a familiar impasse between animal learning theory and cognitive psychology. There are no empirical observations that convincingly rule out either perspective. An account of Tolman's results in terms of place–outcome associations and conditioned place preferences seems unlikely to explain an entire, novel journey to a distant, unseen goal, but chains of stimulus–stimulus associations and the concept of secondary reinforcement can probably be stretched to cover anything.

In lieu of a dispositive empirical result, the main arguments on one side or the other rely on vague notions of parsimony, which in many instances reflect little more than personal or cultural preferences. What some researchers find elegant seems simplistic to others; and what some find rich and rewarding others find unnecessarily complicated. As Tolman[20] (p. 155) put it:

> Why do I want … to complicate things; why do I not want one simple set of laws for all learning? I do not know.… No doubt, any good … [psychiatrist] would be able to trace this back to some sort of nasty traumatic experience in my early childhood.

Modern neuroscience has, for the most part, bypassed the impasse between these two schools of psychology. Radical behaviorism has faded away, and its successor, animal learning theory, often accepts some cognitive variables that intervene between stimuli and responses (Box 4.1). Nevertheless, considerable tension remains between these two theoretical approaches, and this comes to the fore when considering neural representations. For learning theorists, plasticity within associative networks "explains" all (or nearly all) behavior, without any need to invoke map-like representations of locations, objects, or the sequences in which they should be encountered during a journey. In cognitive map theory, the hippocampus (including its homologues in other vertebrates) specializes in exactly these kinds of representations.

There are several ways to resolve this impasse, such as assigning the two competing theories to different brain structures or different computational architectures. Our proposals complement this approach. In Chapter 3 we discussed the advantages that animals gain from reinforcement learning systems; in this chapter, we propose that additional

---

Box 4.1 Model-based reinforcement learning

Model-based reinforcement learning contrasts with model-free learning. The latter depends on stimulus–response–outcome associations based on specific experience. In the former, a representational model is independent of the specific experiences that led to its establishment and the tasks performed during learning. Maze learning serves as the classic example. While learning to navigate through a maze, an animal can acquire a neural representation of the overall structure of the maze: a cognitive map. These models might have been formed while foraging for food, but the animal can later use them to find safe haven, for example. A previously learned sequence of stimulus–response associations or motor commands used while finding food does not necessarily help an animal escape danger, but a memorized model of a foraging field might do so, in the right circumstances. There is a cost, however: an increase in complexity, both of the problem to be solved and of the mechanisms for doing so. Furthermore, when these representations are inaccurate, as must be the case early in learning, their use can impair performance relative to model-free reinforcement learning.

advantages come from having a navigation system. The behavior of vertebrates depends on both for a simple reason: The navigation system evolved after, and augmented, the reinforcement systems. The navigation system and its cognitive maps evolved in early vertebrates because they provided an adaptive advantage over the ancestral condition. Because their prevertebrate ancestors were successful—in their own time—early vertebrates did not "need" cognitive maps, and their existence violates strict parsimony, as the behaviorists of old noticed. The reason for such complexity is that the brain evolved to enhance fitness, not to produce parsimony (see Chapter 1, "Why make it so complicated?").

More recent developments

Research since the mid-1980s has produced many important advances in understanding the neural basis of navigation. Grid cells, boundary cells, and head-direction cells in the medial entorhinal cortex strongly influence hippocampal place cells. It now seems unlikely that place-cell activity depends primarily on sensory inputs that convey constellations of distant cues, as experts once believed. Instead, it appears that distant cues influence the activity of grid cells, boundary cells, and head-direction cells, which in turn affect place-cell activity[35]. In this way, the hippocampus and closely connected regions construct a set of cognitive maps specific to a variety of contexts. These maps contribute to monitoring an animal's progress through a foraging field (grid cells), its current location (place cells), its orientation (head-direction cells), and its location relative to goals.

Although the studies mentioned so far have emphasized distant (extramaze) cues, as opposed to local (intramaze) ones, this bias likely results from the nature of commonly used tasks rather than a fundamental principle. Tasks such as the Morris water maze make it difficult to manipulate local cues. Its circular pool typically lacks identifying landmarks and therefore rats are forced to rely on extramaze cues. When experiments have examined navigation by local cues, such as the subject's distance from the walls of a maze, they revealed that this information also contributes to navigation. Furthermore, when rats could use local features, such as the geometry of a foraging field, they have tended to do so preferentially[36,37]. That said, some neural mechanisms depend on distant cues, such as those that produce head-direction cells[38]. Accordingly, a combination of distant and local cues appears to guide navigation, depending on contexts and task demands.

In addition to distant and local cues, other factors also influence hippocampal function. Early on, O'Keefe[39] emphasized active movement as a major input to place cells, and later research has elaborated this idea. As discussed earlier, for example, whether a rat actively or passively arrives at a location affects place-cell activity[23]. In addition, a rat's upcoming or previous turns within a maze also affect place-cell activity[40,41], indicating the influence of an entire journey as opposed to merely a current location.

One experiment on journey effects[42] involved rats running from varying starting points to a fixed food location for a block of successive trials. The location of the food was then changed for a subsequent block of trials. Figure 4.4(A) shows that good task performance depended on the integrity of the fornix. As shown in Fig. 4.4(B), taken from intact rats, neurons in the hippocampus encoded information about a journey. Specifically, these

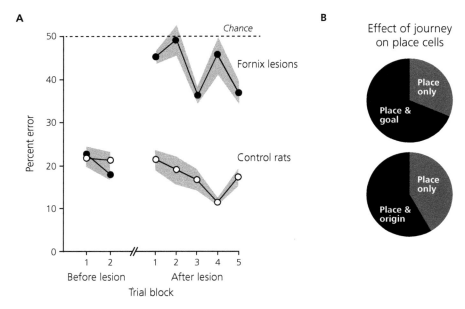

Fig. 4.4 Effect of the journey. (A) Fornix lesions (black circles) caused impairments on a task like the one illustrated in Fig. 4.3(A). In this experiment, the goal location changed from block to block during testing and the starting location varied from trial to trial. Blocks consisted of ten trials, and two groups of rats learned to a criterion of 90% correct choices. One group of rats (black circles) received complete lesions of the fornix; the other group (white circles) underwent sham surgeries. Gray shading indicates the standard error. (B) Pie charts showing the effect of an entire foraging journey on place-cell activity, based on separate analyses. Top, effect of goal location; bottom, effect of origin location. Some neurons in the hippocampus (gray) encoded a rat's location independent of the origin or goal on a given trial, but the origin or goal affected the activity of most place cells (black). From Ferbinteanu J, Shapiro ML. Prospective and retrospective memory coding in the hippocampus. *Neuron* 40:1227–39, © 2003, with permission from Elsevier.

cells showed an influence of the starting and ending locations of individual trials. Thus, in addition to encoding places per se, neurons in the hippocampus differentiate places based on the different origins and goals of a journey[43,44].

Nonspatial representations: terminology and physiology

Up to this point we have emphasized navigation through space. But it has long been recognized that cognitive maps also incorporate objects and odors encountered along a journey. The term "nonspatial" has been applied to features of objects other than their location. In a sense, this term is unfortunate because it is common to include, as "nonspatial," features that depend on spatial analysis but do not indicate locations, such as the size and shape of objects. Nevertheless, because it is so common in the literature, we use the term nonspatial in this way. Likewise, we use the word "scene" for a set of stimulus items and its background. A visual scene, therefore, consists of a set of nonspatial visual stimuli, such as objects or other object-like stimuli, at a set of places within an environment. In the context of vertebrate navigation, this concept needs to be generalized to include olfactory stimuli, along with additional sensory modalities such as electroreception, audition, infrared signals, and somatic sensation, as appropriate to a given species.

Physiological investigations of the hippocampus show that a variety of nonspatial features influence place-cell activity. For example, neurons in the hippocampus, termed landmark-vector cells, have been found to signal spatial location as a vector with its origin at the site of an object[45]. In other experiments, hippocampal neurons encoded locations where an object had appeared in the past, indicating a memory for object–place conjunctions. Knierim and Hamilton[35] review this literature in detail, so we simply note that, contrary to some early conclusions, local nonspatial cues exert a strong influence on place-cell activity. These findings agree with the cognitive map theory insofar as they indicate that the hippocampus houses specialized representations for conjunctions of objects and places that a vertebrate would encounter during a navigational journey.

Virtual reality environments can be used to disentangle the influence of visual and internal inputs that provide navigational information[46]. In these experiments, mice ran on the top of a rotating but otherwise stationary ball as visual stimuli streamed past them, mimicking what occurs as the animals move through space. Visual stimuli could be included or excluded at will. As usual, many hippocampal cells had place fields, as defined in a mouse's initial "excursion" on the ball, and most of these neurons received both visual and internal signals. Roughly half of these cells maintained their place fields in the absence of visual cues, which shows that some combination of proprioceptive and motor-command signals suffice to encode the animal's location. (Later, in Chapter 6, "End effector vector," we discuss an analogous mechanism for the alignment of proprioceptive and visual information underlying reaching movements in primates.)

These findings add weight to the idea that the hippocampus constructs map-like representations[8], including scenes and layouts, from inputs that are nonspatial in the broad sense explained earlier. According to our proposal, representations in the hippocampus reflect a navigational function conserved from early vertebrates, but the original versions of these representations also served as exaptations for derived functions. In humans, these innovations include scene recognition (see Chapter 7, "Humans"), scenario construction (see Chapter 10, "Constructive episodic simulations"), and other emergent traits that developed later (see Chapter 11, "Proposal"), once the hippocampus began to interact with new representational systems (see Chapter 10, "Medial network").

Nonspatial representations: lesion effects

The concept of a cognitive map includes the idea that a foraging vertebrate will encounter a series (or sequence) of vision–place and odor–place conjunctions during a journey. Experiments on rats have demonstrated that hippocampus lesions disrupt the memory of odor or object sequences[47-51]. These findings, and the others related in this section, show how specialized representations that support navigation can be adapted to other kinds of behavior.

In the odor experiments, rats dug into sand-filled cups to obtain a piece of food at the bottom, and the sand in each cup exuded a different odor[47]. After the rats had experienced a sequence of five odors, two scents were selected from the sequence and the rats faced a choice between them (Fig. 4.5A). In this test, the rats could obtain food by choosing the scent that had appeared earlier in the sequence. In a comparison task, rats could obtain food by choosing a novel odor over an odor that had been included in the sequence. As illustrated in Fig. 4.5(B), hippocampus lesions impaired choices based on the sequence of odors but not choices based on odor novelty. These results show that the hippocampus contributes to memories about the order of stimuli, which represent a series of the sort that a vertebrate might encounter during a journey.

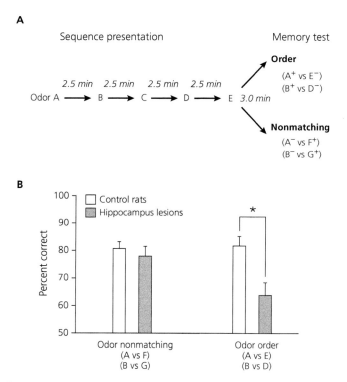

Fig. 4.5 The effect of hippocampus lesions on an odor sequence task. (A) Rats explored scented sand-filled cups to find food, and five distinct odors appeared in a fixed order, several times. After a 3-minute delay period, the rats faced one of two memory tests. In one test (order), they could get food by choosing the scent they had experienced earlier in the sequence (denoted as A+ and B+). In the other test, a nonmatching task, they could get food by choosing an odor (F+ and G+) that differed from all of the samples included in the sequence. (B) Hippocampus lesions affected performance on the order task, but not the nonmatching task. The asterisk (*) indicates a significant effect of the lesion. Reprinted from Fortin NJ, Agster KL, Eichenbaum HB. Critical role of the hippocampus in memory for sequences of events. *Nature Neuroscience* 5:458–62, © 2002 with permission from Macmillan Publishers, Ltd.

A related experiment tested the ability of rats to distinguish two sequences of odors from each other[52]. These rats explored scented cups in two different sequences, labeled A and B (Fig. 4.6A). Sequence-specific odors occurred in positions 1, 2, 5, and 6; common odors appeared in positions 3 and 4. Sequence A thus consisted of items 1A, 2A, 3, 4, 5A, and 6A; sequence B comprised items 1B, 2B, 3, 4, 5B, and 6B. After the rats had learned these two sequences, they were tested on their ability to disambiguate the sequences. To begin the test, the rats were restricted to digging in the first two odor cups of a given sequence (A or B) by lids over the cups belonging to the other sequence. Accordingly, the rats sampled items 1B and 2B, for example, then items 3 and 4. The ability of the rats to uniquely represent

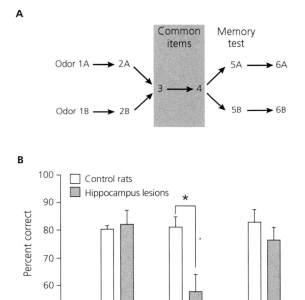

Fig. 4.6 Effect of hippocampus lesions on an odor-sequence task. (A) Rats learned two sequences of odors by exploring cups filled with scented sand. They experienced many repetitions of two different sequences of six odors, sequence A and sequence B, which had common elements for their third and fourth items. The probe test involved choosing between odor 5A and odor 5B after having started with the first four odors from either sequence A or B. In a comparison test, the rats were forced to choose the correct, within-sequence odors for positions 1–5 and they then faced a choice for the odor at position 6. (B) Rats with hippocampus lesions performed poorly on the probe test for position 5, which required them to remember the sequence. In the comparison test, however, they could choose the odor in position 6 correctly after having just smelled the item in position 5, which required only an associative memory linking the odors in positions 5 and 6. The asterisk indicates a significant effect of the lesion. Republished from Agster KL, Fortin NJ, Eichenbaum H. The hippocampus and disambiguation of overlapping sequences. *Journal of Neuroscience* 22:5760–68, © 2002, Society for Neuroscience, with permission.

each sequence was then assessed by measuring the frequency of correct choices on item 5. So upon reaching the fifth item in the sequence that begins with item 1B, the rats were required to choose item 5B, not item 5A. Figure 4.6(B) shows that control rats usually chose correctly, but rats with hippocampus lesions performed near chance levels. These findings reflect another property of the hippocampus homologue that we assume to be conserved from ancestral vertebrates, namely, specialized representations of alternative journeys, each characterized by a unique sequence of odor–place or object–place conjunctions.

Sequence memories might be mediated, in part, by the activity of time cells, neurons in the hippocampus that discharge for brief periods as a rat passes through successive locations[53]. Time, in this sense, refers to relative time within an event or familiar journey. In an object–odor association task, for example, different cells became active for brief periods, in sequence, during different parts of a 10-second period between a sample stimulus and the appearance of choice stimuli. The collective activity of this neuronal population filled the time-gap between these two events[54]. Additional evidence for time cells comes from studies of activity in the hippocampus as animals walk in place on a treadmill[55]. Such experiments have demonstrated that some of these cells encode time independent of location. Most cells had activity that reflected an interaction between spatial and temporal variables, and when the delay period between the sample and choice changed, a temporal recalibration process occurred. This finding suggests that the hippocampus does not encode order or recency per se, but instead encodes an entire temporally extended event, from which vertebrates derive order and recency information. Consistent with this idea, as rats learned trial-unique odor sequences in another experiment, the activity of a neuronal population in the hippocampus reflected the temporal interval between events, and this activity predicted the performance of these rats on the discrimination of relative recency within a sequence of odors[56].

Later, in Chapter 12 ("Hippocampus lesions: effect or no effect"), we review evidence that the hippocampal complex of monkeys plays an essential role in applying a recency strategy to choices that depend on event sequences, and in Chapters 10 and 11 we take up some further derived functions in humans, including the representation of situational contexts, flexible perspectives, and autobiographical events. However, in this chapter we stress a conserved function, one that depends on specialized, map-like representations. These representations guide navigational journeys and include a temporally extended sequence of olfactory and visual stimuli. Once these representations evolved, they could support behaviors based on derivatives of this information, such as sequences and recency. Accordingly, cognitive maps also support the performance of laboratory tasks that require choices among scenes, odors, and sequences, as well as choices based on order, recency, and a context established by such information. Collectively, these capacities have sometimes been categorized as relational memory.

The term relational memory refers to spatial and temporal relations among items in a scene or a series of scenes, including spatial, temporal, and order information[57]. We avoid this term, however, because it can be confused with the concept of relational (and analogical) reasoning, a topic that we take up in Chapter 9 ("Parietal–prefrontal networks").

Terminology aside, this concept concerns an ability anticipated by cognitive map theory: the flexible manipulation and use of representations in the hippocampus, independent of the learning context.

This ability was demonstrated in an experiment in which rats learned arbitrary associations in a training context and then used this knowledge flexibly in probe tests[58]. This task first required learning that two stimuli go together, as follows: Stimulus A was associated with stimulus B, and stimulus 1 was associated with stimulus 2. We abbreviate these relationships as A → B and 1 → 2, respectively, mixing numbers and letters to help keep the two sets of relations separate. Cups filled with scented sand served as stimuli.

To begin with, rats dug through sand with odor A because it was the only cup available, and so it served as the sample stimulus. Later, they learned that after this sample—given the choice between sand with odor B and sand with odor 2—they should choose odor B in order to obtain food (Fig. 4.7A, top half). Likewise, after sniffing odor 1, they

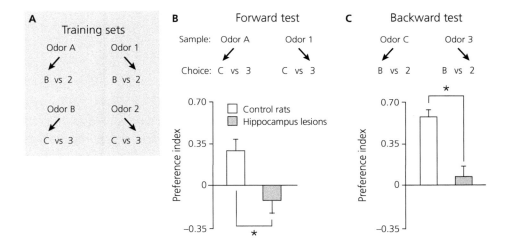

Fig. 4.7 Effect of hippocampus lesions on the memory for paired associates. (A) Rats f rst learned associations among odors. After digging in sand with odor A, the rats faced a choice between two odors, B and 2. The correct choice, B, later served as the cue for selecting odor C. Likewise, rats learned an associative chain: Odor 1 went with odor 2, which went with odor 3. Although rats with hippocampus lesions acquired these odor–odor associations at the same rate as control rats, they were impaired on two tests that require the use of this information in a novel way. (B) A forward test examined memories of the chained associations by presenting the rats with a novel choice: After either odor A or odor 1 they needed to chose between odor C and odor 3. Rats with hippocampus lesions performed poorly, as measured by a preference index [(correct − errors)/(correct + errors)]. Control rats chose correctly on approximately two-thirds of the trials; rats with hippocampus lesions chose correctly on fewer than half of the trials. The asterisk indicates a significant effect of the lesion. (C) A backward test examined associative memories in reverse order compared to what the rats had experienced. Reprinted from Bunsey M, Eichenbaum H. Conservation of hippocampal memory function in rats and humans. *Nature* 379:255–57, © 1996, with permission of Macmillan Publishers, Ltd.

needed to choose odor 2, not odor B. In this way, the rats learned the relations A → B and 1 → 2. Subsequently, the same rats were trained on a linked set of relations: B → C and 2 → 3 (Fig. 4.7A, bottom half). Finally, probe tests examined whether the rats could use their knowledge flexibly, outside the specific context in which they had learned these relations. For example, at the time of the probe test, the rats had previously faced a choice between odor C and odor 3 when stimulus B had been the sample stimulus, but they had never faced the same choice when stimulus A was the sample. In what we call a forward test (Fig. 4.7B, top), the rats had to make this choice. A backward test demonstrated a different kind of flexibility by reversing the sample and choice stimuli. After the rats sniffed odor C as the sample, for example, they needed to choose odor B over odor 2 in order to get some food (Fig. 4.7C, top). Figure 4.7(B, C) shows that control rats used their memories flexibly in both tests, just as rats can use a novel route to reach a spatial goal. Rats with hippocampus lesions had severe impairments on both the forward and backward tests. Note that hippocampus lesions did not impair the initial learning of the odor–odor relations, only the performance on probe tests that required the flexible use of that information at some later time—beyond the training context.

The hippocampus is also necessary for rats to make choices based on the relation between their internal state and a potential goal. In an experiment on this point, hippocampus lesions caused an impairment in choosing between two visual stimuli based on whether the rats were hungry or thirsty[59].

These findings help place the conserved functions of the hippocampus homologue in an ecological context. Navigation refers to more than moving through space, it also involves encountering a sequence of objects, surfaces, landscapes, and layouts at particular times during a journey to a goal.

Nonnavigational functions

Specialized navigation-related representations not only contribute to making choices based on sequences and stimulus relations, they also contribute to other nonnavigational functions. We highlight two types here.

First, the rodent hippocampus plays a role in fear conditioning and anxiety[60–62], which contributes to the avoidance of harm. We return to this function in the next section (see "Septal versus amygdaloid hippocampus"). Second, the hippocampus subserves the social transmission of food preferences. In an experiment that explored this behavior, a demonstrator rat ate some novel food. Later, an observer rat interacted with the demonstrator for a few minutes without any food present. Finally, the observer rat chose between two types of novel foods, including the one previously eaten by the demonstrator. The observer rats usually chose the food previously eaten by the demonstrator, a choice that depended on two odors on the demonstrator's breath: the odor of the ingested food and carbon disulfide[63]. The neuronal and genetic mechanisms underlying these effects are reasonably well understood[64], and it seems likely that carbon disulfide indicated to the observer rat that the demonstrator rat was, at least, still breathing. This is, admittedly, not a particularly high gastronomic standard, but such is a rat's life. Immediately after social exposure, both intact (control) observer rats and observer rats with hippocampus lesions chose the food eaten by the demonstrator rat, as usual[65]. However, after a delay period rats with hippocampus lesions lost this preference, whereas in control rats the preference persisted.

Odors are particularly important in rodent navigation, and so the social transmission of food preferences serves as an example of how navigation-related representations can be adapted to nonnavigational functions. According to our proposal, the hippocampus homologue evolved in response to selective pressures for a mobile life in an aquatic niche. Breathing air for respiration would not begin in earnest for hundreds of millions of years. Eventually, natural selection modified navigational representations to support the social transmission of food preferences, especially when bad breath beats no breath at all.

Septal versus amygdaloid hippocampus

We have said little so far about different parts of the hippocampal complex. In Chapter 2 we explained how the septal–amygdaloid axis became a dorsal–ventral axis in many mammals, including rodents, and a posterior–anterior axis in primates (see Fig. 2.12).

The amygdaloid hippocampus contributes most of the direct connections between the hippocampus and the prefrontal cortex[66,67], and it differs from the septal hippocampus in other ways as well. For instance, the septal hippocampus seems to specialize in the navigational functions commonly studied in the laboratory, such as maze learning. In contrast, the amygdaloid hippocampus has the fear and anxiety functions mentioned earlier (see "Nonnavigational functions")[60,61]. In accord with this idea, brain imaging activations occur in the amygdaloid hippocampus during both fear conditioning and eyeblink conditioning in humans[68].

Both parts of the hippocampus have place fields, although they differ in size. The septal hippocampus has small, finely tuned place fields, usually less than a meter in diameter, whereas the amygdaloid hippocampus has place fields approximately ten times larger[69]. This difference could contribute to small-scale and large-scale navigation, respectively. Furthermore, large place fields might have a role in the generalization of spatial contexts and in remembering places associated with harm or threats. We return to this topic in Chapter 10 ("Septal versus amygdaloid hippocampus") in the context of extended cortical networks that evolved in primates.

The contribution of the amygdaloid hippocampus to fear conditioning and anxiety can be reconciled with a cognitive map function if one considers its large place fields as representations of a large-scale context. From this perspective, the amygdaloid hippocampus seems well suited for representing generally "good" or generally "bad" places over a useful volume of space. The small place fields of the septal hippocampus instead guide navigation that requires high spatial accuracy.

Summary

Rodents, like other vertebrates, engage in navigation to a memorized mixture of places and objects, and they do so in part by using specialized map-like representations that include the sequences and intervals of a journey. We say "in part" because alternative forms of navigation include "snapshot" guidance, which consists of approaching a remembered stimulus or attempting to match a remembered visual scene, and ideothetic guidance, which involves path integration and is sometimes likened to "dead reckoning." The hippocampus homologue probably contributes to these guidance modes as well, especially the latter.

Research on rodents dominates this field, and so we have relied on this literature, but according to our proposal the hippocampus homologue performs its original, conserved function in most vertebrates. Once its specialized representations evolved, however, they became available for other functions and subject to selection. In Chapters 10 and 11 we consider some of these derived traits, but for now we take up navigational functions in monkeys and humans.

Navigation memory in monkeys

The literature on the hippocampus in monkeys has, for the most part, concentrated on memories that seem unrelated to navigation, at first glance. There have been very few experiments in which monkeys have navigated through space like rats in a maze or like monkeys do in their natural habitats. Primate research has focused instead on an attempt to develop a model of human amnesia (see Chapter 12, "The monkey model"), with little reference to the evolutionary adaptations of monkeys or their anthropoid ancestors. Accordingly, the literature on the hippocampus in primates often seems disconnected from the work on rodents.

Recent work has alleviated this contradiction to some extent, in part because of renewed interest in scene memory and open-field foraging. These studies exploit the fact that modern monkeys, like their anthropoid ancestors, make foraging choices based on visual scenes (see Chapter 2, "Visual and behavioral adaptations in anthropoids"). In addition, the use of selective lesions has corrected some misleading reports about the role of the monkey hippocampus in spatial memory, as we explain later (see "A general role in spatial memory?").

Scene memory

Gaffan devised the object-in-place scenes task, which he and his colleagues have used to explore the role of the hippocampus in memories about visual scenes[70,71]. In these experiments, monkeys learned to choose between two object-like stimuli—such as small letters—within a complex background scene, all of which appeared on a video monitor[71]. On a typical trial, two letters appeared at fixed locations within a given scene. Figure 4.8(A) shows an example, with "p" as the correct choice and "g" as the incorrect choice on a particular background. Different letters, in different locations on different backgrounds, were presented from trial to trial. We return to this task in Chapters 8 ("Object-in-place scenes task") and 11 ("Episodic memory"), where we consider whether this task measures episodic memory, but here we focus on some of the structures and pathways necessary for scene learning.

As shown in Fig. 4.8(B), one group of control monkeys learned to make the correct choice after only a few experiences with each scene, which repeats every 20 trials[72].

Both fornix lesions and combined lesions of the temporal stem and the amygdala caused a mild impairment in learning this task (Fig. 4.8C). For reference, the horizontal dashed lines show chance levels of performance (50% correct) and a reduction of the error rate

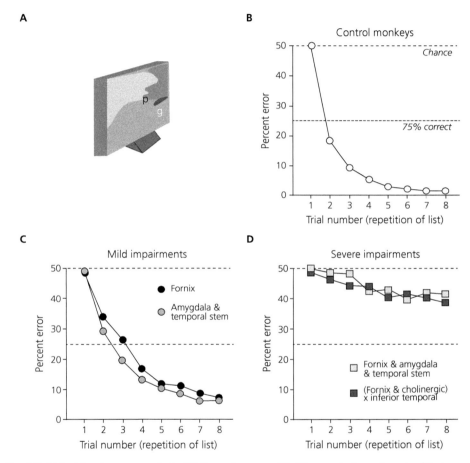

Fig. 4.8 Object-in-place scenes task. (A) Example scene. (B) After control monkeys (unfilled circles) mastered the rules of the task, they learned the correct object-like stimulus in a novel scene after only a few presentations, even though 19 similar object-in-place problems occurred between the presentations of any given scene. (C) Mild impairments followed bilateral lesions of the fornix (black circles) or lesions of the amygdala and temporal stem together (gray circles). (D) The combination of three lesions—to the fornix, the amygdala, and the temporal stem—caused a severe impairment (light gray squares), as did a combination of a unilateral ablation of the inferior temporal cortex in one hemisphere with a unilateral fornix transection and cholinergic lesion in the other (dark gray squares). Adapted from Gaffan D. Against memory systems. *Philosophical Transactions of the Royal Society of London B: Biological Sciences* 357:1111–21, © 2002, by permission of the Royal Society.

by half. On the third presentation of a scene, control monkeys reduced their errors to about 10% (Fig. 4.8B), while monkeys in the two lesion groups made more than twice as many errors (Fig. 4.8C). Monkeys with bilateral lesions in anatomically related regions—including the mammillary bodies[73], anterior thalamus[74], and entorhinal cortex[75]—had comparable impairments, as did monkeys with disconnections of the perirhinal cortex from the fornix[76].

A combined lesion of the fornix, the amygdala, and the white matter tracts in the temporal stem produced a much more severe impairment (Fig. 4.8D). This combination of structures might seem arbitrary, but they go together for a reason. The axons that connect the basal forebrain and midbrain to the temporal lobe travel through three routes: the fornix and fimbria; fibers passing through the amygdala; and the temporal stem. The simultaneous disruption of all three routes caused a severe impairment (Fig. 4.8D, light gray squares). These lesions also disrupted connections between the prefrontal and lateral temporal cortex, a topic we revisit in Chapter 11 ("Modern traits" and "Disconnection"). A similarly severe impairment followed damage to the cholinergic cells of the basal forebrain, combined with a fornix transection in the same hemisphere and an inferior temporal cortex lesion in the opposite hemisphere (Fig. 4.8D, dark gray squares). This result suggests a cholinergic contribution to memory formation, but it might have resulted instead from some less specific effect of this crossed-disconnection lesion. Regardless, these results all show that the hippocampal complex plays an important role in scene memory.

What, readers might ask, does any of this have to do with navigation? Unlike the Morris water maze or the plus-maze task, the object-in-place scenes task does not involve the movement of an animal through space. Instead, the monkeys simply reach to and touch the correct object-like stimulus on a video monitor. Accordingly, no one has ever claimed that this task has anything to do with navigation or foraging. Nevertheless, the object-in-place scenes task draws on the kinds of representations that monkeys need for foraging choices in their natural habitat. In Chapter 2 ("Anthropoids") we explained that, during primate evolution, anthropoids began to travel long distances in search of resources. These animals (or their haplorhine ancestors) evolved several new visual traits, including foveal and trichromatic vision, along with the fine distance analysis that depended on enhancements in stereopsis and depth perception. Accordingly, visual scenes play a crucial role in anthropoid foraging choices, especially for distant resources.

Humans with damage to the fornix, associated with removal of colloid cysts in the third ventricle, performed the object-in-place scenes task like monkeys with fornix transections: They had a mild impairment (see Fig. 11.3). This finding emphasizes a conserved function of the hippocampal complex in monkeys and humans, but it would be a mistake to assume that it has exactly the same functions in these two species. In Chapter 11 ("Episodic memory") we propose that the human hippocampus contributes to some uniquely human traits.

A general role in spatial memory?

Inspired by research on the rodent hippocampus, several monkey experiments have explored whether the hippocampus plays a general role in spatial memory. Unlike the object-in-place scenes task, these experiments bear little relationship to the natural life of anthropoids. Table 4.1 (top three rows) presents some of these results, which at the time they were published seemed to show that the monkey hippocampus has a general spatial memory function. Unfortunately, many of the impairments attributed to the monkey hippocampus during this era resulted instead from inadvertent damage to other structures. In Chapter 12 ("Falsification of the first model") we discuss some similar mistakes, made at about the same time.

In the spatial reversal task, one location (of two possibilities) was designated as correct. After monkeys learned to choose the correct place during one block of trials, the location designated as correct was changed for the next block of trials. Experiments that employed aspiration lesions of the hippocampus suggested that it made a major contribution to this kind of memory[77,78], but these effects depended instead on damage to the underlying parahippocampal cortex. When damage was limited to the hippocampus—in subsequent experiments using selective, excitotoxic lesions—there was no effect on performance of the spatial reversal task[79].

In a test of object–place memories, one object was designated as correct, but only when it occupied a particular place. Two objects appeared at any of several locations: first during the sample phase and again during the test phase. In the test phase, monkeys could obtain food by choosing the object that occupied the same place as it had in the sample presentation[80]. Aspiration lesions of the hippocampus produced a severe impairment on this task[80,81], but—like the spatial reversal task—selective hippocampus lesions had no effect[82], even when monkeys needed to remember several object–place conjunctions simultaneously[83].

Table 4.1 Effects of selective (excitotoxic) versus nonselective (aspiration) lesions on various spatial tasks

Tasks	H	H⁺	PHC
Spatial reversal	–	↓↓	
Object–place association	–	↓↓↓	↓↓↓
Spatial matching: reach	–	↓↓↓	↓↓↓[a]
Spatial nonmatching: open field	↓↓↓		

H, selective excitotoxic lesions of the hippocampus; H⁺, unselective aspiration lesions of the hippocampus, which included additional structures; PHC, lesions of the parahippocampal cortex; ↓↓, moderate impairments; ↓↓↓, severe impairments; –, no impairment. Empty cells indicate a lack of relevant results.

[a] From a variant of the object–place association task, which converted it into a spatial matching task.

For sources, see Murray and Wise[118].

In the spatial matching task, monkeys learned to chose either a previously cued location (according to the matching rule) or to an alternative location (according to the non-matching rule) after a delay period. Like the other false leads in the literature of the 1970s and 1980s, impairments occurred after unselective, aspiration lesions[84], but selective hippocampus lesions left performance intact[85].

Taken together (Table 4.1), traditional laboratory tests of spatial memory provide little evidence that the monkey hippocampus has a spatial memory function in a general sense. Some memory tests that require spatial memory depend on the monkey hippocampus, but some do not. There is a better way to understand the functions of the monkey hippocampus; its specialized representations support foraging choices based on visual scenes—choices that anthropoids make in their natural habitat (see Chapter 2, "Anthropoids"). Some "spatial" tasks draw on these representations, but others do so to a lesser extent, if at all.

One final comment on general spatial analysis: It is tempting to relate reaching movements to an egocentric (intrinsic) coordinate frame, in contrast to navigation, which often depends on an allocentric (extrinsic) frame. For primates, this idea is clearly wrong. As we explain in Chapter 6 ("Coordinate frames and transforms"), posterior parietal and premotor areas represent locations in an extrinsic (allocentric) frame of reference and reaching movements depend on such coordinates. The fact that both premotor–parietal networks and the hippocampus use extrinsic coordinates explains why patients with hippocampus lesions do not have impairments in allocentrically guided reaching[86]. Furthermore, because rodents lack the premotor and posterior parietal areas that evolved in primates (see Chapter 2, "Early primates"), egocentric versus allocentric guidance must be very different in nonprimate species.

Foraging in an open field

A particularly instructive contrast involves the spatial short-interval matching task, which can be tested in two ways. In traditional tests, monkeys reach for their choice during the test phase. As just explained, selective lesions of the hippocampus do not cause a memory impairment in this situation, despite some misleading reports from the earlier literature (Table 4.1, row 3). But in an experimental setting more like natural foraging, the hippocampus makes a crucial contribution to spatial memory (Table 4.1, bottom row)[87].

Tests of spatial memory in an open foraging field have revealed a crucial role for the hippocampus[87]. In one such experiment, monkeys could walk to any of four foraging sites in a large room while on a tether. At each site, an inverted flower pot covered a plate (Fig. 4.9A). Each trial consisted of a sample run, during which monkeys could explore all four sites in order to find the hidden food (Fig. 4.9B). Only one of the four plates had food, which the monkeys consumed. Next, a tether and pulley system allowed the monkeys to be guided back to a cage at one side of the room, after which a delay period ensued. Finally, the monkeys were allowed to choose one (and only one) of the four flower pots. On sample runs, as expected, the monkeys found food on their first choice about 25% of the time, which represents a chance level of performance. Control monkeys

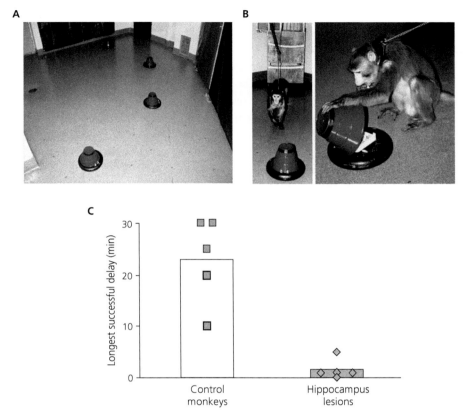

Fig. 4.9 Navigational memory in monkeys. (A) A foraging field. (B) Left: a tethered monkey, with a holding cage in the background. Right: The monkey displaced an inverted flower pot to gain access to food. (C) Effect of hippocampus lesions. In this task, monkeys performed a sample run to find food at one of three possible sites. After a delay period spent in the holding cage, they could obtain additional food at the same site, but they were allowed to explore only one location. After a monkey mastered the task at a delay of 12 seconds, the shortest delay possible, the memory period increased to 30 seconds. If monkeys performed well (83% correct) at that delay, the memory period increased again to 1 minute, then in steps of 1 minute up to 5-minute delays, and finally in steps of 5 minutes up to 30-minute delays. Symbols show the scores of individual monkeys at their longest successful (83% correct) delays. Control monkeys progressed successfully to 10-, 20-, 25-, or 30-minute delays, but monkeys with excitotoxic hippocampus lesions failed at much shorter memory intervals. (B, C) Reproduced from Hampton RR, Hampstead BM, Murray EA. Selective hippocampal damage in rhesus monkeys impairs spatial memory in an open-field test. *Hippocampus* 14:808–18, © 2004, John Wiley & Sons, with permission.

chose the food site first on about 40% of the choice runs, both 5 minutes and 24 hours after the sample run. Monkeys with selective excitotoxic lesions of the hippocampus, in contrast, performed at chance levels during the choice test (not illustrated): a significant impairment.

In a related experiment, monkeys first learned the matching-to-sample rule. During the sample presentation, the monkeys could see trial-unique configurations of three foraging sites in the testing room, with food visible at one of them. During the choice phase, after a delay period during which the monkeys could not see the food, the monkeys were allowed to explore one (and only one) of the three locations. After they learned the matching rule, the interval between the sample presentation and the choice runs was gradually increased until the monkeys could no longer perform the task successfully, defined as 83% correct choices. Most control monkeys performed successfully with delays of 20–30 minutes; most monkeys with selective hippocampus lesions, however, failed at any delay longer than 2 minutes (Fig. 4.9C).

These findings reinforce results from experiments with a monkey-size T-maze (Fig. 4.10A)[88]. In the T-maze task, monkeys began each trial with a run down the maze, but a blockade of one arm forced them into the arm with food: the sample arm. On the test run, the monkeys could choose either arm, but only the arm opposite the sample arm had food. After learning the task, control monkeys made relatively few errors (Fig. 4.10B, unfilled bars) and quickly returned to 90% correct performance. Monkeys with fornix transections (Fig. 4.10B, gray bars), in contrast, made many more errors as they relearned the task to a 90% correct performance level, although most subjects eventually achieved that criterion at a 1-minute delay. Even so, increasing the delay interval to 15 minutes reduced their performance to chance level (Fig. 4.10C, gray circles). Control monkeys could perform at about 80% correct with delays of 15 minutes (Fig. 4.10C, unfilled circles).

In another large-field experiment, monkeys foraged for foods that were located in three of 18 inverted cups set out on a large platform[89]. Monkeys with selective hippocampus lesions learned as quickly as control subjects to choose the locations of the foods when conjunctive color–place cues guided their choices. When the redundant color cues were later removed, however, monkeys with hippocampus lesions performed poorly. This finding points to the use of color–place conjunctions in making foraging choices in a large field.

In a related experiment, monkeys visited opaque boxes in different locations within a large enclosure[90]. Each box contained a different food, and the food type–place conjunctions remained consistent day after day. To pursue the optimal foraging strategy, the monkeys needed to visit each box once and only once, and they typically went to the box with their preferred food first. In another version of this task, colored boxes were used and the conjunctions of food type and color remained constant rather than the conjunctions of food type and place. Compared with control subjects, monkeys with lesions of the hippocampus (sustained in infancy) made more errors, defined as returning to a previously visited box, for both place and color cues. These findings demonstrated a role for the hippocampus in remembering both food type–place and food type–color conjunctions. In addition, after a selective satiation procedure that devalued the preferred food, monkeys with hippocampus lesions continued to choose its box first. In other experimental settings, however, hippocampus lesions had no effect on valuation updating[91], so it seems

A

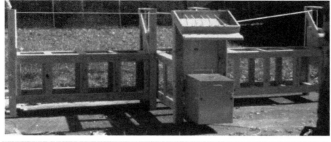

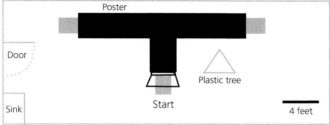

B

C

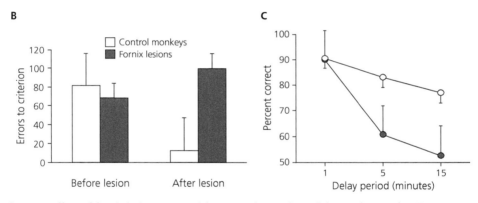

Fig. 4.10 Effect of fornix lesions on spatial memory in monkeys. (A) Top: the monkey T-maze before installation in the testing room. Small cages served as the start box and as goals at the end of each arm. Bottom: view of the T-maze (black), from above, along with the locations of extramaze cues in the testing room. In a sample run, the monkey had no choice but to enter either the left or the right arm of the maze, where it found food in the cage at the end of the arm. The subsequent test run, after a delay period, required the monkey to choose the alternative arm in order to obtain more food: a nonmatching rule. (B) The number of errors to the criterion performance of 90% correct. Error bars show standard error. (C) After the lesion, most of the monkeys could relearn the task at a 1-minute delay (leftmost data points). For these monkeys, increasing the delay period to 15 minutes reduced their performance to chance level (gray circles) but had much less effect on control monkeys (unfilled circles). (A, bottom) Redrawn from Murray EA, Davidson M, Gaffan D, Olton DS, Suomi S. Effects of fornix transection and cingulate cortical ablation on spatial memory in rhesus monkeys. *Experimental Brain Research* 74:173–86, © 1989, with permission of Springer. (B, C) Data from the same source.

likely that the hippocampus associates updated valuations with the food–place and food–color conjunctions that it represents and stores.

In contrast to these results, a different experiment suggested a specialization of the hippocampus for spatial memory[92]. In this study, monkeys could open eight boxes set out in an array, each of which contained food at the beginning of a run. One version of the task involved identical boxes, which differed only in their location; the other used boxes of different colors. In both cases, the most efficient foraging strategy required the monkeys to choose each box once and only once. Contrary to the results summarized earlier[89,90], in this experiment hippocampus inactivations only caused an impairment on the spatial version of the task. Given the positive results (impairments) when redundant color cues were removed from color–place conjunctions[89] and when monkeys needed to remember which color of box was associated with a particular type of food[90], the negative result on the color version of this task probably reflected other variables: the age of the monkeys at time of lesions, the use of temporary inactivations versus permanent lesions, the use of redundant color–place cues versus unique color cues, or the use of conjunctions between color and food type versus color and food availability. The latter two possibilities seem most likely.

Positive results, as usual, carry more weight than negative ones, and so we draw two conclusions from the open-field research: (1) The monkey hippocampus plays a role in foraging based on scenes and locations[87,88,] and (2) it also plays a role in foraging based on nonspatial cues, such as colors, when they are linked either to specific food types[90] or to places with food[89]. In agreement with this conclusion, another experiment showed that selective hippocampus lesions impaired the memory of which objects in a set had been chosen during a block of trials[93].

Summary

The monkey hippocampus contributes to foraging choices that require either navigation through space in an open field or reaching movements that involve choosing object-like stimuli embedded in a spatial scene. It does not, however, function in spatial processing generally. Monkeys with complete, selective lesions of the hippocampus have performed normally on several tests of spatial memory (Table 4.1, top three rows).

Navigation memory in humans

For the most part, we defer a consideration of the human hippocampus to Chapters 10 and 11. Here we mention briefly a selection of findings with close relevance to the rat and monkey research summarized in this chapter.

Imaging

Brain imaging studies have pointed to a role for the human hippocampus in navigation, along with nearby structures such as the subicular, entorhinal, and retrosplenial cortex. In these experiments, activations in these areas correlated with goal proximity, location, and head direction[94,95], as well as with other features relevant to navigation, perspective[96], and landmarks[97]. In another study, brain imaging activations in the human hippocampus correlated with temporal context memory[98,99]. We return to these topics in

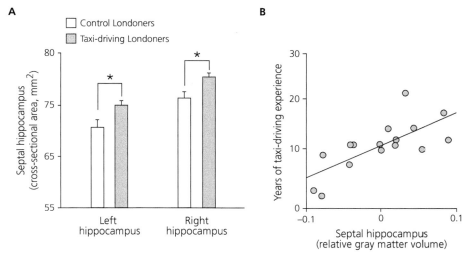

Fig. 4.11 Effect of navigational knowledge on the size of the human hippocampus. (A) Taxi drivers in London have a more extensive knowledge of routes in a complex environment than do other Londoners, and they also have a significantly larger (*) septal hippocampus in both hemispheres. (B) In taxi drivers, the volume of the septal hippocampus correlates with their amount of experience on the job. (A) Redrawn from Maguire EA, Gadian DG, Johnsrude IS, Good CD, Ashburner J, Frackowiak RS, Frith CD. Navigation-related structural change in the hippocampi of taxi drivers. *Proceedings of the National Academy of Sciences U.S.A.* 97:4398–403, © 2000, National Academy of Sciences, U.S.A. (B) From Woollett K, Spiers HJ, Maguire EA. Talent in the taxi: a model system for exploring expertise. *Philosophical Transactions of the Royal Society of London B: Biological Sciences* 364:1407–16, © 2009, by permission of the Royal Society.

Chapter 10 ("Medial network") in the context of some derived properties of an extended hippocampal–navigation system.

The Knowledge

In modern urban life, nothing personifies navigational knowledge better than London taxi drivers. Indeed, their knowledge goes by that exact name: "The Knowledge." These experts have a large septal (posterior) hippocampus relative to other people, including other professional drivers (Fig. 4.11A), and its size increases during decades of practice (Fig. 4.11B)[100–102]. The volume of the hippocampus also predicts the ability to use knowledge about a recently learned spatial layout in order to draw inferences about the relative positions of its landmarks[103].

Maze memory

Some studies of human navigation have used virtual maze tasks, including ones analogous to either the radial-arm maze or the Morris water maze. Hippocampus lesions in humans have caused impairments in learning which arms of a virtual radial maze always had or never had "rewards"[104–106], like some findings in rats[25–30]. However, other studies have revealed differences between the rat and human results. In an experiment like the Morris water maze, lesions of the hippocampus did not cause an impairment of the sort that occurs in rodents, but lesions of the parahippocampal cortex had a modest effect[107].

Topographic maps

Some case studies report that patients with damage to the hippocampus can remember large-scale maps learned prior to their brain injury[108,109]. They can answer questions about how to navigate through topographic features, including the use of alternative routes within a map[108]. Although amnesic patients usually fail to learn new maps, H.M. eventually mastered the floor plan of his house, which he lived in only after his surgery (see Chapter 1, "What happened to Henry?").

Corkin[110] accounts for this spared ability by invoking the thousands of "learning trials" that H.M. had experienced while navigating around his house, over many years. Presumably, areas that represent topographic layouts, such as the parahippocampal and retrosplenial cortex, can support the acquisition of maps without support from an intact hippocampus, although in a way that is usually considered to be slow and inflexible[111-113]. Perhaps the parahippocampal and retrosplenial cortex represent an abstract cognitive map, or a series of such maps, with the hippocampus being required to establish new maps or update previously acquired ones, in either case rapidly and flexibly[114]. As a result, viewpoint-independent representations might depend on the hippocampus, with augmenting areas specializing in similar representations, albeit with less flexibility and less generalization among layouts. We return to this topic in Chapters 10 ("Situational contexts") and 12 ("The summation principle") where we discuss a spared capacity for slow semantic learning in hippocampal amnesia.

Scene memory

Other findings in humans have also provided an important, if indirect, link between the hippocampus and navigation. A study of patients with damage to the hippocampus revealed an impairment in discriminating and learning scenes, but not faces or dot patterns[115]. This impairment resembled the one caused by fornix lesions on the object-in-place scenes task, as discussed earlier for monkeys (see "Scene memory"), although the tasks differed in many ways. In Chapter 7 ("Humans") we deal with the human experiments in more detail, and there we explain that the specialized representations housed in the hippocampus function in both the perception and memory of scenes. Here we emphasize the relationship of scenes to navigation. Although experiments on scene memory in humans did not have overt navigational requirements, the scenes they used look like rooms that people commonly encounter and can move within (Fig. 7.9A). Put in a more formal way, these scenes consisted of conjunctions of objects and surfaces and their arrangement in space, which people can use to guide navigation, at least in principle.

Related studies have emphasized a role for the human hippocampus in the mental construction of scenes. In one such study, patients with hippocampus damage could not construct new, imagined scenarios as well as healthy people[116]. The patients' scenarios were faulty, in part, because their mental imagery lacked the spatial coherence that typically characterizes scenes. We return to this topic in Chapter 10 ("Constructive episodic simulations").

Conclusions

This chapter tackles the hippocampus from an unusual perspective. Topical reviews typically treat the literature in terms of some overarching concept drawn from laboratory or clinical research, such as episodic, spatial, relational, configural, contextual, item-in-context, ideothetic, or associational memory. Instead, we take as our starting point the ideas presented in Chapter 2 about when the hippocampus homologue first arose during evolution, in what kind of animal it developed, and the selective pressures that favored its specialized representations.

According to our proposal, early vertebrates evolved a hippocampus homologue that provided advantages for both foraging and the avoidance of harm, along with other biological needs. In these distant ancestors, just about all behavior involved navigation. Foraging for food and predator avoidance are obvious examples, but temperature regulation and procreation also required navigation. Early vertebrates could only regulate their temperature by moving to cooler or warmer places, and they reproduced by dispersing sperm in relation to deposited eggs. Their navigation system provided these animals with advantages in reaching protected places, remembered resources, moderate temperatures, and breeding spots. The amygdaloid hippocampus, in particular, has functions that reflect this diverse set of behaviors, including autonomic ones[117].

Although convergent evolution remains possible, in view of the comparative data from goldfish, turtles, lizards, several mammals, and a variety of birds (Fig. 4.1A), it seems more likely that the hippocampus and its homologues perform a conserved navigational function:

◆ In goldfish, lesions of the hippocampus homologue have produced a severe impairment in spatial navigation, similar in many respects to the results from mammals in similar circumstances (Fig. 4.1B)[10]. Experiments using a plus-maze like the one illustrated in Fig. 4.3(A)—but wetter—showed that goldfish remembered and returned to a spatial goal when they found themselves at novel starting locations, and they used both novel routes and shortcuts to get there, even without any useful local cues. Moreover, these fish did not depend on any single cue; instead they relied on a general scene or series of scenes[10].

◆ In amniotes, lesions of the medial cortex have impaired navigation in lizards[14] and turtles[15], as illustrated in Fig. 2.7(C).

◆ In rodents, like other vertebrates, a navigational journey involves a sequence of objects, odors, and landscapes at particular intervals. Experiments on rodents have indicated that the hippocampus specializes in map-like representations that guide such journeys. These cognitive maps consist of a temporally extended sequence of olfactory and visual stimuli, among other conjunctive representations.

◆ In anthropoids, experiments on macaque monkeys have demonstrated that their hippocampus uses its specialized visual representations to support navigation in an open field.

◆ In humans, brain imaging and volumetric analyses have provided evidence for a role of the human hippocampal complex in navigation.

In addition to these conserved navigational functions, the hippocampus homologue also contributes to other kinds of behavior, for two related reasons: (1) its specialized representations became subject to selection once they emerged; and (2) the representations needed for navigation can be used for tasks involving choices based on order, recency, and context, as well as for choices among scenes, odors, and sequences. The monkey hippocampal complex, for example, contributes to reaching movements that involve choices among object-like stimuli embedded in a spatial scene (see "Scene memory"). In Chapter 8 ("Event memories") we return to the anthropoid adaptations that underlie this behavior. Likewise, we defer most of our consideration of the human hippocampus to Chapters 7, 10, and 11, where we emphasize derived functions that depend on its interactions with representational systems that evolved in hominins. These innovations include the perception and memory of scenes (see Chapter 7, "Humans") as well as the perception and memory of participating in events (see Chapter 11, "Proposal").

With the advent of ancestral vertebrates, the navigation memory system began to interact with the older systems described in Chapter 3. In Chapter 5 we explore mammalian innovations that manage conflicts within and among these representational systems. Inefficiencies that result from competing representational systems do little harm as long as energy needs remain modest. However, stem mammals adopted a different kind of life.

References

1. Darwin, C. (1839) *The Voyage of the Beagle* (Henry Colburn, London).
2. Shettleworth, S.J. (2010) *Cognition, Evolution, and Behavior* (Oxford University Press, New York).
3. Domjan, M. (2005) *Annu. Rev. Psychol.* **56**, 179–206.
4. Sherry, D.F. and Schacter, D.L. (1987) *Psychol. Rev.* **94**, 439–454.
5. Nadel, L. (1992) *J. Cogn. Neurosci.* **4**, 179–188.
6. Eichenbaum, H. and Cohen, N.J. (2001) *From Conditioning to Conscious Recollection: Memory Systems of the Brain* (Oxford University Press, New York).
7. Tolman, E.C. (1948) *Psychol. Rev.* **55**, 189–208.
8. O'Keefe, J. and Nadel, L. (1978) *The Hippocampus as a Cognitive Map* (Clarendon Press, Oxford).
9. Rodríguez, F., López, J.C., Vargas, J.P., Broglio, C. et al. (2002) *Brain Res. Bull.* **57**, 499–503.
10. Rodríguez, F., López, J.C., Vargas, J.P., Gómez, Y. et al. (2002) *J. Neurosci.* **22**, 2894–2903.
11. Hampton, R.R., Sherry, D.F., Shettleworth, S.J., Khurgel, M. et al. (1995) *Brain Behav. Evol.* **45**, 54–61.
12. Sherry, D.F. and Vaccarino, A.L. (1989) *Behav. Neurosci.* **103**, 308–318.
13. Hampton, R.R. and Shettleworth, S.J. (1996) *Behav. Neurosci.* **110**, 831–835.
14. Day, L.B., Crews, D., and Wilczynski, W. (2001) *Behav. Brain Res.* **118**, 27–42.
15. López, J.C., Vargas, J.P., Gómez, Y., and Salas, C. (2003) *Behav. Brain Res.* **143**, 109–120.
16. Striedter, G.F. (2016) *J. Comp. Neurol.* **524**, 496–517.
17. Patzke, N., Spocter, M.A., Karlsson, K.A., Bertelsen, M.F. et al. (2015) *Brain Struct. Funct.* **220**, 361–383.

18. **Watson, J.B.** (1930) *Behaviorism* (University of Chicago Press, Chicago, IL).

19. **Kohler, W.** (1925) *The Mentality of Apes* (Kegan Paul, Trench, and Trubner, London).

20. **Tolman, E.C.** (1949) *Psychol. Rev.* **56**, 144–155.

21. **Ritchie, B.F.** (1948) Thesis (University of California, Berkeley, CA).

22. **O'Keefe, J.** and **Dostrovsky, J.** (1971) *Brain Res.* **34**, 171–175.

23. **Song, E.Y., Kim, Y.B., Kim, Y.H.,** and **Jung, M.W.** (2005) *Hippocampus* **15**, 8–17.

24. **O'Keefe, J.** and **Conway, D.H.** (1980) *Physiol. Psychol.* **8**, 229–238.

25. **Olton, D.S.** and **Samuelson, R.J.** (1976) *J. Exp. Psychol. Anim. Behav. Process.* **2**, 97–116.

26. **Olton, D.S., Collison, C.,** and **Werz, M.A.** (1977) *Learn. Motiv.* **8**, 289–314.

27. **Olton, D.S.** and **Papas, B.C.** (1979) *Neuropsychologia* **17**, 669–682.

28. **Becker, J.T., Walker, J.A.,** and **Olton, D.S.** (1980) *Brain Res.* **200**, 307–320.

29. **Nadel, L.** and **MacDonald, L.** (1980) *Behav. Neural Biol.* **29**, 405–409.

30. **Sutherland, R.J.** (1985) In: *Electrophysiology of the Archicortex* (eds. Buzsaki, G. and Vanderwolf, C.H.), pp. 255–279 (Akademia Kiado Budapest, Budapest).

31. **Morris, R.G., Garrud, P., Rawlins, J.N.,** and **O'Keefe, J.** (1982) *Nature* **297**, 681–683.

32. **Balleine, B.W.** and **O'Doherty, J.P.** (2010) *Neuropsychopharmacol.* **35**, 48–69.

33. **Holland, P.C.** (2008) *Learn. Behav.* **36**, 227–241.

34. **McDonald, R.J.** and **White, N.M.** (1993) *Behav. Neurosci.* **107**, 3–22.

35. **Knierim, J.J.** and **Hamilton, D.A.** (2011) *Physiol. Rev.* **91**, 1245–1279.

36. **Pearce, J.M., Ward-Robinson, J., Good, M.A., Fussell, C.** et al. (2001) *J. Exp. Psychol. Anim. Behav. Process.* **27**, 329–344.

37. **Hayward, A., McGregor, A., Good, M.A.,** and **Pearce, J.M.** (2003) *Q. J. Exp. Psychol. B* **56**, 114–126.

38. **Zugaro, M.B., Arleo, A., Dejean, C., Burguiere, E.** et al. (2004) *Eur. J. Neurosci.* **20**, 530–536.

39. **O'Keefe, J.** (1976) *Exp. Neurol.* **51**, 78–109.

40. **Wood, E.R., Dudchenko, P.A., Robitsek, R.J.,** and **Eichenbaum, H.** (2000) *Neuron* **27**, 623–633.

41. **Frank, L.M., Brown, E.N.,** and **Wilson, M.** (2000) *Neuron* **27**, 169–178.

42. **Ferbinteanu, J.** and **Shapiro, M.L.** (2003) *Neuron* **40**, 1227–1239.

43. **Shapiro, M.L.** and **Ferbinteanu, J.** (2006) *Proc. Natl. Acad. Sci. USA* **103**, 4287–4292.

44. **Ferbinteanu, J., Shirvalkar, P.,** and **Shapiro, M.L.** (2011) *J. Neurosci.* **31**, 9135–9146.

45. **Deshmukh, S.S.** and **Knierim, J.J.** (2013) *Hippocampus* **23**, 253–267.

46. **Chen, G., King, J.A., Burgess, N.,** and **O'Keefe, J.** (2013) *Proc. Natl. Acad. Sci. USA* **110**, 378–383.

47. **Fortin, N.J., Agster, K.L.,** and **Eichenbaum, H.B.** (2002) *Nat. Neurosci.* **5**, 458–462.

48. **Kesner, R.P., Gilbert, P.E.,** and **Barua, L.A.** (2002) *Behav. Neurosci.* **116**, 286–290.

49. **Dere, E., Huston, J.P.,** and **de Souza Silva, M.A.** (2005) *Brain Res. Brain Res. Protoc.* **16**, 10–19.

50. **Dere, E., Huston, J.P.,** and **de Souza Silva, M.A.** (2007) *Neurosci. Biobehav. Rev.* **31**, 673–704.

51. **Mitchell, J.B.** and **Laiacona, J.** (1998) *Behav. Brain Res.* **97**, 107–113.

52. **Agster, K.L., Fortin, N.J.,** and **Eichenbaum, H.** (2002) *J. Neurosci.* **22**, 5760–5768.

53. **Eichenbaum, H.** (2013) *Trends Cogn. Sci.* **17**, 81–88.

54. **MacDonald, C.J., Lepage, K.Q., Eden, U.T.,** and **Eichenbaum, H.** (2011) *Neuron* **71**, 737–749.

55. **Kraus, B.J., Robinson, R.J., White, J.A., Eichenbaum, H.** et al. (2013) *Neuron* **78**, 1090–1101.

56. **Manns, J.R., Howard, M.W.,** and **Eichenbaum, H.** (2007) *Neuron* **56**, 530–540.

57. **Cohen, N.J.** and **Eichenbaum, H.** (1993) *Memory, Amnesia, and the Hippocampal System* (MIT Press, Cambridge, MA).

58. **Bunsey, M.** and **Eichenbaum, H.** (1996) *Nature* **379**, 255–257.

59. **Kennedy, P.J.** and **Shapiro, M.L.** (2004) *J. Neurosci.* **24**, 6979–6985.

60. Kjelstrup, K.G., Tuvnes, F.A., Steffenach, H.A., Murison, R. et al. (2002) *Proc. Natl. Acad. Sci. USA* **99**, 10825–10830.

61. Bannerman, D.M., Grubb, M., Deacon, R.M., Yee, B.K. et al. (2003) *Behav. Brain Res.* **139**, 197–213.

62. Selden, N.R., Everitt, B.J., Jarrard, L.E., and Robbins, T.W. (1991) *Neuroscience* **42**, 335–350.

63. Galef, B.G., Mason, J.R., Preti, G., and Bean, N.J. (1988) *Physiol. Behav.* **42**, 119–124.

64. Munger, S.D., Leinders-Zufall, T., McDougall, L.M., Cockerham, R.E. et al. (2010) *Curr. Biol.* **20**, 1438–1444.

65. Bunsey, M. and Eichenbaum, H. (1995) *Hippocampus* **5**, 546–556.

66. Blatt, G.J. and Rosene, D.L. (1998) *J. Comp. Neurol.* **392**, 92–114.

67. Cavada, C., Company, T., Tejedor, J., Cruz-Rizzolo, R.J. et al. (2000) *Cereb. Cortex* **10**, 220–242.

68. Knight, D.C., Cheng, D.T., Smith, C.N., Stein, E.A. et al. (2004) *J. Neurosci.* **24**, 218–228.

69. Kjelstrup, K.B., Solstad, T., Brun, V.H., Hafting, T. et al. (2008) *Science* **321**, 140–143.

70. Gaffan, D. (1992) *Eur. J. Neurosci.* **4**, 381–388.

71. Gaffan, D. (1994) *J. Cogn. Neurosci.* **6**, 305–320.

72. Gaffan, D. (2002) *Phil. Trans. R. Soc. B: Biol. Sci.* **357**, 1111–1121.

73. Parker, A. and Gaffan, D. (1997) *J. Cogn. Neurosci.* **9**, 512–521.

74. Parker, A. and Gaffan, D. (1997) *Neuropsychologia* **35**, 1093–1102.

75. Charles, D.P., Browning, P.G.F., and Gaffan, D. (2004) *Eur. J. Neurosci.* **20**, 3157–3164.

76. Gaffan, D. and Parker, A. (1996) *J. Neurosci.* **16**, 5864–5869.

77. Mahut, H. (1971) *Neuropsychologia.* **9**, 409–424.

78. Jones, B. and Mishkin, M. (1972) *Exp. Neurol.* **36**, 362–377.

79. Murray, E.A., Baxter, M.G., and Gaffan, D. (1998) *Behav. Neurosci.* **112**, 1291–1303.

80. Parkinson, J.K., Murray, E.A., and Mishkin, M. (1988) *J. Neurosci.* **8**, 4159–4167.

81. Angeli, S.J., Murray, E.A., and Mishkin, M. (1993) *Neuropsychologia* **31**, 1021–1030.

82. Malkova, L. and Mishkin, M. (2003) *J. Neurosci.* **23**, 1956–1965.

83. Belcher, A.M., Harrington, R.A., Malkova, L., and Mishkin, M. (2006) *Hippocampus* **16**, 361–367.

84. Mahut, H. and Moss, M. (1986) In: *The Hippocampus* (eds. Isaacson, R.L. and Pribram, K.H.), pp. 241–279 (Plenum Press, New York).

85. Murray, E.A. and Mishkin, M. (1998) *J. Neurosci.* **16**, 6568–6582.

86. Shadmehr, R., Brandt, J., and Corkin, S. (1998) *J. Neurophysiol.* **80**, 1590–1597.

87. Hampton, R.R., Hampstead, B.M., and Murray, E.A. (2004) *Hippocampus* **14**, 808–818.

88. Murray, E.A., Davidson, M., Gaffan, D., Olton, D.S. *et al.* (1989) *Exp. Brain Res.* **74**, 173–186.

89. Lavenex, P.B., Amaral, D.G., and Lavenex, P. (2006) *J. Neurosci.* **26**, 4546–4558.

90. Glavis-Bloom, C., Alvarado, M.C., and Bachevalier, J. (2013) *Behav. Neurosci.* **127**, 9–22.

91. Chudasama, Y., Wright, K.S., and Murray, E.A. (2008) *Biol. Psychiat.* **63**, 1084–1091.

92. Forcelli, P.A., Palchik, G., Leath, T., Desjardin, J.T. *et al.* (2014) *Proc. Natl. Acad. Sci. USA* **111**, 4315–4320.

93. Heuer, E. and Bachevalier, J. (2011) *Behav. Neurosci.* **125**, 859–870.

94. Spiers, H.J. and Maguire, E.A. (2007) *Hippocampus* **17**, 618–626.

95. Vass, L.K. and Epstein, R.A. (2013) *J. Neurosci.* **33**, 6133–6142.

96. Doeller, C.F., Barry, C., and Burgess, N. (2010) *Nature* **463**, 657–661.

97. Auger, S.D., Mullally, S.L., and Maguire, E.A. (2012) *PLoS One* **7**, e43620.

98. Hsieh, L.T., Gruber, M.J., Jenkins, L.J., and Ranganath, C. (2014) *Neuron* **81**, 1165–1178.

99. Ezzyat, Y. and Davachi, L. (2014) *Neuron* **81**, 1179–1189.

100. Maguire, E.A., Gadian, D.G., Johnsrude, I.S., Good, C.D. et al. (2000) *Proc. Natl. Acad. Sci. USA* **97**, 4398–4403.

101. Woollett, K. and Maguire, E.A. (2011) *Curr. Biol.* **21**, 2109–2114.

102. Woollett, K., Spiers, H.J., and Maguire, E.A. (2009) *Phil. Trans. R. Soc. B: Biol. Sci.* **364**, 1407–1416.

103. Schinazi, V.R., Nardi, D., Newcombe, N.S., Shipley, T.F. et al. (2013) *Hippocampus* **23**, 515–528.

104. Astur, R.S., Taylor, L.B., Mamelak, A.N., Philpott, L. et al. (2002) *Behav. Brain Res.* **132**, 77–84.

105. Goodrich-Hunsaker, N.J., Livingstone, S.A., Skelton, R.W., and Hopkins, R.O. (2010) *Hippocampus* **20**, 481–491.

106. Goodrich-Hunsaker, N.J. and Hopkins, R.O. (2010) *Behav. Neurosci.* **124**, 405–413.

107. Bohbot, V.D., Kalina, M., Stepankova, K., Spackova, N. et al. (1998) *Neuropsychologia* **36**, 1217–1238.

108. Teng, E. and Squire, L.R. (1999) *Nature* **400**, 675–677.

109. Rosenbaum, R.S., Priselac, S., Kohler, S., Black, S.E. et al. (2000) *Nat. Neurosci.* **3**, 1044–1048.

110. Corkin, S. (2002) *Nat. Rev. Neurosci.* **3**, 153–160.

111. Epstein, R., Graham, K.S., and Downing, P.E. (2003) *Neuron* **37**, 865–876.

112. Epstein, R.A. (2008) *Trends Cogn. Sci.* **12**, 388–396.

113. Kornblith, S., Cheng, X., Ohayon, S., and Tsao, D.Y. (2013) *Neuron* **79**, 766–781.

114. Nadel, L. and Peterson, M.A. (2013) *J. Exp. Psychol. Gen.* **142**, 1242–1254.

115. Mundy, M.E., Downing, P.E., Dwyer, D.M., Honey, R.C. et al. (2013) *J. Neurosci.* **33**, 10490–10502.

116. Hassabis, D., Kumaran, D., and Maguire, E.A. (2007) *J. Neurosci.* **27**, 14365–14374.

117. Swanson, L.W. (2000) *Brain Res.* **886**, 113–164.

118. Murray, E.A. and Wise, S.P. (2004) *Neurobiol. Learn. Mem.* **82**, 178–198.

Chapter 5

The biased-competition memory system of early mammals

Overview

The neocortex evolved in early mammals, along with a high-energy, endo-thermic life that permitted entry into a nocturnal foraging niche. The original neocortex included several agranular prefrontal areas, which used their specialized representations to regulate energy economics through several top-down biases: (1) among neural representations elsewhere that compete to control behavior; (2) toward high-energy foraging when warranted by yet higher-energy expectations; and (3) toward patient foraging when merited by the prediction of specific, high-energy resources in the future. Examples of competing representations include: outcome-directed behaviors versus habits; new, fragile associations versus old, robust ones; and the use of up-to-date versus obsolete contexts. By learning the contexts in which certain representations or foraging strategies should prevail over others—and generating a bias toward them—early mammals could adapt their behavior more effectively than their ancestors could, thereby obtaining and conserving sufficient energy to fuel their costly lives.

A brain the size of a walnut

In a *Far Side®* cartoon by Gary Larson, a human-sized stegosaurus, in the manner of a Royal Air Force officer, addresses a squadron of squamates and other amniotes. "The picture's pretty bleak gentlemen," he intones, "the world's climates are changing, the mammals are taking over, and we all have a brain about the size of a walnut."

That sounds bad: a brain the size of a walnut. No wonder the mammals were taking over. On the other hand, the mammals that were doing the "taking over" had brains considerably smaller than a walnut. Readers might have noticed that in Chapter 2 we placed less emphasis on brain size than discussions of brain evolution commonly do. Analysis of brain size has its place, of course, and an important one. Yet turtle brains and mouse brains do not differ all that much in size, a fact that masks an enormous qualitative difference. Turtle brains, like those of other reptiles, lack a structure that all mammalian brains share: neocortex. As a result, the mammals have "taken over" and other vertebrates have not.

Evolution

Derived traits in mammals

As outlined in Chapter 2 ("Early mammals"), mammals evolved a high-energy life that exploited a nocturnal foraging niche. Many mammalian innovations support either endothermy or high-frequency audition. Adaptations related to endothermy (also known as homeothermy and warm-bloodedness) include hair (pelage), molars (for masticating high-energy foods), and a four-chambered heart (for efficient transfer of oxygen to tissues, also related to high energy needs). Auditory adaptations include external ears (pinnae), inner-ear ossicles, and associated alterations in jaw articulation. Stem mammals also developed mammary glands, of course; otherwise we would call them something else. Other adaptations of the skin, such as sweat and scent glands, function in temperature regulation and communication. The neocortex also emerged some time during the major evolutionary transition that produced early mammals.

Terminology

In this chapter we review evidence that part of the neocortex—areas collectively called the agranular prefrontal cortex—provide a top-down bias among competing behaviors, in part by mediating the competition among and within representational systems that had evolved earlier. Accordingly, we have invented a new name: the biased-competition memory system. The concept of biased competition usually refers to top-down influences over sensory processing[1], often attributed to granular prefrontal areas that evolved in primates (see Chapter 2, "Early primates" and "Anthropoids"). In this chapter we propose that top-down biased competition developed much earlier, in the agranular prefrontal areas shared by all mammals.

We defined the neocortex in Chapter 2, and there we made a special effort to distance our views from those of MacLean and Sanides. According to these often-cited authors, the "transition cortex" or limbic cortex evolved before the more "advanced" neocortical areas. There is no evidence from comparative neuroanatomy to support this idea (see Chapter 2, "Outdated concepts" and "Rings and wrongs"). On the contrary, the comparative evidence indicates clearly that early mammals had homologues of both the "transition" (limbic) areas and the so-called "advanced" areas[2].

As part of our distancing effort, we adopted novel terms for two groups of neocortical areas. With no implications about an evolutionary sequence, we call cortical areas adjacent to allocortex the *ring neocortex* and other parts the *core neocortex* (see Fig. 2.1B). The neocortex thus includes all of the cerebral cortex except allocortical areas: ring neocortex plus core neocortex. Sensory areas make up much of the neocortical core.

The medial part of the ring neocortex includes the infralimbic, prelimbic, anterior cingulate, retrosplenial, and perhaps the medial entorhinal cortex; its lateral component contains the agranular orbitofrontal, agranular insular, perirhinal, and most of the entorhinal cortex (Fig. 5.1B). The agranular prefrontal cortex thus consists of the anterior part of the ring. Not only is the ring neocortex adjacent to allocortex, but it also shares an important characteristic of allocortex: relatively direct projections to the hypothalamus.

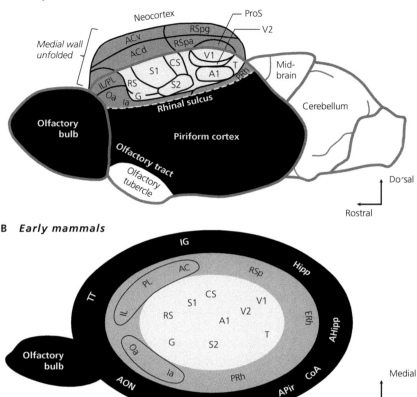

A *Early mammals*

B *Early mammals*

Fig. 5.1 Early mammalian cortex. (A) Reconstruction of an early mammalian brain. Black, allocortex; dark gray, ring neocortex; light gray, core neocortex. The medial neocortex is illustrated as a reflection that maintains continuity with the lateral neocortex. (B) Figurative depiction of an early mammalian brain, in the format of Fig. 2.1(B), showing selected cortical areas. (C) Drawing of the brain of a tenrec, a placental mammal. Note the large proportion of cortex taken up by the lateral allocortex (the piriform area) in (A) and (C). Abbreviations and conventions: A1, primary auditory cortex; ACd and ACv, dorsal (d) and ventral (v) anterior cingulate cortex; AHipp, amygdalohippocampal transition area; AON, anterior olfactory nucleus; APir, amygdalopiriform transition area; CoA, cortical nuclei of the amygdala; CS, caudal somatosensory area; ERh, entorhinal cortex; G, gustatory cortex; Hipp, hippocampal complex; Ia, agranular insular cortex; IG, induseum griseum; IL, infralimbic cortex; Oa, agranular orbitofrontal cortex; PL, prelimbic cortex; PRh, perirhinal cortex; ProS, prostriate cortex; M1, primary motor cortex; RS, rostral somatosensory area; RSpa and RSpg, agranular (a) and granular (g) retrosplenial area; S1, primary somatosensory cortex; S2, secondary somatosensory cortex; T, temporal visual area; TT, tenia tecta; V1, primary visual cortex; V2, secondary visual cortex. (A) Redrawn from Kaas JH. The evolution of brains from early mammals to humans. *Reviews in Cognitive Science* 4:33–45, © 2013, John Wiley & Sons, with permission. (C) Redrawn from Krubitzer L, Künzle H, Kaas J. Organization of sensory cortex in a Madagascan insectivore, the tenrec (*Echinops telfairi*). *Journal of Comparative Neurology* 379:399–414, © 1997, John Wiley & Sons, with permission.

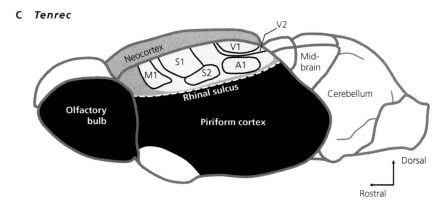

Fig. 5.1 Continued

Early neocortex

Figure 5.1(A) presents a reconstruction of the neocortex in early mammals, based on the areas shared by modern species[2]. The crown members of lineages that branched off early in mammalian history often have brains with relatively little neocortex, as early mammals likely did. For example, the neocortex makes up only 16% of a hedgehog's brain compared with about 74% in anthropoid monkeys. Figure 5.1(C) illustrates the brain of another mammalian species with a small neocortex: the tenrec[3]. The comparative evidence shows that the neocortex began small and enlarged independently in several mammalian lineages.

Advantages of neocortex

The early neocortex, although small, started something big. According to one idea, both the neocortex and allocortex acquire memories, but at different rates[4]. The slower-learning neocortex provides three principal advantages: a larger capacity for memory by virtue of its additional volume; the ability to process and store new specialized representations; and an ability to learn from sporadic events, as opposed to those that occur together in time. As a result, the allocortex (specifically, the hippocampus) better represents current realities and the neocortex better represents the broad statistical regularities of the world, over the long term. This idea underscores a principal theme of this book: New representational systems augment older ones during evolution, and especially during major evolutionary transitions. Augmentation might seem like an unalloyed benefit, but it can create a problem because representational systems can come into conflict.

We propose that the agranular prefrontal cortex contributes to resolving these conflicts. Agranular prefrontal areas emerged among the 20 or so cortical fields that formed the fundamental mammalian inheritance (Fig. 5.1A). New visual, auditory, gustatory, and somatosensory areas of the core neocortex improved the ability of early mammals to represent and store information about stimuli. So, too, did posterior parts of the ring neocortex, such as the perirhinal, entorhinal, and retrosplenial cortex. We return to these nonfrontal areas briefly near the end of this chapter (see "Sensory neocortex") but defer a more detailed consideration of them to Chapters 7 and 10. This chapter focuses instead on the agranular prefrontal cortex and its role in energy management.

Proposal

The agranular prefrontal cortex mediates conflicts: among representations that compete to control behavior; between choices involving high energy expenditure versus energy conservation; and between patient versus urgent foraging. In the ancestors of mammals, representations involving the strongest associations usually controlled behavior because they reached a motor-output threshold faster than competing ones. By generating a top-down bias based on specialized representations of its own, the agranular prefrontal cortex provided early mammals with a mechanism for switching flexibly among foraging strategies—including those guided by relatively weak, recently acquired associations (versus stronger, older ones); current (versus obsolete) contexts; and outcome-directed behaviors (versus habits).

Our proposal used the word "flexibly," which appears commonly in the literature. For example, in Chapter 3 ("Mammals") we mentioned some ways in which mammals react to depleting or diminishing resources more flexibly than other vertebrates. We could continue in that vein, but it would establish little. Experiments purporting to show what a particular species "cannot do" often reflect whether the test (unintentionally) matches a problem that animals face in their natural habitat or fails to do so (equally unintentionally). Given this problem, we do not claim that nonmammalian vertebrates lack a vague trait called "behavioral flexibility." Instead, we suggest that the agranular prefrontal cortex provided early mammals with some advantages in energy management and that these advantages require flexible foraging strategies. Species in other lineages achieve whatever behavioral flexibility they have in some other way.

The findings highlighted in this chapter draw on an extensive neurophysiological and behavioral literature describing the contribution of the agranular prefrontal cortex to adjusting, monitoring, controlling, and enhancing the flexibility of behavior in rodents[5–11]. Instead of attempting a comprehensive review, we select a few studies that shed some light on the adaptive advantages that these areas provide to modern species—in an effort to infer the advantages that they provided to early mammals. Most research on this topic involves rodents, and so this chapter does too. During their independent evolution, both rodents and primates have changed, of course, and neither group resembles their last common ancestor very closely. But for the agranular prefrontal cortex, rodents rule for the time being, although we try to relate the discussion to primates whenever possible.

Connections

Lateral agranular connections

In the spirit of relating the neuroanatomy of rodents and primates, Fig. 5.2(A) shows some connections they share, plotted on a ventral view of the frontal lobe of monkeys. The agranular orbital–insular cortex, also known as the lateral prefrontal cortex in rodents (see

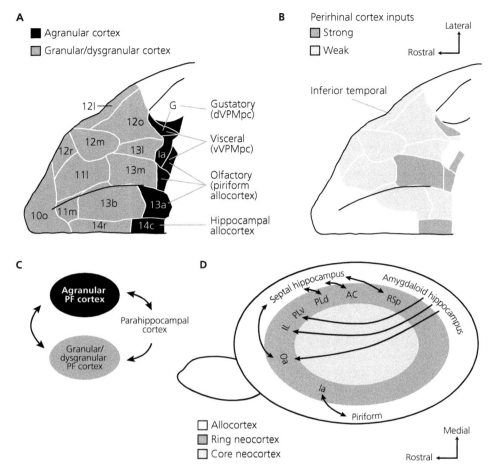

Fig. 5.2 Connections of orbitofrontal cortex. (A) Sensory projections to the agranular (black) orbitofrontal cortex of monkeys, as depicted on a ventral view of the frontal lobe. Rostral is to the left, medial is down. (B) Visual inputs from inferior temporal cortex (indicated by the line) and perirhinal cortex (indicated by shading) to the granular orbitofrontal cortex in monkeys, including relatively weak connections (light shading) and stronger ones (dark shading).
(C) Information flow between the orbitofrontal and parahippocampal areas. (D) Connections between the hippocampus and the agranular prefrontal cortex in rats. Format is as in Fig. 2.1(B), except that ring allocortex is shown in white. Abbreviations: AC, anterior cingulate cortex; dVPMpc and vVPMpc, dorsal (d) and ventral (v) parts of the parvocellular (pc) division of the ventroposteromedial (VPM) nucleus of the thalamus; G, gustatory cortex; Ia, agranular insular cortex; IL, infralimbic cortex; Oa, agranular orbitofrontal cortex; PLd, dorsal part of the prelimbic cortex; PLv, ventral part of the prelimbic cortex; RSp, retrosplenial cortex. (A) Redrawn from Carmichael ST, Price JL. Architectonic subdivision of the orbital and medial prefrontal cortex in the macaque monkey. *Journal of Comparative Neurology* 346:366–402, © 1994, John Wiley & Sons. (B, C) Adapted from Kondo H, Saleem KS, Price JL. Differential connections of the perirhinal and parahippocampal cortex with the orbital and medial prefrontal networks in macaque monkeys. *Journal of Comparative Neurology* 493:479–509, © 2005, John Wiley & Sons.

Table 1.4), receives inputs from several sensory modalities[12]. Olfactory information reaches the lateral prefrontal areas through corticocortical connections from the olfactory bulb; gustatory inputs relay via the brainstem and thalamus to arrive via corticocortical pathways.

The lateral prefrontal cortex also receives some unique sensory inputs (Fig. 5.2) from internal sensors called visceral receptors. They convey itch, warmth, and pain and other homeostatic or metabolic signals, such as those reflecting hypoglycemia, hypoxia, and hypotension, as well as pulmonary, cardiac, and digestive functions[12-18].

Collectively, these three kinds of inputs—olfactory, gustatory, and visceral—place the lateral parts of the agranular prefrontal cortex in a unique position. Olfactory inputs convey information from outside the body, visceral inputs come from the inside, and gustatory inputs provide information about substances entering the body from the outside. These cortical areas therefore process and store information at the heart of foraging. In addition, visual inputs make their way to these areas, especially in primates (Fig. 5.2B). The amygdala and both cholinergic and dopaminergic neurons also send inputs to the lateral prefrontal cortex.

Medial agranular connections

For medial parts of agranular prefrontal cortex, inputs from the hippocampal complex add to those from the amygdala, thalamus, and other sources. Inputs from the hippocampus arrive both directly (Fig. 5.2D) and indirectly via the entorhinal cortex[19,20], among other indirect pathways. We revisit these connections[21], such as the one illustrated in Fig. 5.2(C), in Chapter 11 (see Figs. 11.6 and 11.7).

Projections arising from the medial prefrontal cortex can influence the hippocampus by two main sets of routes: one to the septal hippocampus via the anterior thalamus, the dorsomedial thalamus, or the entorhinal cortex; another to the amygdaloid hippocampus via the nucleus reuniens of the thalamus or the entorhinal cortex[22,23].

Influence on behavior

These connections provide useful information, but they say little about how the agranular prefrontal cortex influences behavior. For placental mammals, traditional thinking invokes projections to the primary motor cortex, but early mammals probably lacked a homologue of this area (Fig. 5.1A). The archetypal architecture of the telencephalon provides greater insight. Figure 5.3 depicts cortex–basal ganglia "loops," which include both the allocortex and neocortex, including the agranular prefrontal cortex. Pallidal outputs from these loops go to the thalamus and then to the cortex, of course, but many also go to brainstem and diencephalic "motor" structures, in the broad sense that includes autonomic, neuroendocrine, and neurosecretory outputs (see Chapter 1, "Brain organization"). Hypothalamic outputs influence all of these unusual "motor" effects, as well as body movements for procreation, foraging, ingestion, and defense. In mammals, the ring neocortex (dark gray in 5.1B and 5.3) adds cortex–basal ganglia "loops" with direct projections to the hypothalamus, like the phylogenetically older "loops" that include the allocortex (black in 5.1B and 5.3)[24].

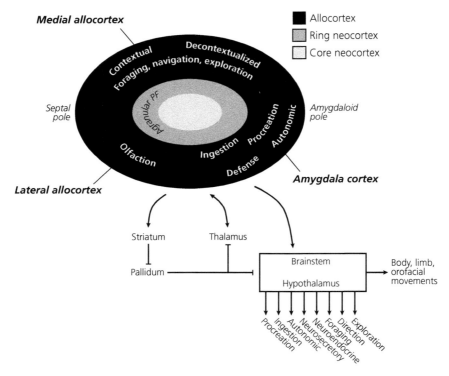

Fig. 5.3 Motor outputs of the telencephalon. Functions for selected allocortical areas, according to the shading convention in Fig. 2.1(B). Excitatory projections are depicted as arrowheads; inhibitory projections are represented by flat line endings.

Figure 5.4 shows autonomic outputs from the ring neocortex and allocortex in rats[25]. The core neocortex influences autonomic outputs less directly than do those two sets of areas. An ability to modulate the balance between energy conservation and energy liberation—the province of the parasympathetic and sympathetic systems, respectively—is a fundamental function of the autonomic nervous system, and the high-energy life that early mammals adopted forever changed the trade-offs involved. So it makes sense that some part of the neocortex regulates that balance, and the ring neocortex seems to perform this function.

This neuroanatomical background sets the stage for the three main parts of this chapter. They deal, respectively, with the medial agranular areas, their interactions with the hippocampus, and the lateral agranular areas (orbital–insular cortex).

Medial agranular areas

A series of experiments have shown that various parts of the medial prefrontal cortex mediate conflicts among competing representations.

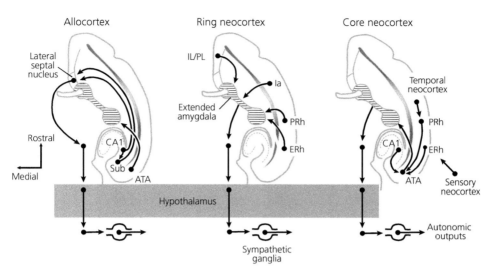

Fig. 5.4 Cortical control of autonomic outputs. Multisynaptic pathways from allocortex and ring neocortex to structures that control autonomic outputs. Hatched area: the extended amygdala. Abbreviations: ATA, amygdaloid cortex transition area; CA1, first cortical field of the hippocampus; ERh, entorhinal cortex; Ia, agranular insular cortex; IL, infralimbic cortex; PL, prelimbic cortex; PRh, perirhinal cortex; Sub, ventral subiculum. Redrawn from Westerhaus MJ, Loewy AD. Central representation of the sympathetic nervous system in the cerebral cortex. *Brain Research* 903:117–27, © 2001, with permission of Elsevier.

Habits versus outcome-directed behavior

A key set of studies demonstrated that two parts of the medial agranular prefrontal cortex, the infralimbic and prelimbic cortex, have different but related functions in rats[26]. Specifically, the infralimbic and prelimbic cortex generate a bias toward habits and outcome-directed behaviors, respectively. The design of these studies made use of the outcome-devaluation procedure described in Chapter 3 ("What happens in instrumental conditioning"), which assesses whether animals make choices based on predicted outcomes. (Recall that we use the term outcome-directed where others use goal-directed.)

Figure 5.5 contrasts the effect of cortical lesions made early in training, as opposed to later, after extensive experience (over-training) had established a habit. In these experiments, rats learned a very simple laboratory behavior: If they pressed one lever (left or right) they got one kind of food; if they pressed the other lever they received a different kind of food. After the rats consumed one of the foods to satiety, they were then allowed to choose one of the levers in extinction, which means that the rats got nothing for pressing either lever. It took the rats a while to recognize this new state of affairs, so their behavior could be measured as they slowly learned that they were wasting their time and effort by pressing a lever.

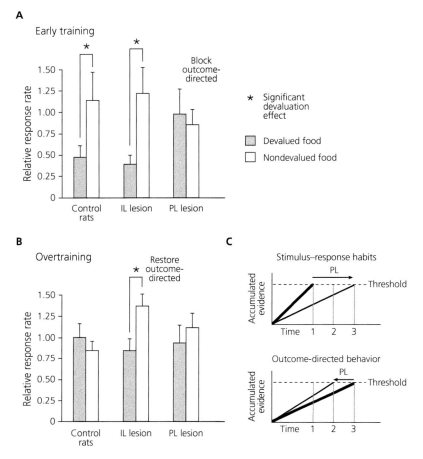

Fig. 5.5 Effects of lesions of the infralimbic and prelimbic cortex on the devaluation effect. (A) Results from relatively inexperienced rats, early in training. The bars show lever-pressing rates, as a proportion of baseline lever pressing in all groups. Error bars: standard error. Asterisks show statistically significant effects on lever pressing of devaluing a food by selective satiation. The unfilled bar shows lever pressing associated with the nondevalued food and the gray bar shows lever pressing associated with the devalued food. Abbreviations: IL, infralimbic cortex; PL, prelimbic cortex. (B) Effects of lesions of the medial prefrontal cortex for over-trained rats, in the format of (A). (C) Top: An imaginary habit network that integrates information about the presence of a stimulus linked to the response that it represents. In the presence of the appropriate stimulus, this network quickly reaches threshold (thick line), at time 1. A suppressive signal from the prelimbic cortex (PL) causes that network to reach its threshold more slowly (thin line), at time 3. Bottom: An enhancing signal from the prelimbic cortex causes the network for an outcome-directed behavior to reach its threshold earlier (thin line) than without the bias (thick line), at time 2. With this top-down bias, an outcome-directed behavior occurs at time 2 (thin line); without the bias, a habit occurs at time 1 (thick line). (A, B) Adapted From Killcross S, Coutureau E. Coordination of actions and habits in the medial prefrontal cortex of rats. *Cerebral Cortex* 13:400–8, © 2003, Oxford University Press, with permission.

Figure 5.5(A) shows results for the early stage of training. Control rats slowed their rate of pressing on the lever that produced the devalued food, and rats with lesions of the infralimbic cortex did the same. Both groups tended to press the lever that produced the normally valued food, a change in behavior called the *devaluation effect* (see Chapter 3, "What happens in instrumental conditioning"). Rats with lesions of the prelimbic cortex did not show this effect. Instead, they tended to press both levers at equal rates, indicating that the lesion rendered their choices insensitive to predicted outcomes. In sum, lesions of the prelimbic cortex, but not the infralimbic cortex, impaired outcome-directed behavior early in training. In terms of affirmative functions, these findings indicate that the prelimbic cortex generates a bias toward outcome-directed behavior.

After over-training, control rats did not show a devaluation effect. The over-trained rats performed habits, meaning that they simply responded in a reflex-like manner to the levers without incorporating predicted outcomes into their choices (Fig. 5.5B, left pair of bars). [In Tolman's felicitous phrase, habits result from an "overdose of repetitions" (Tolman[27], p. 207).] After over-training, lesions of the infralimbic cortex decreased the expression of habits (Fig. 5.5B, middle pair of bars), and so the rats reverted to using predicted outcomes to make their choices. Lesions of the prelimbic cortex had no such effect (Fig. 5.5B, right pair of bars). In a complementary experiment, inactivation (as opposed to a permanent lesion) of the infralimbic cortex also reinstated the devaluation effect, which demonstrates the renewed dominance of outcome-directed behavior[28]. In affirmative terms, these findings indicate that the infralimbic cortex generates a bias toward habits.

This line of research shows that, together, the infralimbic and prelimbic cortex regulate the balance between habits and outcome-directed behavior. In these experiments, rats chose among levers, something that is entirely alien to their natural habitat. In that habitat, however, the same parts of medial prefrontal cortex presumably function to adjust foraging choices based on either sensory inputs alone (habits) or based on a combination of predicted outcomes and sensory inputs (outcome-directed behavior). After rats learn what to do in a given foraging context, other areas establish the relevant representations, and lesions of the prelimbic cortex no longer have such a large effect[29].

Figure 5.5(C) illustrates how this bias might work. As an animal's sensory system accumulates evidence for a stimulus that triggers a response (an S–R habit), at some point the integrated evidence reaches a threshold for action. According to our proposal, the prelimbic cortex either suppresses activity in S–R networks (Fig. 5.5C, top) or accentuates activity in networks that link the same stimulus to both a response and a predicted outcome (Fig. 5.5C, bottom). As a result, the outcome-directed behavior can reach its threshold first. Presumably, the infralimbic cortex has the opposite influence.

For heuristic purposes, Fig. 5.6(A) plots these conclusions onto drawings of a monkey brain, despite the fact that all these results come from rodents. We do this for two reasons: to correct a misunderstanding about homologies and to combine results from the cortex and basal ganglia. The basal ganglia results indicate that a dorsomedial part of the rat striatum subserves outcome-directed behavior and a dorsolateral part subserves

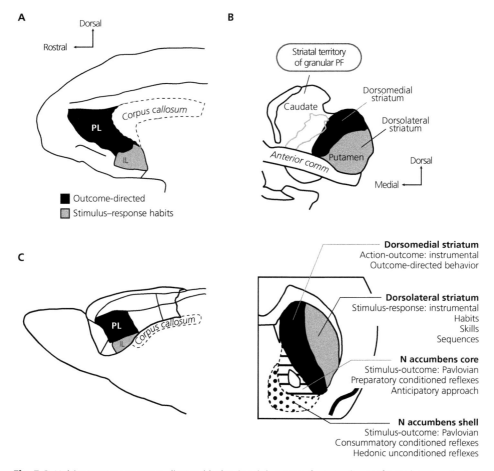

Fig. 5.6 Habits versus outcome-directed behavior. (A) Areas of agranular prefrontal cortex that contribute biases toward habits (gray shading) or outcome-directed behavior (black shading), transposed from the rat results illustrated in (C, left). (B) Striatal nuclei that contribute biases toward habits (gray shading) or outcome-directed behavior (black shading), transposed from the rat results illustrated in (C, right). New granular prefrontal areas evolved in anthropoid primates, which project to the caudate nucleus. (C) Rat results that serve as the basis for (A) and (B). Abbreviations: comm, commissure; IL, infralimbic cortex; PL, prelimbic cortex. (C, right) Redrawn from Yin HH, Ostlund SB, Balleine BW. Reward-guided learning beyond dopamine in the nucleus accumbens: the integrative functions of cortico-basal ganglia networks. *European Journal of Neuroscience* 28:1437–48, © 2008, John Wiley & Sons, with permission.

habits[30–32], much like the prelimbic and infralimbic cortex, respectively. We summarize these findings in Chapter 12 ("Rodents"). Here we simply illustrate the conclusions: for the rodent studies that generated them (Fig. 5.6C) and, by inference, for primates (Fig. 5.6A, B). With these findings in mind, some experts assume that the dorsomedial striatum of rats is homologous with the head of the caudate nucleus of primates[33]. This assumption is understandable, but wrong. The comparative neuroanatomy shows that the development of new parts of the prefrontal cortex in primates led to new cortex–basal ganglia "loops" and new parts of the striatum (see Chapter 2, "New cortical areas"). Like the granular prefrontal cortex, the head of the caudate nucleus is a derived trait of primates. Because rats have no homologue of the head of the caudate nucleus, striatal regions that are homologous to each other in rats and monkeys appear to be shifted laterally and ventrally in primates (Fig. 5.6B)[34]. We revisit this topic in Chapter 12 ("Rodents").

Pavlovian versus instrumental memories

In addition to outcome-directed behaviors and habits, other representations "compete" to control behavior. In Chapter 3 ("What happens in instrumental conditioning") we touched briefly on interactions between Pavlovian and instrumental memories. When Pavlovian memories conflict with instrumental ones, researchers sometimes construe their subjects as "misbehaving." Evidence discussed later in this chapter (see "Competing memories") implicates the medial prefrontal cortex and the hippocampus in mediating the competition between these two kinds of conditioned associations.

Extrinsic versus intrinsic coordinate frames

Another kind of conflict concerns navigation based on extrinsic versus intrinsic coordinates, often called allocentric and egocentric behavior, respectively. In one experiment, extrinsic olfactory guidance was pitted against intrinsic guidance. Some rats learned extrinsic guidance first, whereas others initially learned intrinsic guidance. After learning both guidance rules, inactivation of the medial prefrontal cortex impaired only the one learned most recently[35,36]. This impairment did not result from general "perseveration" because the same lesion had no effect on switching between olfactory stimuli in a reversal task. Taken together, these results suggest a selective impairment on switching between navigational frames.

A related experiment contrasted intrinsic and extrinsic guidance using visual cues[37]. To obtain food in this experiment, rats had to either turn toward a given arm of a plus maze (Fig. 5.7A, upper left) or turn in a given direction relative to their body (Fig. 5.7A, lower right). As we discussed in Chapter 4 ("The cognitive map through history"), the use of extrinsic guidance involves the place rule, like the example in Fig. 4.2. The use of intrinsic guidance involves the "response" rule, although this term can be a little confusing because the place rule might also involve "responses" (to extramaze cues, for example). Accordingly, we prefer to discuss these results in terms of coordinate frames, intrinsic versus extrinsic guidance, instead of "response" versus place rules.

In these experiments, two groups of rats learned both intrinsic and extrinsic guidance rules, but in a different order[37]. Inactivation of the medial prefrontal cortex had no effect on learning to navigate in the second, conflicting coordinate frame, at least not at first. The next day, however, these rats used the more recently learned coordinate frame more poorly than controls, whichever one it was. When faced with competition from older memories, therefore, newer ones appeared to lose the competition. Put another way, older

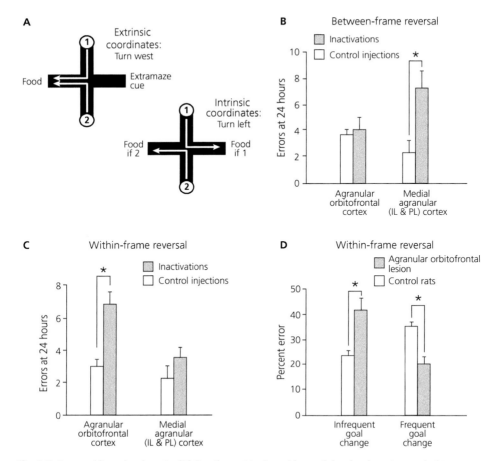

Fig. 5.7 Reversal learning in rats. (A) For the extrinsic-guidance (place) rule, rats needed to turn away from the extramaze cue regardless of starting position (1 or 2). For the intrinsic-guidance ("response") rule, rats executed a motor program as they progressed through the maze. (B) Effects of lesions of the agranular prefrontal cortex on reversals between coordinate frames. (Recall that we use the term lesion for any manipulation that disrupts the function of a brain structure.) (C) Effects of lesions of the agranular prefrontal cortex on reversal of goals within a given coordinate frame. (D) Effect of lesions of the agranular orbitofrontal cortex on reversals within an extrinsic coordinate frame, from a different experiment than (A–C). In an eight-arm radial-arm maze, rats began at one of three starting points and learned to find food at a particular extrinsic location. Then the location of the food was changed either frequently (three to seven trials per goal location) or infrequently (more than 20 trials per goal location). (B, C) Adapted from Young JJ, Shapiro ML. Double dissociation and hierarchical organization of strategy switches and reversals in the rat PFC. *Behavioral Neuroscience* 123:1028–35, © 2009, American Psychological Association, with permission. (D) Adapted from Riceberg JS, Shapiro ML. Reward stability determines the contribution of orbitofrontal cortex to adaptive behavior. *Journal of Neuroscience* 32:16402–9, © 2012, Society for Neuroscience, with permission.

memories appeared to cause proactive interference that made it difficult to use newer memories after some time (a day or so) had elapsed.

Subsequent experiments[38] confirmed these results and extended them by showing that rats with inactivations confined to the prelimbic cortex had impairments in retaining the new rule after switching between intrinsic and extrinsic coordinate frames (Fig. 5.7D). This lesion did not affect switching within a given coordinate frame, however (Fig. 5.7C). Thus the prelimbic cortex does not seem to underlie switching among choices per se, a conclusion that agrees with the results from the olfactory reversal task mentioned earlier. Instead, this agranular prefrontal area seems to be necessary for generating a bias toward one navigational guidance rule or another[38] and for learning the context for using newly learned, fragile memories to guide behavior, as opposed to older, robust ones[37]. In the next section ("New versus old memories") we examine this conflict in more detail.

In a separate experiment, neuronal activity in the prelimbic and infralimbic cortex signaled a transition between guidance rules[37]. Discharge rates increased earlier in the prelimbic cortex than in the infralimbic cortex as rats learned a new guidance rule, and only appeared in the infralimbic cortex after the rats had learned to switch between the two coordinate frames proficiently. These findings support the idea that these areas mediate the competition between guidance rules and also that the infralimbic cortex generates a bias toward habits.

New versus old memories

The infralimbic cortex contributes to other top-down biases as well. One example involves extinction learning. As explained in Chapter 3, extinction generally masks older behaviors rather than "erasing" the representations underlying them. Accordingly, older representations, which predict that a particular outcome will occur, compete with newer ones that predict the opposite.

Sometimes, after extinction learning has occurred, animals express the original, masked representations again, a phenomenon called spontaneous recovery or reinstatement depending on the details[39]. (Recovery occurs as a function of time while reinstatement follows presentations of the outcome alone.) In one experiment, lesions of the infralimbic cortex had no effect on extinction learning per se (Fig. 5.8A), but did alter the subsequent re-expression of the original memories. Compared with control subjects, rats with lesions of the infralimbic cortex showed greater spontaneous recovery (Fig. 5.8B) and reinstatement (Fig. 5.8C) at an early stage of training[40]. As extinction strengthened with over-training, the lesion-induced impairment became less pronounced[41]. These findings indicate that an intact infralimbic cortex generates a bias toward newer representations at a time when they remain relatively weak. Without the influence of this area rats behave less flexibly, as if bound to their older, better-established representations.

Additional experiments have shown that this influence is a general one and not unique to extinction learning. In one study, the infralimbic cortex was found to make a similar contribution when a given stimulus participated in conflicting associations. An example from Pavlovian learning involved conditioned inhibition[42], and one from instrumental

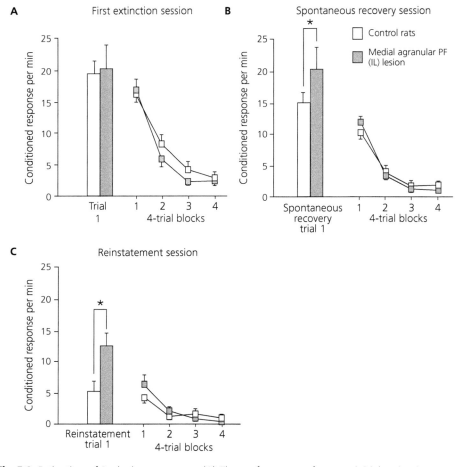

Fig. 5.8 Extinction of Pavlovian responses. (A) The performance of rats on initial extinction training. (B) Effect of medial prefrontal cortex lesions on spontaneous recovery during the next day's testing session (bars), followed by additional extinction training. (C) Effect of medial prefrontal cortex lesions on reinstatement, which followed presentation of the outcome. Adapted from Rhodes SEV, Killcross S. Lesions of rat infralimbic cortex enhance recovery and reinstatement of an appetitive Pavlovian response. *Learning and Memory* 11:611–6, © 2004, reproduced with permission from John Wiley & Sons.

conditioning involved reversal learning[11]. In both cases, when a new behavior conflicted with an older one, the infralimbic cortex provided a bias toward the new. Similar results have come from the study of fear conditioning, for both the acquisition and retention of freezing responses[43].

From these experiments, the infralimbic cortex seems to emit a top-down bias toward newer, fragile behaviors, and this influence becomes especially prominent when previously established memories interfere with newer ones. Its bias toward habits (Fig. 5.5B) is difficult to reconcile with this idea, however, because habits usually involve old, sturdy representations and not new, fragile ones. Perhaps the later-developing S–R habits can be viewed as newer memories subject to proactive interference from the initial outcome-directed (S–R–O) memories. Other functions of the infralimbic cortex also seem to violate a simple summary in terms of a bias toward new behaviors. In a study of Pavlovian trace conditioning in monkeys, the conditioned and unconditioned stimuli were separated by a stimulus-free delay period. Lesions of the infralimbic cortex blocked the sustained autonomic arousal that otherwise occurred during this delay period, although autonomic responses during the stimulus period developed normally[44]. Similar results have been reported for trace cardiovascular conditioning in rats with medial prefrontal cortex lesions[45]. Perhaps these findings reflect the fact that in natural foraging the disappearance of resources (or stimuli linked to them) often indicates that they have ceased to be available. In the trace-conditioning experiment, the short-term memory of a recent conditioned stimulus conflicted with the sensory state during the delay period, during which the monkeys saw no conditioned stimulus. Perhaps the infralimbic cortex generated a bias toward the memory-driven response (arousal) during the delay period, as opposed to the sensation-driven one (no arousal). Regardless, like a bias toward habits, these results do not seem to be consistent with a bias toward new behaviors. So perhaps the infralimbic cortex generates several biases, including some that regulate autonomic outputs based on memories, some that favor habits, and some that serve to overcome proactive interference and thus favor newer memories over older ones.

Learned versus innate behaviors

In addition to the biases discussed thus far, lesions of the medial prefrontal cortex have also impaired the ability of rats to surmount innate behaviors.

In a matching-to-position experiment, rats were required to overcome an innate trait known as spontaneous alternation or spontaneous exploration, in which they tend to avoid a recently explored location. After a sample trial, the rats needed to choose between two foraging locations. To obtain food, they had to return to the location that contained food on the sample trial. Despite their innate tendency toward spontaneous alternation, control rats mastered the matching-to-position task readily. A combined lesion of the prelimbic and infralimbic cortex, however, caused an impairment on this task[46]. Importantly, this lesion did not have the same effect on the nonmatching-to-position task, which rewards spontaneous alternation. These findings suggest that the medial prefrontal cortex regulates competition between learned and innate behaviors as well as among learned behaviors.

Competing cost estimates

When animals choose among actions, they need to take into account both costs and benefits. Experiments usually focus on two kinds of costs: effort and delay.

Another part of the medial prefrontal cortex, the anterior cingulate cortex, contributes to biasing behaviors according to effort costs[47–49]. In one experiment, rats chose between a larger and a smaller amount of food, and control rats readily climbed over a demanding barrier in order to obtain the larger amount. Rats with lesions of the anterior cingulate cortex, however, contented themselves with the smaller outcome, which was less costly but also less valuable. Rats with these lesions would only climb over the barrier when the size of the larger food outcome increased dramatically[47]. Rats with lesions of the anterior cingulate cortex seem to overestimate effort costs relative to benefits. Recast in terms of affirmative functions, these findings indicate that an intact anterior cingulate cortex biases animals toward greater energy expenditure in order to obtain a highly valuable outcome, which can be described as an increase in effort tolerance.

Some evidence indicates that the anterior cingulate cortex exerts this bias specifically when animals face a choice among two or more options. When rats simply needed to make a single action to gain access to food, such as pressing a lever, lesions of this area had little effect[48]. This finding demonstrates that damage to the anterior cingulate cortex does not render rats unmotivated. Instead, it seems to become important when animals need to overcome a tendency to conserve energy. Recent work on primates has extended this idea to the cognitive effort needed to solve challenging problems[50].

In a neurophysiological experiment, cells in the anterior cingulate cortex were found to encode different kinds of costs separately. Only a few of these neurons encoded value in the way expected for a general cost–benefit analysis, which would combine effort and delay costs. Most cells instead selectively encoded one or the other[51]. Neurons in two parts of the granular frontal cortex, the dorsolateral prefrontal cortex and the granular orbitofrontal cortex, encoded delay costs with little encoding of effort costs, and cingulate motor areas had the opposite characteristics. These results point to specializations for different cost factors, with medial prefrontal areas emphasizing effort costs and lateral prefrontal areas stressing delay costs. We return to the latter later (see "Lateral agranular areas").

Summary

Table 5.1 summarizes the biases generated by the medial agranular areas. The anterior cingulate cortex provides a bias toward greater energy expenditure, which makes sense in terms of mammalian evolution. Mammals adapted to a high-energy, endothermic life from an ancestral state that depended on extracting energy from external sources, as ectothermic (cold-blooded) animals do today. The expenditure of relatively high levels of energy for yet higher energy gains—effort tolerance—represents a fundamentally mammalian way of life (and, convergently, an avian one as well).

Infralimbic and prelimbic areas contribute top-down biases of a different kind. They appear to work in tandem to bias behavior:

◆ when extrinsic factors (sensory stimuli), alone, guide choices (S–R habits), as opposed to when a combination of extrinsic factors and intrinsic ones guide choices (outcome-directed behaviors);

◆ when extrinsic and intrinsic coordinate frames compete to guide navigation;

◆ when foraging choices depend on newer, weaker behaviors as opposed to older, stronger ones that generate proactive interference;

◆ when learned behaviors conflict with innate ones;

Table 5.1 Behavioral biases from agranular prefrontal areas

Region	Area	Bias	Balance
Medial agranular prefrontal cortex	Anterior cingulate	◆ Toward high-cost–high-benefit actions (effort tolerance)	◆ Expenditure versus conservation of energy
	Prelimbic	◆ Toward choices based on predicted outcomes versus habits (choices dependent solely on external stimuli) ◆ Toward choices in new guidance frames (extrinsic versus intrinsic, for example)	◆ Exploitation versus exploration ◆ Internal versus external contexts ◆ Older, stronger versus newer, weaker memories
	Infralimbic	◆ Toward habits ◆ Toward choices based on new, fragile memories ◆ Toward maintaining autonomic outputs based on predicted (but unseen) outcomes	
Lateral agranular prefrontal cortex	Agranular orbitofrontal	◆ Toward delayed high-value resources when no cue bridges a delay period ◆ Toward recently successful choices (within a guidance frame) when outcomes change infrequently ◆ Toward valuable specific outcomes	◆ Patient versus urgent foraging ◆ Specific versus general foraging
	Agranular insular	◆ Toward delayed high-value resources (contrast effects)	

◆ and, as we discuss later (see "Competing memories"), when Pavlovian approach behavior competes with instrumental responses.

Although Table 5.1 summarizes the biases generated by medial agranular areas, it says nothing about the specialized representations stored there. The experiment on switching between guidance rules, summarized earlier (see "Extrinsic versus intrinsic coordinate frames"), exemplifies this distinction, which can be characterized as one between process and knowledge[52]. In this case, the *process* corresponds to a "downstream" bias and the *knowledge* consists of the representations that these areas store. The experiments in question show that the prelimbic cortex provides a bias that enables rats to stick with a recently successful guidance rule, despite interference from a competing rule that they had acquired first. The question is: What specialized representations trigger this bias? Whatever they are, they do not underlie the ability to learn a guidance rule in the first place or to learn rule–outcome associations in a general sense. Rats with lesions of the prelimbic cortex can do both. Instead, these representations seem to encode associations between the recent success of a guidance rule and the recent positive affect associated with this success, information that the amygdala probably provides. Likewise, the association between a rule and recent success might differ by location or some other aspect of context, information that the hippocampus could provide. If we apply these ideas to the medial prefrontal cortex, as a whole, its specialized representations appear to consist of knowledge about the recent success of a behavior or guidance rule, the affective concomitants of this success, and the behavioral context in which these successes occurred.

This idea points to a role for inputs from the amygdala and the hippocampus in establishing the specialized representations stored and processed in the medial prefrontal cortex. We addressed some likely contributions of the amygdala in Chapter 3 ("What happens in Pavlovian conditioning" and "What happens in instrumental conditioning"); we now bring the hippocampus into the discussion.

Medial prefrontal–hippocampus interactions

Lesion studies in rodents have demonstrated that the hippocampus and medial prefrontal cortex need to interact in order to establish and retrieve certain kinds of representations.

Object–place, object–order conjunctions

Some of the key experiments have involved cross-disconnection lesions, a procedure explained in Chapter 1 ("Lesion effects"). In one such experiment, removal of the hippocampus in one hemisphere was combined with removal of either the medial prefrontal cortex or the perirhinal cortex in the other hemisphere[53]. As a control procedure, lesions were made in the same hemisphere.

Figure 5.9(A) shows the stimulus arrangement for two tests of memory, both of which yielded negative results in these experiments (no impairment). In the top row, rats inspected a sample array that consisted of two identical objects. In a subsequent test, they demonstrated their prior experience with the sample object by exploring the novel object (arrow), a behavior described earlier as spontaneous exploration or spontaneous alternation. In the bottom row of Fig. 5.9(A), the novel aspect of the stimulus array was the fact that one object appeared at a novel place (arrow) during the test compared with the sample. Disconnecting the medial prefrontal cortex or the perirhinal cortex from the hippocampus did not affect the performance of the rats on either of these tests (not illustrated)[53], which shows that the subjects could still detect the novelty of objects and their locations.

The same disconnection lesions, in contrast, caused a severe impairment on similar tasks that involved either object–place or object–order conjunctions. In Fig. 5.9(B, C), schematics of the stimulus arrays for both tasks appear above the results. For the object-in-place task (Fig. 5.9B), the same four objects appeared during the sample and test phases, but two of them exchanged locations. Rats with lesions confined to one hemisphere performed this task normally, but those with crossed-disconnection lesions had a severe impairment. The temporal-order task yielded a similar result (Fig. 5.9C). These

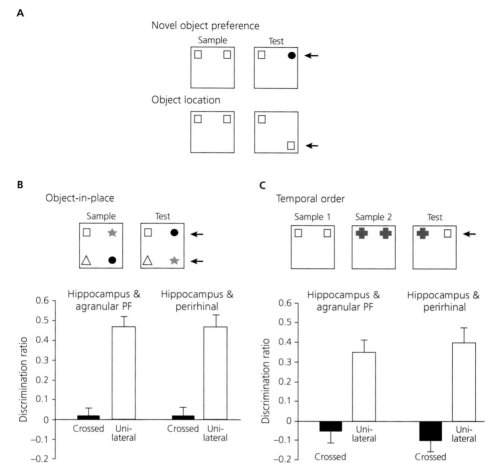

Fig. 5.9 Spontaneous exploration in rats. (A) Depiction of the arena and stimuli used in two tasks, each with the sample period to the left and the test period to the right. The arrows show the novel stimulus or location in the test phase for each task. (B) Effects of unilateral and crossed-disconnection (crossed) lesions of the hippocampus and either the medial agranular prefrontal cortex (left) or the perirhinal cortex (right) on the object-in-place task, illustrated immediately above the bar plots. The arrows show the object–location conjunctions having relatively greater novelty. The bars represent the relative frequency of spontaneous exploration of the novel conjunctions versus the familiar conjunctions. Error bars: standard error. (C) Results from the temporal-order task in the format of (B). Adapted from Barker GR, Warburton EC. When is the hippocampus involved in recognition memory? *Journal of Neuroscience* 31:10721–31, © 2011, Society for Neuroscience, with permission.

findings show that the hippocampus must interact with the medial prefrontal cortex and the perirhinal cortex, two parts of the neocortical ring, in order for rats to use object–place and object–order conjunctions to guide foraging choices.

Object–place–context conjunctions

In a related experiment, rats began each sample run at the origin of an E-maze[54]. From this vantage point, they saw two objects, each in a particular place, and the texture of the maze floor established a context. Later, the rats saw one of the two objects again, along with a novel one. Control rats tended to spend more time with the novel object: spontaneous exploration again. By manipulating objects, places, and maze-floor contexts, these variables could be studied alone or in various combinations. Lesions of the fornix, which disrupted connections between the medial prefrontal cortex and the hippocampal complex (among other structures), reduced spontaneous exploration when it required object–place–context conjunctions, although the rats recognized the objects normally[55]. The effects of fornix lesions in other studies has ruled out an impairment in either place or contextual representations alone[55]. Taken together, these findings suggest that hippocampus–prefrontal interactions support integrated object–place–context memories or that some other fornix-mediated connection does so. Recall from Chapter 4 ("Scene memory") that fornix lesions in monkeys caused an impairment in choosing an object-like stimulus embedded in a background scene.

Context information provided by the hippocampus

Crossed-disconnection and fornix lesions disrupt hippocampus–prefrontal interactions in both directions and throughout each postsurgical test session. Optogenetic inactivations, in contrast, can specifically eliminate interactions in the hippocampus-to-prefrontal cortex direction, as well as during specific parts of each session.

In one experiment using this method, mice first learned to perform a T-maze version of the spatial nonmatching-to-position task[56,57], as explained earlier (see "Learned versus innate behaviors"). A sample run revealed the location of food in one arm of the maze, and, after a delay, the mice could find food only in the other arm of the maze during a choice run. (Fornix lesions caused an impairment on this task in monkeys, as illustrated in Fig. 4.10.) After training, the investigators used optical stimulation to inactivate inputs from the hippocampus to the medial prefrontal cortex during the sample run, the choice run, or throughout the task. Inactivation during the sample run impaired performance, but inactivation at other times did not. Sample-run inactivation also disrupted the discharge synchrony between neurons in the medial prefrontal cortex and the amygdaloid (ventral) hippocampus, which was highest during sample runs, especially for correct choices. On trials without inactivation of inputs from the hippocampus, the location of the sample could be decoded from neuronal activity in the medial prefrontal cortex. On trials with these inactivations, the location of the sample could not be decoded.

These results show that inputs to the medial prefrontal cortex from the hippocampus conveyed information about object–place conjunctions in this experiment. Once the medial prefrontal cortex established these representations, which occurred during the sample run, inputs from the hippocampus were no longer needed[56].

A related experiment made use of an elevated plus-maze to manipulate anxiety[58]. This type of maze has wall-free arms that provoke anxiety, in contrast to more protected, tunnel-like arms. Although this anxiety has been interpreted in terms of a fear of falling, the more likely explanation involves the vulnerability of fossorial rodents to predation in an open, unfamiliar foraging field, as opposed to tunnels or familiar fields. Inactivation of inputs from the hippocampus to the medial prefrontal cortex increased the amount of time that mice spent in the wall-free, anxiety-provoking arms. At the same time, neural oscillations in the theta range (4–7 cycles per second) were affected by the inactivation; theta-band oscillations in the hippocampus and medial frontal cortex became less synchronized with each other, and similar changes occurred at the neuronal level. In a safe, familiar field, the same inactivation had no such effects. These findings suggest that inputs from the hippocampus to the medial prefrontal cortex convey contexts that affect behaviors related to predation risks.

Competing memories

In another crossed-disconnection experiment[59], a rat faced a wall with five holes arrayed horizontally. On each trial, a light came on for 500 ms at the back of one of the holes, and the rat had five seconds to poke its snout into the illuminated hole. If it did, food appeared elsewhere in the testing box. Once they had learned this task, control rats usually made one nose-poke in the correct hole and pivoted to obtain the food in about 1.5 seconds. This task was originally called a serial reaction time task, but because that name implies a repeated sequence, we call it the five-choice task instead.

A surgical disconnection of the amygdaloid (ventral) hippocampus and the medial prefrontal cortex (Fig. 5.10A) caused two impairments in this experiment: a weak tendency to perform a nose-poke between trials (not illustrated), and an unnecessary double-poke into the correct hole before pivoting to retrieve the food. The frequency of double-pokes increased to about 60% of the trials over a series of testing sessions (Fig. 5.10B, solid line).

These findings have been interpreted in terms of "behavioral inhibition," failures of which are said to lead to "compulsive" or "impulsive" behaviors. To understand these findings in an ecological context, however, we need to go beyond these concepts. First, the idea that the prefrontal cortex or any part of it functions mainly in behavioral inhibition conflicts with a great deal of evidence[60-65]. Second, it is apparent from Fig. 5.10(B) that the full impairment did not appear immediately after the lesion, as one would expect after the removal of an "inhibitory center." Instead, the learning curve illustrated in Fig. 5.10(B) demonstrates that the rats in these experiments learned a new way of performing the task after the lesion. Third, interpretations in terms of psychiatric concepts, such as impulsivity and compulsivity, have little relevance to the natural life of rats. By considering

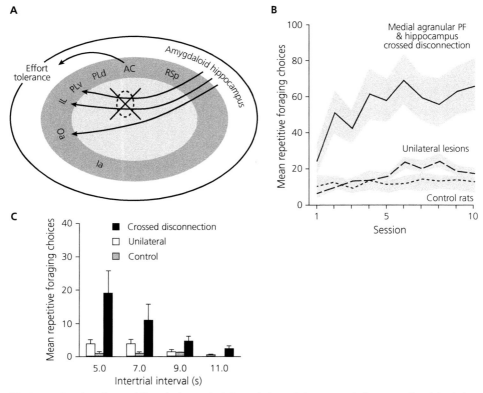

Fig. 5.10 The visually cued five-choice task. (A) Depiction of the crossed-disconnection (×) of the hippocampus from the medial prefrontal cortex, in the format of Figure 2.1B. (B) Effect of the disconnection lesion on the mean frequency of an extra nose-poke. Shading: standard error. (C) Effect of increasing the intertrial interval on the mean frequency of an extra nose-poke. Error bar: standard error. (B) Adapted from Chudasama Y, Doobay VM, Liu Y. Hippocampal-prefrontal cortical circuit mediates inhibitory response control in the rat. *Journal of Neuroscience* 32:10915–24, © Society for Neuroscience, 2012, with permission. (C) Redrawn from Chudasama Y, Doobay VM, Liu Y. Hippocampal-prefrontal cortical circuit mediates inhibitory response control in the rat. *Journal of Neuroscience* 32:10915–24, © 2012, Society for Neuroscience.

these results in an evolutionary context, instead, we can understand them in terms that are important to the success of these animals—and of mammals generally. Instead of a battle between behavioral inhibition and impulsivity, these results reflect two advantages provided to mammals by the medial agranular cortex: (1) regulating the competition between Pavlovian and instrumental memories (see Chapter 3, "What happens in instrumental conditioning") and (2) balancing effort costs with predicted energy gains.

◆ On the first point, consider the fact that Pavlovian associations between beneficial outcomes and either places (holes) or stimuli (lights) conflicted with instrumentally conditioned responses in this version of the five-choice task. Pavlovian approach behavior would have produced a tendency to nose-poke into a "good" place or to move toward the visual cue; instrumental conditioning favored an optimal cost–benefit solution that maximized the reward rate: one nose-poke and a quick turn to obtain the food. As explained earlier (see "Habits versus outcome-directed behavior"), the infralimbic cortex promotes instrumentally acquired habits and the prelimbic cortex promotes instrumental outcome-directed behaviors. After the crossed-disconnection lesion in this experiment, the infralimbic and prelimbic areas that remained intact lost a key input and so their influences surely diminished. This factor alone would have pushed the rats toward Pavlovian approach behavior and away from the instrumentally conditioned response: "misbehavior," "errors," "impulsivity," and "compulsivity," at least as some see it.

♦ On the second point, the results suggest that the same crossed-disconnection lesion disrupted cost–benefit optimization. Viewed in terms of foraging behavior, the lesioned rats could hardly be described as severely impaired, much less deranged or "mentally ill." They simply made an unnecessary nose-poke and thus foraged suboptimally most of the time, which cost them a little more effort and some extra time— about 1 second longer to obtain food. The observation that the lesioned rats increased the number of extra nose-pokes over the first few testing sessions (Fig. 5.10B) indicates that they learned a new balance between estimated costs and benefits. So, too, does the finding that increasing the intertrial interval reduced the impairment (Fig. 5.10C). The relative cost of a 1-second delay in obtaining food decreased as the intertrial interval lengthened.

Thus, in addition to disrupting Pavlovian–instrumental biases, medial prefrontal–hippocampus disconnections interfered with biases that optimize cost–benefit trade-offs. In the absence of the usual influences from the infralimbic and prelimbic cortex, an intact bias from the anterior cingulate cortex (see "Competing cost estimates") promoted a degree of tolerance for wasteful nose-pokes.

Current versus obsolete contexts

A recent neurophysiological and behavioral study has revealed some additional aspects of medial prefrontal–hippocampus interactions[66]. These experiments employed an item-in-context task that required rats to dig into small cups to obtain food. The test items consisted of an odor plus the color and texture of the nonfood material in the cups. A context was established by placing the same two test items in boxes with different wallpaper patterns. To obtain food, rats learned to choose one item in the context of the first box (and its wallpaper), but they needed to choose the other item in the context of the second box (and its wallpaper). For example, to get food the rats had to choose cumin-scented sand over some other scent in a box with striped wallpaper. Neural activity was then recorded in the hippocampus before and after pharmacological inactivation of the medial prefrontal cortex.

Although inactivation of the medial prefrontal cortex had little effect on place coding in the hippocampus, it affected the encoding of item–context conjunctions. During the inactivations in this experiment, neurons in the hippocampus that normally signaled only one of two items in a given box came to signal both. This finding supports the idea that the medial prefrontal cortex biases representations of item–context conjunctions in the hippocampus, either by suppressing otherwise valuable item–context representations when they are encountered in a wrong or obsolete context[67], by enhancing one of several competing item–context representations in the correct or up-to-date context, or both. The same inactivations also impaired task performance, which supports the idea that a top-down bias from the medial prefrontal cortex contributes importantly to the behavior.

In a follow-up study, rats explored the context boxes before any items were placed inside[68]. At that time, theta rhythms in the septal (dorsal) hippocampus preceded those in the amygdaloid (ventral) hippocampus, which might have reflected the transfer of context information or perhaps a transition from a small-scale to a large-scale context. After gaining some experience in a particular context box, theta activations in the amygdaloid (ventral) hippocampus, in turn, preceded similar oscillations in the medial prefrontal cortex, consistent with a transfer of context information in that direction. Finally, as the rats explored items in a given context box, theta activations in the medial prefrontal cortex preceded those in the septal hippocampus, as expected for a top-down bias.

In accord with this idea, a neurophysiological experiment in humans found an increase in theta-band coherence between the agranular parts of the medial prefrontal cortex and the hippocampus. Intriguingly, this increased coherence occurred selectively as subjects learned transitive inferences. These results suggested an enhancement in the level of cooperation between the hippocampus and the medial agranular cortex when subjects first integrated individual associations in order to draw a transitive inference[69].

Summary

Prefrontal cortex–hippocampus interactions epitomize what happens when a new representational system augments existing ones. The ancestors of mammals lacked neocortex, and so they lacked a medial prefrontal cortex. Once these areas evolved, however, the hippocampus could supply them with its specialized representations, such as object–place and object–order conjunctions, which convey information about behavioral contexts. In return, the medial prefrontal cortex could use its own specialized representations to generate a bias among competing representations in the hippocampus, such as those involving up-to-date item–context conjunctions versus obsolete ones.

Interactions between the prefrontal cortex and the hippocampus also contribute to regulating the competition between instrumental and Pavlovian memories, as well as to optimizing cost–benefit trade-offs (see "Competing memories").

Almost all of these findings come from rodents, which, unlike primates, only have the agranular parts of the medial prefrontal cortex (see Chapter 2, "Early primates"). However, these areas have retained their connections with the hippocampus in primates (see Chapter 11, "Prefrontal cortex–hippocampus connections"), and we assume that the results in rodents reflect conserved mammalian traits.

Lateral agranular areas

The lateral prefrontal cortex of early mammals included the agranular insular and agranular orbitofrontal cortex: orbital–insular cortex. A series of experiments have shown that these areas represent the specific sensory features of outcomes, such as tastes, smells, and visceral sensations, and thereby play a key role in learning linkages between stimuli and specific outcomes. This knowledge then contributes to a top-down bias that balances "patient" with "urgent" foraging.

Contrast effects

The results of one experiment suggested that rats with lesions of the agranular insular cortex have impairments in recalling tastes. Rats first learned that pressing one lever produced a certain food item, whereas pressing another lever produced a different kind of food[70]. After devaluing one of these two foods, the lesioned rats behaved like control rats: They shifted to the lever producing the alternative, normally valued food. When lever presses ceased to produce any food—the extinction procedure—control rats continued to press the lever associated with the more highly valued food until they stopped pressing the levers altogether. Lesioned rats, in contrast, pressed the two levers equally often until the lever-pressing response was extinguished. This finding indicates that, if they hadn't seen the food recently, the lesioned rats had trouble recalling the specific taste or smell of the food associated with each lever. Another observation led to a similar conclusion; lesions of agranular insular cortex blocked the expression of the mouth and face movements that rats made in anticipation of unpalatable foods or fluids[71,72].

In a related experiment, rats showed a bias against consuming a low-value resource when they could expect a high-value option to come along later, a behavior called the anticipatory contrast effect. In this experiment, rats sampled a fluid with a relatively low concentration of sucrose and then chose whether to continue consuming it or to abstain until a higher-energy (and sweeter) option appeared later. Lesions of the agranular insular cortex eliminated the anticipatory contrast effect[73], so rats with these lesions tended to satiate themselves on the low-value option. Such lesions also blocked the successive negative contrast effect[74], which we described in Chapter 3 ("Mammals") as a derived mammalian trait. Both of these effects involved the rejection of low-energy resources based on the expectation of a specific, high-value resource. The ability to retrieve representations of specific, high-value tastes or smells could have contributed to both of these contrast effects.

Delay tolerance versus intolerance

The remaining part of the lateral prefrontal cortex, the agranular orbitofrontal cortex, biases behavior based on delay costs, among other functions. In an experiment contrasting effort and delay costs, rats had to choose between the two arms of a T-maze[49]. One choice yielded a small amount of some resource immediately, and the other led to a larger amount after a delay. These experiments resembled those on the anticipatory contrast effect, but differed in that the rats could not sample the early, low-value option; they needed to choose in advance. And, like the results on the anticipatory contrast effect, lesions of the lateral prefrontal cortex—in this case of the agranular orbitofrontal cortex— caused an impairment. In both cases, the choices of lesioned rats revealed a degree of delay intolerance (impatience or "impulsivity") compared with control rats. When recast in terms of affirmative functions, these results suggest that the lateral agranular cortex, including its orbitofrontal component, promotes delay-tolerant (patient) foraging. A bias toward patient foraging probably provided advantages to early mammals by maximizing energy consumption in a stable mixture of low- and high-value resources.

Other results, however, have supported the opposite conclusion[75-77]. In these studies, rats with lesions of the orbitofrontal cortex had more delay tolerance (patience) than usual. These findings contradict a simple interpretation of orbitofrontal lesion effects as abnormal impulsivity and indicate instead that the orbitofrontal cortex sometimes promotes delay-intolerant (urgent) foraging. One study attempted to reconcile these conflicting conclusions by appealing to individual differences[78]. Several technical factors might also have contributed to the discrepancy, such as the presentation of equal delay costs at the beginning of each test session and the presence or absence of reward-predictive cues during the delay periods. Indeed, the pattern of findings across studies suggests that the orbitofrontal cortex is necessary for signaling expected outcomes when no external cues bridge a delay period[49], but not when such cues predict an outcome[78,79]. Taken together, these results suggest that the agranular orbitofrontal cortex represents expected outcomes and sometimes uses these representations to generate a bias toward patient or urgent foraging depending on an individual's proclivity and the availability of external cues, among other factors.

In addition to individual differences, species differences can also affect the trade-off between patient and urgent foraging. Two species of New World monkeys, cotton-top tamarins and common marmosets, both consume many foods in their natural habitat, but tamarins eat more insects and marmosets consume more tree gum. Tree gum oozes out slowly and reliably and remains available for a long time. Insects move, often quickly, and so their availability can decrease rapidly. In accord with their dietary preferences, one experiment revealed that gum-loving marmosets had a high level of delay tolerance, and tamarins had very little[80,81]. Assuming that the agranular orbitofrontal cortex plays a conserved role across mammals, relatively small adjustments in its biasing functions can adapt foraging strategies to the dietary preferences of a given species (or an individual). Both patient and urgent foraging strategies can provide advantages in certain circumstances, depending on the dynamics of preferred and fallback resources.

Reversals within a guidance frame

Earlier we discussed experiments in which rats learned to switch between two guidance rules: extrinsic (place) rules to intrinsic ("response") rules or vice versa (see "Extrinsic versus intrinsic coordinate frames"). Inactivation of the prelimbic cortex had no effect on learning a new rule but markedly impaired the retention of that rule a day later (Fig. 5.7B, right)[37,38]. Rats with these inactivations tended to revert to the first-learned rule, presumably because it generated proactive interference with rules learned later. Despite this impairment in switching across guidance rules, the same rats, with the same inactivations of the prelimbic cortex, acquired and retained reversals within either guidance frame normally (Fig. 5.7C, right). Inactivations of the orbitofrontal cortex had the opposite effect. At least for the first few reversals, rats with these inactivations retained a newly acquired goal poorly *within* a given coordinate frame (Fig. 5.7C, left), but behaved normally for reversals *across* intrinsic and extrinsic guidance rules (Fig. 5.7B, left).

Similar results have come from compound discrimination learning. In these experiments, rats had to choose between cups with different combinations of covering materials and digging media, and reversals could be either within or across stimulus dimensions[82]. In this case, nonspatial information provided the guidance frame rather than spatial coordinates.

The impairment that followed lesions of the orbitofrontal cortex also depended on the frequency of reversals[83]. For infrequent reversals, the lesions impaired performance; for highly frequent reversals, the same lesion improved performance (Fig. 5.7D). Recast in terms of affirmative functions, these findings suggest that the orbitofrontal cortex provides an advantage when foraging outcomes change relatively rarely, as exemplified by infrequent reversals within a coordinate frame. In a rat's natural habitat, infrequent goal changes correspond to relatively stable resource conditions in a foraging field, and under such conditions foraging choices probably depend on similarly stable stimulus–outcome representations in the orbitofrontal cortex.

This idea also explains why rats with lesions of the orbitofrontal cortex outperformed control subjects during frequent reversals. Rats with such lesions lost many of their stimulus–outcome representations. With their intact medial prefrontal cortex, they could apply a win–stay strategy unencumbered by obsolete stimulus–outcome representations in the orbitofrontal cortex, which—because they depend on averages over several foraging choices—cannot keep up with frequent reversals. This finding further highlights the importance of competition among representations in the control of behavior, and in this case rats benefited when stimulus–outcome representations lost that competition.

Stimulus–outcome predictions

In support of this idea, another experiment found that rats with lesions of the agranular orbitofrontal cortex more often chose or approached devalued stimuli than did control rats[84–86], which suggested a problem with predicting outcomes based on these stimuli. Likewise, neural activity in this area encoded several features of outcomes, most notably their specific sensory attributes such as taste and smell[87]. In contrast to their disruption of stimulus–outcome memories, lesions of the agranular orbitofrontal cortex left choices based on action–outcome associations intact[88].

Based on these results and others, the idea has arisen that the orbitofrontal cortex (including its agranular part) represents stimulus–outcome associations, whereas the medial prefrontal cortex (and especially the anterior cingulate cortex) represents action–outcome associations[89–91]. We call this idea the stimulus–action dichotomy; it has gained support from studies of Pavlovian contingency degradation, Pavlovian-to-instrumental transfer (PIT), and the differential-outcomes effect in rats[88,92].

The agranular orbitofrontal cortex plays a particularly important role in linking stimuli with the sensory features of outcomes[93,94]. In one experiment, rats learned to expect a particular ("first") food item after a "first" visual stimulus[95]. Later, rats saw this stimulus along with a second visual stimulus, after which a second food item followed. As explained in Box 3.1, the first stimulus fully predicted the first food item, and so rats could not learn the association between the second stimulus and the first food item. They could, however, learn the association between the second stimulus and the second food item. Rats pressed a lever to obtain that second, highly rated food, but did so less frequently after devaluation of that food. This finding demonstrates that they anticipated the specifics of the second food item. Lesions of the agranular orbitofrontal cortex impaired the ability of rats to learn the relationship between the second stimulus and the second food[95]. Because the two foods differed in their taste and smell, this result points to a role for this cortical area in linking sensory cues with the specific features that distinguish potential outcomes from each other.

Relation to primates

The stimulus–action dichotomy has been extended to primates[90]. As we explained in Chapter 2 ("Early primates"), the prefrontal cortex of primates includes both the agranular areas that all mammals share and the granular areas that evolved in primates. So the question becomes: Does the stimulus–action dichotomy, as established for the agranular prefrontal cortex of rodents, apply to the granular prefrontal areas of primates?

Some evidence from monkeys suggests that the answer is no. In one experiment, lesions of the granular orbitofrontal cortex caused an impairment on an *action*–outcome task[96] (see Fig. 6.10); in another, lesions of the anterior cingulate cortex caused an impairment in *object* reversal learning[97]. Furthermore, a number of neurophysiological studies have demonstrated that neurons in the anterior cingulate cortex of monkeys encode the value of visual stimuli[98–100], and brain imaging results in humans have provided support for these findings[101,102]. So the primate anterior cingulate cortex does not seem to be completely specialized for action–outcome associations, and, likewise, the primate orbitofrontal cortex does not seem to have functions specific to stimulus–outcome associations.

Our proposals suggest a way to reconcile these apparent contradictions. In monkeys, the stimulus–outcome[65,103] and action–outcome[96] devaluation tasks both involved a special kind of stimulus as the outcome: a particular food item. Through its interactions with the amygdala, the granular orbitofrontal cortex provides access to the updated value of an outcome's specific sensory features (see Chapter 6, "Orbitofrontal–amygdala interactions"). Furthermore, in monkeys the visual features of these outcomes predominate because of the primate adaptations discussed in Chapter 2 ("Early primates" and "Anthropoids"). According to one view, then, the primate orbitofrontal cortex is indeed specialized for stimulus–outcome memories, as the stimulus–action dichotomy supposes, but in the case of the action–outcome result[96] the stimulus in question was the food item that served as the outcome, especially its visual features. In this case, an action–food object conjunction, represented in the primate orbitofrontal cortex, served as the equivalent of a "stimulus" that accessed the current value of the predicted outcome.

The contribution of the anterior cingulate cortex to object reversal learning in monkeys[97] could also reflect primate specializations. As we explain in Chapter 6, primates evolved a new representational system for grasping and manipulating objects in a visual frame of reference. Accordingly, in the case of the object reversal task[97] perhaps the object information was bound into conjunctions with the actions that could be performed with that object, a concept known as an *affordance* (see Chapter 6, "Affordances"). From this perspective, the impairment on object reversals caused by lesions of the anterior cingulate cortex reflected a problem with affordance–outcome memories, even though the experiment did not require grasping or manipulating objects. In this case, an object–action conjunction, represented in the anterior cingulate cortex, served as the equivalent of an "action" for action–outcome memories.

Summary

The reason for holding on to the stimulus–action dichotomy, despite evidence from monkeys that seems to contradict it, stems from the evolutionary perspective adopted in this book. The stimulus–action dichotomy reflects something fundamental to the life of mammals. The transition from a low-energy, ectothermic life to a high-energy, endothermic one benefited from two capacities: (1) the ability to pursue net energy gains even though they require relatively high energy expenditures, which depends on action–outcome associations; and (2) the ability to make choices that favor higher-energy outcomes even though other outcomes are available, which depends on stimulus–outcome associations.

Table 5.1 summarizes the biases generated by the lateral agranular areas, collectively called the orbital–insular cortex. Efficient foraging requires an accurate prediction of specific outcomes, along with a varying degree of tolerance for delay costs. In some circumstances, the orbital–insular areas provide a bias toward delay tolerance (patient foraging), especially when better outcomes can be expected later. In other circumstances, a bias toward delay intolerance (urgent foraging) is more advantageous. Stimulus–outcome memories also underlie choices made within a guidance frame—intrinsic versus extrinsic frames, for example—especially in foraging fields with moderate levels of resource stability (characterized by low-frequency reversals in the laboratory).

Sensory neocortex

The chapter has concentrated on the rostral part of the ring neocortex: the agranular prefrontal cortex. But early mammals also evolved the caudal ring neocortex as well as the core neocortex (Fig. 5.1B). We touch on these areas only briefly because their adaptive advantages and specialized representations seem relatively straightforward.

In the caudal ring neocortex, the perirhinal and parahippocampal areas contribute to object representations and the representations of spatial layouts, respectively. We deal with the perirhinal cortex in detail in Chapter 7 ("The perception–memory dichotomy"). The retrosplenial cortex contributes to transforming spatial information between intrinsic and extrinsic coordinate frames and to representing spatial layouts[104,105]. The entorhinal cortex plays a role in representing the progression of an animal through space, among other functions. In Chapter 10 ("A medial network") we take up the idea that the medial parts of the posterior ring—including the retrosplenial, parahippocampal, and medial entorhinal cortex—augment the navigation system.

Many parts of the core neocortex have sensory functions, and this is especially true for the areas inherited from early mammals. The primary visual cortex is homologous in mammals and modern reptiles[106], but seems to be the exception. The remaining core neocortical areas evolved *de novo* in mammals. They process and store specialized sensory representations, including visual–auditory and visual–somatosensory conjunctions, along with conjunctions restricted to a single sensory modality.

Conclusions

Advantages

Early mammals were endothermic (warm-blooded) animals that consumed much more energy than their ancestors did: perhaps ten-fold more. In the ancestral condition, the strongest representations usually prevailed because they reached a threshold for producing motor outputs faster than those based on weaker associations (Fig. 5.5C). The kinds of memories that controlled behavior therefore changed only slowly.

Accordingly, early mammals benefited from brain mechanisms that could quickly overcome well-established—but obsolete—representations that would otherwise control behavior. They also benefitted from an ability to surmount the ancestral tendency to conserve energy when greater exertion yielded a net energy gain, as well as from a capacity for rejecting lower-value options in favor of patient foraging for higher-value ones—depending on circumstances as well as on differences among species and individuals.

The proposal in this chapter says that a particular part of the neocortex provided these advantages: the agranular prefrontal cortex. By learning which representations and guidance rules should predominate in a given context and generating a top-down bias that favored them, early mammals could gather enough energy to generate heat internally and thereby circumvent their ancestors' need to absorb energy from warm surroundings. As a result of these and other adaptations—such as those involved in energy extraction and conservation (molars and hair, for example)—early mammals could forage nocturnally and in other cool conditions.

Walnut brains and nutty ideas

In the *Far Side*® cartoon mentioned earlier (see "A brain the size of a walnut"), a stegosaurus lamented his lame brain: just 80 grams in a 3-million-gram body. A typical macaque monkey, in contrast, has a larger brain in a body of just a few thousand grams. The stegosaurus expressed concern about whether animals with a walnut-sized brain could ward off the coming "age of mammals." He should have worried more about the neocortex.

In Chapter 2 ("Outdated concepts") we mentioned the fascination of popular science with "reptilian brains." A recent example from the Canadian Broadcasting Corporation went like this:

> The "lizard brain" is a catch-all term for the areas of our brain that developed between 500 million and 150 million years ago and are primarily responsible for instinct, emotion and recording memories, as well as visceral feelings that influence or even direct our decisions.
>
> The neocortex, on the other hand, is the area of our brain responsible for reason, language, imagination, abstract thought and consciousness. Scientists say the neocortex has only been around for two or three million years.
>
> Luksic and Howell (2014)[107]

Even the stegosaurus would have known better, and he had a brain the size of a walnut. Although "scientists say" many astounding things, it is doubtful that any of them has ever claimed an origin for neocortex as recently as 2–3 million years ago, given that 200 million is closer to the truth.

Most research on top-down biased competition concentrates on the sensory representations that underlie perception[1]. In this chapter we have proposed that the prefrontal cortex also directs a top-down bias toward representations that compete to control behavior. Representations of actions also compete with each other, as we explain in Chapter 6.

References

1. Desimone, R. and Duncan, J. (1995) *Annu. Rev. Neurosci.* **18**, 193–222.
2. Kaas, J.H. (2013) *Wiley Interdiscip. Rev. Cogn. Sci* .**4**, 33–45.
3. Krubitzer, L., Künzle, H., and Kaas, J. (1997) *J. Comp. Neurol.* **379**, 399–414.
4. McClelland, J.L., McNaughton, B., and O'Reilly, R. (1995) *Psychol. Rev.* **102**, 419–457.
5. Narayanan, N.S., Cavanagh, J.F., Frank, M.J., and Laubach, M. (2013) *Nat. Neurosci.* **16**, 1888–1895.
6. Narayanan, N.S. and Laubach, M. (2008) *J. Neurophysiol.* **100**, 520–525.
7. Newman, L.A., Creer, D.J., and McGaughy, J.A. (2015) *J. Physiol. Paris* **109**, 95–103.
8. Durstewitz, D., Vittoz, N.M., Floresco, S.B., and Seamans, J.K. (2010) *Neuron* **66**, 438–448.
9. Robbins, T.W. (2000) *Exp. Brain Res.* **133**, 130–138.
10. Brown, V.J. and Bowman, E.M. (2002) *Trends Neurosci.* **25**, 340–343.
11. Chudasama, Y. and Robbins, T.W. (2003) *J. Neurosci.* **23**, 8771–8780.
12. Ray, J.P. and Price, J.L. (1992) *J. Comp. Neurol.* **323**, 167–197.
13. Yaxley, S., Rolls, E.T., and Sienkiewicz, Z.J. (1990) *J. Neurophysiol.* **63**, 689–700.
14. Zhang, Z.H., Dougherty, P.M., and Oppenheimer, S.M. (1998) *Brain Res.* **796**, 303–306.
15. King, A.B., Menon, R.S., Hachinski, V., and Cechetto, D.F. (1999) *J. Comp. Neurol.* **413**, 572–582.
16. Craig, A.D. (2002) *Nat. Rev. Neurosci.* **3**, 655–666.
17. Saper, C.B. (2002) *Annu. Rev. Neurosci.* **25**, 433–469.

18. Drewes, A.M., Dimcevski, G., Sami, S.A., Funch-Jensen, P. et al. (2006) *Exp. Brain Res.* **174**, 443–452.

19. Barbas, H. and Blatt, G.J. (1995) *Hippocampus* **5**, 511–533.

20. Muñoz, M. and Insausti, R. (2005) *Eur. J. Neurosci.* **22**, 1368–1388.

21. Kondo, H., Saleem, K.S., and Price, J.L. (2005) *J. Comp. Neurol.* **493**, 479–509.

22. Aggleton, J.P. (2011) *Neurosci. Biobehav. Rev.* **36**, 1579–1596.

23. Prasad, J.A. and Chudasama, Y. (2013) *J. Neurosci.* **33**, 8494–8503.

24. Swanson, L.W. (2000) *Brain Res.* **886**, 113–164.

25. Westerhaus, M.J. and Loewy, A.D. (2001) *Brain Res.* **903**, 117–127.

26. Killcross, S. and Coutureau, E. (2003) *Cereb. Cortex* **13**, 400–408.

27. Tolman, E.C. (1948) *Psychol. Rev.* **55**, 189–208.

28. Coutureau, E. and Killcross, S. (2003) *Behav. Brain Res.* **146**, 167–174.

29. Ostlund, S.B. and Balleine, B.W. (2005) *J. Neurosci.* **25**, 7763–7770.

30. Yin, H.H., Knowlton, B.J., and Balleine, B.W. (2004) *Eur. J. Neurosci.* **19**, 181–189.

31. Yin, H.H., Ostlund, S.B., Knowlton, B.J., and Balleine, B.W. (2005) *Eur. J. Neurosci.* **22**, 513–523.

32. Yin, H.H., Knowlton, B.J., and Balleine, B.W. (2006) *Behav. Brain Res.* **166**, 189–196.

33. Balleine, B.W. and O'Doherty, J.P. (2010) *Neuropsychopharmacol.* **35**, 48–69.

34. Wise, S.P. (2008) *Trends Neurosci.* **31**, 599–608.

35. Ragozzino, M.E., Wilcox, C., Raso, M., and Kesner, R.P. (1999) *Behav. Neurosci.* **113**, 32–41.

36. Ragozzino, M.E., Kim, J., Hassert, D., Minniti, N. et al. (2003) *Behav. Neurosci.* **117**, 1054–1065.

37. Rich, E.L. and Shapiro, M.L. (2007) *J. Neurosci.* **27**, 4747–4755.

38. Young, J.J. and Shapiro, M.L. (2009) *Behav. Neurosci.* **123**, 1028–1035.

39. Bouton, M.E. (2006) *Learning and Behavior: A Contemporary Synthesis* (Sinauer, Sunderland, MA).

40. Rhodes, S.E. and Killcross, S. (2004) *Learn. Mem.* **11**, 611–616.

41. Lebron, K., Milad, M.R., and Quirk, G.J. (2004) *Learn. Mem.* **11**, 544–548.

42. Rhodes, S.E.V. and Killcross, A.S. (2007) *Eur. J. Neurosci.* **26**, 2654–2660.

43. Sierra-Mercado, D., Padilla-Coreano, N., and Quirk, G.J. (2011) *Neuropsychopharmacol.* **36**, 529–538.

44. Rudebeck, P.H., Putnam, P.T., Daniels, T.E., Yang, T. et al. (2014) *Proc. Natl. Acad. Sci. USA* **111**, 5391–5396.

45. Frysztak, R.J. and Neafsey, E.J. (1994) *Brain Res.* **643**, 181–193.

46. Dias, R. and Aggleton, J.P. (2000) *Eur. J. Neurosci.* **12**, 4457–4466.

47. Walton, M.E., Bannerman, D.M., and Rushworth, M.F. (2002) *J. Neurosci.* **22**, 10996–11003.

48. Schweimer, J. and Hauber, W. (2005) *Learn. Mem.* **12**, 334–342.

49. Rudebeck, P.H., Walton, M.E., Smyth, A.N., Bannerman, D.M. et al. (2006) *Nat. Neurosci.* **9**, 1161–1168.

50. Shenhav, A., Botvinick, M.M., and Cohen, J.D. (2013) *Neuron* **79**, 217–240.

51. Hosokawa, T., Kennerley, S.W., Sloan, J., and Wallis, J.D. (2013) *J. Neurosci.* **33**, 17385–17397.

52. Wood, J.N. and Grafman, J. (2003) *Nat. Rev. Neurosci* .**4**, 139–147.

53. Barker, G.R. and Warburton, E.C. (2011) *J. Neurosci.* **31**, 10721–10731.

54. Eacott, M.J. and Easton, A. (2010) *Neuropsychologia* **48**, 2273–2280.

55. Easton, A., Zinkivskay, A., and Eacott, M.J. (2009) *Hippocampus* **19**, 837–843.

56. Spellman, T., Rigotti, M., Fusi, S., Gogos, J. et al. (2014) Program no. 358.11. *2014 Neuroscience Meeting Planner* (Society for Neuroscience, Washington, DC). Online.

57. Spellman, T., Rigotti, M., Ahmari, S.E., Fusi, S. et al. (2015) *Nature* **522**, 309–314.

58. Padilla, N., Pierce, G.M., Blackman, D., Spellman, T. et al. (2014) Program no. 358.20. *2014 Neuroscience Meeting Planner* (Society for Neuroscience, Washington, DC). Online.

59. Chudasama, Y., Doobay, V.M., and Liu, Y. (2012) *J. Neurosci.* **32**, 10915–10924.

60. Passingham, R.E. and Wise, S.P. (2012) *The Neurobiology of the Prefrontal Cortex* (Oxford University Press, Oxford).

61. Walton, M.E., Behrens, T.E., Buckley, M.J., Rudebeck, P.H. et al. (2010) *Neuron* **65**, 927–939.

62. Rudebeck, P.H. and Murray, E.A. (2008) *J. Neurosci.* **28**, 8338–8343.

63. Murray, E.A. and Rudebeck, P.H. (2013) *Front. Neurosci.* **7**, 112.

64. Chudasama, Y., Kralik, J.D., and Murray, E.A. (2007) *Cereb. Cortex* **17**, 1154–1159.

65. Rudebeck, P.H., Saunders, R.C., Prescott, A.T., Chau, L.S. et al. (2013) *Nat. Neurosci.* **16**, 1140–1145.

66. Navawongse, R. and Eichenbaum, H. (2013) *J. Neurosci.* **33**, 1002–1013.

67. Depue, B.E. (2012) *Neurosci. Biobehav. Rev.* **36**, 1382–1399.

68. Place, R.J., Farovik, A., and Eichenbaum, H. (2014) Program no. 560.12. *2014 Neuroscience Meeting Planner* (Society for Neuroscience, Washington, DC). Online.

69. Backus, A.R., Szebényi, S., Schoffelen, J.M. *et al.* (2014) Program no. 82.10. *2014 Neuroscience Meeting Planner* (Society for Neuroscience, Washington, DC). Online.

70. Balleine, B.W. and Dickinson, A. (2000) *J. Neurosci.* **20**, 8954–8964.

71. Holland, P. (1998) *Neuropharmacol.* **37**, 461–469.

72. Kiefer, S.W. and Orr, M.R. (1992) *Behav. Neurosci.* **106**, 140–146.

73. Kesner, R.P. and Gilbert, P.E. (2007) *Neurobiol. Learn. Mem.* **88**, 82–86.

74. Lin, J.Y., Roman, C., and Reilly, S. (2009) *Behav. Neurosci.* **123**, 810–814.

75. Winstanley, C.A., Dailey, J.W., Theobald, D.E.H., and Robbins, T.W. (2004) *Neuropsychopharmacol.* **29**, 1331–1343.

76. Winstanley, C.A., Theobald, D.E., Cardinal, R.N., and Robbins, T.W. (2004) *J. Neurosci.* **24**, 4718–4722.

77. Kheramin, S., Body, S., Mobini, S., Ho, M.Y. et al. (2002) *Psychopharmacol.* **165**, 9–17.

78. Zeeb, F.D., Floresco, S.B., and Winstanley, C.A. (2010) *Psychopharmacol.* **211**, 87–98.

79. Mariano, T.Y., Bannerman, D.M., McHugh, S.B., Preston, T.J. et al. (2009) *Eur. J. Neurosci.* **30**, 472–484.

80. Stevens, J.R., Hallinan, E.V., and Hauser, M.D. (2005) *Biol. Lett.* **1**, 223–226.

81. Stevens, J.R., Rosati, A.G., Ross, K.R., and Hauser, M.D. (2005) *Curr. Biol.* **15**, 1855–1860.

82. McAlonan, K. and Brown, V.J. (2003) *Behav. Brain Res.* **146**, 97–103.

83. Riceberg, J.S. and Shapiro, M.L. (2012) *J. Neurosci.* **32**, 16402–16409.

84. Gallagher, M., McMahan, R.W., and Schoenbaum, G. (1999) *J. Neurosci.* **19**, 6610–6614.

85. Pickens, C.L., Saddoris, M.P., Setlow, B., Gallagher, M. et al. (2003) *J. Neurosci.* **23**, 11078–11084.

86. Pickens, C.L., Saddoris, M.P., Gallagher, M., and Holland, P.C. (2005) *Behav. Neurosci.* **119**, 317–322.

87. Schoenbaum, G., Chiba, A.A., and Gallagher, M. (1998) *Nat. Neurosci.* **1**, 155–159.

88. Ostlund, S.B. and Balleine, B.W. (2007) *J. Neurosci.* **27**, 4819–4825.

89. Rushworth, M.F., Behrens, T.E., Rudebeck, P.H., and Walton, M.E. (2007) *Trends Cogn. Sci.* **11**, 168–176.

90. Rudebeck, P.H., Behrens, T.E., Kennerley, S.W., Baxter, M.G. et al. (2008) *J. Neurosci.* **28**, 13775–13785.

91. Camille, N., Tsuchida, A., and Fellows, L.K. (2011) *J. Neurosci.* **31**, 15048–15052.

92. McDannald, M.A., Saddoris, M.P., Gallagher, M., and Holland, P.C. (2005) *J. Neurosci.* **25**, 4626–4632.

93. Gremel, C.M. and Costa, R.M. (2013) *Nat. Commun.* **4**, 2264.

94. Keiflin, R., Reese, R.M., Woods, C.A., and Janak, P.H. (2013) *J. Neurosci.* **33**, 15989–15998.

95. Burke, K.A., Franz, T.M., Miller, D.N., and Schoenbaum, G. (2008) *Nature* **454**, 340–344.

96. Rhodes, S.E.V. and Murray, E.A. (2013) *J. Neurosci.* **33**, 3380–3389.

97. Chudasama, Y., Daniels, T.E., Gorrin, D.P., Rhodes, S.E.V. et al. (2012) *Cereb. Cortex* **23**, 2884–2898.

98. Kennerley, S.W., Behrens, T.E., and Wallis, J.D. (2011) *Nat. Neurosci.* **14**, 1581–1589.

99. Rudebeck, P.H., Mitz, A.R., Chacko, R.V., and Murray, E.A. (2013) *Neuron* **80**, 1519–1531.

100. Cai, X. and Padoa-Schioppa, C. (2012) *J. Neurosci.* **32**, 3791–3808.

101. Landmann, C., Dehaene, S., Pappata, S., Jobert, A. et al. (2007) *Cereb. Cortex* **17**, 749–759.

102. Marsh, A.A., Blair, K.S., Vythilingam, M., Busis, S. et al. (2007) *NeuroImage* **35**, 979–988.

103. Baxter, M.G., Parker, A., Lindner, C.C., Izquierdo, A.D. et al. (2000) *J. Neurosci.* **20**, 4311–4319.

104. Ranganath, C. and Ritchey, M. (2012) *Nat. Rev. Neurosci.* **13**, 713–726.

105. Nadel, L. and Peterson, M.A. (2013) *J. Exp. Psychol. Gen.* **142**, 1242–1254.

106. Hall, J.A., Foster, R.E., Ebner, F.F., and Hall, W.C. (1977) *Brain Res.* **130**, 197–216.

107. Luksic, N. and Howell, T. (2014) CBC News. http://www.cbc.ca/news/politics/why-our-brains-aren-t-built-for-democracy-1.2784220.

Part III

Primate augmentations

As primate evolution unfolded, new representational systems emerged and old ones changed. In Chapter 6 we take up primate innovations, including a suite of cortical areas for visually guided movement. In the subsequent two chapters we discuss anthropoid innovations. In Chapter 7 we explain that the posterior parietal and temporal areas of early primates developed into a feature system. Then, in Chapter 8, we examine new granular prefrontal areas that gave rise to a goal system.

The manual-foraging memory system of early primates

Overview

As early primates adapted to a life confined to the fine branches of trees, new premotor and posterior parietal areas stored memories about how to reach toward, grasp, and manipulate objects, including foods and food-bearing branches. The first granular prefrontal areas also emerged in these animals. They directed the search for and attention to items of value in the fine-branch niche and updated the valuation of predicted outcomes to reflect current biological needs. Inferior temporal areas provided these prefrontal areas with specialized visual representations. We call this suite of adaptations the manual-foraging system, although it also performs many other functions. In early primates, this system used vision to find, keep track of, choose, and obtain valuable items in a cluttered and unsteady environment. In humans, its representations subserve the "autopilot" control of reaching.

H.M.'s long-lost hobby

In a study of motor learning, H.M. performed a task that required him to grasp a robot's handle and move it to a visual goal. To do this, he needed to overcome a complex pattern of powerful and unpredictable forces generated by the robot[1]. Testing required several sessions, and H.M.'s impairment prevented him from remembering his previous performance, of course. For example, on the first day of testing—a mere 4 hours after his initial practice session—H.M. returned from a break and claimed that he had never before seen the robotic apparatus. Yet when he sat down in front of it, he knew how to perform the task without any additional instructions.

As H.M. held the robot's handle and moved it around, he would launch into an extended explanation about how the task reminded him of hunting birds, a hobby of his youth. Day after day, the experimenters listened patiently as H.M. recounted the details of his boyhood adventures in Rhode Island, the birds he had seen, the rifles he had owned, and the pleasures he had taken in hunting. He would repeat these stories, almost verbatim, three or four times an hour, accomplishing little more than delaying data collection and exasperating the people trying to run the experiment.

Despite these frustrations, H.M. had grasped an important concept along with the robot's handle. Shooting a flying bird involves calculating metrics such as distance, direction, and speed, culminating in a shot aimed at a particular angle or distance ahead of a moving target. As H.M. recognized implicitly, reaching requires similar computations, typically without the slightest ability to articulate any of these impressive mathematical feats. Importantly, these computations depend on a form of memory: stored representations of the mathematical transforms needed to achieve a goal.

In this chapter we explain that the specialized representations that H.M. used for his hobby—along with those underlying other visually guided movements—descended from early primates. Simply put, H.M.'s long-lost hobby depended on his most remote primate heritage.

Evolution

Along with several visual innovations, early primates evolved a modified way of reaching for and grasping food, all the while stabilizing themselves on the flimsy branches of trees and shrubs (see Chapter 2, "Early primates"). Figure 6.1(A) shows an artist's conception of a stem primate (*Carpolestes*), emphasizing its grasping hands and feet, which set the stage for a leaping–grasping, hindlimb-dominated form of locomotion in early true primates (euprimates).

The appearance of several new cortical areas accompanied developments in vision and locomotion. New premotor and posterior parietal areas emerged, along with inferior and superior temporal areas and two new granular parts of the prefrontal cortex: the granular orbitofrontal cortex and the caudal prefrontal cortex (see Chapter 2, "Early primates"). Figure 6.2(A) illustrates a selection of these areas as components of cortex–basal ganglia "loops," along with some connections among them. Each new cortical area, along with older ones like the perirhinal cortex, has its own cortex–basal ganglia "loops."

The idea that primates developed new cortical areas and new ways of guiding movements remains controversial, but few comparative neuroanatomists share these doubts[2]. Critics cite the fact that rodents and other mammals make dexterous movements, as primates do, reach and manipulate objects, and have cortical areas that share many properties with the new cortical areas that emerged in primates[3]. Why, then, do we consider visually guided movement and the areas underlying them to be primate innovations?

A general answer is that visually guided movements depend on primate innovations *in primates*. Other mammalian lineages have evolved similar mechanisms in parallel. Common inheritance contributes, as well, but less than usually supposed. The fact that rats, cats, and raccoons, among other mammals, reach and manipulate objects says little about the history of these capacities in primates. The development of several new areas— in posterior parietal, premotor, temporal, and prefrontal cortex—changed forever how primates make their way in the world. These mechanisms, of course, built on some ancestral traits. Tree shrews, the sister group of primates, appear to have some form of the primate parietal–motor network[4], but other mammals have much less. So when we treat

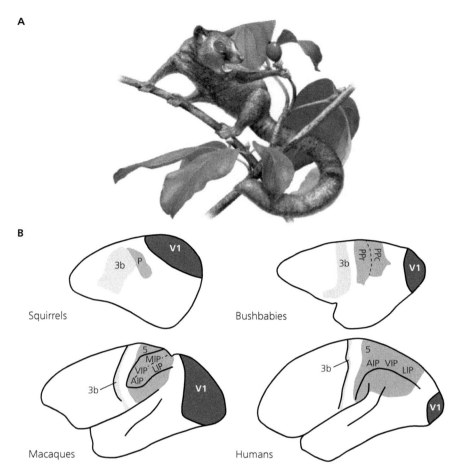

Fig. 6.1 A stem primate reaching for a stem and a comparison of posterior parietal areas among selected mammals. (A) A reconstruction of *Carpolestes*, a plesiadapiform primate (see Fig. 2.10). (B) The parietal cortex in a rodent (squirrels), a strepsirrhine (bushbabies), and two anthropoids (humans and macaques). Rostral is to the left, dorsal is up. Abbreviations: 3b and 5 correspond to specific parietal areas; AIP, anterior intraparietal area; LIP, lateral intraparietal area; MIP, medial intraparietal area; P, parietal cortex; PPc, caudal posterior parietal cortex; PPr, rostral posterior parietal cortex; V1, primary visual cortex; VIP, ventral intraparietal area. (A) Reproduced in grayscale from Sargis EJ. Primate origins nailed. *Science* 298:1564–5, © 2002, reprinted with permission from the American Association for the Advancement of Science. (B) Adapted from Krubitzer L, Padberg J. Evolution of association pallial areas: parietal association areas in mammals. In *Encyclopedic Reference of Neuroscience*, ed. AB Butler, pp. 1225–31, © 2009, with permission of Springer.

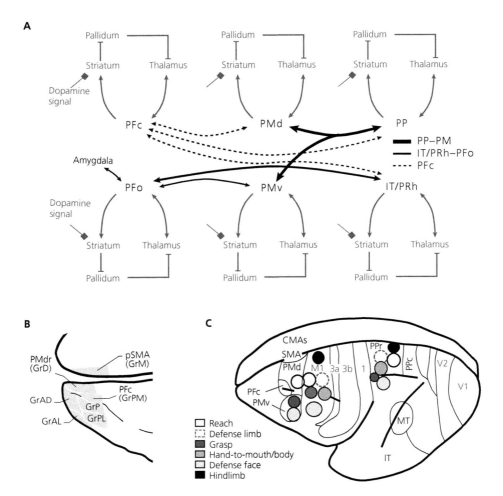

Fig. 6.2 New cortical areas and connections in primates. (A) New cortex–basal ganglia "loops" of early primates and the cortical areas they included. Three major sets of connections are designated by thick solid lines, thin solid lines, and dashed lines, respectively, as indicated by the key to the right. (B) The granular prefrontal areas (gray shading) in bushbabies, a representative strepsirrhine. (C) Regions in the brain of a strepsirrhine from which electrical stimulation evokes coordinated movements. Abbreviations: 3a, 3b, and 1 correspond to specific parietal areas; CMAs, cingulate motor areas; GrAD, anterodorsal granular cortex; GrAL, anterolateral granular cortex; GrD, dorsal granular cortex; GrM, medial granular cortex; GrP, posterior granular cortex; GrPL, posterolateral granular cortex; GrPM, posteromedial granular cortex; IT, inferior temporal cortex; MT, middle temporal cortex; PFc, caudal prefrontal cortex; PFo, granular orbitofrontal cortex; PMd, dorsal premotor cortex; PMdr, rostrodorsal premotor cortex; PMv, ventral premotor cortex; PP, posterior parietal cortex; PPc, caudal posterior parietal cortex; PPr, rostral posterior parietal cortex; PRh, perirhinal cortex; pSMA, pre-supplementary motor area; SMA, supplementary motor area; ST, superior temporal cortex; V1, primary visual cortex; V2, secondary visual cortex. (B) From Figure 2.3 in Passingham RE, Wise SP. *The Neurobiology of the Prefrontal Cortex*, © 2012, Oxford University Press. Reproduced with permission of OUP. (C) Adapted from Stepniewska I, Gharbawie OA, Burish MJ, Kaas JH. Effects of muscimol inactivations of functional domains in motor, premotor and posterior parietal cortex on complex movements evoked by electrical stimulation. *Journal of Neurophysiology* 111:1100–19, © 2014, The American Physiological Society, reprinted with permission.

these new areas as primate innovations, we leave open the possibility that some of these traits emerged somewhat earlier, in the last common ancestor of tree shrews and primates.

The heart of the manual-foraging system consists of its new posterior parietal and premotor areas. A comparative analysis indicates that many mammals have small cortical fields that might be homologous to some of the parietal[5] and premotor areas in primates, but not many[6-10]. Figure 6.1(B), for example, illustrates a posterior parietal area in a squirrel[7]. Rats have a similar area, and a premotor area as well, maybe two. The few, small posterior parietal and premotor areas of rodents need not be homologous with the like-named areas in primates; they might be rodent specializations. After all, rodents and primates have evolved separately for tens of millions of years, and primates are not alone in their ability to evolve new cortical areas. Remple et al.[10] concluded, for example, that the posterior parietal area in rats has more in common with the somatosensory areas of anthropoids than with the anthropoid posterior parietal cortex.

This point aside, primates have many more areas in both the premotor and posterior parietal cortex than rodents do (Fig. 6.1B). More importantly, they also have many more areas than the last common ancestor of primates and rodents, marked by the asterisk in Fig. 1.6. A similar conclusion applies to the last common ancestor of primates and tree shrews, the sister group of primates. As mentioned earlier, tree shrews have elements of the manual-foraging system[4], but they appear to lack the elaborate, multi-area organization observed in the posterior parietal and premotor cortex of primates[10]. In this context, Fang et al.[11] (p. 331) described the connections among posterior parietal and premotor areas in the bushbaby, a strepsirrhine primate, and compared these traits with previous studies of tree shews. In their view:

> the evidence suggests that the rather complex framework for sensorimotor processing … in [bushbabies] is similar to that seen in anthropoid primates. Thus, this framework likely emerged with or before early primates, but not … [as early as] the common ancestors of tree shrews … and primates, insofar as tree shrews have a much simpler cortical system.

Figure 6.2(B, C) illustrates some of the new primate areas in the bushbaby, emphasizing movements of importance in their natural habitat, such as feeding, reaching, grasping, and defensive actions. We take up this topic later (see "Action modules"). Figure 6.3 traces derived primate traits from an ancestral condition: the inheritance from early placental mammals (Fig. 6.3A)[6]. The areas and connections in black indicate the innovations of early primates (Fig. 6.3B) and anthropoids (Fig. 6.3C).

An evolutionary perspective places two ideas in a new light: one regarding habits, the other regarding the dorsal visual stream. First, the prevailing view of memory systems lumps reaching, grasping, and manipulating objects with stimulus–response habits. The rationale for this view seems to be little more than exclusion from the kinds of memories lost in human amnesia. An evolutionary perspective treats these behaviors, instead, as specific adaptations to a once-new foraging niche. This idea has little in common with the concept of a habit that comes from animal learning theory: the product of prolonged instrumental conditioning (see Chapter 3, "What happens in instrumental conditioning"). Second, evolutionary ideas help resolve a controversy about the dorsal visual stream. One school of thought claims that it functions in spatial perception and attention[12], another

A Early placental mammals

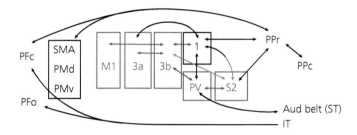

B Primate elaboration

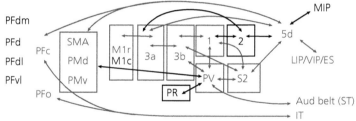

C Anthropoid elaboration

Fig. 6.3 New cortical areas and connections in early primates and anthropoids. (A) Parietal and frontal areas in early placental mammals and selected connections (arrows). The figure omits the prefrontal areas discussed in Chapter 5, among others. (B) New areas and connections of early primates (black) that elaborated the ancestral traits (gray). (C) Additional elaborations in anthropoid primates (black), along with their ancestral state (gray). Abbreviations: 3a, 3b, 1, 2, and 5d correspond to specific parietal areas; Aud, auditory cortex; A1, primary auditory cortex; ES, extrastriate visual cortex; LIP, lateral intraparietal area; M1, primary motor cortex; M1c, caudal primary motor cortex; M1r, rostral primary motor cortex; MIP, medial intraparietal area; PFc, caudal prefrontal cortex; PFd, dorsal prefrontal cortex; PFdl, dorsolateral prefrontal cortex; PFdm, dorsomedial prefrontal cortex; PFo, granular orbitofrontal cortex; PFvl, ventrolateral prefrontal cortex; PM, posteromedial somatosensory cortex; PMd, dorsal premotor cortex; PMdr, rostrodorsal premotor cortex; PMd, dorsal premotor cortex; PMdr, rostrodorsal premotor cortex; PMv, ventral premotor cortex; PPc, caudal posterior parietal cortex; PPr, rostral posterior parietal cortex; PR, rostral parietal somatosensory cortex; PV, posterior ventral somatosensory cortex; R, rostral somatosensory cortex; S1, primary somatosensory cortex; S2, secondary somatosensory cortex; VIP, ventral intraparietal area. Adapted from Krubitzer L. In search of a unifying theory of complex brain evolution. *Annals of the New York Academy of Sciences* 1156:44–67, © 2009, New York Academy of Sciences, with permission.

that it uses vision to control action[13]. We expand on this topic in Chapter 8 ("How versus where is neither here nor there"), but for now we simply state our conclusions:

- The emphasis on visually guided action results from interactions between the posterior parietal cortex and frontal areas that evolved in early primates.

- The emphasis on spatial perception and attention results from interactions between the posterior parietal cortex and frontal areas that evolved much later, in anthropoids.

Connections

Like Fig. 6.3(C), Fig. 6.4(A) uses black type for anthropoid innovations and gray type for areas that anthropoids inherited from earlier primates. This chapter focuses on cortical developments in early primates; anthropoid innovations are dealt with in Chapters 7 and 8. In general, the more rostral parts of the premotor cortex connect with the more caudal parts of the posterior parietal cortex. [For simplicity, a great deal is omitted in Fig. 6.4(A), including medial premotor areas and local connections among premotor and posterior parietal areas.]

Figure 6.4 also illustrates some connections of the new granular prefrontal areas of early primates: the caudal prefrontal cortex (Fig. 6.4B) and granular orbitofrontal cortex (Fig. 6.4C) (see Chapter 2, "Early primates"). The connections of these areas in strepsirrhines generally agree with those in anthropoids[9,14,15], so they probably represent a common inheritance from early euprimates. Note that these two parts of the granular prefrontal cortex have dramatically different connections. The caudal prefrontal cortex, which includes the frontal eye fields, has connections with both middle- and low-order visual areas, along with parts of the superior temporal and posterior parietal cortex. The granular orbitofrontal cortex shares only a few of these pathways. The connections that it does have are summarized later (see "Properties of the granular orbitofrontal cortex").

The anatomy of the orbital and caudal prefrontal cortex seems generally similar from primate to primate, although we note here some differences that become important later in this chapter (see "Influence of the orbitofrontal cortex on premotor areas"). In anthropoid primates, the granular orbitofrontal cortex has few, if any, direct connections with the premotor cortex. Instead, it relays information to premotor areas mainly via the dorsolateral and ventrolateral parts of the prefrontal cortex[16,17]. In strepsirrhines, in contrast, the granular orbitofrontal cortex has direct connections with the ventral premotor cortex, and it appears to project directly to the posterior parietal cortex as well (see Figs. 14 and 20B of Fang et al.[11], the anatomical descriptions of Preuss and Goldman-Rakic[14], and Fig. 12 of Stepniewska et al.[15]).

The manual-foraging system as a whole

Preuss[18,19] first proposed that the new cortical areas of early primates evolved as adaptations to the fine-branch niche (see Chapter 2, "Early primates"). In recognition of primate specializations for foraging in this niche, predominantly with a grasping hand, we have

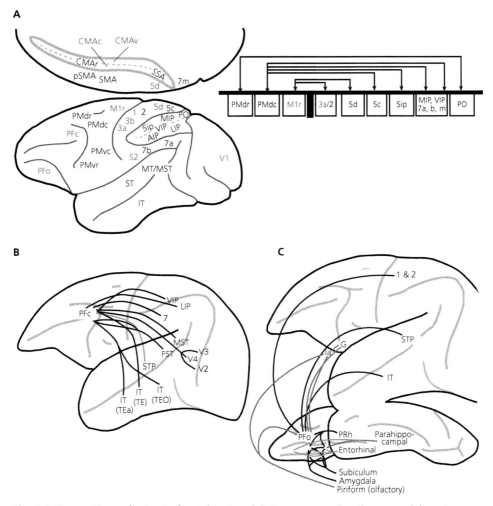

Fig. 6.4 Connections of primate frontal cortex. (A) Areas composing the manual-foraging system (black type) in macaque monkeys, a representative anthropoid. The chart to the right shows selected connections among the areas depicted in the drawing. The black bar denotes the fundus of the central sulcus. (B), (C) Connections of the prefrontal areas that emerged in early primates, depicted in macaque monkeys, a representative anthropoid. (B) Connections of the caudal prefrontal cortex. Each line indicates a reciprocal corticocortical connection. (C) Connections of the granular orbitofrontal cortex, in the format of (B). Abbreviations: 3a, 3b, 1, 2, 5c, 5d, 5ip, 7, 7a, 7b, and 7m correspond to specific parietal areas; AIP, anterior intraparietal area; CMAs, cingulate motor areas; FST, fundal area of the superior temporal sulcus; G, gustatory cortex; Ia, agranular insular cortex; IT, inferior temporal cortex; LIP, lateral intraparietal area; M1, primary motor cortex; M1c, caudal primary motor cortex; M1r, rostral primary motor cortex; MIP, medial intraparietal area; MST, medial superior temporal cortex; MT, middle temporal area; PFc, caudal prefrontal cortex; PFo, granular orbitofrontal cortex; PMdc, caudodorsal premotor cortex; PMdr, rostrodorsal premotor cortex; PMvc, caudoventral

devised a new name for these adaptations: the manual-foraging system. This label leaves out many functions of the new cortical areas, such as controlling movements of the head, eyes, mouth, face, and hindlimbs, as well as defensive and socially relevant actions. It does serve, however, to emphasize a particularly important set of primate innovations and the selective pressures that favored them.

Challenges

It is easy to underestimate the computational problems posed by the niche invaded by early primates. Simplified laboratory settings make the visuomotor life of primates seem relatively easy: a few visual stimuli, a bar to press, a handle to move, and so forth. A different view emerges from an appreciation of the ecological context in which early primates evolved.

To guide the movements required in the fine-branch niche, early primates needed to solve a host of computational problems, some specific to that niche:

◆ Eye, head, and body movements can change a goal's location in retinal coordinates, and the head and body move a lot on flimsy branches. Indeed, several primate specializations involve the ability to track an object with smooth pursuit eye movements, which keeps the object at a constant retinal coordinate as the object, head, or body moves.

◆ The physics of the limb require different movements depending on the postural orientation of the arm, even for a given hand position and goal.

◆ When reaching through a thicket of branches, the hand cannot always head directly toward a goal.

◆ The removal of food items from their attachments, while perching on an unstable substrate, takes precisely calibrated forces, as does grasping a food-bearing branch and pulling it toward the mouth.

◆ Once the hand contains an item, its combined mass changes the torques needed to move the hand to a goal. When an item weighs either more or less than expected, or a branch is stiffer or more compliant, the motor system needs to adapt its commands.

Fig. 6.4 Continued
premotor cortex; PMvr, rostroventral premotor cortex; PO, parietal–occipital visual area; PRh, perirhinal cortex; pSMA, pre-supplementary motor area; SSA, supplementary sensory area; S1, primary somatosensory cortex; S2, secondary somatosensory cortex; SMA, supplementary motor area; SS, somatosensory cortex; ST, superior temporal cortex; STP, superior temporal polysensory cortex; TE, a temporal area, part of the inferior temporal cortex; TEa, anterior part of area TE; TEO, occipital part of area TE; V1, primary visual cortex; V2, secondary visual cortex; V2...V4, extrastriate visual areas; VIP, ventral intraparietal area. (A) From Shadmehr R, Wise SP. *The Computational Neurobiology of Reaching and Pointing*, © 2005, published by The MIT Press. (B) Figure 5.2 in Passingham RE, Wise SP. *The Neurobiology of the Prefrontal Cortex*, © 2012, Oxford University Press. Reproduced with permission of OUP. (C) Figure 4.2 in the same source. Reproduced with permission of OUP.

Add to all of this the fact that the brain controls movements with signals that travel relatively slowly down axons (compared, for example, with wires); that it depends on muscles that take tens of milliseconds to generate force after receiving a motor command; that many of these factors change as an animal grows, strengthens, or weakens; and that the brain needs to use somatosensory feedback that arrives after a substantial transmission delay, sometimes amounting to several hundred milliseconds. It takes a book to explain how primates solve all of these problems; fortunately, there is one[20].

Equally fortunately, readers do not need to endure an entire book to understand this chapter. A few points suffice as background: (1) visually guided actions depend on large parts of the neocortex, many of which evolved in early primates; (2) each reaching movement depends on memories stemming from previous movements; (3) reaching in primates occurs in a visual, extrinsic, allocentric frame of reference, based on retinal coordinates; and (4) the same computations used for reaching with the hand also apply to other visually guided actions, including defensive maneuvers, locomotion, tool use, and pointing-like movements, including those involved in H.M.'s long-lost hobby.

Proposal

In response to selective pressures imposed by the fine-branch niche, early primates developed the manual-foraging system, which stores the specialized representations needed to find, choose, keep track of, evaluate, reach, grasp, detach, and manipulate food items, as well as to bring foods and food-bearing branches to the mouth. The same system supports hindlimb, head, and orofacial movements, defensive actions, and communicative gestures. It depends in large part on primate-specific cortical areas, including most of the premotor and posterior parietal cortex, two parts of the granular prefrontal cortex, and new visual areas in the inferior temporal cortex.

The last sentence of this proposal refers to a suite of new cortical areas that provide the principal neural adaptations underlying the manual-foraging system:

♦ New posterior parietal and premotor areas compute and store the coordinate transforms needed for visually guided movements. These calculations require neural representations that are modified after each movement in order to adjust future movements. Similar representations adjust ongoing movements.

♦ New inferior temporal areas, along with the older perirhinal cortex, interact with granular parts of the orbitofrontal cortex to represent the visual features of predicted outcomes, including foods, and update the valuation of these features in accord with current biological needs.

♦ Both the posterior parietal and inferior temporal areas, along with lower-order visual areas, interact with the caudal prefrontal cortex, which searches for and maintains attention on valuable items. The posterior parietal areas provide information about metric features of the visual world, such as the number of items, distances, locations, order, durations, and speeds; the ventral and occipital visual areas provide their specialized representations of the world's qualitative, attribute features, including color, shape, glossiness, translucence, and visual texture.

In the remainder of this chapter, we take up these three topics, in turn.

Parietal–premotor networks

Parietal–premotor networks use and adapt specialized neural representations to correct errors in visually guided movements: some for ongoing movements, some for future movements. Evidence from disorders of the basal ganglia implicates cortex–basal ganglia "loops" in correcting ongoing movements; the effects of cerebellar disease indicate that cortex–cerebellar "loops" adjust future movements[21].

Coordinate frames and transforms

Parietal–premotor networks transform visual information into the metrics of movement, with their various subdivisions specialized for different coordinate frames and different kinds of movement. For primates, many of these movements involve the arm, hand, head, and eyes. Shadmehr and Wise[20] explain the basics of coordinate frames and transforms, and interested readers can consult original sources for updates[22–34].

Three points exemplify the general principles:

◆ The lateral intraparietal area (LIP) encodes visual stimuli in terms of salience[35] and eye movements intended to fixate salient stimuli[36–38]. According to neurophysiological evidence, LIP uses a body-centered coordinate frame for its computations[31,39–41], and it exerts a motor influence via connections with the caudal prefrontal cortex and the superior colliculus[42].

◆ The medial intraparietal area (MIP), also known as the parietal reach region, represents the locations of visual stimuli in a retinal coordinate frame[23,43] and signals the metrics of movements needed to reach these locations[32–34,44,45]. MIP exerts an influence over movements through its connections with the dorsal premotor cortex[46,47].

◆ The anterior intraparietal area (AIP) encodes key features of objects to be grasped[48], such as orientation and size[49], using an object-centered coordinate frame. AIP exerts its motor influence via projections to ventral premotor areas[50].

Evidence from inactivation experiments has provided support for the latter point. In these studies, inactivation of parietal and motor areas impaired hand function, especially for the accurate and fine control of the fingers. Inactivation of the primary motor cortex caused such effects, of course[51–55], but so did inactivations of the ventral premotor cortex[56] and the anterior intraparietal area[52,57], which impaired the grasping and manipulation of objects. These findings indicate that dorsal components of the parietal–premotor network subserve reaching movements and that ventral parts function in grasp and manipulation, with some oculomotor and head control mixed in. Accordingly, several coordinate frames function in parallel for particular kinds of movement.

The fundamental ideas about parietal–premotor computations stem from theoretical work that began in the 1980s[58–61]. We can only touch on this vast literature here, but Fig. 6.5 illustrates the basic concepts.

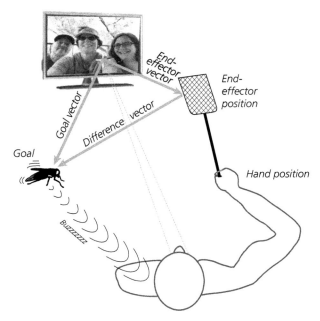

Fig. 6.5 Reaching vectors. While watching the three authors of this book on a flat-screen television, a person (viewed from above) plans to swat a loudly buzzing horsefly. Dashed lines: the orientation of gaze. White plus sign: the fixation point. Gray arrows: vectors computed by the manual-foraging system. Adapted from Shadmehr R, Wise SP. *The Computational Neurobiology of Reaching and Pointing*, © 2005, published by The MIT Press.

The posterior parietal cortex uses sensory inputs to estimate two important coordinates: the location of "the thing that moves," such as the hand, and the location of the goal of that movement. To illustrate the origin of this coordinate frame, Fig. 6.5 depicts the head and arm of a person watching the three authors on television, with the visual fixation point indicated by a plus sign on the screen.

Although visual reference frames are often called "eye coordinates" or "eye-centered coordinates," it is important to recognize that these terms refer to a coordinate frame based on retinal signals, not on the eyes per se. The distinction is important because sensory signals from the two retinas combine for stereoscopic vision, which underlies depth perception. Accordingly, the critical coordinate frame has three dimensions, with its origin somewhere "out there" in space—not centered on the eyes, which remain firmly anchored in the head. Like all coordinate systems, the one that guides reaching movements consists of axes and an origin, and in this case the origin is a point at some distance from the animal's head. In primates that have a fovea, such as anthropoids, the origin of this coordinate system probably corresponds to the fixation point, but other origin points are also possible, in theory.

Likewise, a coordinate frame centered on "the thing that moves" often goes by terms like "hand coordinates" or "hand-centered coordinates." These terms apply perfectly well to many situations, but the term end-effector applies more generally. Primates usually use their hands as end-effectors, but "the thing that moves" can be some other part of the body or something held in the hand. Figure 6.5 portrays a fly swatter, not the hand, as the end-effector. The horsefly serves, unwittingly and almost certainly unwillingly, as the goal.

The manual-foraging system estimates the location of both the end-effector and the goal in an extrinsic coordinate frame based on vision. The ability to represent the location of any sort of end-effector explains why this mechanism generalizes so readily to the use of tools, such as fly swatters. Furthermore, the goal neither needs to be visible nor at the location of the stimulus that guides movement. The goal might be located acoustically, and it might be at some place offset from the location of the stimulus. To swat a moving fly, for example, the swatter should be aimed at some point in advance of the fly's current location. But to begin with, we consider a simpler situation: aiming for a gigantic, but stationary, horsefly. In this scenario, the fly somehow senses impending doom and initiates an escape plan by beating its wings in a way that generates a loud buzz prior to takeoff.

Goal vector

Figure 6.5 depicts a vector from the fixation point to the goal, called the goal vector. Gaffan and Hornak[62] reported something important about its representation in the brain. In their experiment, monkeys learned to choose one object-like stimulus on a video monitor among five stimuli arrayed horizontally. After lesions that disconnected the posterior visual cortex from the frontal cortex, the monkeys made errors when they should have chosen a stimulus contralateral to the fixation point. This finding shows that the posterior cortex of both hemispheres contains representations of potential goals in the contralateral half of visual space, relative to the current fixation point, and that these visual areas promote the selection of a goal through interaction with the frontal cortex.

Figure 6.6(C) depicts several ways of estimating the location of a goal. The current location of a visible (or audible) goal is the most obvious, and for that reason can be called standard mapping. The term mapping refers to an algorithm that transforms a stimulus into a goal location. Standard mapping works well for stationary goals, when the stimulus is also the target of action. For example, one might look directly at a sessile fly to swat it. To swat a moving fly, however, the location of the goal needs to be estimated on the basis of its speed and direction. The term transformational mapping refers to this kind of calculation. Figure 6.6(C) also depicts two additional kinds of nonstandard mapping: one for arbitrary relationships between a stimulus and a goal, and another for the absence of any current stimulus (internally generated goals).

End-effector vector

Earlier we said that the posterior parietal cortex uses "sensory inputs" to estimate the location of the end-effector. We avoided saying "visual inputs" because the manual-foraging system uses more than that. The posterior parietal cortex also receives signals from sensory transducers in muscles and, to a lesser extent, in skin and joints. These signals, called proprioceptive inputs, enable posterior parietal areas to align information

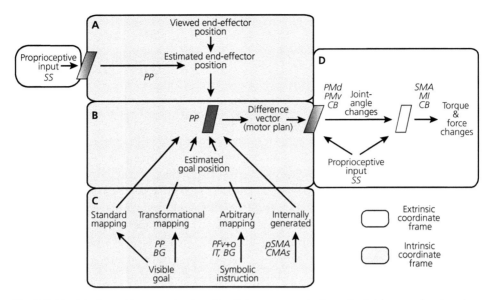

Fig. 6.6 Model of reaching in primates. Parallelograms symbolize adaptable neural networks. Shading indicates transformations between intrinsic (dark) and extrinsic (light) coordinates. (A) One network stores memories about the alignment of proprioceptive input with visually sensed end-effector locations. (B) A second network computes the difference vector. (C) Additional networks generate spatial goals in a variety of ways. (D) Other networks use memories about the physics of the world and limb to transform the difference vector into joint-angle changes and forces. Abbreviations: BG, basal ganglia; CB, cerebellum; CMAs, cingulate motor areas; IT, inferior temporal cortex; M1, primary motor cortex; PFo, granular orbitofrontal cortex; PFv, ventral prefrontal cortex; PMd, dorsal premotor cortex; PMv, ventral premotor cortex; PP, posterior parietal cortex; PRh, perirhinal cortex; pSMA, pre-supplementary motor area; SMA, supplementary motor area; SS, somatosensory cortex. From Shadmehr R, Wise SP. *The Computational Neurobiology of Reaching and Pointing*, © 2005, published by The MIT Press.

about muscle lengths and joint angles with the location of the end-effector as sensed visually. Figure 6.6(A) illustrates this convergence.

With experience, neural networks learn the relationship between proprioceptive signals and the end-effector locations sensed visually at the same time. As a result, the manual-foraging system can estimate the location of an end-effector in an extrinsic, visual coordinate frame—even without vision of the hand. Proprioceptive representations come in handy for reaching in the dark and, more generally, for reaching to a goal while maintaining visual fixation on a target. Together, these memories align visual and proprioceptive information to estimate the location of the end-effector in visual coordinates. [Recall from Chapter 4 ("Nonspatial representations: terminology and physiology") that something similar occurs in the hippocampus.] Figure 6.5 labels the distance and direction from the fixation point to the end-effector as the "end-effector vector."

Work by Rushworth et al.[63,64] provided evidence that certain parts of the posterior parietal cortex—specifically areas 5d, 7b, and MIP—play a necessary role in estimating the initial location of the end-effector. In their experiment, monkeys reached from several starting hand locations to a fixed goal. After a combined lesion of the three areas just mentioned, the monkeys reached accurately in the dark, provided that their hands always started in the same place. They also reached the goal accurately in the light, even when their hands started in different places. When their initial hand locations varied, however, and they could not see their hands in the dark, the lesioned monkeys reached inaccurately. Lesions of other parts of the posterior parietal cortex, specifically areas 7a and the LIP cortex, caused impairments in reaching to goals in the light. These findings show that dorsal parts of the posterior parietal cortex estimate current end-effector locations based on proprioceptive information.

Note that the posterior parietal cortex does not simply sense the location of an end-effector. It actively aligns visual and proprioceptive information by computing the necessary mathematical transforms to make these inputs agree. Such transforms require memory, and, like other memories, they depend on specialized representations that adapt with experience. The role of these representations has been demonstrated in people wearing special eyeglasses or goggles with prisms that shifted the location of the end-effector and goal on the retina but had no effect on proprioceptive signals. This perturbation caused a misalignment between vision and proprioception, which led to errors in reaching. After seven to ten reaches, the relevant representation gradually adapted to the new (visually shifted) condition. Removal of the prisms then generated a new error, this time of the same magnitude as the original one but in the opposite direction. These *after-effects* also persisted for several reaches, until practice restored the original transform.

Difference vector

So far, we have said that the posterior parietal cortex estimates the location of both the end-effector and the goal, and that it does so in extrinsic, retinal coordinates (Fig. 6.6A, C). In Fig. 6.6(B), these estimations come together in the form of a difference vector, a resultant of vector subtraction (Fig. 6.5). The difference vector corresponds to a movement plan, but note what happens as a result of vector subtraction: the origin of the vector shifts from the fixation point to the end-effector.

At first glance, the difference vector seems to suggest that the brain plans movements in a hand- or end-effector-centered coordinate space. Psychophysical evidence, however, shows that the difference vector is initially encoded in extrinsic, retinal coordinates, like the goal and end-effector vectors. Several findings support this conclusion:

♦ In one experiment, subjects viewed distorted visual feedback[65]. As a result, they could make movements that were perfectly straight in either visual or actual coordinates, but not both. In these conditions, the subjects made reaching movements that had a small arc in actual space, so that the visual feedback showed a straight trajectory. This finding demonstrates the dominance of extrinsic visual coordinates.

◆ In another experiment, subjects reached to an acoustic goal. In doing so, they made the same subtle errors (overshoots) as they did when reaching to a visual goal using peripheral vision[66]. These errors make sense for vision because the peripheral retina lacks the high spatial acuity of the fovea. But auditory localization should not have suffered from the same inaccuracy. The fact that it did indicates that the motor system transforms acoustic locations into visual coordinates.

◆ In a third study, congenitally blind subjects made straighter reaching movements than sighted people did[67]. The reason is that sighted people suffer from minor distortions of vision that become incorporated into their motor plans. Congenitally blind people have never experienced such distortions and so make straighter movements.

◆ Finally, neurophysiological studies have monitored neurons in the manual-foraging system as they recalculated motor plans, just before or after every saccadic eye movement[68,69]. This updating occurred even when neither the end-effector nor the target had moved, in which case there was no need to change or recalculate the motor plan. The motor system nevertheless recomputed the difference vector, presumably because the saccade caused the locations of the goal and end-effector to fall on new retinal coordinates.

All these results, and others[20], support the conclusion that the parietal–premotor networks encode the difference vector in an extrinsic, visual frame of reference.

The plan for a reaching movement requires more than a simple two-dimensional vector specifying a distance and direction, of course. The specialized literature deals in detail with the variety of motor commands that can occur for a given difference vector. To begin with, the fly-plagued television-watcher in Fig. 6.5 can swat at the fly with his elbow up or down. This change in initial posture alters the motor commands needed to reach the goal even before the swatter moves. Another factor involves the smoothness of movement; the motor system minimizes dramatic jerks of the limb in favor of smooth acceleration and deceleration. Limiting the activation of muscles opposing the desired changes in joint angle, called coactivation, can also be significant. Of all of the relevant factors, the most important involve minimizing the error at the end of the movement or along its path, and generating a movement as straight as possible in visual coordinates. The motor system has additional constraints, such as the principle called Fitts' law: with faster movements comes a decrease in accuracy, and vice versa. So it takes a sizable swatter to hit the fly because accuracy will suffer at high movement speeds. A slower movement would be more accurate, but a skillful horsefly would be long gone.

Like the alignment between proprioceptive and visual information, the difference vector is more than a computation: it involves stored representations. There are many ways to reach a goal—slow and careful, fast and loose, curved to avoid obstacles, with zigs and zags to show off, and so forth. These variations are called control policies[70], and many motor memories involve such policies. The need to develop control policies that avoid visible obstacles might explain, at least in part, why the manual-foraging system encodes difference vectors in visual coordinates.

For a given difference vector and control policy, the manual-foraging system needs to transform sensory stimuli into joint-angle changes, muscle forces, and torques. As depicted in Fig. 6.6(D), these motor outputs necessarily use intrinsic, body-based coordinates because they depend on the geometry of the limb. The requisite coordinate transforms involve memories, called *internal models* in the motor-control literature. Although motor-control experts do not usually refer to them as memories, that is what they are: stored, experienced-based representations. In this case, they incorporate the physics of the limb, objects held in the hand, and interactions within the limb, among other factors. These representations consist of the spatial and motor transforms needed for a given difference vector and control policy, and, like the explicit memories of human cognitive psychology, a particular sensory context can lead to their retrieval[71]. In a sense, internal models resemble the cognitive maps discussed in Chapter 4. Both internal models and cognitive maps reflect stored information: about the way in which the body interacts with the outside world and about the layout of that world, respectively.

The memories that compose internal models come in two forms: those for transforming motor commands into movements, called forward models, and those for transforming desired movements into motor commands, called inverse models. Inverse models, likewise, come in two varieties: those for joint-angle changes, called inverse kinematics, and those for forces, called inverse dynamics.

Factors such as arm posture, the weight of a grasped object, and forces imposed on the limb alter the changes in joint angle and forces needed to reach a goal. As a result, movements often have a degree of error. Accordingly, internal models need to adapt from movement to movement, much like the prism adaption described earlier (see "End-effector vector"). Every movement causes a small adjustment in the internal models, until movements conform to both the difference vector and the control policy. Put another way, these adjustments update memories in the form of visuomotor transforms, and every movement changes the state of these memories in a way that affects subsequent movements. Internal models thus persist over many movements, albeit with modification, and so a given movement depends on previous ones. Visual goals, in contrast, can change from movement to movement, and the target for one movement can be independent of the others.

Autopilot control

Not only do manual-foraging memories reduce errors from movement to movement, they also reduce errors during ongoing movements, a mechanism called "autopilot control" in humans. In an experiment by Desmurget et al.[72], human subjects reached to a spot of light. Whenever a spot appeared, the subjects made a saccadic eye movement to look at it and began to reach to the same location, which served as a visual goal. On occasion, the spot jumped to a new location during the saccade, which prevented the subjects from noticing its shift. Nevertheless, the subjects quickly and smoothly adjusted their ongoing reaching movement and reached to the goal's new location. Later, however, they denied both that the stimulus had moved and that their reaching movement had deviated from the original plan[73]. When the subjects were instructed to reach to the original goal even if the light spot jumped, they could not resist making the automatic adjustment.

The posterior parietal cortex plays an especially important role in this "autopilot" function[72,74-76]. When repetitive transcranial magnetic stimulation (rTMS) disrupted neural processing in this brain region, subjects could not adjust their reaching movement when the goal jumped[72]. Stimulation of the primary motor cortex had no such effect. In parallel experiments, patients with bilateral lesions of the posterior parietal cortex could reach to a goal that never moved, but failed to show the autopilot adjustment when a goal jumped[76]. These patients reached directly to the initial location of the goal and then made a second movement to correct the error.

The ability to smoothly adjust movements in progress depends, in part, on the continuous recalculation of the difference vector as the movement unfolds. Whenever a goal moves or jumps to a new location, the difference vector changes accordingly, and the movement continues until the length of that vector reaches zero. Because goals usually remain visible throughout a reaching movement, their locations do not require memory, but each motor command does. It depends on a stored representation of the appropriate visuomotor transform, which converts the difference vector into joint-angle changes and forces.

Prior experience can also correct ongoing movements in another way. Figure 6.7 presents an idea about how this might work. Forward models transform motor commands—called either efference copy or corollary discharge—into a neural simulation of the proprioceptive feedback that should return during the movement, taking neural and physical delays into account. These simulations depend on experienced-based estimates of expected feedback, and they correspond to a series of predicted limb configurations as the movement unfolds. As a result of these predictions, corrections need not wait until the end of a movement, and so reaching movements can be adjusted in flight.

Experimental evidence from people with Huntington's disease points to the basal ganglia as an important component of the forward model and of autopilot adjustments. In the early stages of the disease most of the pathology is confined to the striatum, and this is especially true for carriers of the Huntington's gene who have yet to develop overt symptoms. In tests of both diagnosed patients and asymptomatic gene carriers, the subjects performed reaching movements that diverged from those of healthy subjects about 300 ms after the beginning of movement, at the time when feedback would first arrive[77]. At this point in the movement, their actions became inefficient and jerky, especially as they got closer to the goal. These findings show that both the patients and asymptomatic gene carriers have a significant impairment in adjusting ongoing movements.

In Chapter 12 ("If not habits, what?") we return to these findings and develop the idea that the concept of a forward model better summarizes the general function of the basal ganglia than the popular notion that it subserves habits.

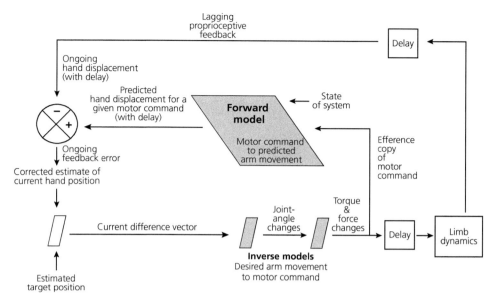

Fig. 6.7 Forward models. Neural networks compute the feedback that should occur for a given motor command, in order to correct ongoing movements. Format as in Fig. 6.6. Adapted from Fig. 4 of Wise SP, Willingham DT. Motor skill learning. In: *Encyclopedia of Neuroscience*, ed. LR Squire, vol. 5, pp. 1057–66. Academic Press, © 2009, Elsevier, reprinted with permission.

Action modules

At another level of analysis, parietal–premotor networks subserve what might be called action modules. Sustained electrical stimulation of the motor, premotor[78–81], and posterior parietal[82,83] cortex evokes movement patterns resembling reaching, grasping, feeding, and defensive movements, among others, such as locomotion.

Figure 6.8(A) shows the layout of action modules in the frontal cortex of an anthropoid primate; and Fig. 6.8(C) shows an example in which direct cortical stimulation brings a monkey's hand to its mouth, as in feeding. Figure 6.2(C) illustrates the locations of various action modules in both the frontal and posterior parietal cortex of a strepsirrhine primate.

In these experiments, posterior parietal and motor areas that have direct connections with each other usually produced the same coordinated action patterns when stimulated[15,82–86]. These areas appear to have a hierarchical organization, as revealed by the finding that inactivation of the primary motor cortex blocked the outputs caused by stimulation of either the premotor or posterior parietal cortex[86].

The action module that corresponds to feeding-like movements in monkeys coincides roughly with the ventral premotor area. Nudo and Masterton[87,88] identified this area as a source of corticospinal projections in several primates, but not in any other mammal. Their neuroanatomical analysis also showed that its size correlates with an arboreal life,

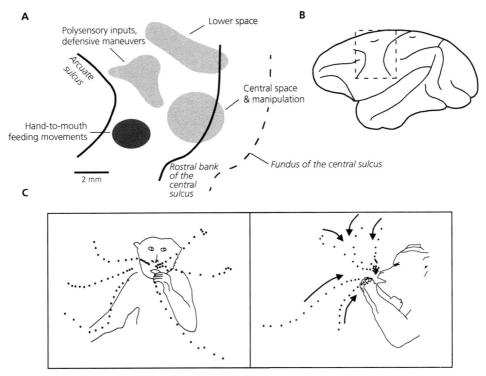

Fig. 6.8 Coordinated movements. (A) Frontal areas in macaque monkeys from which sustained electrical stimulation evoked coherent actions. (B) The dashed box shows the location of (A). (C) Each dot shows the hand's position as sustained electrical stimulation of the cortex produced a movement of the monkey's hand to its mouth, as occurs in feeding movements. (A) Courtesy of Michael Graziano, reproduced from Wise SP. The evolution of ventral premotor cortex and the primate way of reaching. In: *The Evolution of Primate Nervous Systems*, eds. TM Preuss, JH Kaas, pp. 157–66, © 2007, Elsevier, reprinted with permission. (C) Reproduced from Graziano MS, Taylor CS, Moore T, Cooke DF. The cortical control of movement revisited. *Neuron* 36:349–62, © 2002, with permission from Elsevier.

as opposed to manual dexterity, hand–eye coordination, or other factors. Connections of the ventral premotor cortex with both the primary motor cortex and the posterior parietal cortex are roughly similar across a broad diversity of primates—including strepsirrhines, platyrrhines, and catarrhine monkeys[89–94]—which provides further support for the idea that the ventral premotor cortex is an innovation of early primates. Unlike other motor and premotor areas, the corticospinal projections emanating from the ventral premotor cortex terminate mainly in the rostral segments of the cervical spinal cord[95], which contain motor neurons controlling the head, shoulder, and respiration. The ventral premotor cortex also projects to the facial nucleus in the brainstem, which controls the lower face, lip, and jaw[96,97]. Collectively, these outputs suggest a role in controlling coordinated movements of the head and mouth. Furthermore, experimental inactivation of the ventral premotor area has induced impairments in adjusting the configuration of the hand to the size of objects[56]. Taken together with the neuroanatomy that suggests a role in coordinated head, mouth, and breathing movements, this finding supports the idea that the ventral premotor cortex plays a role in all of the movements required for hand-to-mouth feeding.

Tree shrews, the sister group of primates, have similar interactions between the posterior parietal and the primary motor cortex[4], and so this basic pattern of organization probably arose in their last common ancestor.

Affordances

A different level of analysis involves the concept of affordances (see Chapter 5, "Relation to primates"). Just as there are many ways to reach from one place to another, a given object can elicit many different actions. According to Gibson[98], vision should be viewed in an ecological context. Rather than considering vision in the context of perceptual representations, a Gibsonian perspective emphasizes the actions associated with visual inputs. An object's affordances include anything that an agent can do to it or with it, and the same idea applies to surfaces such as slopes and stairs. Many of the adaptations of early primates relate to the affordances of objects and obstacles in the fine-branch niche.

Evidence from humans shows that lesions of the posterior parietal cortex disrupt movements related to an object's affordances, including both manipulation and reaching movements. Tool use, for example, can be badly impaired, even in patients who have no serious weakness or other low-level motor disorder. Neurologists diagnose ideational apraxia when these patients cannot use pantomime to demonstrate the use of tools, although they can name them accurately. Lesions around the intraparietal sulcus, and especially those that include the dorsal parts of the posterior parietal cortex, can also cause an impairment called optic ataxia, in which patients cannot make effective goal-directed reaching movements[99,100]. Like apraxia, ataxia leaves the ability to recognize objects intact.

Tests in one influential patient, known as D.F., showed the opposite pattern of preserved and impaired functions. She had a large bilateral lesion of the temporal cortex near its occipital boundary, along with a smaller parietal lesion, also near the occipital cortex, in the left hemisphere[101–103]. Unlike patients with optic ataxia, who can recognize objects, D.F. had a severe impairment in doing so, a disorder called visual agnosia. Despite this disability, D.F. could make visually guided movements pretty effectively. She was able to adopt a hand configuration appropriate to the affordances of an object, such as its size and shape, although she could not report much about these metrics. Furthermore, she was able to orient her hand correctly to penetrate a rectangular slot, although she could not make a similar movement to signal the slot's perceived orientation to someone else.

These findings indicate that parietal–premotor networks plan visually guided movement in terms of object affordances. In patients with optic ataxia and ideational apraxia these mechanisms function poorly, if at all. In patients like D.F., they remain relatively intact despite extensive disruption of the visual pathways that support the identification and naming of objects. We address the latter functions in Chapter 9 ("Temporal–prefrontal networks").

Affordance competition

Yet another level of analysis involves the competition among affordances. That statement sounds abstract, but the principle is simple: look at an object or apparatus and choose what to do with it. A typical experiment involves several potential goals for a reaching movement, and the subject needs to choose among them—something like the situation depicted in Fig. 6.5, but with several horseflies. Cisek[104] presents a model of parietal–premotor interactions for reaching, in which each of several potential goals automatically elicits the requisite visuomotor transforms. These transforms, of course, correspond to long-term visuomotor memories. Collectively, they convert an object's location and affordances into the metrics of action: speeds, directions, torques, forces, and control policies. According to Cisek's model, the manual-foraging system specifies and prepares the metrics of several motor plans simultaneously prior to a choice being made among them.

Neurophysiological experiments have provided support for the idea that parietal–premotor networks plan two or more actions at the same time[105]. In one study, a spatial goal was designated first, and only later did the monkey receive a signal indicating whether to reach to that goal with the left or right arm. Neurons in the premotor cortex encoded both arm movements simultaneously as soon as the goal appeared, long before the monkey could choose which movement to make[106]. The same goes for other kinds of limb movements and saccades. Indeed, abundant evidence has shown that the motor system represents several potential goal locations simultaneously[48,107–116].

Cisek's[104] model appears to clash with some traditional ideas. *Stage* or *goods* models[117] treat the choice among potential goals as a separate and early stage of neural processing, sometimes called the "cognitive" or "decision" stage. However, according to Cisek's *affordance-competition* model, the manual-foraging system specifies the *metrics* of potential movements first, then an assessment of their relative value leads to a choice among them (Fig. 6.9A). According to stage or goods models, relative valuations lead to the choice of a goal first, followed by a motor plan (metrics) that will achieve that goal (Fig. 6.9B).

A neurophysiological study has provided support for the affordance-competition model[118]. In this experiment, cells in the posterior parietal and premotor cortex encoded the metrics for two potential movements as soon as two visible goals appeared. Only later did the activity of these cells begin to reflect the relative value of the two options.

Figure 6.9 contrasts the two models using the terms value and cost in a general sense, but choices reflect several such decision variables. Potential variables (or situational dimensions) include stimulus salience, the costs of physical effort and neural processing, the magnitude and probability of reward, delays in obtaining the expected benefits, and the updated subjective value of a predicted outcome, among other variables that define what is sometimes called a state space—all of which are encoded by neurons in the manual-foraging system[35,119–122].

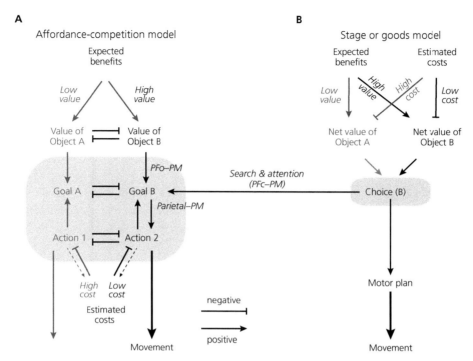

Fig. 6.9 Contrasting models of choices. (A) An affordance-competition model. (B) A stage or goods model. Gray shading: parietal–premotor networks. Abbreviations: PFo, granular orbitofrontal cortex; PFc, caudal prefrontal cortex; PM, premotor cortex. Adapted from Cisek P. Making decisions through a distributed consensus. *Current Opinion in Neurobiology* 22:927–36, © 2012, Elsevier, with permission.

To understand these models in an evolutionary perspective, we need to extend the discussion beyond parietal–premotor networks to incorporate another primate innovation: the granular orbitofrontal cortex.

Temporal–orbitofrontal networks

Stage and goods models gain support from the fact that people can make choices even when the metrics of action are impossible to specify. Goals, in this sense, can be *metrically abstract*. People can, for example, choose an apple over a banana without any information about where either might appear in the future. Spatial goals can also be abstract, such as when they involve relative location[123]. One can, for example, decide to choose the leftmost point in a spatial array before it appears on a computer monitor. This leftmost point has no concrete coordinates at the time of the choice because there is no way of knowing where the array will pop up on the monitor.

The specialized literature often treats the stage and affordance-competition models as opposing and incompatible ideas. Instead, according our proposal, they reflect related evolutionary developments in early primates. The stage or goods mechanism depends on the granular orbitofrontal cortex, a primate innovation, and only it can deal with choices among metrically abstract goals. The affordance-competition mechanism depends on parietal–premotor networks, another primate innovation, and it is limited to choices among metrically concrete goals. These two networks are coordinated through the influence of the granular orbitofrontal cortex on parietal–premotor networks. To discuss that interaction, however, we first need to consider interactions between the granular orbitofrontal cortex and the amygdala.

Orbitofrontal–amygdala interactions

In Chapter 3 ("What happens in instrumental conditioning") we discussed the role of the amygdala in updating the valuations of behavioral outcomes and their features. Here we take up the interaction between the amygdala and a cortical area that evolved in early primates: the granular orbitofrontal cortex (see Chapter 2, "Early primates"). As with lesions of the amygdala, lesions of the granular orbitofrontal cortex have little or no effect on the appetite or food preferences of monkeys, but they do affect the choices among objects[124,125] or actions[126] based on updated valuations, as discussed in Chapter 5 ("Relation to primates"). Figure 6.10 illustrates some of the relevant results.

The devaluation task assesses the ability to make choices based on the updated valuations of predicted outcomes. In one version of this task, introduced in Chapter 3 ("What happens in instrumental conditioning"), monkeys first learned several object–food pairings, with two different kinds of foods. In this initial phase of the devaluation task, some objects were paired with food item A and others with food item B. Figure 6.10(B) depicts the association of a cubic object with a blackberry. The monkeys later faced a probe test in which they chose—on a series of trials—between two objects. For every choice, one of the objects was associated with food A and the other with food B. The monkeys received a food item by selecting either object; there was no wrong choice. In the baseline condition, the subjects' choices usually reflected their food preferences. In the next stage of the experiment, the monkeys consumed one of the foods to satiety, after which they faced additional probe tests. Control monkeys shifted their choices toward the objects associated with the alternative (unsated) food, but monkeys with lesions of the granular orbitofrontal cortex or of the amygdala did so much less frequently, if at all (Fig. 6.10, left)[125]. Crossed disconnections of the orbitofrontal cortex in one hemisphere and the amygdala in the other produced the same result[124]. So, too, did an experiment involving a choice between two actions. In this case, the monkeys chose between "tap" and "hold" actions performed on a touch screen, and these two actions were associated with different food outcomes. As mentioned in Chapter 5 ("Relation to primates"), lesions of the granular orbitofrontal cortex caused an impairment on this task as well (Fig. 6.10, right)[126]. In Chapter 3 ("What happens in instrumental conditioning") we explained that inactivation of the amygdala before selective satiation blocked the devaluation effect but inactivation afterwards did not[127]. The results of these experiments support three conclusions: (1) the amygdala and the granular orbitofrontal cortex need to interact in order to update the

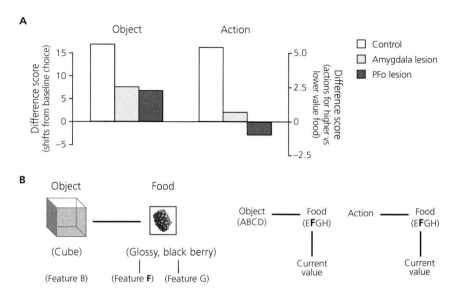

Fig. 6.10 Effects of lesions on devaluation effects. (A) Effect of bilateral lesions of the amygdala or granular orbitofrontal cortex (PFo) on two versions of the devaluation task, one involving a choice between two objects, the other involving a choice between two actions. (B) Depiction of feature conjunctions that represent the cue and an outcome. Letters A–D in (B) indicate sensory features of objects. Letters E–H in (B) indicate sensory features of a predicted food outcome. (A) Adapted From Murray EA, Rhodes SEV. Monkeys without an amygdala. In *Living Without an Amygdala*, eds. DG Amaral, R Adolphs, pp. 252–87, © 2016. Reprinted with permission of Guilford Press.

valuation of object–outcome or action–outcome conjunctions; (2) this process occurs as monkeys become sated (selectively) on a food that will serve as a predicted outcome during future probe tests; and (3) neither the amygdala nor its interactions with the orbitofrontal cortex is needed later, during the probe tests, when monkeys use these updated valuations to make choices.

Figure 6.10(B) illustrates how this mechanism might work. As we explain in Chapter 7, neurons in the lateral temporal cortex represent conjunctions of visual features at various levels of complexity (see Fig. 7.3A, B). The perirhinal cortex, for example, represents visual feature conjunctions at the level of natural objects. According to our proposal, the primate orbitofrontal cortex also represents natural objects, but in its case conjoined with some additional features, such as smell and taste, as well as the neural equivalent of a valuation, such as "highly desirable." Figure 6.10(B) depicts this valuation feature as a "current value" conjoined with specific sensory features of a food outcome. In this example, the glossiness of a blackberry is linked to the valuation "highly desirable." When faced with a choice between two objects or two actions, the one associated with a representation of a predicted outcome that includes the valuation feature "highly desirable" wins. However, as a monkey consumes blackberries to satiety, the amygdala gradually downgrades this valuation from "highly desirable" to "desirable," then neutral, "mildly disagreeable," and finally "disgusting." These subjective assessments apply to both incentive motivation (wanting a particular outcome) and hedonic motivation (liking that outcome). In probe tests that take place after the satiation procedure, an object or action elicits the same outcome representation as it did prior to satiation, but now that representation includes an updated valuation dimension. Predicted visual features that were previously associated with the value "highly desirable" are now linked to "disgusting." The choice is obvious. After the valuation updating has occurred, the amygdala does not contribute all that much until the value of an outcome changes again—as it inevitably will.

These findings indicate that the advantage provided to primates by their orbitofrontal–amygdala interactions involves updating the valuations of predicted outcomes, especially their visual features, in accord with current biological needs. When the granular orbitofrontal cortex first evolved in early primates, it allowed them to link a nonfood object or an action with the visual features of predicted food outcomes, along with their current value, without having to relearn the relevant associations. Expressed in terms of conjunctive representations and the example illustrated in Fig. 6.10(B), the granular orbitofrontal component of the manual-foraging system stores representations such as cube–glossy blackberry or tap–glossy blackberry that also have a valuation dimension or can access that valuation. Interactions with the amygdala update the valuation feature based on an animal's current state, which provides advantages in terms of the nutritional benefits conferred by dietary diversity.

Against this conclusion, some research has pointed to a more general role for the granular orbitofrontal cortex in learning and updating stimulus–outcome associations, such as those measured in tasks with changing reward probabilities or choice–outcome reversals (also known as object reversals). These conclusions come mainly from findings based on aspiration lesions of the granular orbitofrontal cortex[128,129]. A more recent experiment made use of more selective, excitotoxic lesions of the granular orbitofrontal cortex, which spared fibers passing through or near this area. These lesions had no effect on the learning of object reversals[125] or a task involving changing reward probabilities[130]. For reversal learning, the same study showed that a lesion aimed at cutting fibers in the subcortical white matter—a procedure that left most of the granular orbitofrontal cortex intact—caused the impairment, rather than damage to the granular orbitofrontal cortex per se. These findings point to a specific role of the granular orbitofrontal cortex in updating valuations of the features of predicted outcomes, rather than in learning about stimulus–outcome or choice–outcome likelihoods. A nearby area, namely the ventrolateral prefrontal cortex, probably mediates the updating of predicted outcomes in terms of reward probabilities[130,131]. In Chapter 8 ("Credit assignment") we return to this topic.

Taken together, these results point to interactions among the inferior temporal and perirhinal cortex, the granular orbitofrontal cortex, and the amygdala as playing a crucial role in updating the valuation of predicted outcomes in accord with current biological needs.

Properties of the granular orbitofrontal cortex

We have already discussed some connections of the granular orbitofrontal cortex. Figure 6.4(C) shows a selection of this area's corticocortical connections, mainly from outside the frontal lobe. Figure 5.2(A) emphasizes olfactory, gustatory, and visceral inputs; Fig. 5.2(B) shows some visual inputs; and Fig. 5.2(C) illustrates connections with the parahippocampal cortex. Figure 6.2(A, lower left) illustrates dopaminergic inputs to striatal components of this area's cortex–basal ganglia "loops," along with connections between the amygdala and cortical components of the same circuits[132]. These illustrations come from macaque monkeys, but, as discussed earlier, they probably reflect the neuroanatomy of early primates fairly well.

Taken together, these connections place the primate orbitofrontal cortex in a unique position among cortical areas. They provide it with most of the information needed for choosing among potential objects[117] and actions[104]. Like other cortex–basal ganglia "loops," those involving the orbitofrontal cortex receive input from the midbrain dopaminergic neurons indicating whether a choice has produced the predicted outcome, less than that, or more (see Fig. 3.4C). As explained earlier (see "Orbitofrontal–amygdala interactions"), the interactions of this area with the amygdala update the valuation of predicted outcomes. The visual attributes of outcomes are of particular importance to primates (see Fig. 5.2B), but taste and smell also play a major role (see Fig. 5.2A).

Figure 6.10(B) depicts the features of outcomes with letters (E, F, G, and H). In the natural habitat of primates, foraging choices often depend on subtle sensory distinctions, exemplified by the glossiness of a berry (feature F in the figure). According to our proposal, the inferior temporal and perirhinal cortex provide such information to the granular orbitofrontal cortex, which transforms these features into biases among potential goals and actions.

Figure 6.11 illustrates a possible mechanism for the influence of granular orbitofrontal areas over parietal–premotor action modules. Padoa-Schioppa[117] and several other researchers[133–136] review the literature on the granular orbitofrontal cortex from a neuroeconomics perspective, so we present only one experiment as an example. In this experiment, monkeys faced a choice between visual stimuli, each of which comprised a number of colored squares. Each color corresponded to a differently flavored juice, and the number of squares indicated the volume that would be available if chosen. Padoa-Schioppa[117] called these stimulus arrays "offers" by analogy with human economics. In the example shown in Fig. 6.11, the monkeys were indifferent to an offer of four drops of juice C versus two drops of juice B (horizontal line). Indifference indicates that the two choices have approximately equal value. Obviously, colored squares on a video monitor have no value per se. However, they can elicit the memories of valuable outcomes previously associated with the squares.

According to Padoa-Schioppa[137], these experiments show that neurons in the granular orbitofrontal cortex encode the value of an offer, the value of a choice, and the chosen juice, presumably in terms of taste (Fig. 6.11). It is clear enough, in general terms,

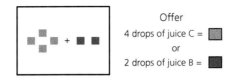

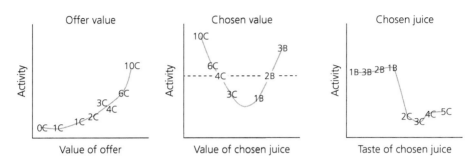

Fig. 6.11 Neuronal mechanisms for encoding value. Top: Visual display on a monitor screen. Bottom: Encoding properties of cells in the granular orbitofrontal cortex. Each data point shows the activity of an orbitofrontal cortex neuron for a certain numbers of drops (0–10) of a given kind of juice: juice B or juice C. The horizontal dashed line indicates an indifference point in neural activity. Adapted from Padoa-Schioppa C. Neuronal origins of choice variability in economic decisions. *Neuron* 80:1322–36, © 2013, with permission from Elsevier.

how these neural signals could generate the choice of a goal in stage or goods models (Fig. 6.9B). The most valuable offer somehow prevails over less valuable ones, becomes the chosen offer (choice B in Fig 6.9B), and leads to the chosen juice. A question remains about how neural activity in the granular orbitofrontal cortex can contribute to a choice among goals and actions.

Influence of the orbitofrontal cortex on premotor areas

The problem is that the orbitofrontal cortex cannot really "do" anything, at least not in any direct way. Not only does the anatomy of cortex–basal ganglia "loops" indicate that the granular orbitofrontal cortex has little in the way of direct motor outputs, but a neurophysiological experiment showed that cells in that area did not represent actions or spatial goals prior to movement[138]. Accordingly, the orbitofrontal cortex must influence actions indirectly, predominantly through corticocortical routes.

According to one version of the affordance-competition model, a biasing signal goes from the granular orbitofrontal cortex to the premotor areas. This bias favors one among two or more competing motor plans, each one specified by parietal–premotor networks. A possible mechanism for this influence involves areas that have connections with both the granular orbitofrontal and premotor areas, which Fig. 6.12(B) places in ovals labeled "granular PFvl, dl." It is likely that other prefrontal areas also mediate these influences, and we expect differences among primates due to the emergence of new prefrontal areas in anthropoids (see Chapters 2 and 8). In anthropoids, the dorsolateral prefrontal cortex seems to mediate interactions between the granular orbitofrontal cortex and premotor cortex. In Fig. 6.12(B), one oval represents the conjunction of a glossy berry and a position to the right of the current hand position; the other represents a dull berry to the left. Neurophysiological studies have provided plentiful evidence of neurons that encode conjunctions of stimulus features and locations[139], even with no relevance to the task[140,141]. Figure 6.12(A) illustrates the respective difference vectors.

In this example, we assume that a foraging primate knows from memory that glossy berries have a sweet taste whereas dull berries taste bitter. In other words, the visual feature "glossiness" is associated with a specific sensory outcome. Once activated by its preferred

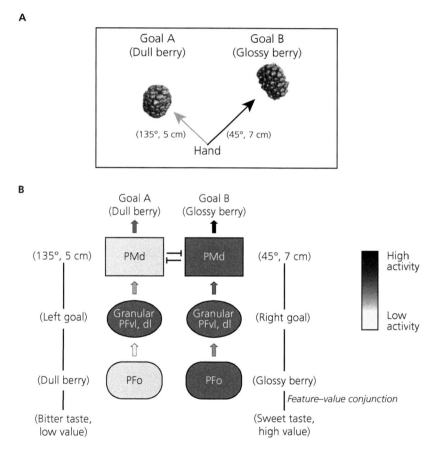

Fig. 6.12 Value-based biasing. (A) Depiction of alternative hand movements to two berries. (B) Pathways for transmitting updated valuation signals from the granular orbitofrontal (PFo) cortex to the dorsal premotor cortex (PMd) via other parts of the granular prefrontal (PF) cortex, such as the ventrolateral (PFvl) and dorsolateral (PFdl) prefrontal areas. Lines between PMd networks symbolize mutual inhibition.

feature conjunction, both prefrontal ovals could transmit value-related signals from the granular orbitofrontal cortex to the premotor areas[16], much like a switch flipped to the "on" position allows electrical current to pass through a circuit. In the example illustrated in Fig. 6.12, the monkey sees both a dull berry to the left and a glossy berry to the right, so both ovals have high levels of activity. The high predicted-outcome valuations associated with the glossy berry can then pass from the granular orbitofrontal to the premotor cortex through the ovals, with greater activity for the more valuable goal. As a result, the motor plan for a rightward movement reaches threshold first, the monkey reaches to the right, and thereby obtains the glossy, sweet-tasting berry.

Two additional possibilities deserve mention. In early primates, like modern strepsirrhines[11,14,15], the granular orbitofrontal cortex might have had direct connections with the ventral premotor cortex. Perhaps anthropoids lost this connection after their new granular prefrontal areas emerged. In addition, the inferior temporal, perirhinal, and orbitofrontal cortex might have influenced the premotor cortex via the amygdala. A projection from these cortical areas to the amygdala is well established[132], and a projection from the amygdala to the premotor cortex exists in macaque monkeys[142]. Given the sparse distribution of its terminals, however, it could be a vestigial form of a once-important pathway, one that became less significant after new prefrontal areas evolved and created new corticocortical routes to the premotor cortex.

In stage or goods models, the granular orbitofrontal cortex has to work in a different way, leading first to the choice of a metrically abstract goal. This process leads nowhere, however, unless the animal later finds that goal through some sort of search mechanism. Another primate innovation, the caudal prefrontal cortex, helps primates do that.

Caudal prefrontal networks

According to our proposal, primates evolved a new mechanism for choosing a food item and then searching for it based on the memory of past "offerings" by the fine-branch niche. As always, an evolutionary development of this kind is not necessary for successful foraging, but it could provide an advantage by conserving time and concentrating effort on the most valuable options. In this context, we can view the two models depicted in Fig. 6.9 as analogous to two strategies for buying produce. One approach involves going to a market specifically to get blackberries, having already chosen them over the alternatives (the goods model); the other requires one to survey the options available at the market and choose whatever seems best (the affordance-competition model). For the former, the caudal prefrontal cortex contributes to a search function through its interactions with the visual areas of cortex (Figs. 6.2A, 6.3B, and 6.4B). Presumably, these search functions involve a top-down biased-competition mechanism[143] of the sort discussed in Chapter 5, aimed at finding an item that has already been selected.

Results from cortical-stimulation studies have provided support for this idea. In one experiment, cells in extrastriate visual areas responded more robustly to stimuli at particular locations after electrical stimulation of the caudal prefrontal cortex, and inactivation of the caudal prefrontal cortex caused an impairment in detecting a light in peripheral visual space[144].

Search also works in a different way, one more related to the concept of bottom-up attention. One glossy berry among several dull ones is said to "pop out" and attract attention. "Pop out," in this sense, involves the search for salient items among the clutter of a complex visual world. In an experiment by Sato and Schall[145], for example, neurons in the caudal prefrontal cortex increased their activity when a visual stimulus "popped out" because it differed in color from other stimuli that appeared at the same time. Neurons in this area signaled the location of the "pop-out" stimulus shortly after it appeared, even when the monkey needed to make a saccade away from that stimulus to a different spatial goal. Later, most of these cells encoded the location of the goal.

These results support the idea that the caudal prefrontal cortex functions in both top-down and bottom-up attention, including both its overt and covert varieties[146]. Overt attention involves eye movements to fixate an attended item; covert attention consists of orienting attention to an item without fixating it.

Both the caudal prefrontal and posterior parietal cortex contribute to visual search. During relatively simple "pop-out" searches, such as those that involved a single stimulus feature, cells in area LIP encoded the goal before cells in the caudal prefrontal cortex did. During more complex searches, which involved visual conjunctions, activity in the caudal prefrontal cortex encoded the goal first[147]. Findings of this kind support the idea that the caudal prefrontal cortex plays a role in search and attention and exerts its influence through interactions with more posterior cortical areas. They also point to complex interactions between top-down and bottom-up attention.

In terms of stage or goods models (Fig. 6.9B), the rarity of a valuable resource, such as a glossy blackberry, would cause black glossiness to "pop out" of the clutter as soon as such a stimulus comes into view. At that point, a metrically abstract goal would become metrically concrete, and the motor plan for a movement to that stimulus would reach its threshold rapidly. This process would avoid the delay required to "read in" an estimated value of that choice, as posited by the affordance-competition model. In a sense, the prior selection of a metrically abstract goal combined with attentional biases from the caudal prefrontal cortex to sensory areas—the quest for a glossy blackberry—preempts the influence of later valuation signals.

The attentional functions of the caudal prefrontal cortex can contribute to competition among motor plans in another way as well. For simplicity, we have considered only one goal at a time. Accordingly, the choice of one potential goal implies the suppression of others. In natural conditions, however, movements to future goals can be planned even as the pursuit of a current goal progresses. After the choice of one goal, the "losers" of the most recent competition can continue to attract attention and become a subsequent goal. In this way, the caudal prefrontal cortex empowers primates to keep track of the "runners-up" in a value-based competition, especially in terms of their locations, and pursue them with minimal delay. Planned sequences have similar characteristics.

Conclusions

As early primates adapted to the small-branch niche, they developed a suite of new cortical areas, including new posterior parietal, premotor, temporal, and prefrontal areas, many of which exploited enhancements in vision. The development of the fovea and trichromatic vision remained for the future, but their frontally directed eyes allowed early primates to see in dim light, in depth, and around obstacles over a large part of visual space. A leaping–grasping, hindlimb-dominated mode of locomotion freed the forelimbs for manual foraging and a hand-to-mouth feeding technique.

Their new posterior parietal and premotor areas used extrinsic, retinal coordinates to store and adapt the representations needed to reach for, grasp, and manipulate items, as well as to adjust ongoing movements; their caudal prefrontal cortex directed the search for and attention to valuable items distributed among the fine branches; and their granular orbitofrontal cortex updated the valuation of predicted outcomes, especially for the visual features of those outcomes. Along with the visual areas that provided this information, the premotor, posterior parietal, caudal prefrontal, and granular orbitofrontal cortex composed the manual-foraging memory system, which provided early primates with the ability to choose valuable items in accord with current biological needs, keep track of their locations, and produce the forces required to obtain them while moving around, often quickly, on unsteady branches.

In humans, visually guided movements occur without any awareness of the knowledge and computations that underlie them. People know about categories of berries (Fig. 6.10), for example, and the events involved in gathering them, but not the specialized representations that transform the location of a berry into movements that bring their fingers exactly to it and grasp it with the precise force needed to detach but not bruise it. To account for this lack of awareness, popular science sometimes invokes the concept of "muscle memory." But the vertebrate brain does not "outsource" visuomotor memories to the limbs. Some protostomes seem to adopt that approach[148], but in vertebrates the representations guiding such skilled actions reside in the brain. In primates, recently evolved parts of the neocortex store these transforms, and they take up a considerable proportion of it. Accordingly, the manual-foraging system serves as a straightforward example of a cognitive module in the brain, as this term is commonly used in evolutionary psychology: a cognitive adaptation that evolved at a specific time and place, in response to particular selective pressures. Were it not for the fact that we cannot communicate motor memories to each other, except in the form of mathematics and attendant descriptions[20], this example of a cognitive module should settle any controversy about their existence.

This chapter began with an anecdote about H.M., and some readers might think that the connection with memory ends there. After all, given the way that the term memory is usually used in psychology, it doesn't seem to apply to visually guided movements. In information theory and computer science, however, memory simply corresponds to stored information. Accordingly, visually guided reaching depends on a form of memory: specialized neural representations that compute transforms among sensory and motor coordinate frames. A suite of new cortical areas evolved in early primates to store and adapt these representations, along with those underlying attention to and choices among objects and actions in the fine-branch niche. These innovations set the stage for elaborations and augmentations as primates diversified, which we explore in Chapters 7–10.

References

1. **Shadmehr, R., Brandt, J.,** and **Corkin, S.** (1998) *J. Neurophysiol.* **80**, 1590–1597.

2. **Kaas, J.H.** (2013) *Wiley Interdiscip. Rev. Cogn. Sci.* **4**, 33–45.

3. **Whishaw, I.Q.** (2003) *Behav. Brain Res.* **146**, 31–41.

4. **Baldwin, M.K., Cooke, D.F.** and **Krubitzer, L.** (2016) *Cereb. Cortex* pii: bhv329 [Epub ahead of print].

5. **Wilber, A.A., Clark, B.J., Forster, T.C., Tatsuno, M.** et al. (2014) *J. Neurosci.* **34**, 5431–5446.

6. **Krubitzer, L.** (2009) *Ann. NY Acad. Sci.* **1156**, 44–67.

7. **Krubitzer, L.** and **Padberg, J.** (2009) In: *Encyclopedic Reference of Neuroscience* (ed. Butler, A.B.), pp. 1225–1231 (Springer, Berlin).

8. **Cooke, D.F., Goldring, A., Recanzone, G.H.,** and **Krubitzer, L.** (2014) In: *The Visual Neurosciences* (eds. Chalupa, L.M. and Werner, J.), pp. 1049–1063 (MIT Press, Cambridge, MA).

9. **Wu, C.W.H., Bichot, N.P.,** and **Kaas, J.H.** (2000) *J. Comp. Neurol.* **423**, 140–177.

10. **Remple, M.S., Reed, J.L., Stepniewska, I., Lyon, D.C.** et al. (2007) *J. Comp. Neurol.* **501**, 121–149.

11. **Fang, P.C., Stepniewska, I.,** and **Kaas J.H.** (2005) *J. Comp. Neurol.* **490**, 305–333.

12. **Ungerleider, L.G.** and **Mishkin, M.** (1982) In: *Analysis of Visual Behavior* (eds. Ingle, J., Goodale, M.A. and Mansfield, R.J.W.), pp. 549–586 (MIT Press, Cambridge, MA).

13. **Milner, A.D.** and **Goodale, M.A.** (2007) *The Visual Brain in Action* (Oxford University Press, Oxford).

14. **Preuss, T.M.** and **Goldman-Rakic, P.S.** (1991) *J. Comp. Neurol.* **310**, 507–549.

15. **Stepniewska, I., Cerkevich, C.M., Fang, P.C.,** and **Kaas, J.H.** (2009) *J. Comp. Neurol.* **517**, 783–807.

16. **Takahara, D., Inoue, K., Hirata, Y., Miyachi, S.** et al. (2012) *Eur. J. Neurosci.* **36**, 3365–3375.

17. **Barbas, H.** and **Pandya, D.N.** (1989) *J. Comp. Neurol.* **286**, 353–375.

18. **Preuss, T.M.** (1993) In: *Primates and Their Relatives in Phylogenetic Perspective.* (ed. MacPhee R.D.), pp. 333–362 (Plenum, New York).

19. **Preuss, T.M.** (2007) In: *Evolution of Nervous Systems* (eds. Kaas, J.H. and Preuss, T.M.), pp. 2–34 (Elsevier, New York).

20. **Shadmehr, R.** and **Wise, S.P.** (2005) *The Computational Neurobiology of Reaching and Pointing* (MIT Press, Cambridge, MA).

21. **Wise, S.P.** and **Willingham, D.T.** (2009) In: *Encyclopedia of Neuroscience* (ed. Squire, L.R.), vol. **5**, pp. 1057–1066 (Academic Press, Oxford).

22. **Chang, S.W.** and **Snyder, L.H.** (2010) *Proc. Natl. Acad. Sci. USA* **107**, 7951–7956.

23. **Chang, S.W., Papadimitriou, C.,** and **Snyder, L.H.** (2009) *Neuron* **64**, 744–755.

24. **Batista, A.P., Santhanam, G., Yu, B.M., Ryu, S.I.** et al. (2007) *J. Neurophysiol.* **98**, 966–983.

25. **Blohm, G., Keith, G.P.,** and **Crawford, J.D.** (2009) *Cereb. Cortex* **19**, 1372–1393.

26. **Bremner, L.R.** and **Andersen, R.A.** (2012) *Neuron* **75**, 342–351.

27. **Crawford, J.D., Henriques, D.Y.,** and **Medendorp, W.P.** (2011) *Annu. Rev. Neurosci.* **34**, 309–331.

28. Marzocchi, N., Breveglieri, R., Galletti, C., and **Fattori, P.** (2008) *Eur. J. Neurosci.* **27**, 775–789.

29. McGuire, L.M. and **Sabes, P.N.** (2009) *Nat. Neurosci.* **12**, 1056–1061.

30. McGuire, L.M. and **Sabes, P.N.** (2011) *J. Neurosci.* **31**, 6661–6673.

31. Mullette-Gillman, O.A., Cohen, Y.E., and **Groh, J.M.** (2005) *J. Neurophysiol.* **94**, 2331–2352.

32. Pesaran, B., Nelson, M.J., and **Andersen, R.A.** (2006) *Neuron* **51**, 125–134.

33. Cui, H. and **Andersen, R.A.** (2007) *Neuron* **56**, 552–559.

34. Cui, H. and **Andersen, R.A.** (2011) *J. Neurosci.* **31**, 18130–18136.

35. Leathers, M.L. and **Olson, C.R.** (2012) *Science* **338**, 132–135.

36. Mazzoni, P., Bracewell, R.M., Barash, S., and **Andersen, R.A.** (1996) *J. Neurophysiol.* **76**, 1439–1456.

37. Gold, J.I. and **Shadlen, M.N.** (2007) *Annu. Rev. Neurosci.* **30**, 535–574.

38. Roitman, J.D. and **Shadlen, M.N.** (2002) *J. Neurosci.* **22**, 9475–9489.

39. Colby, C.L. and **Duhamel, J.R.** (1996) *Brain Res. Cogn. Brain Res.* **5**, 105–115.

40. Colby, C.L., Duhamel, J.R., and **Goldberg, M.E.** (1996) *J. Neurophysiol.* **76**, 2841–2852.

41. Snyder, L.H., Batista, A.P., and **Andersen, R.A.** (1998) *J. Neurophysiol.* **79**, 2814–2819.

42. Paré, M. and **Wurtz, R.H.** (2001) *J. Neurophysiol.* **85**, 2545–2562.

43. Buneo, C.A., Jarvis, M.R., Batista, A.P., and **Andersen, R.A.** (2002) *Nature* **416**, 632–636.

44. Kalaska, J.F. and **Crammond, D.J.** (1995) *Cereb. Cortex* **5**, 410–428.

45. Pesaran, B., Nelson, M.J., and **Andersen, R.A.** (2008) *Nature* **453**, 406–409.

46. Johnson, P.B., Ferraina, S., Bianchi, L., and **Caminiti, R.** (1996) *Cereb Cortex.* **6**, 102–119.

47. Wise, S.P., Boussaoud, D., Johnson, P.B., and **Caminiti, R.** (1997) *Annu. Rev. Neurosci.* **20**, 25–42.

48. Baumann, M.A., Fluet, M.C., and **Scherberger, H.** (2009) *J. Neurosci.* **29**, 6436–6448.

49. Nakamura, H., Kuroda, T., Wakita, M., Kusunoki, M. et al. (2001) *J. Neurosci.* **21**, 8174–8187.

50. Fluet, M.C., Baumann, M.A., and **Scherberger, H.** (2010) *J. Neurosci.* **30**, 15175–15184.

51. Brochier, T., Boudreau, M.J., Paré, M., and **Smith, A.M.** (1999) *Exp. Brain Res.* **128**, 31–40.

52. Kermadi, I., Liu, Y., Tempini, A., and **Rouiller, E.M.** (1997) *Somat. Mot. Res.* **14**, 268–280.

53. Matsumura, M., Sawaguchi, T., Oishi, T., Ueki, K. et al. (1991) *J. Neurophysiol.* **65**, 1542–1553.

54. Rouiller, E.M., Yu, X.H., Moret, V. et al. (1998) *Eur. J. Neurosci.* **10**, 729–740.

55. Schieber, M.H. and **Poliakov, A.V.** (1998) *J. Neurosci.* **18**, 9038–9054.

56. Fogassi, L., Gallese, V., Buccino, G., Craighero, L. et al. (2001) *Brain* **124**, 571–586.

57. Gallese, V., Murata, A., Kaseda, M., Niki, N. et al. (1994) *NeuroReport* **5**, 1525–1529.

58. Bullock, D. and **Grossberg, S.** (1988) In: *Dynamic Patterns in Complex Systems* (eds. Kelso, J.A.S., Mandell, A.J. and Shlesinger, M.F.) (World Scientific Publishers, Singapore).

59. Cisek, P., Grossberg, S., and **Bullock, D.** (1998) *J. Cogn. Neurosci.* **10**, 425–444.

60. Burnod, Y., Baraduc, P., Battaglia-Mayer, A., Guigon, E. et al. (1999) *Exp. Brain Res.* **129**, 325–346.

61. Andersen, R.A. and **Buneo, C.A.** (2002) *Annu. Rev. Neurosci.* **25**, 189–220.

62. Gaffan, D. and **Hornak, J.** (1997) *Brain* **120**, 1647–1657.

63. Rushworth, M.F.S., Nixon, P.D., and **Passingham, R.E.** (1997) *Exp. Brain Res.* **117**, 292–310.

64. Rushworth, M.F.S., Nixon, P.D., and **Passingham, R.E.** (1997) *Exp. Brain Res.* **117**, 311–323.

65. Wolpert, D.M., Ghahramani, Z., and **Jordan, M.I.** (1995) *Exp. Brain Res.* **103**, 460–470.

66. Pouget, A., Ducom, J.C., Torri, J., and **Bavelier, D.** (2002) *Cognition* **83**, B1–B11.

67. Sergio, L.E. and **Scott, S.H.** (1998) *Exp. Brain Res.* **122**, 157–164.

68. Heiser, L.M. and **Colby, C.L.** (2006) *J. Neurophysiol* .**95**, 2751–2767.

69. Duhamel, J.-D., Colby, C.L., and **Goldberg, M.E.** (1992) *Science* **255**, 90–92.

70. Ijspeert, A.J., Nakanishi, J., and **Schaal, S.** (2002) *Proc IEEE Int. Conf. on Robotics and Automation*, pp. 1398–1403.

71. Wainscott, S.K., Donchin, O., and Shadmehr, R. (2005) *J. Neurophysiol.* **93**, 786–800.

72. Desmurget, M., Epstein, C.M., Turner, R.S., Prablanc, C. et al. (1999) *Nat. Neurosci.* **2**, 563–567.

73. Day, B.L. and Lyon, I.N. (2000) *Exp. Brain Res.* **130**, 159–168.

74. Prablanc, C. and Martin, O.J. (1992) *Neurophysiology* **67**, 455–469.

75. Desmurget, M., Pelisson, D., Rossetti, Y., and Prablanc, C. (1998) *Neurosci. Biobehav. Rev.* **22**, 761–788.

76. Grea, H., Pisella, L., Rossetti, Y., Desmurget, M. et al. (2002) *Neuropsychologia* **40**, 2471–2480.

77. Smith, M.A., Brandt, J., and Shadmehr, R. (2000) *Nature* **403**, 544–549.

78. Cooke, D.F. and Graziano, M.S.A. (2004) *J. Neurophysiol.* **91**, 1648–1660.

79. Graziano, M. (2006) *Annu. Rev. Neurosci.* **29**, 105–134.

80. Graziano, M.S., Taylor, C.S., and Moore, T. (2002) *Neuron* **34**, 841–851.

81. Graziano, M.S., Taylor, C.S., Moore, T., and Cooke, D.F. (2002) *Neuron* **36**, 349–362.

82. Gharbawie, O.A., Stepniewska, I., Qi, H., and Kaas, J.H. (2011) *J. Neurosci.* **31**, 11660–11677.

83. Stepniewska, I., Fang, P.C., and Kaas, J.H. (2005) *Proc. Natl. Acad. Sci. USA* **102**, 4878–4883.

84. Stepniewska, I., Fang, P.C., and Kaas, J.H. (2009) *J. Comp. Neurol.* **517**, 765–782.

85. Stepniewska, I., Friedman, R.M., Gharbawie, O.A., Cerkevich, C.M. et al. (2011) *Proc. Natl. Acad. Sci. USA* **108**, E725–E732.

86. Stepniewska, I., Gharbawie, O.A., Burish, M.J., and Kaas, J.H. (2014) *J. Neurophysiol.* **111**, 1100–1119.

87. Nudo, R.J. and Masterton, R.B. (1988) *J. Comp. Neurol.* **277**, 53–79.

88. Nudo, R.J. and Masterton, R.B. (1990) *J. Comp. Neurol.* **296**, 559–583.

89. Kaas, J.H. (2004) *Anat. Rec. A Discov. Mol. Cell Evol. Biol.* **281**, 1148–1156.

90. Dum, R.P. and Strick, P.L. (2005) *J. Neurosci.* **25**, 1375–1386.

91. Preuss, T.M., Stepniewska, I., and Kaas, J.H. (1996) *J. Comp. Neurol.* **371**, 649–675.

92. Lu, M.-T., Preston, J.B., and Strick, P.L. (1994) *J. Comp. Neurol.* **341**, 375–392.

93. Gharbawie, O.A., Stepniewska, I., Burish, M.J., and Kaas, J.H. (2010) *Cereb. Cortex* **20**, 2391–2410.

94. Burish, M.J., Stepniewska, I., and Kaas, J.H. (2008) *J. Comp. Neurol.* **507**, 1151–1168.

95. Dum, R.P. and Strick, P.L. (2005) In: *Motor Cortex in Voluntary Movements* (eds. Riehle, A. and Vaadia, E.), pp. 3–47 (CRC Press, Boca Raton, FL).

96. Morecraft, R.J., Louie, J.L., Herrick, J.L., and Stilwell-Morecraft, K.S. (2001) *Brain* **124**, 176–208.

97. Morecraft, R.J., Cipolloni, P.B., Stilwell-Morecraft, K.S., Gedney, M.T. *et al.* (2004) *J. Comp. Neurol.* **469**, 37–69.

98. Gibson, J.J. (1979) *The Ecological Approach to Visual Perception* (Houghton Mifflin, Boston, MA).

99. Critchley, M. (1953) *The Parietal Lobes* (Edward Arnold, London).

100. Rondot, P., de Recondo, J., and Dumas, J.L. (1977) *Brain* **100**, 355–376.

101. Goodale, M.A., Milner, A.D., Jakobson, L.S., and Carey, D.P. (1991) *Nature* **349**, 154–156.

102. James, T.W., Culham, J., Humphrey, G.K., Milner, A.D. et al. (2003) *Brain* **126**, 2463–2475.

103. Milner, A.D. and Goodale, M.A. (1993) In: *Progress in Brain Research* (eds. Hicks, T.P., Molotchnikoff, S. and Ono, T.), pp. 317–337 (Elsevier, Amsterdam).

104. Cisek, P. (2012) *Curr. Opin. Neurobiol.* **22**, 927–936.

105. Cisek, P. and Kalaska, J.F. (2010) *Annu. Rev. Neurosci.* **33**, 269–298.

106. Hoshi, E. and Tanji, J. (2006) *J. Neurophysiol.* **95**, 3596–3616.

107. Basso, M.A. and Wurtz, R.H. (1998) *J. Neurosci.* **18**, 7519–7534.

108. Bastian, A., Riehle, A., Erlhagen, W., and Schoner, G. (1998) *NeuroReport* **9**, 315–319.

109. Bastian, A., Schoner, G., and Riehle, A. (2003) *Eur. J. Neurosci.* **18**, 2047–2058.

110. Cisek, P. and Kalaska, J.F. (2005) *Neuron* **45**, 801–814.

111. Klaes, C., Westendorff, S., Chakrabarti, S., and Gail, A. (2011) *Neuron* **70**, 536–548.

112. McPeek, R.M. and Keller, E.L. (2002) *J. Neurophysiol.* **87**, 1805–1815.

113. Platt, M.L. and Glimcher, P.W. (1997) *J. Neurophysiol.* **78**, 1574–1589.

114. Powell, K.D. and Goldberg, M.E. (2000) *J. Neurophysiol.* **84**, 301–310.

115. Schall, J.D. and Bichot, N.P. (1998) *Curr. Opin. Neurobiol.* **8**, 211–217.

116. Scherberger, H. and Andersen, R.A. (2007) *J. Neurosci.* **27**, 2001–2012.

117. Padoa-Schioppa, C. (2011) *Annu. Rev. Neurosci.* **34**, 333–359.

118. Pastor-Bernier, A. and Cisek, P. (2011) *J. Neurosci.* **31**, 7083–7088.

119. Dorris, M.C. and Glimcher, P.W. (2004) *Neuron* **44**, 365–378.

120. Gold, J.I. and Shadlen, M.N. (2000) *Nature* **404**, 390–394.

121. Kim, S. and Lee, D. (2011) *Biol. Psychiatr.* **69**, 1140–1146.

122. Platt, M.L. and Glimcher, P.W. (1999) *Nature* **400**, 233–238.

123. Yamagata, T., Nakayama, Y., Tanji, J., and Hoshi, E. (2012) *J. Neurosci.* **32**, 12934–12949.

124. Baxter, M.G., Parker, A., Lindner, C.C., Izquierdo, A.D. et al. (2000) *J. Neurosci.* **20**, 4311–4319.

125. Rudebeck, P.H., Saunders, R.C., Prescott, A.T., Chau, L.S. et al. (2013) *Nat. Neurosci.* **16**, 1140–1145.

126. Rhodes, S.E.V. and Murray, E.A. (2013) *J. Neurosci.* **33**, 3380–3389.

127. Wellman, L.L., Gale, K., and Malkova, L. (2005) *J. Neurosci.* **25**, 4577–4586.

128. Jones, B. and Mishkin, M. (1972) *Exp. Neurol.* **36**, 362–377.

129. Izquierdo, A., Suda, R.K., and Murray, E.A. (2004) *J. Neurosci.* **24**, 7540–7548.

130. Rudebeck, P.H. and Murray, E.A. (2014) Program no. 206.10. *2014 Neuroscience Meeting Planner* (Society for Neuroscience, Washington, DC). Online.

131. Rudebeck, P.H., Saunders, R.C., Lundgren, D., and Murray, E.A. (2015) Program no. 176.09. *2015 Neuroscience Meeting Planner* (Society for Neuroscience, Washington, DC). Online.

132. Amaral, D.G., Price, J.L., Pitkanen, A., and Carmichael, S.T. (1992) In: *The Amygdala: Neurobiological Aspects of Emotion, Memory and Mental Dysfunction* (ed. Aggleton, J.P.), pp. 1–66 (Wiley-Liss, New York).

133. Abe, H., Seo, H., and Lee, D. (2011) *Ann. NY Acad. Sci.* **1239**, 100–108.

134. Morrison, S.E. and Salzman, C.D. (2011) *Ann. NY Acad. Sci.* **1239**, 59–70.

135. Schultz, W., O'Neill, M., Tobler, P.N., and Kobayashi, S. (2011) *Ann. NY Acad. Sci.* **1239**, 109–117.

136. Wallis, J.D. and Kennerley, S.W. (2010) *Curr. Opin. Neurobiol.* **20**, 191–198.

137. Padoa-Schioppa, C. (2013) *Neuron* **80**, 1322–1336.

138. Wallis, J.D. and Miller, E.K. (2003) *Eur. J. Neurosci.* **18**, 2069–2081.

139. Kim, J.N. and Shadlen, M.N. (1999) *Nat. Neurosci.* **2**, 176–185.

140. Genovesio, A., Tsujimoto, S., and Wise, S.P. (2011) *J. Neurosci.* **31**, 3968–3980.

141. Chen, N.H., White, I.M., and Wise, S.P. (2001) *Exp. Brain Res.* **139**, 116–119.

142. Avendaño, C., Price, J.L., and Amaral, D.G. (1983) *Brain Res.* **264**, 111–117.

143. Desimone, R. and Duncan, J. (1995) *Annu. Rev. Neurosci.* **18**, 193–222.

144. Armstrong, K.M. and Moore, T. (2007) *Proc. Natl. Acad. Sci. USA* **104**, 9499–9504.

145. Sato, T.R. and Schall, J.D. (2003) *Neuron* **38**, 637–648.

146. Passingham, R.E. and Wise, S.P. (2012) *The Neurobiology of the Prefrontal Cortex* (Oxford University Press, Oxford).

147. Buschman, T.J. and Miller, E.K. (2007) *Science* **315**, 1860–1862.

148. Sumbre, G., Gutfreund, Y., Fiorito, G., Flash, T. et al. (2002) *Science* **293**, 1845–1848.

Chapter 7

The feature memory system of anthropoids

Overview

Anthropoid primates and their haplorhine ancestors adapted to diurnal foraging, with the fovea and trichromacy among their visual innovations. Along with these developments, the posterior parietal and temporal cortex elaborated into the feature memory system, commonly known as the dorsal and ventral streams. The parietal parts of this system specialized in representing the metrics of resources, such as their distances and amounts; the temporal areas specialized in representing the visual and acoustic signs of resources, especially at a distance. In addition to these anthropoid innovations, the feature system incorporated sensory areas that had evolved in early mammals, such as the perirhinal and primary visual cortex, as well as posterior parietal and temporal areas that had emerged in early primates. In anthropoids, the feature system functioned along with the navigation system to underpin perceptions and memories that supported distance foraging.

Perception, action, and actuality

> The knowledge we use when we see has come from millions of years of interacting with objects .... The main lesson of illusions is that perceptions are not tied to object reality. Perceptions are guesses—predictive hypotheses—of what may be out there. They are our most intimate reality; yet as for any hypotheses, they may be wrong ....
>
> Gregory[1] (p. 21)

How can we interact with the world effectively if, as Gregory says, our perceptions are divorced from "object reality"? The Ebbinghaus illusion serves as an instructive example[2]. When small disks surround a bigger one, we perceive the central disk as larger than it actually is (Fig. 7.1C, top left). Likewise, when large disks surround a smaller one, the central shape seems smaller than the reality (Fig. 7.1C, top right). In an experiment using such stimuli, when the sizes of the two central disks were adjusted until they both seemed to be the same size, the one surrounded by large circles became bigger than the one surrounded by small circles (Fig. 7.1 C, bottom). Later, when subjects reached to the central disks to pick them up, they separated their thumb and index finger more for the larger disk than for the smaller one, despite the illusion of equal size (Fig. 7.1D)[2]. This finding and others like it[3–10] show that visually guided actions reflect "object realities" better than perception does.

Accurate movements and inaccurate perceptions both result from the evolutionary history of specialized representational systems, which arose at different times, in different

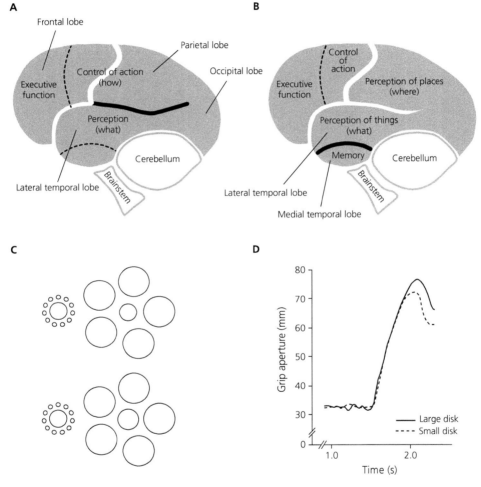

Fig. 7.1 Illusions. (A) Depiction of the perception–action dichotomy. (B) Depiction of the perception–memory dichotomy. (C) The Ebbinghaus size-contrast illusion. In the top half, the central disks had equal diameters, but people perceived the left central disk as larger. In the bottom half, the right central disk had a larger diameter, but people perceived the two central disks as congruent. (D) Hand aperture as subjects reached toward the edge of two central disks that they perceived as congruent. (C, D) Adapted from Aglioti S, DeSouza JFX, Goodale MA. Size-contrast illusions deceive the eye but not the hand. *Current Biology* 5:679–85, © 1995, Elsevier, with permission.

ancestors, and in response to different selective pressures. Visually guided movements depend on the manual-foraging system of early primates (see Chapter 6), which represents the metrics of graspable objects and must do so with exquisite accuracy. Visual perception tolerates inaccuracies because it depends on sensory areas that evolved in anthropoids, ancestors that sometimes made foraging choices based on relative quantities and qualities. Such judgments do not require absolute accuracy for the items being compared.

Because this chapter deals with visual perception, one aspect of the prevailing view becomes particularly pertinent. It treats a cortical area that we consider to be part of the feature system, the perirhinal cortex, as a "memory area" that lacks perceptual functions. Accordingly, a good deal of the discussion in this chapter focuses on this area, which brings in another so-called "memory" area, the hippocampus: a key part of the navigation system discussed in Chapter 4. For ease of reference, we call the idea that the cortex has segregated "perception" and "memory" areas the perception–memory dichotomy, and the thick line in Fig. 7.1(B) depicts the boundary between the two.

A similar concept distinguishes "perception" areas from those involved in the control of actions. It assigns visual perception to the inferior temporal cortex and visually guided action to the posterior parietal cortex[5,6]. We call this idea the perception–action dichotomy, and the thick line in Fig. 7.1(A) depicts the boundary between "perception" and "action" areas.

Both ideas remain popular, but, as Gregory says, like "any hypotheses, they may be wrong." The perception–memory dichotomy is wrong in two ways. Not only do the "memory areas" also have perceptual functions (see "The perception–memory dichotomy"), but the "perception areas" also have memory functions (see "Perception and memory"). The perception–action dichotomy is also wrong if interpreted literally. Many cortical areas classed as "perception areas" also contribute to the selection of action. Visual attributes such as color and shape can guide actions[10], and in Chapter 8 ("Arbitrary mapping" and "Conditional motor learning") we explain how the inferior temporal cortex contributes directly to this class of visually guided movements.

The two dichotomies depicted in Fig. 7.1(A, B) do not derive from fantasy, however. They represent an understandable misreading of the evidence, which stems in part from a reluctance to take evolution into account. The thick line in Fig. 7.1(B) indicates something important, all right, but it is not a boundary between "perception areas" and "memory areas." Instead, it separates a sensory area that evolved in early mammals, the perirhinal cortex (see Chapter 2, "Early mammals"), from inferior temporal areas that evolved in early primates and became especially prominent in anthropoids (see Chapter 2, "Early primates" and "Anthropoids"). The thick line in Fig. 7.1(A) also indicates a significant boundary. It separates sensory areas representing metrics, such as number, distance, and duration, from those representing qualitative attributes, such as color, shape, and visual texture[11-14]. Both the thick lines in Fig. 7.1 reflect evolutionary developments in our anthropoid ancestors as they adapted to life in their time and place.

Evolution

In Chapter 2 ("Anthropoids") we explained some of the changes that occurred in the brains and bodies of anthropoids after their divergence from other haplorhines. For the purposes of the present chapter, the most important developments involved vision and the elaboration of the posterior parietal and temporal cortex. In Chapter 8 we explore additional cortical developments in anthropoids, focusing on their new granular prefrontal areas. Figure 7.2(A) (left) shows the key anthropoid areas, shaded in dark gray.

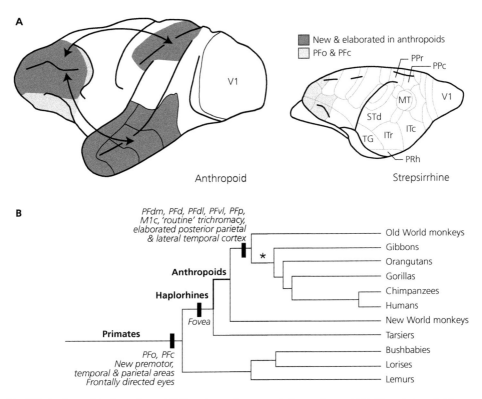

Fig. 7.2 Anthropoid adaptations. (A) Drawings of representative anthropoid (left) and strepsirrhine (right) brains, from a macaque and a bushbaby, respectively. Dark shading indicates the feature and goal systems in anthropoids; light shading marks prefrontal parts of the manual-foraging system. (B) Cladogram of primates, with emphasis on visual adaptations. The asterisk marks the last common ancestor of the ape–human lineage. Abbreviations: ITc, caudal inferior temporal cortex; ITr, rostral inferior temporal cortex; MT, middle temporal area; PFc, caudal prefrontal cortex; PFd, dorsal prefrontal cortex; PFdl, dorsolateral prefrontal cortex; PFdm, dorsomedial prefrontal cortex; PFo, granular orbitofrontal cortex; PFp, polar prefrontal cortex; PFvl, ventrolateral prefrontal cortex; PPc, caudal posterior parietal cortex; PPr, rostral posterior parietal cortex; PRh, perirhinal cortex; STd, dorsal superior temporal cortex; V1, primary visual cortex. Note that many of the innovative traits of Old World primates evolved in parallel in New World monkeys. (A) Cortical field boundaries on the right from Wong P, Kaas JH. Architectonic subdivisions of neocortex in the Galago (*Otolemur garnetti*). *Anatomical Record* 293:1033–69, © 2010, Wiley-Liss, Inc.

Figure 7.2(B) presents a cladogram emphasizing visual adaptations. As we explained in Chapters 2 ("Early primates" and "Anthropoids") and 6 ("Evolution"), many posterior parietal and temporal areas first appeared during the evolution of early primates, and both regions became larger and more elaborate during anthropoid evolution. Figures 6.1(B) and 6.3 illustrate some anthropoid developments in the posterior parietal areas, and similar augmentations occurred in the temporal cortex. As Kaas[15] (p. 1243) puts it, citing Felleman and Van Essen[16]:

> In Old World monkeys, over 30 visual areas have been proposed … and these primates have greatly expanded regions of visual cortex in the temporal and parietal lobes compared to most New World monkeys and all prosimians.

In the epigraph to this chapter (see "Perception, action, and actuality") we quoted Gregory as saying that our knowledge of the visual world comes from a long history of interacting with objects. That makes sense for objects, which people and other primates grasp and manipulate (see Chapter 6). But combinations of colors and shapes can also serve as signs of resource availability, often distant ones[17]. Sensory signs, like cues in the laboratory, cannot be grasped or manipulated in the way that nearby objects can. The same goes for relative quantities. Grivets grasp grapes, not greener or greater. The grivet—an Old World monkey species—can, of course, grasp green objects, including grapes, and can choose a greener grape over a less green one or a greater number of grapes over a lesser number. But neither grivets nor any other primate can literally grasp relations such as greener or greater.

With their foveas and the habit of foraging in daylight, evolving anthropoids saw much more than their ancestors could, especially in distant places. Stimuli that served as cues about distant resources did not require an accurate representation to provide an advantage to our anthropoid ancestors.

Proposal

With these ideas in mind, we advance the following proposal:

> *The feature memory system evolved in anthropoid primates, which foraged over large distances in daylight. A dorsal component of this system incorporated the posterior parietal areas of early primates, which specialized in visuomotor metrics (see Chapter 6). This region enlarged and elaborated in anthropoids, and its specialized representations came to support the perception and memory of visual metrics, such as number, distance, order, and duration. A ventral component of the feature system incorporated the temporal areas of early primates, along with sensory areas that evolved in early mammals, such as the perirhinal cortex. Like the dorsal component, the ventral one also enlarged and elaborated in anthropoids, and its specialized representations came to support the perception and memory of visual and acoustic signs, which indicated the presence and location of resources. As a whole, the feature system provided evolving anthropoids with advantages in making foraging choices at a distance and served as an exaptation for social signaling.*

The name *feature system* is merely a shorthand, of course, as we explained in Chapter 1 ("What did evolution produce?"). Other representational systems encode and store sensory features, so it might seem strange to apply this name to a limited set of cortical areas. According to our proposal, these areas developed specialized representations of the metrics and attributes of visual and auditory stimuli, and it is to these features that the name refers. As such, we could have entitled this chapter "The metrics–attributes memory system of anthropoids," and we invite readers to take the simpler term, "feature," in that way. The crucial part, however, is the last word: anthropoids. By any name, the specialized representations processed and stored in the feature system include important anthropoid innovations, intermixed among various kinds of representations that they inherited from early mammals, early primates, and their haplorhine ancestors.

Although the cortical areas comprising the feature system have been the subject of many reviews, only rarely have these discussions taken evolution or the lives of anthropoids into account[18,19]. According to the standard account, the occipital–parietal component of the feature system corresponds to a dorsal visual stream, which functions as the "where" system; the occipital–temporal component corresponds to a ventral stream, which functions as the "what" system[20]. Monosyllabic minimalisms of this kind are sometimes useful, but in this case they promote two misconceptions:

- The word "what" implies that the temporal cortex functions principally in the perception of objects. An evolutionary perspective indicates an additional role, one that involves the perception and memory of signs that indicate the location and availability of distant resources. We return to this topic in Chapter 8 ("Arbitrary categorization") in the context of temporal–prefrontal networks.

- The word "where" implies that the posterior parietal cortex mainly represents locations. As we explain later (see "Metrics"), its function is better understood as representing a wide variety of metrics, including distance, number, order, and duration, among others, with a particular emphasis on relational metrics.

Attributes

Our proposal implies that, sometime during anthropoid evolution, an enlarged and elaborated inferior temporal cortex added new kinds of representations to those available in the ancestral condition. In previous chapters we have dealt with new brain structures such as the hippocampus homologue of early vertebrates (see Chapter 4), the neocortex of early mammals (see Chapter 5), and new cortical areas in early primates (see Chapter 6). In each case, we advanced a proposal that spelled out some advantages provided by the specialized representations supported by these structures. For anthropoids, however, we defer most of this discussion to Chapter 8, which focuses on the prefrontal cortex. Accordingly, Chapters 7 and 8 should be considered together in this regard. The reason is that the contributions of the temporal cortex depend, in part, on its interactions with the new granular prefrontal areas that evolved in anthropoids. In this chapter, we concentrate instead on the feature system in isolation from the prefrontal cortex, beginning with the temporal cortex and the ventral visual stream.

The standard account of the ventral visual stream posits a series of processing stages (Fig. 7.3). So much has been written about this aspect of the anthropoid visual system that we only touch on a few, selected points here. From left to right in Fig. 7.3(A) this processing pathway includes the primary visual (striate) cortex, a number of extrastriate areas, the inferior temporal cortex, and the perirhinal cortex. Figure 7.3(B) illustrates how four visual features, indicated by the letters A–D, combine in various ways:

◆ Low-level representations involve elemental features and simple conjunctions.

◆ Mid-level representations involve feature conjunctions that are more complex than low-order features but less complex than whole objects.

◆ High-level representations involve complex conjunctions of features that often correspond to whole objects or their equivalent among other kinds of stimuli.

Despite the impression left by Fig. 7.3 we do not mean to imply that the information flows in only one direction, from left to right as depicted in the figure. Although neuronal responses in the perirhinal cortex depend on the features encoded by neurons in the inferior temporal cortex[21], representations in the inferior temporal cortex depend on inputs from the perirhinal (and entorhinal) cortex[22,23]. These interactions reflect modern conditions. Before primates evolved, the perirhinal cortex could not have depended on inputs from the inferior temporal cortex because the latter did not exist in anything like its present form.

As mentioned earlier, the standard view of the ventral visual stream holds that the inferior temporal cortex functions as a stage in an "object–analyzer" pathway. This line of thinking, however, neglects some important aspects of anthropoid evolution. In Chapter 2 ("Anthropoids") we explained that ancestral anthropoids not only needed to deal with objects that they could recognize, grasp, and manipulate, but also with distant cues and signs of resources. Color is a particularly important aspect of distance foraging, and combinations of colors and shapes probably played a key role in choices among distant foraging goals. Lesion evidence supports the idea that the inferior temporal cortex

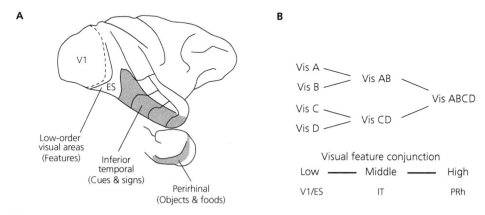

Fig. 7.3 Feature conjunctions in the occipital and temporal cortex of macaque monkeys. (A) Lateral view of a monkey brain. Rostral is to the right. (B) Conjunctions of visual (Vis) features A, B, C, and D, from low- to high-order visual areas. Abbreviations: ES, extrastriate visual areas; IT, inferior temporal cortex; PRh, perirhinal cortex; V1, primary visual cortex.

functions in distinguishing among colors but not among objects or other object-like stimuli[24]. From an evolutionary perspective, the fact that most mammals can recognize objects without an elaborate inferior temporal cortex suggests that it has some different function.

Object analysis is an important part of the function of the ventral stream, of course, but it need not involve the inferior temporal cortex. Multiple feedforward and feedback projections bypass the intermediate stages originally proposed for the ventral stream. Some primary and extrastriate visual areas project directly to the perirhinal cortex, for example, without relaying information via the inferior temporal cortex[25]. As a result of these connections, object recognition pathways can, in principle, bypass the inferior temporal cortex, although some dependency seems to have developed in anthropoids[21].

Another perspective also points to a role for the inferior temporal cortex apart from object analysis. Some researchers have proposed the existence of as many as four visual processing pathways extending from the primary and extrastriate visual areas into the inferior temporal cortex, many of which have little to do with the foveal processing that underlies object identification. The dorsal part of the inferior temporal cortex specializes in representing the lower part of the visual field; the ventral inferior temporal cortex is biased toward the upper visual field; and a ventral part of area V4 specializes in representing the peripheral visual field[25]. None of this has much to do with object identification. Furthermore, cortex in the ventral bank and fundus of the superior temporal sulcus specializes in motion processing, not object identification. In this context, the idea that the inferior temporal cortex functions "for the purpose" of object identification requires a thorough reconsideration.

This reconsideration leads to a straightforward, if unconventional, conclusion: The inferior temporal cortex does not function exclusively or even primarily as a way-station toward object perception, identification, or recognition. Instead, it processes and stores new, specialized kinds of feature conjunctions, which evolved in ancestral anthropoids in response to the selective pressures of their time and place. Its mid-level feature conjunctions might improve the ability to identify objects to some extent, but their principal adaptive advantage is to represent the signs of distant resources.

Rather than devoting this chapter to the specialized representations that developed in the inferior temporal cortex, we refer readers to a recent volume on visual neuroscience[26], which considers the neurophysiology and psychophysics of glossiness, visual texture, color contrast, spatial frequency, stereopsis, color–shape conjunctions, face recognition, and so forth. Although these topics are important, they are not crucial for understanding the conceptual issues addressed in this chapter. By putting such topics aside, we can focus on a narrower set of specialized representations, in the perirhinal cortex and the hippocampus, which underlie both the perception and memory of objects and scenes. The perception–memory dichotomy[27] (see "Perception, action, and actuality") conflicts directly with this idea, of course, and so it serves as the focal point of this chapter. Later, we address whether sensory areas, such as the inferior temporal cortex, also have memory functions (see "Perception and memory"). First, however, we tackle the perception–memory dichotomy from a different angle, asking the opposite question: Do the so-called "memory areas" also have perceptual functions? This question has particular importance for the feature system because one of its key components, the perirhinal cortex, is usually grouped with the hippocampus as part of the so-called "medial temporal lobe memory system."

The perception–memory dichotomy

The prevailing doctrine and its discontents

According to the perception–memory dichotomy, memory depends on the "medial temporal lobe" and perception depends on the sensory areas of cortex. From a neurophysiological perspective, a rigid dichotomy between "perception" and "memory" areas seems implausible. It implies that neurons encoding object features for perception somehow refrain from playing any role in remembering those same objects. Likewise, neurons in "memory areas"—sometimes only a few millimeters away—somehow avoid making any contribution to perception, despite encoding a great deal of information about sensory inputs. Despite these dubious assumptions, the perception–memory dichotomy remains popular, in large part because it emerged from a simple observation. H.M. and other amnesic patients have severe memory impairments but relatively intact perceptual abilities, at least when tested in the standard ways (see "Traditional perception measures"). Proponents of the prevailing view also cite, as support for their ideas, two sets of experimental results from monkeys, which readers can find in reports by Buffalo et al.[28,29]:

- When monkeys had to choose between two stimuli that reappeared trial after trial, with no intervening stimuli (Fig. 8.8B, left), lesions of the perirhinal cortex caused a substantial impairment during testing the next day, but lesions of the inferior temporal cortex did not.

- When monkeys had to choose between two stimuli that reappeared only after several intervening trials involving different stimuli (see Fig. 8.8B, right), lesions of the inferior temporal cortex caused an impairment, but lesions of the perirhinal cortex did not.

These two tasks are usually called serial discrimination learning and concurrent discrimination learning, respectively, but we use different terms. We call the former the *single-pair task* and the latter the *multiple-pair task* in order to highlight the key procedural difference between them. Proponents of the perception–memory dichotomy consider the single-pair procedure to be a "memory task" and the multiple-pair procedure to be a "perception task." In Box 7.1 we explain why.

Given that lesions of the perirhinal cortex cause an impairment on the single-pair ("memory") task but not on the multiple-pair ("perception") task, it seems to follow that the perirhinal cortex functions in memory but not perception[29]. Likewise, lesions of the inferior temporal cortex cause an impairment on the so-called "perception task" and not on the "memory task," so it seems to function in perception but not memory[28–30]. Because

Box 7.1 Discriminating among discrimination tasks

The prevailing view of memory systems assumes that the single-pair task, also known as serial discrimination learning, is a "memory task" because it does not depend very much on perception. First, monkeys always chose between two grossly different stimuli in these experiments, which differed along so many dimensions—of color, shape, and size—that the monkeys could easily tell them apart. Second, monkeys had to recall the correct choice the next day or after several days.

In contrast, the multiple-pair task, also known as concurrent discrimination learning, is assumed to be a "perception task" because it requires distinctions among many stimuli, to the point that this factor is thought to determine the monkey's overall performance.

So when experiments showed that lesions of the perirhinal cortex impaired performance on the single-pair task and not the multiple-pair task they seemed to support an exclusive role for this cortical area in memory. Likewise, a selective impairment on the multiple-pair task after lesions of the inferior temporal cortex seemed to support an exclusive role for this cortical area in perception.

To be fair, advocates of the perception–memory dichotomy interpreted some additional results as support for their ideas as well. Reducing memory requirements by shortening a memory period should convert a "memory" task into a "perception" task. In accord with this assumption, lesions of the inferior temporal cortex impaired performance on memory tasks with brief delays, including short-interval matching tasks and spontaneous visual recognition, as measured by preferential viewing[29,30].

However, these results have little persuasive power. First, they depend to a large extent on two negative results: (1) Lesions of the perirhinal cortex did not cause an impairment on the multiple-pair task[29] and (2) lesions of the inferior temporal cortex did not affect performance on the single-pair task[28,29]. Conclusions based on negative results are inherently weak because they require acceptance of the null hypothesis based on a failure to reject it: a well-known statistical fallacy. Second, these experiments did not tax perception in a systematic way, as the feature-ambiguity experiments did[20,35–37]. And third, labels like "memory task" and "perception task" mask something more important: the stimulus material used in these experiments.

Results from other discrimination tasks (see Figs. 7.4 and 7.5) showed that the perirhinal cortex has memory functions and that the inferior temporal cortex has perceptual functions, as the prevailing view maintains. However, in addition, carefully designed discrimination tasks have demonstrated conclusively that the perirhinal cortex also has perceptual functions (see "Feature ambiguity") and that the inferior temporal cortex also has memory functions (see "Perception and memory"), as the prevailing view denies.

H.M. and other amnesic patients are said to have intact perceptual abilities—wrongly, as we explain later (see "Humans")—these monkey data fall neatly into line with the perception–memory dichotomy.

The key issue, however, is whether names like "perception task" and "memory task" accurately identify what the subjects in these experiments need to do. We have direct information from H.M. that they do not. If the multiple-pair procedure makes discrimination learning into a "perception task," then H.M. should have performed it well. Instead, he had a severe impairment on this task[31]. Of course, no one knows whether people and monkeys perform the multiple-pair task in the same way, but this finding certainly raises doubts about the assumption that it taxes perception independent of memory.

Given that some experts interpret the monkey experiments of Buffalo et al.[28,29] as support for the perception–memory dichotomy, and because this interpretation conflicts with our proposal, we need to ask how this doctrine arose in the first place. The answer involves a crucial variable in discrimination-learning experiments—a factor not captured by terms such as serial, concurrent, single-pair, multiple-pair, memory, or perception. The issue turns on the nature of the stimuli used in such experiments[32–34], and more specifically the extent to which stimuli share visual features: a concept called feature ambiguity or feature overlap[32]. Once this factor is taken into account, we can understand the specialized representations of each cortical area as an evolutionary innovation that provided an advantage to one of our ancestors.

Monkeys

Feature ambiguity

Natural objects often have many features in common, such as various combinations of colors and shapes. The more features in common, the higher the overlap among stimulus features. Because of feature overlap, the identification of objects requires the representation of a large set of features. Cortical neurons encode conjunctions of these features, and these unique feature conjunctions differentiate stimuli with high levels of feature overlap. We focus on qualitative visual features here, which we call attributes. The same principles, however, probably also apply to visual metrics and other sensory modalities.

The concepts of feature ambiguity and feature overlap are important for understanding the functions of the ventral stream[20,35–37] (Fig. 7.3A, B), and a consideration of brain evolution helps clarify the issues involved. In Chapters 2 and 5 we explained that the perirhinal cortex emerged in early mammals. By representing feature conjunctions at the level of natural objects, it functioned to disambiguate the objects that these animals encountered during foraging. As such, the perirhinal cortex has always been part of a visual processing pathway. (Some experts have taken its somatosensory inputs, for example, to contradict the classification of the perirhinal cortex as a visual area[38]. We see no conflict, however, between the multimodal character of the perirhinal cortex and its place in a visually dominated feature system; it seems a natural progression to add yet more features to the representation of objects.)

Experiments that place the perirhinal cortex securely within the ventral visual stream required subjects to discriminate pairs of stimuli with high feature overlap, little feature overlap, or intermediate properties (Fig. 7.4). Saksida and Bussey summarize this line of research in detail[32,37], so we present only a brief overview here, beginning with three experiments.

The first type of experiment used compound stimuli, each consisting of two images, to manipulate feature ambiguity. Figure 7.4(A, left) shows two stimuli that share all of the features in their top halves. Despite this ambiguity, subjects needed to choose the left stimulus to obtain food. This task used four pairs of compound stimuli: AB+, CD+, CB−, and AD−, where + indicates the correct choice. The name biconditional applies to this task because the correct choice had to meet two conditions (A and B, in this example, or C and D). A name of this type provides little help in understanding the results, but the concepts of feature overlap and ambiguity help a great deal. Because no single set of features determined the correct choice, the monkeys needed to represent feature conjunctions in order to disambiguate the compound stimuli. The key point of the experiment was its contrast between conditions of high feature ambiguity (Fig. 7.4A) and low feature ambiguity (not illustrated). In the former, every component image appeared equally often in both correct and incorrect choices. In the latter, each component image appeared in either correct choices or incorrect choices, but never both.

In the second feature-ambiguity experiment, a morphing algorithm mixed the features of two stimuli to varying degrees. In these experiments, subjects first learned which of two normal images to choose (Fig. 7.4B, top row). The subjects then used these memories to choose between stimuli with morphing-induced feature ambiguity (Fig. 7.4B, second and third rows). Notably, this task involved the discrimination of a single pair of images.

In the third kind of feature-ambiguity experiment, subjects learned the transverse patterning task. A given stimulus always served as both the correct and incorrect choice in equal proportions (Fig. 7.4C). For example, the monkey needed to choose the image with the flag on some trials (top row) and to avoid it on other trials (bottom row).

These three experiments yielded similar results[39,40]. Lesions of the perirhinal cortex caused impairments when monkeys needed to choose between stimuli with high levels of feature ambiguity, but not when they made otherwise identical choices between stimuli with little feature ambiguity. Figure 7.5(A) shows that lesions of the perirhinal cortex caused a significant impairment in the biconditional task under conditions of high feature ambiguity; Fig. 7.5(B) documents the severe impairment for conditions of high feature ambiguity in the morphing task; and Fig. 7.5(C) illustrates the impairments on the transverse patterning task. These findings demonstrated that the amount of feature overlap in the stimulus material explained the effects of perirhinal cortex lesions, not labels such as "memory" or "perception" tasks. Furthermore, they indicated that the earlier findings on discrimination tasks by Buffalo et al.[28,29]—which were interpreted as reflecting roles for the inferior temporal cortex and the perirhinal cortex in "perception" and "memory," respectively—also resulted from the stimulus material used.

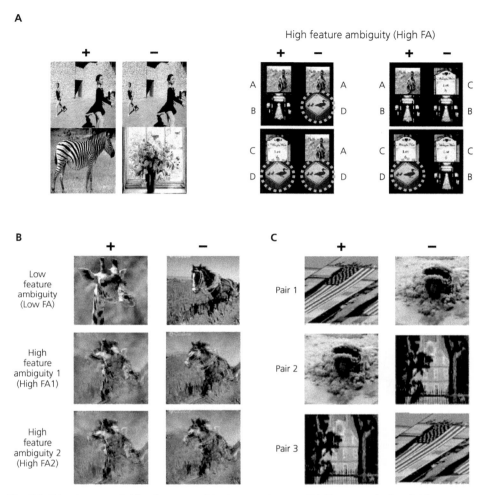

Fig. 7.4 Stimulus material for feature-ambiguity experiments. (A) Compound stimuli. The monkeys needed to choose the left compound stimulus in each set to receive a reward (+). The alternative choice produced no reward (–). (B) Morphed stimuli. The top pair shows the picture that the monkeys needed to choose (left) and avoid (right). The next two rows represent stimuli with various mixtures of features taken from the two pictures in the top row. (C) Transverse patterning. Each row represents one of three possible trial types. Adapted from Murray EA, Bussey TJ, Saksida LM. Visual perception and memory: a new view of medial temporal lobe function in primates and rodents. *Annual Review of Neuroscience* 30:99–122, © 2007, Annual Reviews. Reproduced with permission of Annual Reviews, http://www.annualreviews.org.

Selective lesions of the hippocampus did not cause a significant impairment in any of the feature-ambiguity tasks. In fact, for the transverse patterning task (Figs. 7.4C and 7.5C), hippocampus lesions led to an improvement in performance compared with control monkeys[33]. This finding probably resulted from reducing the interference generated by strategies mediated by the hippocampus. Even a modest tendency to make a choice based on the location of a stimulus within a visual scene, for example, will interfere with performance on the transverse patterning task. In Chapter 4 ("Scene memory") we explained that the hippocampal complex contributes to such choices. The finding that the

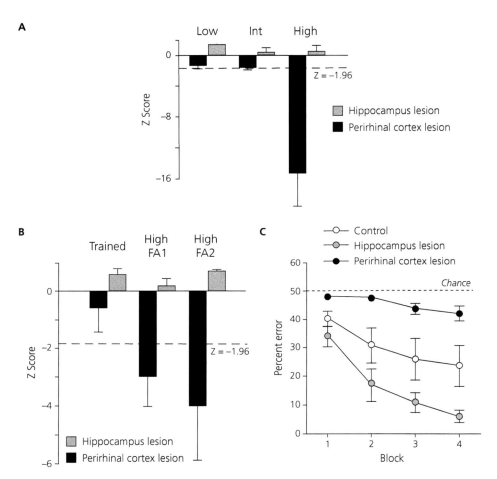

Fig. 7.5 Results from the feature-ambiguity experiments in monkeys. (A) Results from the compound-stimulus experiment (Fig. 7.4A). The dashed horizontal line shows the level of impairment that reached statistical significance. The abscissa indicates the level of feature ambiguity from low, through intermediate (Int), to high levels. (B) Results from the morphing experiment (Fig. 7.4B). Abbreviations: FA1, feature ambiguity at one high level of morphing; FA2, feature ambiguity at another, higher level. Format as in (A). (C) Results from the transverse patterning experiment (Fig. 7.4C), averaged over blocks. Error bars: standard error. Adapted from Murray EA, Bussey TJ, Saksida LM. Visual perception and memory: a new view of medial temporal lobe function in primates and rodents. *Annual Review of Neuroscience* 30:99–122, © 2007, Annual Reviews. Reproduced with permission of Annual Reviews, http://www.annualreviews.org.

hippocampus interferes with a perirhinal cortex function provides a strong indication that the various components of the so-called "medial temporal lobe memory system" have different functions, reflecting their specialized representations.

Critics of the feature-ambiguity experiments have suggested that the key results depended on either learning or memory. The experiment with morphed stimuli, described earlier, ruled out this objection. In this task, monkeys first learned to discriminate a single pair of stimuli with a low level of feature ambiguity, which they did easily. They then performed a probe test that involved a high level of ambiguity. The probe test (Fig. 7.5B) thus evaluated the ability of monkeys to distinguish stimuli with a high level of feature ambiguity on a small number of trials, which precluded learning effects. Furthermore, an analysis of the behavioral data confirmed that the monkeys did not exhibit learning during the performance of this task. In all three feature-ambiguity tasks, stimuli with high and low levels of ambiguity had the same memory requirements, which ruled out any objection in terms of memory load. Later in this chapter, we explain that the same arguments apply to studies in humans (see "Humans")[41].

A related task eliminated entirely the requirement to remember stimuli from trial-to-trial. In this task, monkeys needed to choose the odd stimulus out among several images[42]. In an example trial, monkeys saw a face from several different angles, along with the face of a different individual. The latter served as the odd stimulus out. Lesions of the perirhinal cortex caused impairments on this task even though the correct choice depended entirely on stimuli that subjects viewed simultaneously. In this task, subjects did not need to remember stimuli from trial to trial as in standard visual discrimination learning. Again, the concept of feature ambiguity accounts for these results without relying on specialized cognitive processes—perception versus memory—in different parts of the cortex.

Discrimination tasks that use stimuli with extensive feature overlap are difficult, of course, but task difficulty cannot explain the results either. In these and other experiments, monkeys with lesions of the perirhinal cortex could still learn difficult discriminations, including: those involving very small differences in the size, shape, and color of visual stimuli; images of objects rotated in various ways (but not previously viewed from that particular perspective); and images degraded by visual noise[40,42,43].

Summary

Taken together, these findings demonstrate that the perirhinal cortex represents feature conjunctions in support of both perception and memory. Later, we summarize findings demonstrating that sensory areas of cortex function in memory as well as perception (see "Perception and memory"). Together, these findings rule out both aspects of the perception–memory dichotomy.

There is an important qualification, however. The perirhinal cortex has perception and memory functions only for representations at a particular level of complexity[32]. When experiments use stimuli that are too simple[28,29] other cortical areas can handle the task. The perirhinal cortex, therefore, provides a very specific adaptive advantage: neural representations at the level of natural objects. The evolutionary history of this area, and the millions of years of interacting with objects that led to its properties, explains why it represents some levels of feature overlap and not others. This conclusion does not mean that laboratory experiments need to use naturalistic, three-dimensional stimuli, only that researchers should choose stimulus material carefully, taking into account the evolutionary adaptations of their research subjects.

Rodents

Research in rodents also supports the idea that the perirhinal cortex functions in visual perception, along with memory. In addition to tasks like those used in monkey research, rodent experiments often involve the exploration of objects in a foraging field. The field usually contains a novel object among familiar ones, and rats tend to spend more time exploring the former.

Conserved traits

Many results from rodents resemble those from monkeys. For example, in experiments that minimize the importance of positional and contextual cues, hippocampus lesions had no effect on object memory for periods of 48 hours[44]. These findings show that the hippocampus plays a minor role, if any, in object memory per se, in agreement with the most reliable results from monkeys (see Chapter 12, "Hippocampus lesions: small effect or no effect?").

Rodent research also reveals the effects of lesions of the perirhinal cortex, in isolation or combined with damage to either the entorhinal cortex, postrhinal cortex, or both. (The postrhinal cortex is probably homologous with the parahippocampal cortex of primates, or at least a part of it.) These lesions have consistently caused an impairment on short-interval matching tasks in rodents[45-47], as they have in monkeys[48] (see Chapter 12, "Falsification of the first model"). Likewise, rats with lesions of the perirhinal cortex (or combined lesions of the perirhinal and postrhinal cortex) had impairments on tasks that used stimuli with high levels of feature ambiguity. For example, perirhinal cortex lesions caused impairments in making odd-stimulus-out judgments among stimuli with high levels of feature ambiguity[49,50], and the degree of the impairment depended on the amount of feature overlap[49,51]. Importantly, these lesions caused significant impairments even without a substantial delay period[49,50,52], which agrees with results from monkeys that had combined lesions of the perirhinal and entorhinal cortex[53].

False recognition

In typical tests of object memory in rodents, a foraging field contains two different objects: one novel and one familiar. In an experiment by McTighe et al.[54], the field contained two identical objects instead. Rats first explored a sample pair of objects and, after an hour or so, they then saw either the familiar pair again or two versions of a novel object. As already mentioned, when rats choose between one novel and one familiar object they spend more time with the former: spontaneous exploration. Likewise, in the

McTighe et al. version of the task, control rats spent more time exploring a pair of novel objects than they did a familiar pair. After perirhinal cortex lesions, however, the rats spent the same amount of time with both pairs. This result could have occurred for either of two reasons:

◆ In forgetting, lesioned rats might have treated familiar objects as novel and therefore spent an abnormally long time exploring them.

◆ In false recognition, lesioned rats might have treated novel objects as familiar and therefore spent an abnormally short time with them.

McTighe et al. obtained a clear-cut result: Lesions of the perirhinal cortex caused false recognition. At first glance, this finding seems perplexing. Why would removal of an area that represents objects cause false recognition?

One possibility is that lesions of the perirhinal cortex removed the representations of natural objects, which rendered their subjects susceptible to interference from other sensory features. Figure 7.6 illustrates this idea, based on a replication in mice of results originally obtained in rats. The left column depicts the sample presentation, which applies to all three rows of the figure. The mice first saw two versions of the sample object and encoded its features both as elements {A, B, and C} and as a unique conjunction {ABC}. The top row depicts intact mice as they remember both the elemental features and the unique conjunction during the delay period. On some trials, the mice saw the sample objects again during the test phase. Control subjects recognized the object-unique feature conjunctions and treated the objects as familiar.

The middle row shows the effect of perirhinal cortex lesions, which led to false recognition. But how could the animals "recognize" an object they had never seen? The reason was that during the delay period the mice saw many low-order visual features in their cage, and the novel objects probably shared one or more of them. Figure 7.6 designates one such feature as {D}. According to this interpretation, control mice recognized the novelty of objects by contrasting what they saw with the object representations that they had in memory, based on unique feature conjunctions such as {ABC}. If an object was not represented in memory, the mice would have known that the stimulus pair was novel and treated it as such. Lesions of the perirhinal cortex removed these representations, which prevented the lesioned mice from recognizing that the stimuli were novel. As a result, feature {D} led to false recognition, a form of interference.

Visual isolation during the delay period prevented false recognition (Fig. 7.6, bottom row). This sensory restriction restored normal exploratory behavior by protecting animals with perirhinal cortex lesions from low-order visual features, thus eliminating the interference from feature {D}. Later, we discuss a similar result for humans, which involved both false recognition and protection from interference (see "Feature-ambiguity effects").

The prevailing view

These results agree remarkably well with our evolutionary account of the function of the perirhinal cortex. Yet, in contrast to these findings, Clark et al.[55] concluded that rats with

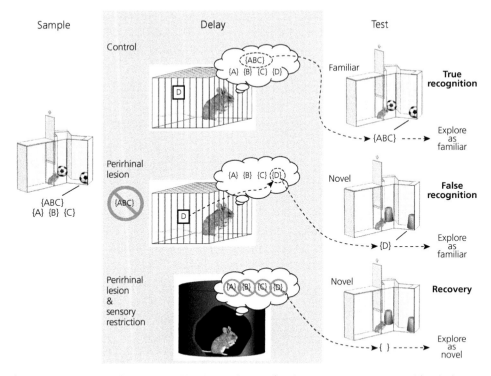

Fig. 7.6 Spontaneous object recognition in a rodent. Left column: A mouse saw two identical objects as a sample. {ABC} represents a conjunction of features at a high level of complexity; {A}, {B}, and {C} each indicate an elemental feature. Middle column (shaded): conditions during a delay period in control animals (top), lesioned animals placed in their home cage during the delay period (middle), and lesioned animals placed in a dark box during the delay period (bottom). The cloud shows the feature or features that the animal remembered during the delay period, including a feature in the cage: feature {D}. Right column: In the test phase, the mouse saw two identical objects, either the same ones as during the sample (familiar) or different ones (novel). The features in brackets represent the features or feature conjunctions used by the animal in choosing an exploration strategy. The null bracket, { }, indicates that the mouse did not recognize, truly or falsely, any of the item's features. Mouse and cage drawings from Romberg C, McTighe SM, Heath CJ, Whitcomb DJ, Cho K, Bussey TJ, Saksida LM. False recognition in a mouse model of Alzheimer's disease: rescue with sensory restriction and memantine. *Brain* 135:2103–14, © 2012, Oxford University Press, with permission.

lesions of the perirhinal cortex have normal perception of stimuli with a high degree of feature overlap. In their experiment, rats learned to discriminate one pair of stimuli, after which they underwent 150 trials with morphed stimuli. After lesions of the perirhinal cortex, the rats were then retrained with the same stimuli and presented with the morphed images again. This experiment yielded a negative result (i.e., there was no lesion-induced change in behavior), which Clark et al. interpreted as ruling out a role for the perirhinal cortex in perception.

Beyond the inherent weakness of negative results, the experimental design had important shortcomings, especially its use of stimulus material consisting of elongated images with their most distinctive features at the ends. The amount of functional feature overlap among such images could not be evaluated without knowing where the subjects attended within each stimulus. These experiments neither monitored nor controlled selective attention. Occlusion of one quadrant of an object, a procedure used in these experiments, did little to solve this problem although it did provide some useful data. After occlusion, a drop-off in performance showed that these rats used at least some of the occluded features to perform the task, and not the integrated feature conjunction.

Another factor was also important. The initial learning of the task required more than 10,000 trials, which revealed that the task used by Clark et al. was much more difficult than the ones used in the monkey or rodent experiments discussed earlier in this chapter (see "Monkeys" and "Rodents"). A high level of task difficulty often indicates an excessively artificial laboratory task, one too far afield from the problems that animals face in natural conditions. Artificiality occurs to some extent in every laboratory task, of course. However, in this extreme case the results probably reflected a mismatch between the stimulus material used and the objects that rodents encounter during natural foraging.

A more recent paper from the same laboratory also argued against a role for the perirhinal cortex in perception. Hales et al.[56] reported that lesions of both the hippocampus and perirhinal cortex decreased the normal preference for exploring the odd stimulus during the odd-stimulus-out task. Neither lesion affected traditional discrimination learning. The authors concluded that control rats relied on long-term memory to perform the odd-stimulus-out task because they moved among the stimuli slowly. It is more likely, however, that an impairment on a task requiring stimulus comparisons reflected a problem with perception. The finding that damage to the hippocampus also caused an impairment does not mean that the task is a "memory task" or that the perirhinal cortex is a "memory area," merely that the task required the specialized representations of both the perirhinal cortex (for objects) and the hippocampus (for navigation among objects). The negative result on discrimination learning simply followed from the unconstrained nature of such tasks and the ability of subjects to solve them in many different ways (see Chapter 12, "First attempts").

Summary

The perirhinal cortex evolved in early mammals (see Chapter 2, "Early mammals" and Chapter 5, "Evolution"), and its specialized representations provided advantages in distinguishing among the objects that they encountered during foraging. When experiments use stimulus material with a level of feature overlap typical of natural objects—and prevent animals from solving the task by using low-order features—lesions of the perirhinal cortex cause impairments. The evidence from rodents, therefore, supports that from monkeys: both demonstrate that the perirhinal cortex contributes directly to perception and memory.

Humans

In humans, the perception–memory dichotomy has taken an especially strong form. Given the inclusion of the hippocampus and perirhinal cortex in the "medial temporal lobe memory system," a perceptual role for either area might seem unlikely[38,57–60]. Reports of reasonably good perception after lesions of the so-called "memory areas" align with such views, and when neuropsychologists observe perceptual difficulties in patients with damage to these areas they tend to ascribe these impairments to concomitant cortical damage elsewhere, such as in the fusiform gyrus[61–63].

Recently, this attitude has changed, for two reasons. First, feature-ambiguity experiments, like those used with monkeys, have pointed to a role for the human perirhinal cortex in perception as well as memory. Second, these and other experiments have revealed that both the perirhinal cortex and the hippocampus support specialized forms of perception and memory. As explained earlier for monkeys (see "Feature ambiguity"), the functions of the perirhinal cortex and the hippocampus reflect their specialized representations: the former for object-level conjunctions, the latter for the kinds of representations useful for navigation (along with other functions that draw on these representations). We now take up these topics, in turn.

Feature-ambiguity effects

In experiments most like those on monkeys, patients with lesions that included the perirhinal cortex learned to discriminate among stimuli with variable levels of feature overlap. These experiments used the multiple-pair procedure described earlier. As Fig. 7.7 illustrates, four types of stimulus material—blobs, barcodes, bugs, and beasts—produced broadly similar results, which closely resembled the effects of selective lesions of the perirhinal cortex in monkeys (Fig. 7.5A, B). For each kind of stimulus, the patients had the largest impairment when stimuli had a high degree of feature ambiguity, with little or no impairment for highly distinct, low-ambiguity stimuli[64].

The attribution of these impairments to the perirhinal cortex deserves a comment. As well as damage to the perirhinal cortex, these patients had evidence of involvement of the septal (posterior) and amygdaloid (anterior) hippocampus, entorhinal cortex, amygdala, and anterior temporal cortex[65]. It is for this reason that we use the label "perirhinal cortex and hippocampus+" in Figs. 7.7–7.9 and 7.11, with emphasis on the (+). Fortunately, the impairment in these patients was remarkably similar to that caused by selective lesions of the perirhinal cortex in monkeys. Accordingly, the results in combination bolster an interpretation in terms of perirhinal cortex function.

Similar considerations apply to patients with semantic dementia. In a test illustrated in Fig. 7.8(A, B), patients with this degenerative disorder also had an impairment in the multiple-pair discrimination task, and this impairment was specific to stimuli with a high degree of feature ambiguity[66]. In Chapter 9 ("Anatomy of semantic dementia") we discuss the brain areas affected in semantic dementia, but for now we simply note that the damage includes the perirhinal cortex[67,68]. Like monkeys with selective lesions of the perirhinal cortex (Fig. 7.5A, B), patients with semantic dementia had specific impairments

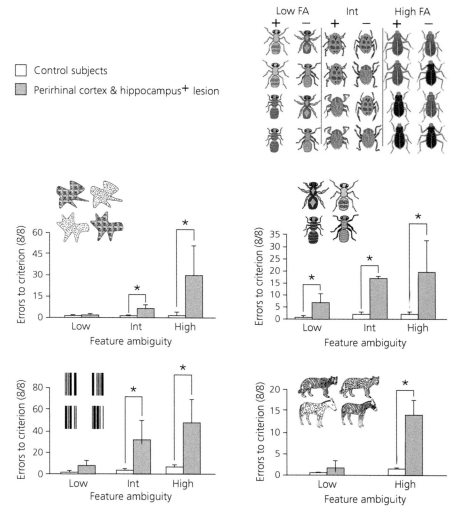

Fig. 7.7 Blobs, bugs, barcodes, and beasts. Top: one of the stimulus types, bugs, divided into stimulus pairs, each with a correct (+) and incorrect (–) choice. The degree of feature overlap varied from low, through intermediate (Int), to high levels. Bottom: effect of lesions of the perirhinal cortex, hippocampus, and nearby areas on feature ambiguity tasks. Top left, blobs (complex shapes with different fills); bottom left, barcodes; top right, "bugs" (arthropods); bottom right, "beasts" (animals). Asterisks denote statistically significant impairments. Redrawn from Barense MD, Bussey TJ, Lee ACH, Rogers TT, Davies RR, Saksida LM, Murray EA, Graham KS. Functional specialization in the human medial temporal lobe. *Journal of Neuroscience* 25:10239–46, © 2005, Society for Neuroscience, with permission.

in identifying and distinguishing certain stimuli with high levels of feature ambiguity. Stimuli with lower levels of feature overlap did not cause these patients any difficulty, also like the monkey results. Figure 7.8(C) summarizes these results, adding data from patients with static (as opposed to degenerative) lesions that included the perirhinal cortex (triangles), like the results illustrated in Fig. 7.7.

Figure 7.8(D) shows results from a different experiment, one that used the odd-stimulus-out task. Patients with semantic dementia had perceptual impairments both for pictures of familiar objects and for novel object-like stimuli constructed from shapes and shadings (called greebles). Again, these patients showed perceptual impairments in high-ambiguity conditions but not in low-ambiguity conditions, as did patients with static lesions (Fig. 7.8E).

Perhaps the most comprehensive analysis of feature ambiguity comes from a study by Barense et al.[69]. In their experiment, two stimuli appeared simultaneously: These stimuli consisted of blobs similar to those illustrated in Fig. 7.7, but with two shapes, one inside the other. The subjects then indicated by button presses whether two stimulus items matched each other perceptually. Three feature dimensions defined each blob: inner shape, outer shape, and fill; and the two stimuli on every trial differed from each other in either one or three dimensions. When the stimuli differed in just one dimension they shared more features and therefore served as a high feature-ambiguity condition. When they differed along three dimensions, feature overlap was low.

In the high-ambiguity condition, control subjects shifted their gaze among locations within a blob much more than from blob to blob. This finding demonstrated that they analyzed the ambiguous stimuli in their entirety, rather than by serial comparison of isolated features from blob to blob. Furthermore, brain imaging studies revealed greater activation in the perirhinal cortex for high-ambiguity than for low-ambiguity conditions, independent of task difficulty[69]. Patients with lesions that included the perirhinal cortex had a significant impairment on this task[70].

False recognition[71] and interference in memory contributed to this impairment, like the findings summarized earlier for rodents (see "False recognition"). Patients with lesions that included the perirhinal cortex performed progressively worse as trials built up during a testing session, which was probably a result of trial-to-trial interference[69]. The presentation of perceptually distinct colored stimuli between trials with high-ambiguity blobs served to reduce interference and restored performance to normal levels.

Representational specializations

If, among the so-called "memory areas" of the "medial temporal lobe," only the perirhinal cortex has a perceptual function, the prevailing view might survive simply by eliminating this area from its model of memory. Empirical contradictions go much deeper than that, however. A number of studies demonstrate that—like damage to the perirhinal cortex—damage to the hippocampus impairs both perception and memory, a conclusion that comes from tests of recognition memory[72,73], discrimination learning[74], and performance of the odd-stimulus-out task[65]. Lee et al.[75] and Graham et al.[34] review these and

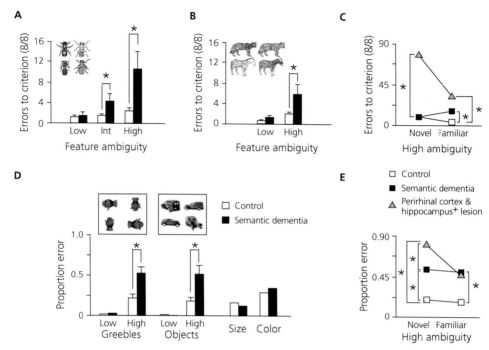

Fig. 7.8 Effect of feature overlap on two tasks in two patient groups. (A–C) Multiple-pair discrimination learning. (D, E) The odd-stimulus-out task. (A, B) Patients with semantic dementia (black bars) performed as well as healthy subjects (unfilled bars) for familiar stimuli with low levels of feature overlap. For bugs (A) and beasts (B), high levels of feature ambiguity led to perceptual impairments. (C) For patients with semantic dementia (black squares), discrimination impairments were specific to familiar stimulus material, such as bugs and beasts, and were not seen for novel stimuli, such as barcodes and blobs. Patients with lesions like those from Fig. 7.7 (gray triangles) had large impairments for both kinds of stimuli. Note that the control data point for the novel stimuli had the same value as for patients with semantic dementia and so is not visible in the plot. (D) For the odd-stimulus-out task, greebles are object-like stimuli consisting of combinations of shapes and surfaces. Patients with semantic dementia had a significant impairment in high- but not low-ambiguity conditions for both this novel stimulus material and drawings of familiar objects. Size and color perception were unaffected in these patients. (E) Results on the odd-stimulus-out task from semantic dementia patients (black squares) and patients with static lesions that included the perirhinal cortex (gray triangles). Asterisks denote statistically significant impairments. Adapted from Barense MD, Rogers TT, Bussey TJ, Saksida LM, Graham KS. Influence of conceptual knowledge on visual object discrimination: insights from semantic dementia and MTL amnesia. *Cerebral Cortex* 20:2568–82, © 2010, Oxford University Press, with permission.

complementary findings in detail, so we discuss only some of these results here. Not only does the hippocampus play a role in perception, but it does so in a particular cognitive domain: for visual scenes, but not for faces or spatial patterns[73].

Figure 7.9 illustrates some representative results, based on the odd-stimulus-out task. We explained earlier (see "Feature ambiguity") that this task has no significant memory

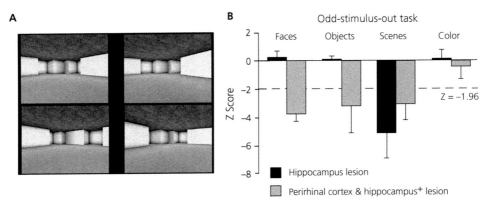

Fig. 7.9 Odd-stimulus-out task. (A) Scenes used in the odd-stimulus-out task. The lower, left scene is the odd one out. (B) Scores on four versions of the odd-stimulus-out task. Bars extending below the dashed line indicate statistically significant impairments. Note that the data in (B) came from two different experiments, one involving repeated stimuli and the other using trial-unique stimuli. The plus sign (+) after hippocampus indicates that additional structures were included in the lesion. From Lee AC, Barense MD, Graham KS. The contribution of the human medial temporal lobe to perception: bridging the gap between animal and human studies. *Quarterly Journal of Experimental Psychology, B* 58:300–25, © 2005, Taylor & Francis, with permission. www.tandfonline.com.

component beyond the need to remember the rule: choose the stimulus that is unlike the others in an array of items (Fig. 7.9A). Note that in the odd-stimulus-out experiments with monkeys there was an initial learning component, but in the human studies no prior training occurred before testing, which involved trial-unique stimuli. In this experiment, one group of subjects was characterized by selective, partial lesions of the hippocampal complex; the other group by lesions that included the hippocampus and neocortical areas near it, most notably the perirhinal cortex—like the patients whose results are illustrated in Fig. 7.7.

Like H.M., subjects in both lesion groups performed normally on traditional neuropsychological measures of perception. Such observations, of course, led to the perception–memory dichotomy in the first place. Tasks using scenes as stimulus material, however, revealed perceptual impairments in both patient groups, consistent with their hippocampus lesions[75]. Figure 7.9(A) shows some of the scenes used in these experiments, which looked like a room one might navigate through, perhaps to reach a door. As Fig. 7.9(B) (black bars) illustrates, patients with lesions restricted to the hippocampus, although impaired on the odd-stimulus-out task for scene stimuli, did not have the same difficulties for faces, object-like pictures, or colored squares.

Patients with more extensive damage, which included the perirhinal cortex, had more pervasive perceptual difficulties. Figure 7.9(B) (gray bars) documents their impairments on many versions of the odd-stimulus-out task, including for faces and objects. These patients performed the color version of the odd-stimulus-out test normally, however, which shows that they understood the requirements of the task, and that, like the monkeys, they could perform difficult perceptual discriminations when the stimulus material did not tap representations thought to be dependent upon either the perirhinal cortex or the hippocampus. In addition to the odd-stimulus-out task, perception and memory was tested with a matching task that had no delay period, and these experiments yielded similar results. We direct readers to two reviews[34,75] for the details of these experiments.

A report by Mundy et al.[70] generalized these findings by incorporating perceptual learning into the mix. According to the prevailing view, because such learning establishes implicit (procedural) knowledge, the perirhinal cortex and the hippocampus should not be involved. By pre-exposing subjects to stimulus material of three kinds—complex scenes, faces, or dot patterns (Fig. 7.10A)—Mundy et al. could measure the performance benefits that follow perceptual learning. They found that hippocampus damage impaired the learning of sensory discriminations for scenes but not for faces or dot patterns (Fig. 7.11A, middle; Fig. 7.11B, left). This lesion also caused the loss of a reaction-time benefit for previously viewed scenes, while retaining faster responses for previously seen faces and dot patterns (Fig. 7.11B, right). Lesions that included the perirhinal cortex[76] led to impairments in both scene and face learning, but not in dot-pattern learning (Fig. 7.11A, right; Fig. 7.11C). These patients performed as well or better than healthy subjects in their preserved cognitive domains (Fig. 7.11A, left; gray shading in Fig. 7.11B, C).

Results from four brain imaging experiments reinforced the idea that the hippocampus and perirhinal cortex house different and specialized representations. The first showed activations in the hippocampus for scenes and in the perirhinal cortex for faces (Fig. 7.10B)[70]. The second used multivariate pattern classifiers to decode activation in the hippocampus and perirhinal cortex. Multivoxel decoding in the hippocampus distinguished among scenes but not objects[77]; in contrast, multivoxel decoding in the perirhinal cortex distinguished among objects but not scenes[78]. The third compared the discrimination of viewpoints—the angles from which subjects saw a scene, face, or object—that were either easy or difficult to distinguish from one another. This study revealed a significant difficulty-related difference in activation for scenes in the hippocampus and for faces and objects in the perirhinal cortex[79]. The fourth involved the odd-stimulus-out task with objects and faces that differed in familiarity. Greater activation occurred in the perirhinal cortex, but not in the hippocampus, when subjects perceived objects and faces as familiar, compared to unfamiliar stimuli[80]. Importantly, this result did not depend on how well the subjects remembered the stimuli, which rules out an interpretation in terms of long-term memory or incidental learning[81].

Studies that contrast the impairments seen in Alzheimer's disease and semantic dementia also support the idea that the hippocampus and perirhinal cortex process and store different, specialized representations. In Chapter 9 ("Anatomy of semantic dementia") we explain that these two patient groups differ in many respects, but especially in the degree of degeneration in the septal (posterior) hippocampus. The hippocampus (and especially the septal hippocampus), is severely atrophied in Alzheimer's

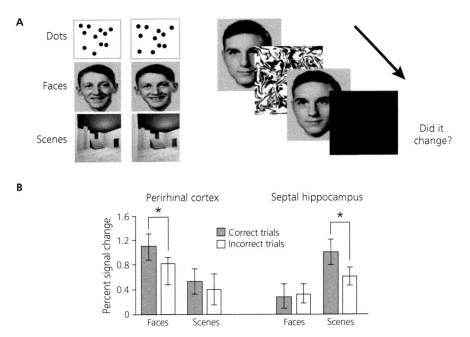

Fig. 7.10 The dots, faces, and scenes tasks. (A) Examples of stimulus items used in perception tasks. In these experiments, pre-exposure to the stimuli resulted in perceptual learning, which aided subsequent task performance. Subjects reported whether the stimulus was the same or different in a series of stimulus presentations. (B) Brain imaging activations for the faces and scenes tasks, with a comparison between correct versus incorrectly discriminated trials. From Mundy ME, Downing PE, Dwyer DM, Honey RC, Graham KS. A critical role for the hippocampus and perirhinal cortex in perceptual learning of scenes and faces: complementary findings from amnesia and fMRI. *Journal of Neuroscience* 33:10490–502, © 2013, Society for Neuroscience, with permission.

disease, whereas patients with semantic dementia typically have greater damage to the perirhinal cortex. In the trial-unique, odd-stimulus-out task discussed earlier (see "Feature-ambiguity effects"), patients with Alzheimer's disease had impairments in oddity judgments about scenes, as opposed to faces, whereas the reverse was true for patients with semantic dementia[82,83].

Taken together, this literature demonstrates differential contributions to scene and object–face perception by two distinct representational systems: the former involving the hippocampus and the navigation system (see Chapter 4); the latter involving the perirhinal cortex and the feature system.

Artificial networks

Computational models also support the ideas presented here. A model by Cowell et al.[84,85] simulated lesions in an connectionist network trained to discriminate inputs. Different

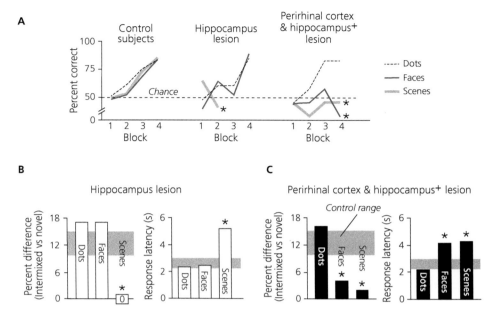

Fig. 7.11 Perceptual learning. (A) Learning of the three tasks depicted in Fig. 7.10(A) in control subjects and in two patients: one with a lesion of the hippocampus, the other with combined damage to the hippocampus, perirhinal cortex, and nearby areas. (B) Performance accuracy and response speed in the patient with the hippocampus lesion compared with the standard error observed in healthy control subjects (gray shading). The bars indicate the difference in the percentage of correct responses for intermixed novel and pre-exposed stimuli, taken together, versus novel stimuli. (C) Data for the patient with the larger lesion. Format as in (B). Asterisks indicate significant differences from control subjects. From Mundy ME, Downing PE, Dwyer DM, Honey RC, Graham KS. A critical role for the hippocampus and perirhinal cortex in perceptual learning of scenes and faces: complementary findings from amnesia and fMRI. *Journal of Neuroscience* 33:10490–502, © 2013, Society for Neuroscience, with permission.

layers of the model generated conjunctions with increasing complexity from lower layers to higher layers (Fig. 7.3B). Removal of the lower layers impaired the discrimination of inputs with small amounts of feature ambiguity; removal of higher layers did so for inputs with large amounts. These models prove a principle: We can understand the experimental results from monkeys, rodents, and humans without relying on the perception–memory dichotomy.

Cowell et al. drew an analogy between the middle layers of their network and the inferior temporal cortex. Likewise, they related the higher layers to the perirhinal cortex. They also postulated a yet higher layer that added more dimensions to conjunctive representations and might correspond to the hippocampus. In biological systems, these additional dimensions probably involve contextual, temporal, and layout-related features[84]. Figure 9.7(C) illustrates this pathway in the context of another one that includes the perirhinal cortex: a pathway that sends conjunctive representations to the prefrontal cortex, which adds dimensions related to outcomes, goals, and actions (see Chapter 9, "Conclusions").

A related computational model by Elfman et al.[86] explained why some brain imaging studies have seemed to support a role for the hippocampus in memory but not perception. The authors showed that the hippocampus became activated in a graded manner for tasks that are usually interpreted in terms of perception, but in a step-wise, threshold-like manner during tasks typically thought of as taxing memory. The graded patterns resulted from the similarity among stimuli used in the former kind of test, which resulted in pattern completion. In tasks thought to tax memory, pattern completion only occurred some of the time, and so the activations appeared at a particular threshold[87]. Depending on the level of feature overlap and the statistical threshold set for detecting activations, these properties could create the false impression of activation specific to "memory tasks."

Traditional perception measures

We still need to explain why patients with lesions of the hippocampus and the perirhinal cortex seem, on the surface, to have preserved perceptual abilities. Our explanation is that standard neuropsychological tests of perception place little demand on the specialized, conjunctive representations that these cortical areas process and store[88]. Tests such as copying a complex drawing, for example, can be performed using feature-by-feature comparison, and are not, therefore, dependent upon conjunctive representations in either area. The same goes for other common tests of perception, such as counting dots and identifying letters. The specialized representations of the hippocampus and the perirhinal cortex—for complex scenes and commonly encountered objects, respectively—can only be revealed by tests that match their specializations.

When we say that the perirhinal cortex represents conjunctions at the level of natural objects[89], the word *level* has more importance than the word *object*. In humans, the perirhinal cortex mediates perceptions and memories of much more than objects per se. We have already mentioned its role in representing faces (Figs. 7.9B, 7.10B, and 7.11) and it also seems to contribute to the representation of semantic categories. In one study, the perirhinal cortex showed greater activation when people distinguished semantic items with high levels of feature ambiguity, such as lambs versus sheep, than when they did so for more distinctive (low-ambiguity) items, such as snakes versus pigs[90]. These findings indicate that the perirhinal cortex represents conjunctions with high amounts of feature overlap for both visual and semantic items. Auditory conjunctions, however, appear to be processed separately for the most part[91].

The fact is that any kind of stimulus—even those that are not objects—can have feature overlap that happens to be at the same level as that seen among natural objects. According to our proposal, the perirhinal cortex functions at this level because of its origins in stem mammals and the advantages they gained from disambiguating the objects in their world. Homologues of the perirhinal cortex have subsequently adapted to the life of modern mammals, including humans.

Summary

Experimental results from humans, like those from monkeys and rodents, have ruled out the perception–memory dichotomy and have pointed instead to a different idea, one that aligns with our evolutionary perspective. The perirhinal cortex and hippocampus evolved to process and store specialized representations, which in both cases provided a particular ancestor with competitive advantages. The perirhinal cortex evolved in early mammals, and it specialized in conjunctive representations at the level of natural objects; a homologue of the hippocampus evolved in early vertebrates, and it specialized in representing complex scenes and spatial layouts that reflect its ancestral role in navigation (see Chapter 4, "Scene memory"). Box 7.2 relates some testimony from a patient supporting the latter conclusion. For both the perirhinal cortex and the hippocampus, a specialization for a particular kind of representation accounts for the data much better than does a specialization for memory.

Not only does the dominant view of memory reject a role for the hippocampus in perception, but its concept of "memory" is limited to explicit (declarative) forms. The evidence points to a broader role for the hippocampus: (1) perception in addition to memory; and (2) implicit memory in addition to explicit memory. In fact, the hippocampus plays a necessary role in implicit scene perception[65,92], implicit scene memory[93], and implicit perceptual learning (Fig. 7.11)[34,82] in addition to explicit memory. In Chapter 11 we take up the topic of explicit memory, and so we defer further consideration of the implicit–explicit distinction until then.

Box 7.2 A patient's introspection

Graham et al.[34] (p. 832) quote a patient with damage restricted to the hippocampus, who once explained her symptoms as follows:

> The areas of my life that I find most challenging are when I am given a series of directions, remembering my way around somewhere (familiar or unfamiliar), how I got into a building and how I can get out of it again, driving somewhere not only for the first time, but many times, remembering where I left my car and how I got into the car park in the first place, which way to turn out of a car park to get home …. Whichever angle I look, everything looks the same.
>
> I would prefer not to call my experiences "memory problems," they are not. This is a total misrepresentation of the damage I have. What I experience are "orientational problems".

The patient discerned from her symptoms the fundamental distinction between navigation via snapshot memory and via a cognitive map, describing the former as clearly as in any professional writing:

> I check my position at regular intervals. I literally take mental photos by stopping, turning round and taking a visual snapshot. When it is time to find my way back, I rely on my mental snapshots. I think my visual memory is good and it compensates for the reduced spatial memory I have.

Metrics

So far this chapter has dealt with attribute features, but the feature system of anthropoids also has areas specialized for metric representations, which include parameters such as number, speed, distance, duration, and relative location.

Posterior parietal cortex

We begin with a particularly important metric: order. Neurophysiological experiments in monkeys have shown that cells in the posterior parietal cortex encode the place of an item in an ordered sequence[94,95], and lesions of these areas impaired the performance of tasks requiring order information[96]. (In Chapter 8, "Neurophysiology," we discuss impairments on order tasks after lesions of the granular prefrontal cortex[97,98].)

Posterior parietal cortex neurons also encode another metric: ordinal number. Figure 7.12(A) illustrates the activity of cells in area 5, a part of the posterior parietal cortex that encoded the number of movements made by monkeys. In this task, monkeys either pushed or turned a handle on each trial, and the task required that they make the same movement five trials in succession. After five handle turns, for example, the monkeys had to switch to pulling the handle for five trials. The black line in Fig. 7.12(A) shows the activity of a neuronal population that encoded the third movement in this sequence. The

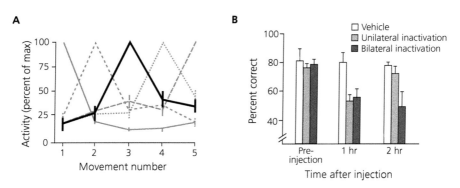

Fig. 7.12 Representation of a metric in area 5 of the posterior parietal cortex. Monkeys made one of two movements for five consecutive trials, then switched to the alternative for five trials. (A) The activity of five populations of cells after trial onset and prior to a "go" signal that initiated a movement. The black line illustrates a neuronal population that encoded the third movement in the sequence. Gray lines show different neuronal populations. Each population had a preference for either the first, second, third, fourth, or fifth movement. For each population, the activity was normalized to the maximum. Error bars: standard error. (B) Performance before and after inactivations of area 5, either unilaterally (light gray) or bilaterally (dark gray) for two time points after inactivation. Unfilled bars represent control (vehicle) injections. Error bars: standard error. (A) Reprinted from Sawamura H, Shima K, Tanji J. Numerical representation for action in the parietal cortex of the monkey. *Nature* 415:918–22, © 2002, with permission from Macmillan Publishers Ltd. (B) Adapted from Sawamura H, Shima K, Tanji J. Deficits in action selection based on numerical information after inactivation of the posterior parietal cortex in monkeys. *Journal of Neurophysiology* 104:902–10, © 2010, Macmillan Publishers Ltd.

gray lines show four additional neuronal populations, one each for the other four movements[99]. In accord with these data, inactivation of the area containing these cells caused an impairment on this task, which was especially severe after bilateral inactivations (Fig. 7.12B)[96].

Figure 7.13(A) illustrates a different metric: relative length. In this experiment, monkeys saw two line segments, usually of different lengths. This stimulus array served as a sample for the short-interval matching task. After a delay period, the monkeys then saw a series of additional displays, and to receive a reward they had to press a switch when the proportion of the two lines matched that of the sample. In the trial illustrated in Fig. 7.13(A), the sample consisted of two lines: one four units in length, the other two units. So the monkeys needed to press the switch whenever the line proportion had a ratio of 2-to-1. Figure 7.13(B) shows the activity of a neuron from the posterior parietal cortex (area 7) that encoded relative length[100]. Specifically, when the monkey saw the test stimulus, the highest level of activity occurred for line-segment ratios of 3-to-4 in this particular neuron.

Other neurophysiological experiments have demonstrated that posterior parietal neurons encode a wide variety of metrics, and in Chapter 8 ("Neurophysiology") we explain that cells in the prefrontal cortex do so as well[101-104]. These metrics include the number of items in a stimulus array[105], the absolute length of line segments[105], and abstract spatial categories such "above" or "below"[106], as well as other spatial categories[107] and both duration and distance[103,104,108-112]. Although number and duration have an especially large literature[95,111,113], it seems likely that the posterior parietal cortex of monkeys processes and stores metrics of most, if not all, kinds.

Neurons in these areas also reflect metric-based task rules, such as one that says to choose a larger number of items over a smaller number. Figure 7.13(C) shows the activity of a neuron that encoded such a rule, and neurons in these areas also encoded analogous rules for the length of line segments, such as one that instructed a choice of the shorter of two lines[100,114-116].

We could relate additional instances of such coding, but these examples suffice to demonstrate that the anthropoid posterior parietal cortex encodes much more than spatial locations. Although often referred to as a "where" system (Fig. 7.1B), the dorsal visual stream has a much broader function than that.

Foraging

No one doubts that anthropoid primates use qualitative attributes of the visual world to make foraging choices, such as colors and visual textures. However, the use of metric features requires some documentation. Accordingly, several field and laboratory studies have investigated whether anthropoids use relational metrics in making foraging choices.

Numerosity has received the most attention. Anthropoids easily learn to make choices based on the number of items in a particular part of visual space[117,118], as do other primates[119]. In some circumstances, anthropoids prefer to make choices based on other

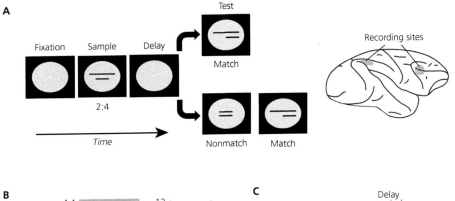

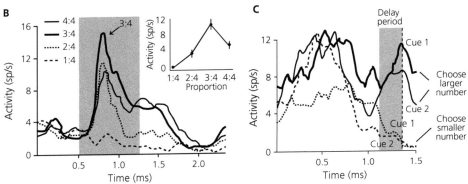

Fig. 7.13 The encoding of relational metrics in the prefrontal and posterior parietal cortex. (A) A short-interval matching task that used a pair of line segments as the sample. The monkey made a choice based on the ratio of the two lengths. This sample stimulus had a ratio of 2-to-4. The brain drawing to the right shows the areas studied (shading). (B) The activity of a neuron in the posterior parietal cortex during the task shown in (A). The measured interval corresponded to the shaded period, relative to the onset of the test stimulus (0 ms). This cell preferred length ratios of 3-to-4 (heavy line). The inset shows the mean number of spikes per second (sp/s) and the standard error for different length ratios. (C) The activity of a prefrontal cortex neuron during a relative-number task. On each trial, one of four cues appeared: two of the cues indicated that the monkeys needed to choose the greater quantity in a choice between arrays with different numbers of items, and two cues provided the opposite instruction. During the delay period, this neuron preferred trials when the goal was the larger number of items (continuous lines) compared with the smaller number (dashed lines). (A, B) Redrawn from Vallentin D, Nieder A. Representations of visual proportions in the primate posterior parietal and prefrontal cortices. *European Journal of Neuroscience* 32:1380–7, © 2010, with permission from John Wiley & Sons. (C) Redrawn from Bongard S, Nieder A. Basic mathematical rules are encoded by primate prefrontal cortex neurons. *Proceedings of the National Academy of Sciences U.S.A.* 107:2277–82, © 2010, with permission.

kinds of quantitative information, such as average density of items or other summed measures[120,121], but they can use number to the exclusion of other metrics. Macaque monkeys can also apply abstract rules based on relative numerosity, such as learning to choose the larger number of items in one sensory context and the smaller number in a different context[115,117,118]. As for other foraging-related metrics, common marmosets make foraging choices based both on the distance to an item and nearer–farther distinctions[122]; baboons and capuchin monkeys use above–below distinctions[123,124]; and macaques make choices based on relative distance, with astoundingly steep discounting functions[125-128]. In one such study, it required a nine-fold increase in food quantity to induce monkeys to move 15 feet rather than 10 feet[127]!

Conclusions

Perception and memory

Perception and memory do not map onto different parts of the cerebral cortex as depicted in Fig. 7.1(B). Instead, cortical fields that the prevailing view designates as "memory areas" also contribute to perceptions involving their specialized representations. We have concentrated on this "half" of the perception–memory dichotomy, but its other "half" is equally problematic: Areas classed as "perception areas" also store memories.

We point here to just four of many[129] results that support this conclusion. First, Chapter 6 ("Goal vector") discussed evidence from a lesion study in monkeys which showed that posterior sensory areas house memories for potential goals contralateral to the fixation point[130].

Second, in a brain imaging experiment[131], subjects first made perceptual judgments about famous people, locations, and the recency of object use. For several sensory areas, multivariate pattern classifiers were trained on the activations that occurred during these sessions, for later use. In the next phase of the experiment, the subjects learned arbitrary associations between pairs of these stimuli: a paired-associate task. Finally, in a subsequent imaging session, the subjects saw a stimulus, waited through a delay period, saw a second stimulus, and reported whether it was a member of a pair with the first. For cortical activations that occurred during the paired-associate task, the multivariate pattern classifiers could decode the kind of stimulus held in memory during the delay period, even though the classifiers had been trained on the perceptual task. These classifiers can only work if perception and memory draw on common representations—in this case, memories activated during the delay period.

Third, similar pattern classifiers could decode line orientations maintained in memory in areas V1–V4 of the human visual cortex, and these activations closely resembled perceptual responses[132].

Fourth, a study of gene expression in the secondary visual cortex (V2) of rats showed that proteins regulating an intracellular signaling pathway converted temporary stimulus memories, which usually dissipated in less than an hour, into memories that persisted for months[133]. Cells expressing this regulatory protein were located in layer 6, and an excitotoxic lesion of this layer eliminated the long-term memories of these visual stimuli.

Vision and streams

With rare exceptions[18,19], discussions of the visual processing streams have neglected the evolutionary and ecological context that produced them. According to our proposal, as anthropoids became large, far-ranging, diurnal foragers (see Chapter 2, "Anthropoids"), enhanced representations of visual metrics and the qualitative signs of resources provided these animals with advantages in making foraging choices at a distance. Although we have not dealt with them here, similar representations supported social interactions as well, such as those involving face recognition and postural gestures.

The emergence of the fovea (in haplorhines) and trichromatic vision (in catarrhines), along with other enhancements in vision, changed forever the information available to the anthropoid brain. The feature system exploited these developments by storing new kinds of representations. Representations differ from area to area in the kinds of conjunctive representations that they process and store: each adapted to a particular kind of information important to that particular species. Different species have their own sets of areas and therefore varying capacities for representing particular conjunctions. All mammals can process and store visual information of the kind represented in the V1 (striate) and V2 cortex, as well as at the level of natural objects, as represented in the perirhinal cortex. In addition to these conserved traits, anthropoids developed new and elaborated areas in the posterior parietal and lateral temporal cortex, which make up the bulk of their feature system. This evolutionary sequence implies that the "mid-level" feature conjunctions represented in the inferior temporal cortex (Fig. 7.3B) evolved long after both the high-level representations of the perirhinal cortex and the low-order representations of the V1 and V2 cortex (see Chapter 2, "Early primates"). Furthermore, all of these specialized areas evolved long after the hippocampal homologue (see Chapter 2, "Early amniotes"). Theories that posit an ordered hierarchy from low-order visual areas to the hippocampus[84] need to address an evolutionary history indicating that the highest of these levels evolved most remotely in vertebrate history and mid-levels evolved most recently. As new representational systems arose, they altered the functions of older ones, mainly through interactions with them.

In the epigraph of this chapter (see "Perception, action, and actuality"), we quoted Gregory's statement that the "main lesson of [visual] illusions is that perceptions are not tied to object reality." But some aspects of vision are. Vision-for-action, for example, cannot tolerate illusions. In Chapter 6 we explained that, as part of the manual-foraging system, parietal–premotor networks use visuomotor memories for interacting with objects and other affordances in the world. Box 7.3 depicts vision-for-action in action by illustrating the properties of a premotor cortex neuron, one that encoded the location of a remembered visual stimulus when it served as the target of a reaching movement, but not when it served solely as a spatial matching stimulus (Fig. B.1 in Box 7.3). Reaching for, grasping, and manipulating objects require a metric accuracy tied very tightly to object reality.

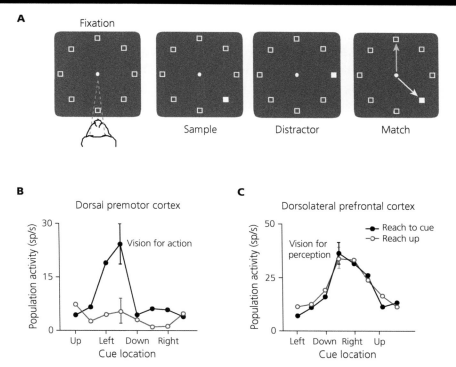

Box 7.3 Vision-for-action versus vision-for-perception at the neuronal level

A

Fixation

Sample

Distractor

Match

B Dorsal premotor cortex

Population activity (sp/s)

Vision for action

Up   Left   Down   Right
Cue location

C Dorsolateral prefrontal cortex

Population activity (sp/s)

Vision for perception

● Reach to cue
○ Reach up

Left   Down   Right   Up
Cue location

Fig. B.1 Vision-for-action and vision-for-perception in neuronal activity. (A) In this experiment, the monkey began each trial by fixating a light spot at the center of a circular array of light-emitting diodes. On each trial, one of the lights turned on as the sample for the short-interval (spatial) matching task. After some number of distractor (nonmatching) stimuli, the monkey made a reaching movement immediately after the match stimulus appeared. Two rules were alternated in blocks: The monkey either reached to the matching stimulus (white arrow) or to the top location regardless of where the sample and match had appeared (gray arrow). (B) A vision-for-action cell from the dorsal premotor cortex. This neuron encoded the sample and match stimuli only when they served as the target of movement, with a preference for stimuli down and to the left of the fixation point. (C) A vision-for-perception neuron from the dorsolateral prefrontal cortex. This cell had the same activity regardless of where the monkey reached, with a preference for cues down and to the right. The directions on the abscissa differ in (B) and (C) in order to normalize the plots to the maximum. From di Pellegrino G., Wise SP. Visuospatial versus visuomotor activity in the premotor and prefrontal cortex of a primate. *Journal of Neuroscience* 13:1227–43, © 1993, republished with permission of the Society for Neuroscience.

Figure B.1(B) illustrates the activity of a vision-for-action neuron, located in the dorsal premotor cortex[137]. In this experiment, the monkey needed to follow one of two rules, which alternated in blocks of trials. For both rules, the monkey had to detect a spatial matching stimulus. When a match occurred, the monkey then made a reaching movement that differed depending on the rule. According to one rule, the monkey needed to reach to the matching stimulus in order to obtain a reward (Fig. B.1A, white arrow); for the other rule, the monkey needed to reach to a fixed location (gray arrow), regardless of the matching cue's location.

Most cells in the dorsal premotor cortex encoded the location of a matching stimulus when it served as a goal for movement (Fig. B.1B, black circles) but not (or to a lesser extent) when the monkey simply detected a match (unfilled circles), even for the same cue locations. This property reflects the role of premotor areas in vision-for-action. In contrast, results in Fig. B.1(C) come from a neuron in the granular prefrontal cortex. Cells there encoded stimulus location regardless of the movement that it triggered. Neurons encoding vision-for-action and vision-for-perception coexist, intermixed, in the granular prefrontal cortex[138], but the dorsal premotor cortex is highly specialized for controlling visually guided movements[137].

Vision-for-perception, in contrast, involves relational analysis of attributes and metrics in the world. The feature system does not require absolute accuracy to provide an adaptive advantage, as long as it gets the relative values right: more here, less there; something a little glossier than something else. According to this account, perceptual illusions result in part from the adaptations of our anthropoid ancestors and the kinds of foraging choices that they made.

Audition and streams

Efforts to integrate auditory parts of the superior temporal cortex[134,135] into the ventral stream also suffer from a neglect of evolution. Some discussions invoke the concept of "auditory objects"[136], but the idea of acoustic *signs* makes more sense from an evolutionary perspective[17]. Of course, objects can make noises, but this does not validate the concept of an "acoustic object." Of more relevance to the life of anthropoids is the fact the sounds made by feeding animals serve as signs of resources. Boisterous birds with a diurnal, frugivorous feeding habit can indicate the location of fruit, for example (see Chapter 2, "Anthropoids"). As anthropoids began to diversify and travel long distances in pursuit of resources, their superior temporal cortex served as an adaptation for improved foraging choices based on acoustic cues. Experts in audition regularly relate their monkey findings to human language, but our common anthropoid ancestor could not have known that some of their descendants would jabber and prattle one day. In their time and place—in the face of predation risks and the need for distant, volatile resources—they had more pressing problems. Food speaks a language that all anthropoids understand.

The feature system of anthropoids supports perceptions and memories of the world, based on specialized, conjunctive representations. Another set of anthropoid innovations uses these representations to generate goals in an innovative way, as we explain in Chapter 8.

References

1. Gregory, R.L. (2001) *Nature* **410**, 21.
2. Aglioti, S., DeSouza, J.F.X., and Goodale, M.A. (1995) *Curr. Biol.* **5**, 679–685.
3. Goodale, M.A., Milner, A.D., Jakobson, L.S., and Carey, D.P. (1991) *Nature* **349**, 154–156.
4. Bridgeman, B. (1992) *Theory Psychol.* **2**, 73–88.
5. Milner, A.D. and Goodale, M.A. (1993) In: *Progress in Brain Research* (eds. Hicks, T.P., Molotchnikoff, S. and Ono, T.), pp. 317–337 (Elsevier, Amsterdam).
6. Milner, A.D. and Goodale, M.A. (2007) *The Visual Brain in Action* (Oxford University Press, Oxford).
7. Milner, A.D. (1995) *Neuropsychologia* **33**, 1117–1130.
8. Boussaoud, D., di Pellegrino, G., and Wise, S.P. (1996) *Behav. Brain Res.* **72**, 1–15.
9. Passingham, R.E. and Toni, I. (2001) *NeuroImage* **14**, S125–S131.
10. Lebedev, M.A. and Wise, S.P. (2002) *Behav. Cogn. Neurosci. Rev.* **1**, 108–129.
11. Gagin, G., Bohon, K.S., Butensky, A., Gates, M.A. et al. (2014) *J. Vision* **14**, 12.
12. Lafer-Sousa, R. and Conway, B.R. (2013) *Nat. Neurosci.* **16**, 1870–1878.
13. Bell, A.H., Hadj-Bouziane, F., Frihauf, J.B., Tootell, R.B. et al. (2009) *J. Neurophysiol.* **101**, 688–700.
14. Nishio, A., Goda, N., and Komatsu, H. (2012) *J. Neurosci.* **32**, 10780–10793.
15. Kaas, J.H. (2014) In: *The New Visual Neurosciences* (eds. Warner, J. and Chalupa, L.), pp. 1233–1246 (MIT Press, Cambridge, MA).
16. Felleman, D.J. and Van Essen, D.C. (1991) *Cereb. Cortex* **1**, 1–47.
17. Passingham, R.E. and Wise, S.P. (2012) *The Neurobiology of the Prefrontal Cortex* (Oxford University Press, Oxford).
18. Paré, M. and Dorris, M.C. (2011) In: *Oxford Handbook of Eye Movements* (eds. Liversedge, S.P., Gilchrist, I., and Everling, S.), pp. 257–278 (Oxford University Press, Oxford).
19. Kaas, J.H., Gharbawie, O.A., and Stepniewska, I. (2011) *Front. Neuroanat.* **5**, 34.
20. Ungerleider, L.G. and Mishkin, M. (1982) In: *Analysis of Visual Behavior* (eds. Ingle, J., Goodale, M.A. and Mansfield, R.J.W.), pp. 549–586 (MIT Press, Cambridge, MA).
21. Hirabayashi, T., Takeuchi, D., Tamura, K., and Miyashita, Y. (2013) *Science* **341**, 191–195.
22. Hirabayashi, T., Takeuchi, D., Tamura, K., and Miyashita, Y. (2013) *Neuron* **77**, 192–203.
23. Higuchi, S. and Miyashita, Y. (1996) *Proc. Natl. Acad. Sci. USA* **93**, 739–743.
24. Buckley, M.J., Gaffan, D., and Murray, E.A. (1997) *J. Neurophysiol.* **77**, 587–598.
25. Kravitz, D.J., Saleem, K.S., Baker, C.I., Ungerleider, L.G. et al. (2013) *Trends Cogn. Sci.* **17**, 26–49.
26. Warner, J. and Chalupa, L. (2014) *The New Visual Neurosciences* (MIT Press, Cambridge, MA).
27. Squire, L.R. (2009) *Neuron* **61**, 6–9.
28. Buffalo, E.A., Ramus, S.J., Clark, R.E., Teng, E. et al. (1999) *Learn. Mem.* **6**, 572–599.
29. Buffalo, E.A., Ramus, S.J., Squire, L.R., and Zola, S.M. (2000) *Learn. Mem.* **7**, 375–382.
30. Mishkin, M. (1982) *Phil. Trans. R. Soc. Lond. B: Biol. Sci.* **298**, 83–95.
31. Hood, K.L., Postle, B.R., and Corkin, S. (1999) *Neuropsychologia* **37**, 1375–1386.
32. Bussey, T.J. and Saksida, L.M. (2007) *Hippocampus* **17**, 898–908.

33. Saksida, L.M., Bussey, T.J., Buckmaster, C.A., and Murray, E.A. (2007) *Cereb. Cortex* **17**, 108–115.

34. Graham, K.S., Barense, M.D., and Lee, A.C. (2010) *Neuropsychologia* **48**, 831–853.

35. Murray, E.A. and Bussey, T.J. (1999) *Trends Cogn. Sci.* **3**, 142–151.

36. Bussey, T.J. and Saksida, L.M. (2002) *Eur. J. Neurosci.* **15**, 355–364.

37. Murray, E.A., Bussey, T.J., and Saksida, L.M. (2007) *Annu. Rev. Neurosci.* **30**, 99–122.

38. Suzuki, W.A. (2010) *Trends Cogn. Sci.* **14**, 195–200.

39. Bussey, T.J., Saksida, L.M., and Murray, E.A. (2002) *Eur. J. Neurosci.* **15**, 365–374.

40. Bussey, T.J., Saksida, L.M., and Murray, E.A. (2003) *Eur. J. Neurosci.* **17**, 649–660.

41. Barense, M.D., Gaffan, D., and Graham, K.S. (2007) *Neuropsychologia* **45**, 2963–2974.

42. Buckley, M.J., Booth, M.C.A., Rolls, E.T., and Gaffan, D. (2001) *J. Neurosci.* **21**, 9824–9836.

43. Hampton, R.R. and Murray, E.A. (2002) *Behav. Neurosci.* **116**, 363–377.

44. Forwood, S.E., Winters, B.D., and Bussey, T.J. (2005) *Hippocampus* **15**, 347–355.

45. Mumby, D.G. and Pinel, J.P.J. (1994) *Behav. Neurosci.* **108**, 11–18.

46. Aggleton, J.P., Keen, S., Warburton, E.C., and Bussey, T.J. (1997) *Brain Res. Bull.* **43**, 279–287.

47. Winters, B.D., Forwood, S.E., Cowell, R.A., Saksida, L.M. et al. (2004) *J. Neurosci.* **24**, 5901–5908.

48. Baxter, M.G. and Murray, E.A. (2001) *Hippocampus* **11**, 201–203.

49. Bartko, S.J., Winters, B.D., Cowell, R.A., Saksida, L.M. *et al.* (2007) *J. Neurosci.* **27**, 2548–2559.

50. Bartko, S.J., Winters, B.D., Cowell, R.A., Saksida, L.M. et al. (2007) *Learn. Mem.* **14**, 821–832.

51. Eacott, M.J. and Norman, G. (2004) *J. Neurosci.* **24**, 1948–1953.

52. Norman, G. and Eacott, M.J. (2004) *Behav. Brain Res.* **148**, 79–91.

53. Eacott, M.J., Gaffan, D., and Murray, E.A. (1994) *Eur. J. Neurosci.* **6**, 1466–1478.

54. McTighe, S.M., Cowell, R.A., Winters, B.D., Bussey, T.J. et al. (2010) *Science* **330**, 1408–1410.

55. Clark, R.E., Reinagel, P., Broadbent, N.J., Flister, E.D. et al. (2011) *Neuron* **70**, 132–140.

56. Hales, J.B., Broadbent, N.J., Velu, P.D., Squire, L.R. et al. (2015) *Learn. Mem.* **22**, 83–91.

57. Stark, C.E.L. and Squire, L.R. (2000) *Learn. Mem.* **7**, 273–278.

58. Suzuki, W.A. (2009) *Neuron* **61**, 657–666.

59. Squire, L.R., Wixted, J.T., and Clark, R.E. (2007) *Nat. Rev. Neurosci.* **8**, 872–883.

60. Squire, L.R., Shrager, Y., and Levy, D.A. (2006) *Learn. Mem.* **13**, 106–107.

61. Levy, D.A., Shrager, Y., and Squire, L.R. (2005) *Learn. Mem.* **12**, 61–66.

62. Shrager, Y., Gold, J.J., Hopkins, R.O., and Squire, L.R. (2006) *J. Neurosci* .**26**, 2235–2240.

63. Kim, S., Jeneson, A., van der Horst, A.S., Frascino, J.C. et al. (2011) *J. Neurosci.* **31**, 2624–2629.

64. Barense, M.D., Bussey, T.J., Lee, A.C.H., Rogers, T.T. et al. (2005) *J. Neurosci.* **25**, 10239–10246.

65. Lee, A.C., Bussey, T.J., Murray, E.A., Saksida, L.M. et al. (2005) *Neuropsychologia* **43**, 1–11.

66. Barense, M.D., Rogers, T.T., Bussey, T.J., Saksida, L.M. et al. (2010) *Cereb. Cortex* **20**, 2568–2582.

67. Davies, R.R., Graham, K.S., Xuereb, J.H., Williams, G.B. et al. (2004) *Eur. J. Neurosci.* **20**, 2441–2446.

68. Davies, R.R., Halliday, G.M., Xuereb, J.H., Kril, J.J. et al. (2009) *Neurobiol. Aging* **30**, 2043–2052.

69. Barense, M.D., Groen, I.I., Lee, A.C., Yeung, L.K. et al. (2012) *Neuron* **75**, 157–167.

70. Mundy, M.E., Downing, P.E., Dwyer, D.M., Honey, R.C. et al. (2013) *J. Neurosci.* **33**, 10490–10502.

71. Yeung, L.K., Ryan, J.D., Cowell, R.A., and Barense, M.D. (2013) *J. Exp. Psychol. Gen.* **142**, 1384–1397.

72. Bird, C.M., Shallice, T., and Cipolotti, L. (2007) *Neuropsychologia* **45**, 1160–1171.

73. Taylor, K.J., Henson, R.N., and Graham, K.S. (2007) *Neuropsychologia* **45**, 2428–2438.

74. Graham, K.S., Scahill, V.L., Hornberger, M., Barense, M.D. et al. (2006) *J. Neurosci.* **26**, 7547–7554.

75. Lee, A.C., Barense, M.D., and Graham, K.S. (2005) *Q. J. Exp. Psychol. B* **58**, 300–325.

76. Lee, A.C. and Rudebeck, S.R. (2010) *J. Cogn. Neurosci.* 22, 2823–2835.
77. Bonnici, H.M., Kumaran, D., Chadwick, M.J., Weiskopf, N. et al. (2012) *Hippocampus* 22, 1143–1153.
78. Libby, L.A., Hannula, D.E., and Ranganath, C. (2014) *J. Neurosci.* 34, 14233–14242.
79. Barense, M.D., Henson, R.N., Lee, A.C., and Graham, K.S. (2010) *Hippocampus* 20, 389–401.
80. Barense, M.D., Henson, R.N., and Graham, K.S. (2011) *J. Cogn. Neurosci.* 23, 3052–3067.
81. O'Neil, E.B., Cate, A.D., and Kohler, S. (2009) *J. Neurosci.* 29, 8329–8334.
82. Lee, A.C., Buckley, M.J., Gaffan, D., Emery, T. et al. (2006) *J. Neurosci.* 26, 5198–5203.
83. Lee, A.C., Levi, N., Davies, R.R., Hodges, J.R. et al. (2007) *Neuropsychologia* 45, 2135–2146.
84. Cowell, R.A., Bussey, T.J., and Saksida, L.M. (2010) *Hippocampus* 20, 1245–1262.
85. Cowell, R.A., Bussey, T.J., and Saksida, L.M. (2010) *J. Cogn. Neurosci.* 22, 2460–2479.
86. Elfman, K.W., Aly, M., and Yonelinas, A.P. (2014) *Hippocampus* 24, 1672–1686.
87. Aly, M., Ranganath, C., and Yonelinas, A.P. (2013) *Neuron* 78, 1127–1137.
88. Farah, M.J. (2004) *Visual Agnosia* (MIT Press, Cambridge, MA).
89. Erez, J., Cusack, R., Kendall, W., and Barense, M.D. (2016) *Cereb. Cortex* 26, 2271–2282.
90. Clarke, A. and Tyler, L.K. (2014) *J. Neurosci.* 34, 4766–4775.
91. Barense, M.D., Erez, J., Ma, H., and Cusack, R. (2014) *Cogn. Affect. Behav. Neurosci.* 14, 336–353.
92. Lee, A.C., Buckley, M.J., Pegman, S.J., Spiers, H. et al. (2005) *Hippocampus* 15, 782–797.
93. Chun, M.M. and Phelps, E.A. (1999) *Nat. Neurosci.* 2, 844–847.
94. Ninokura, Y., Mushiake, H., and Tanji, J. (2004) *J. Neurophysiol.* 91, 555–560.
95. Roitman, J.D., Brannon, E.M., and Platt, M.L. (2007) *PLoS Biol.* 5, e208.
96. Sawamura, H., Shima, K., and Tanji, J. (2010) *J. Neurophysiol.* 104, 902–910.
97. Petrides, M. (1991) *Proc. R. Soc. B: Biol. Sci.* 246, 299–306.
98. Petrides, M. (1995) *J. Neurosci.* 15, 359–375.
99. Sawamura, H., Shima, K., and Tanji, J. (2002) *Nature* 415, 918–922.
100. Vallentin, D. and Nieder, A. (2010) *Eur. J. Neurosci.* 32, 1380–1387.
101. Genovesio, A., Tsujimoto, S., and Wise, S.P. (2006) *J. Neurophysiol.* 95, 3281–3285.
102. Genovesio, A., Tsujimoto, S., and Wise, S.P. (2009) *Neuron* 63, 254–266.
103. Yumoto, N., Lu, X., Henry, T.R., Miyachi, S. et al. (2011) *PLoS One* 6, e19168.
104. Sakurai, Y., Takahashi, S., and Inoue, M. (2004) *Eur. J. Neurosci.* 20, 1069–1080.
105. Tudusciuc, O. and Nieder, A. (2009) *J. Neurophysiol.* 101, 2984–2994.
106. Merchant, H., Crowe, D.A., Robertson, M.S., Fortes, A.F. et al. (2011) *Front. Syst. Neurosci.* 5, 69.
107. Crowe, D.A., Goodwin, S.J., Blackman, R.K., Sakellaridi, S. et al. (2013) *Nat. Neurosci.* 16, 1484–1491.
108. Berdyyeva, T.K. and Olson, C.R. (2010) *J. Neurophysiol.* 104, 141–159.
109. Schneider, B.A. and Ghose, G.M. (2012) *PLoS Biol.* 10, e1001413.
110. Janssen, P. and Shadlen, M.N. (2005) *Nat. Neurosci.* 8, 234–241.
111. Leon, M.I. and Shadlen, M.N. (2003) *Neuron* 38, 317–327.
112. Nieder, A., Freedman, D.J., and Miller, E.K. (2002) *Science* 297, 1708–1711.
113. Diester, I. and Nieder, A. (2007) *PLoS Biol.* 5, e294.
114. Bongard, S. and Nieder, A. (2010) *Proc. Natl. Acad. Sci. USA* 107, 2277–2282.
115. Vallentin, D., Bongard, S., and Nieder, A. (2012) *J. Neurosci.* 32, 6621–6630.
116. Eiselt, A.K. and Nieder, A. (2013) *J. Neurosci.* 33, 7526–7534.
117. Brannon, E.M. (2006) *Curr. Opin. Neurobiol.* 16, 222–229.

118. Brannon, E.M. and Terrace, H.S. (2000) *J. Exp. Psychol. Anim. Behav. Process.* **26**, 31–49.

119. Merritt, D.J., MacLean, E.L., Crawford, J.C., and Brannon, E.M. (2011) *Front. Psychol.* **2**, 23.

120. Stevens, J.R., Wood, J.N., and Hauser, M.D. (2007) *Anim. Cogn.* **10**, 429–437.

121. Beran, M.J., Evans, T.A., and Harris, E.H. (2008) *Anim. Behav.* **75**, 1793–1802.

122. MacDonald, S., Spetch, M.L., Kelly, D.M., and Cheng, K. (2004) *Learn. Motiv.* **35**, 322–347.

123. Depy, D., Fagot, J., and Vauclair, J. (1999) *Behav. Process.* **48**, 1–9.

124. Spinozzi, G., Lubrano, G., and Truppa, V. (2004) *J. Comp. Psychol.* **118**, 403–412.

125. Poti, P. (2000) *Anim. Cogn.* **3**, 69–77.

126. De Lillo, C., Spinozzi, G., Truppa, V., and Naylor, D.M. (2005) *J. Comp. Psychol.* **119**, 155–165.

127. Kralik, J.D. and Sampson, W.W. (2012) *Behav. Process.* **89**, 197–202.

128. Sayers, K. and Menzel, C.R. (2012) *Anim. Behav.* **84**, 795–803.

129. D'Esposito, M. and Postle, B.R. (2015) *Annu. Rev. Psychol.* **66**, 115–142.

130. Gaffan, D. and Hornak, J. (1997) *Brain* **120**, 1647–1657.

131. Lewis-Peacock, J.A. and Postle, B.R. (2008) *J. Neurosci.* **28**, 8765–8771.

132. Harrison, S.A. and Tong, F. (2009) *Nature* **458**, 632–635.

133. Lopez-Aranda, M.F., Lopez-Tellez, J.F., Navarro-Lobato, I., Masmudi-Martin, M. et al. (2009) *Science* **325**, 87–89.

134. Romanski, L.M., Averbeck, B.B., and Diltz, M. (2005) *J. Neurophysiol.* **93**, 734–747.

135. Romanski, L.M. and Averbeck, B.B. (2009) *Annu. Rev. Neurosci.* **32**, 315–346.

136. Poremba, A., Malloy, M., Saunders, R.C., Carson, R.E. et al. (2004) *Nature* **427**, 448–451.

137. di Pellegrino G. and Wise, S.P. (1993) *J. Neurosci.* **13**, 1227–1243.

138. Lebedev, M.A., Douglass, D.K., Moody, S.L., and Wise, S.P. (2001) *J. Neurophysiol.* **85**, 1395–1411.

Chapter 8

The goal memory system
of anthropoids

Overview

The goal memory system depends on granular prefrontal areas that emerged in anthropoid primates. As anthropoids diversified, they became larger animals, with extensive home ranges, long lives, high energy requirements, and large brains. They foraged in daylight, faced a serious threat of predation, and needed to cope with shortfalls in necessary resources. The ancestral reinforcement learning mechanisms produced too many unproductive and costly foraging choices, in part because such learning is cumulative, based on an average over several events. The goal system reduced the frequency of errors by generating goals based on: (1) the representation of single goal-related events; (2) new attribute and metric contexts provided by the feature system; and (3) abstract strategies that transferred solutions from familiar problems to novel ones. By reducing foraging errors, the goal system provided an advantage in adapting to the highly volatile resources on which anthropoids came to depend.

Flourens and his hens

> The earliest experiments on the frontal areas were those of the French neurologist Flourens (1824), who ... attributed to the frontal lobes, acting in harmony with the rest of the brain, the higher perceptual, associative and executive functions of the mind.
>
> Fulton[1] (p. 447)

Some ideas about the frontal lobe have flourished forever, it seems. Flourens' ideas in the early nineteenth century, echoed by Fulton in the 1940s, could pass as fashionable today. Never mind that he based his conclusions on the study of a hen, and hens do not have a homologue of the frontal lobes. Perceptual, associative, and executive functions: The primate prefrontal cortex contributes to all of those and more, but this chapter advances a different idea about its fundamental function:

> the generation
> of goals in a novel way
> to augment old ways

Passingham and Wise[2], recognizing that a haiku wouldn't do, develop this idea at book length, arguing that the granular prefrontal cortex accumulates specialized representations of behavioral goals—including the contexts, actions, and outcomes associated with these goals. Put another way, the new anthropoid prefrontal areas function as a goal system, which specializes in knowledge about "what to do." Its goals correspond to objects and places that serve as targets of action.

The proposal of Passingham and Wise[2] resembles previous ideas about prefrontal cortex function, such as those emphasizing multiple demand cognition[3,4], supervisory attention[5,6], strategic and rule-guided behavior[7], and memories of "what to do" and "how to act" in various circumstances[8–10]. Indeed, it would be surprising if any idea about the prefrontal cortex seemed completely novel, if for no other reason than that every conceivable possibility has been advanced at some time or another over the past couple of centuries.

Some previous proposals about the prefrontal cortex can be rejected, however, including those claiming that its principal function is either behavioral inhibition[11,12], working memory[13], or "perception–action cycles"[14]. The prefrontal cortex contributes to these processes, of course, but it has many other functions as well, including top-down attention, categorization, decision making, subjective valuation, the application of abstract rules and strategies, behavioral planning, and sequential behavior. The problem with a list like this is that it fails to capture the fundamental or overarching function of the primate prefrontal cortex, something that ties everything together. In addition, these lists tend to emphasize cognitive processes at the expense of stored knowledge[9]. An understanding of the prefrontal cortex requires both.

Evolution

In Chapters 2 ("Anthropoids") and 7 ("Evolution") we discussed anthropoid evolution, including derived traits such as the fovea (inherited from stem haplorhines), enhanced depth perception, and trichromatic vision, along with the development of new granular prefrontal areas: the dorsomedial, dorsal, dorsolateral, ventrolateral, and polar prefrontal cortex (see Fig. 1.3).

The first anthropoids were small animals with a diurnal foraging habit and a leaping–grasping form of locomotion. Foraging in the daytime has many advantages, but it also enhances the risk of predation. As they diversified, various anthropoid species increased in size and adopted quadrupedal locomotion, moving long distances through the trees. In part because of their larger size, these animals came to rely on the products of angiosperm trees, such as fruits and tender leaves. Their diet included other items, of course, such as insects, but only angiosperms could provide sufficient nutrition[15]. These resources had a highly patchy distribution, with valuable items scattered over a large and dangerous home range. Each species of angiosperm tree produced fruits that ripened at different times in different places, with dramatic variation within an anthropoid's home range: from year to year and over other time spans. In some years, a given stand of trees could fail to produce

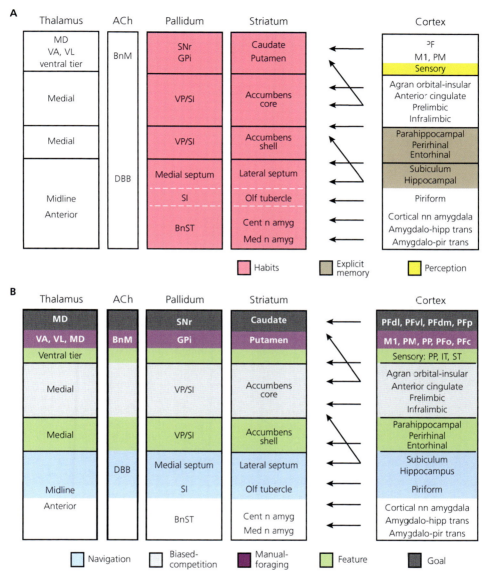

Plate 1 From Fig. 2.3. Cortex–basal ganglia modules as memory systems. (A) The prevailing view of memory systems. The color code is shown at the bottom. This version applies the "habit" system to the basal ganglia as a whole, as recognized in its extended sense. Most research on habits focuses on the dorsal basal ganglia. (B) The evolution accretion model. Format and abbreviations as in the legends of Figs. 2.1 and 2.2. Additional abbreviations: MD, mediodorsal nucleus; VA, ventroanterior nucleus; VL, ventrolateral nucleus. Adapted from Murray EA, Wise SP. What, if anything, is the medial temporal lobe, and how can the amygdala be part of it if there is no such thing? *Neurobiology of Learning and Memory* 82:178–98, © 2004, Elsevier, with permission.

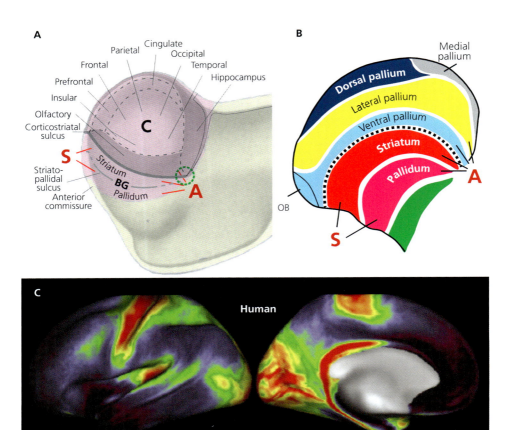

Plate 2 (A) and (B) from Fig. 2.8. (A) Location of cortical areas in the embryonic human brain. Rostral is to the left. The green dashed circle shows the region that becomes the frontotemporal junction, which includes the piriform cortex as it makes a transition with the cortical nuclei of the amygdala. (B) Telencephalic regions expressing diagnostic patterns of developmental regulatory genes. Abbreviations: A, amygdala; BG, basal ganglia; C, neocortex; OB, olfactory bulb; S, septal nuclei. (C) Expansion of the lightly myelinated granular prefrontal cortex in hominins from structural brain imaging. Blue–purple areas have lighter myelination; red–orange areas are highly myelinated. (A) Reprinted from Swanson LW. Cerebral hemisphere regulation of motivated behavior. *Brain Research* 886:113–64, © 2000, Elsevier, with permission. (B) Modified from Puelles L, Kuwana E, Puelles E, Bulfone A, Shimamura K, Keleher J, Smiga S, Rubenstein JL. Pallial and subpallial derivatives in the embryonic chick and mouse telencephalon, traced by the expression of the genes dlx-2, Emx-1, Nkx-2.1, Pax-6, and Tbr-1. *Journal of Comparative Neurology* 424:409–38, © 2000, John Wiley & Sons, with permission. (C) Reproduced from Glasser MF, Goyal MS, Preuss TM, Raichle ME, Van Essen DC. Trends and properties of human cerebral cortex: correlations with cortical myelin content. *NeuroImage* 93P2:165–75, © 2014, Elsevier, with permission.

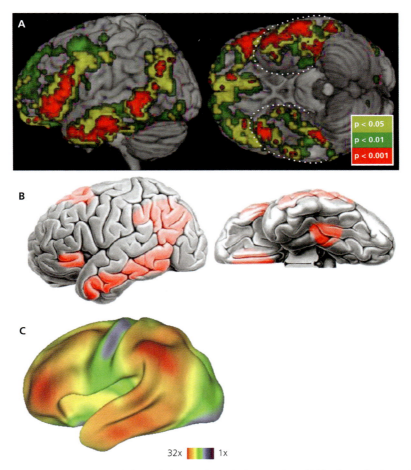

Plate 3 Brain imaging, semantic knowledge, and cortical expansion. (A) Red voxels show the highest activation for a set of semantic memory tasks versus control tasks that required the matching of scrambled images. Other colors indicate lower *p*-values for activations, as shown in the key (lower right). (B) Semantic memory network in pink based on a meta-analysis of brain imaging studies. (C) Map of regional cortical expansion in humans based on established homologies, ranging from the same extent as in macaque monkeys (1×, blue) to more than 30-fold larger (32×, red). (A) From Visser M, Jefferies E, Embleton KV, Lambon Ralph MA. Both the middle temporal gyrus and the ventral anterior temporal area are crucial for multimodal semantic processing: distortion-corrected fMRI evidence for a double gradient of information convergence in the temporal lobes. *Journal of Cognitive Neuroscience* 24:1766–78, © 2012, The MIT Press Journals. Reprinted by permission of MIT Press Journals. (B) From Binder JR, Desai RH, Graves WW, Conant LL. Where is the semantic system? A critical review and meta-analysis of 120 functional neuroimaging studies. *Cerebral Cortex* 19:2767–96, © 2009, Oxford University Press, with permission. (C) From Van Essen DC and Dierker DL. Surface-based and probabilistic atlases of primate cerebral cortex. *Neuron* 56:209–225, © 2007, with permission from Elsevier.

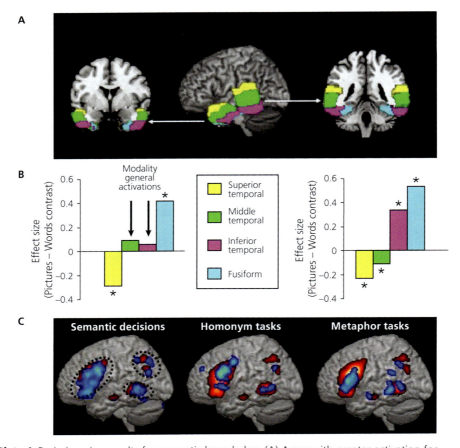

Plate 4 Brain imaging results for semantic knowledge. (A) Areas with greater activation for words, as opposed to pictures, were observed in superior and middle parts of the temporal lobe, and the reverse occurred in the inferior and medial parts of the temporal lobe. Domain-general areas (green and purple regions of interest in the anterior temporal lobe, left brain slice) did not show a difference between words and pictures (green and purple bars on the left plot), although they had high levels of activation for both. The figure neglects hemispheric differences. (B) Effect size for words versus pictures. The left plot corresponds to the imaging slice above it, and likewise for the right plot. Asterisks indicate significant difference in activation for pictures versus words. (C) Areas in red and orange were activated more for tasks demanding high levels of semantic control than for tasks that require relatively low levels. The activations during three tasks—one semantic, one phonological, and one metaphorical—appear in blue, superimposed on the areas activated by high levels of semantic control. (A, B) From Visser M, Jefferies E, Embleton KV, Lambon Ralph MA. Both the middle temporal gyrus and the ventral anterior temporal area are crucial for multimodal semantic processing: distortion-corrected fMRI evidence for a double gradient of information convergence in the temporal lobes. *Journal of Cognitive Neuroscience* 24:1766–78, © 2012, The MIT Press Journals. Reprinted by permission of MIT Press Journals. (C) Reproduced from Noonan KA, Jefferies E, Visser M, Lambon Ralph MA. Going beyond inferior prefrontal involvement in semantic control: evidence for the additional contribution of dorsal angular gyrus and posterior middle temporal cortex. *Journal of Cognitive Neuroscience* 25:1824–50, © 2013, The MIT Press Journals. Reprinted by permission of MIT Press Journals.

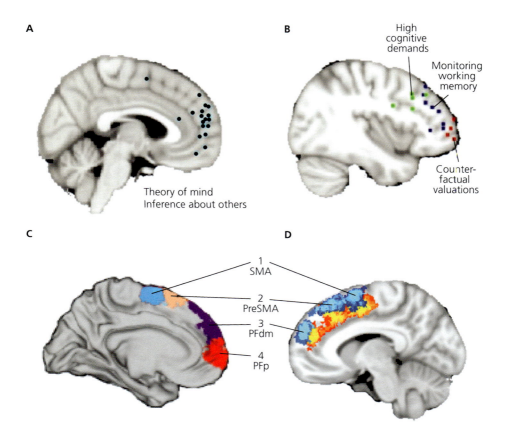

Pate 5 (A) Meta-analysis of brain imaging activations related to a theory of mind and inferences about other people, as synthesized by Amodio DM and Frith CD (Meeting of minds: the medial frontal cortex and social cognition. *Nature Reviews Neuroscience* 7:268–77, © Macmillan, 2006). (B) Meta-analysis of peak activations for tasks involving the monitoring of items in working memory, multiple cognitive demands, and the relative valuations of chosen and foregone behavioral options (see text for sources). Note that this imaging level is much more lateral than the one in (A). The designated areas correspond to the dorsolateral prefrontal cortex (purple and green) and the lateral part of the polar prefrontal cortex (red). (C), (D) Clusters based on imaging tractography for two analyses of the medial frontal cortex. Abbreviations: PreSMA presupplementary motor area; SMA, supplementary motor area; PFdm, the dorsomedial prefrontal cortex; PFp, the polar prefrontal cortex. Reproduced from Sallet J, Mars RB, Noonan MP, Neubert FX, Jbabdi S, O'Reilly JX, Filippini N, Thomas AG, Rushworth MF. The organization of dorsal frontal cortex in humans and macaques. *Journal of Neuroscience* 33:12255–74, © 2013, Society for Neuroscience, 2013, with permission.

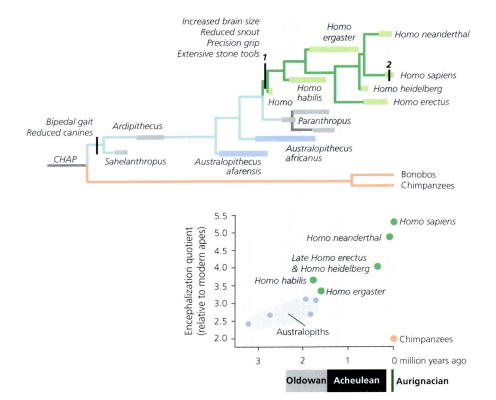

Plate 6 From Figs. 10.2 and 11.1(C). Comparison of encephalization quotients and a figurative cladogram of hominins. The sets of traits labelled by the numerals 1 and 2 refer to the sets of derived cognitive traits that are listed at the bottom of Fig. 11.1(C). The thick parts of the cladogram lines indicate the range of fossil specimens for the species in question. CHAP, chimpanzee–human ancestral population. The formal names of fossil humans, *Homo neanderthalensis* and *Homo heidelbergensis*, have been shortened to *Homo neanderthal* and *Homo heidelberg*, respectively. Both parts of the figure were adapted from plots presented by Klein RG. *The Human Career*, © 2009, University of Chicago Press.

fruit at all, and, at best, only a small proportion of trees in an anthropoid's home range produced anything nutritious at any given time. So any shortfall in the products of angiosperm trees must have caused severe challenges, especially to relatively large anthropoids. In this context, reducing the frequency of unproductive foraging choices would have provided an important selective advantage.

Passingham and Wise[2] propose that the new prefrontal areas reduce errors through event- and strategy-based mechanisms for choosing foraging goals. According to this idea, the goal system establishes representations of goals in conjunction with the context, actions, and outcomes that occur along with them. When a context recurs, even if it has happened only once or twice, these conjunctive representations include a goal linked to that context, an action that achieves the goal, and a specific outcome.

Processing pathways

The new anthropoid prefrontal areas sit atop three information-processing pathways (Fig. 8.1), analogous to the one illustrated in Fig. 7.3 and in one instance an extension of it (see Fig. 9.7C). From medial to lateral, they involve goals and actions, sensory contexts, and outcomes[2]. By integrating this information, the prefrontal cortex can create conjunctive representations of contexts, goals, actions, and outcomes in a way that other areas cannot.

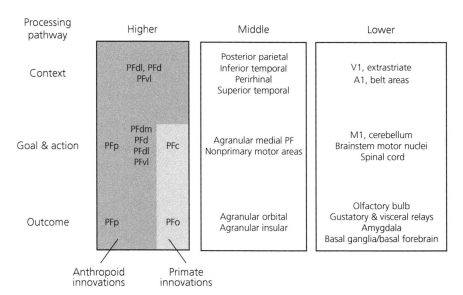

Fig. 8.1 Processing pathways involving the goal system. Abbreviations: A1, primary auditory cortex; M1, primary motor cortex; PFc, caudal prefrontal cortex; PFd, dorsal prefrontal cortex; PFdm, dorsomedial prefrontal cortex; PFdl, dorsolateral prefrontal cortex; PFo, granular orbitofrontal cortex; PFp, polar prefrontal cortex; PFvl, ventrolateral prefrontal cortex; PM, several premotor areas; V1, primary visual cortex.

Context pathway

The context pathway extends the ventral and dorsal streams into the granular prefrontal cortex. Context, in this sense, refers mainly to the metrics and attributes of items in the environment, such as objects. It is important to bear in mind that this meaning of context differs from the common one in the hippocampus literature, which refers to integrated scenes and backgrounds.

The inferior temporal, superior temporal, and perirhinal cortex project to the ventrolateral and granular orbitofrontal cortex[16–18]; posterior parietal areas send inputs to the dorsal and dorsolateral prefrontal cortex[19,20]. As we explained in Chapter 7, the former group of areas represent objects and the sensory signs of resources (attributes); the latter represent metrics such as relative numbers, durations, distances, order, and locations.

Goal and action pathway

The goal and action pathway involves connections of the granular prefrontal cortex with premotor, posterior parietal, and anterior cingulate areas. Premotor areas provide the prefrontal cortex with information about actions; and the prefrontal cortex generates a top-down bias on the premotor cortex (see Chapter 6, "Affordance competition"). The granular orbitofrontal cortex plays a particularly pivotal role in these interactions because of its representations of specific predicted outcomes and their current valuations (see Chapter 6, "Orbitofrontal–amygdala interactions"). In monkeys, neurons in the granular orbitofrontal cortex do not represent actions prior to movement[21], so they probably exert their influence via connections with the dorsolateral, dorsal, ventrolateral, and dorsomedial prefrontal cortex (see Fig. 1.3)[22–26] through the following routes:

- The dorsolateral prefrontal cortex has connections with dorsal premotor areas, many via the dorsal prefrontal cortex[27].

- The ventrolateral prefrontal cortex has connections with ventral premotor areas[27–29], as well as multisynaptic connections with the dorsal premotor cortex[27].

- The dorsomedial prefrontal connects with the anterior cingulate cortex and the cingulate motor areas[30].

Because no granular prefrontal areas project to either the spinal cord[31,32] or the primary motor cortex[27,28,33–35], they must exert their influence on action indirectly. Neuroanatomists now dismiss older ideas that focused on funneling information from the prefrontal cortex through the basal ganglia to the motor areas. This concept has been replaced with the idea of parallel cortex–basal ganglia "loops" (see Chapter 2, "Rings and loops")[36,37]. Some connections link such "loops" to each other at subcortical levels[38], but, even taking this idea into account, the most likely route for the granular prefrontal cortex to influence behavior involves corticocortical connections.

Outcome pathway

The outcome pathway has both visual and nonvisual components. The inferior temporal and perirhinal cortex send information to the granular orbitofrontal cortex about the visual features of outcomes; agranular orbital–insular areas provide it with olfactory, gustatory, and visceral information[39]. As a result of these convergent inputs, neurons in the granular orbitofrontal cortex represent conjunctions of outcome features, including sight–smell, sight–taste, and smell–taste (flavor) combinations[40].

The three processing pathways operate independently, to an extent, and some integration occurs prior to their convergence on the prefrontal cortex. Nevertheless, the larger importance of these processing pathways lies in their cooperative functions when combined in the granular prefrontal cortex. No one today denies specializations among prefrontal areas—each part has a unique pattern of connections, after all[2]—but the quest for localizing functions has sometimes obscured their collective, integrated contribution to behavior[41]. Intrinsic connections within the primate prefrontal cortex promote a degree of integration that other areas cannot match. By bringing together high-level information about contexts, goals, actions, and outcomes, the primate prefrontal cortex has all of the information needed for generating goals of a sophisticated nature[2].

Proposal

The goal memory system depends on granular prefrontal areas that first appeared in anthropoid primates. These areas reduced foraging errors by generating goals in three new and related ways: (1) from representations of sensory contexts that were unavailable to their ancestors; (2) from representations of single goal-related events (concrete context–goal–action–outcome conjunctions, which serve as goal exemplars); and (3) from representations of abstract context–goal–action–outcome conjunctions (behavioral rules and strategies).

In the remainder of this chapter, we take up these three aspects of goal generation in turn, followed by a consideration of how these developments augmented the ancestral condition. According to our proposal, all of these functions involve conjunctive representations of goals, contexts, actions, and outcomes: the specialized representations of the new anthropoid prefrontal areas. When a context recurs, the goal associated with it can be retrieved, as can the associated action and a predicted outcome. Once retrieved, these representations influence behavior mainly via a bias on the manual-foraging system[42-44] (see Chapter 6, "Affordance competition").

These two aspects of goal generation—conjunctive representations and top-down biases—complement each other. Respectively, conjunctive representations and top-down biases correspond to knowledge and process[9], and both depend on the unique pattern of connections that characterizes the anthropoid prefrontal cortex. Conjunctive representations result from its ability to integrate context, goal, action, and outcome information[2]; the top-down bias depends on its connections with premotor and other posterior cortical areas.

New contexts

Once the new anthropoid prefrontal areas evolved, they could draw on the enhanced sensory representations of contexts provided by the feature system, including both metric and attribute features. As we explained in Chapter 7, the feature system that evolved in anthropoids augmented the ancestral condition with some additional sensory representations. Among these developments, the dorsal visual stream represents metric (quantitative) features such as relative number, distance, direction, speed, duration, and order, and the ventral stream represents (qualitative) attributes such as color, shape, visual texture, glossiness, and translucence.

Metric features

Neuropsychology

Passingham and Wise[2] review neuropsychological, brain imaging, and neurophysiological findings that point to a role for the dorsal and dorsolateral prefrontal cortex in goal choices based on sensory metrics. They propose that this set of areas:

> generates goals based on a current context that can include the location, duration, distance, number, rate, and order of recent events, especially visual events. It uses these features, such as spatial and temporal order, to generate both concrete and abstract goals, as well as sequences of such goals. When necessary, it prospectively encodes these goals until an attempt can be made to achieve them and in this way defeats interference from irrelevant events.
>
> Passingham and Wise[2] (p. 193)

In an experiment that provided support for this proposal, monkeys needed to choose among 25 opaque doors, each of which concealed a piece of food[45]. We described other experiments of this type in Chapter 4 ("A general role in spatial memory?"). Like those experiments, the optimal foraging strategy required monkeys to choose each door once and only once. Macaque monkeys with lesions of the dorsolateral prefrontal cortex performed this task less efficiently than control subjects, and experiments on marmosets produced the same result[46]. These results indicate that lesions of the dorsolateral prefrontal cortex disrupt orderly foraging.

Studies of the delayed response task have tended to dominate this line of research. In most versions of this task, monkeys have needed to choose a transiently cued location after a delay period, out of two possibilities. Experiments of this type have spanned more than eight decades, and lesions of the dorsolateral prefrontal cortex have consistently caused permanent and severe impairments, often reducing monkeys to chance performance for as long as testing continued[47–49]. Most interpretations of this result have invoked the concept of spatial working memory, but good performance of the task also requires the application of an abstract rule. The reason is that in all of these experiments the same set of locations was cued trial after trial, and so the accumulated events caused massive interference to build up in memory. Accordingly, the monkeys needed to use a particular rule: "choose the location of the *most recent* spatial cue" or, in terms of order, "choose the location of the *last* cue." Although this aspect of the task has rarely been recognized, the spatial delayed response task has always depended on a metrics-based rule, one based on the order or recency of sensory cues. In agreement with this account, lesions of the dorsolateral prefrontal cortex have also caused an impairment in either rule memory[50] or, according to an alternative interpretation of the same data, top-down attention based on rules.

The delayed alternation task requires monkeys to switch between two spatial goals from trial to trial. In these experiments, therefore, monkeys had to use their memory of the most recently rewarded location to choose their next goal, despite the fact that both potential goals had been correct in the recent past and equally so over the long run. In experiments too numerous to mention here, lesions of the dorsolateral prefrontal cortex have caused a severe and permanent impairment on this task, much like their effects on the delayed response task.

In contrast to the serious impairments on these two tasks, monkeys with the same lesions could learn the spatial reversal task normally[51,52] or with only a mild impairment[49]. In this task, one location was designated as correct for a block of consecutive trials. Later, the alternative location was designated as correct for another block of trials. The reinforcement learning systems could solve this problem by updating place–outcome associations. According to our proposal, lesions of the dorsolateral prefrontal cortex caused impairments on the delayed response and delayed alternation tasks because both tasks required the memory of a single event to choose a goal and because that event was crucial to implementing a metric rule—one based on the order in which spatial cues occurred or their relative recency. The reinforcement learning systems could not solve these two problems because all potential goal locations took on the same average value over several trials.

Brain imaging

A large brain-imaging literature on the primate prefrontal cortex emphasizes working memory. The working memory theory of the prefrontal cortex has four formulations, which occur in various combinations:

- The prefrontal cortex has some working memory functions.
- Only the prefrontal cortex functions in working memory.
- The prefrontal cortex functions solely in working memory.
- All of the prefrontal cortex functions in working memory.

The first formulation is correct; the other three are wrong. Passingham and Wise[2] give the details, which a more recent report supports[53], but even without empirical refutation an evolutionary perspective casts doubt on the second one. It implies that an area specific to anthropoids functions as the sole working memory mechanism in these species[13] despite the fact other species have working memory without this area[54]. This is not impossible, but it is not very likely either.

Furthermore, brain imaging results that seem to reflect working memory for stimulus items have alternative interpretations. The *n*-back task serves as a typical example. In one version of this task, a stimulus three events in the past determined the current goal. For example, after a sequence of visually presented letters—O, I, N, K—the correct goal was "I." The cortical activations that occurred during this task could therefore have reflected the memory of event order rather than (or in addition to) the stimulus items.

In another experiment[55], subjects saw a series of spatial cues. After a 6-second delay period, they then had to report whether a second sequence matched the first one or, according to an alternative response rule, they had to point to the cue locations in their original order. The first test required working memory and not goal planning because the subjects could not anticipate which response rule they would have to follow. The second test required some combination of working memory and goal planning. If activation of the dorsolateral prefrontal cortex mainly reflected working memory, significant activation should have occurred during both tests, but it did so only during the second. A related experimental design used two successive delay periods rather than two separate tests, and it yielded the same conclusion[56].

The lack of significant activation in the first test, despite a requirement for (retrospective) spatial working memory, suggests to some experts that the dorsolateral prefrontal cortex specializes in the prospective memory of pending goals. However, as we explained in Chapter 1 ("Methods"), brain imaging methods do not have sufficient sensitivity to support conclusions based on negative results. The most that we can conclude from the brain imaging findings is that they point to a role for the dorsolateral prefrontal cortex in some combination of retrospective working memory and the prospective coding of future goals.

Neurophysiology

Neurophysiological experiments in monkeys have found that some neurons in the dorsolateral prefrontal cortex encode retrospective memories, whereas others encode prospective memories—for both spatial[57] and nonspatial[58,59] goals. Stated more generally, the dorsolateral prefrontal cortex represents both metric contexts (including the retrospective memory of cues) and goals (including prospective plans held in memory). According to Passingham and Wise[2], the prefrontal cortex generates these goals on the basis of such contexts, a process that cannot be performed by other cortical areas. In support of this idea, neurons in the dorsolateral prefrontal cortex have been found to encode a wide variety of metrics: a sequence of goals[60-62]; the temporal order of stimuli[63]; stimulus durations[64-70]; conjunctions of order and stimulus attributes[71,72]; conjunctions of order and relative distance[73]; conjunctions of order and relative duration[74]; conjunctions of outcomes and times[75]; the number of dots in a stimulus array[76]; the length of line segments[76]; abstract spatial categories such above or below[77]; and rules based on spatial categories[78]. [In Chapter 7 ("Metrics") we discussed metric representations in the posterior parietal cortex, which provides this information to the granular prefrontal areas.]

Once metric information reaches the dorsolateral prefrontal cortex, its neurons represent various conjunctions of contexts, goals, actions, and outcomes. Neurons in this area have been found to encode conjunctions of: goals and outcomes[79-81]; outcomes and actions[21,82]; goals and actions[81]; qualitative attributes and actions[83,84]; abstract rules and actions[85]; combinations of stimulus attributes[86]; attributes, strategies, and goals[87]; and attributes and locations[88]. All of these representations could contribute to goal generation, as well as to top-down attention directed toward objects and places of value[8,89,90]. In addition, activity in the dorsolateral prefrontal cortex has been reported to represent categories of contexts and categories of goal sequences[60,91,92]; decision variables such as the quantity and probability of expected rewards (outcomes)[84,93,94]; and the use of abstract problem-solving strategies[87] or rules[79,85,95,96] to generate goals. Cells with mixed and dynamically adapting selectivity seem to be particularly important in this regard because they can adapt to a wide variety of circumstances[97].

"How" versus "where" is neither here nor there

As we noted in Chapters 6 ("Evolution") and 7 ("Perception, action, and actuality"), the posterior parietal cortex functions both in the perception of metrics[98] and in visually guided movement[99–101]. In monosyllabic terms, the question seems to be whether it functions as part of a "where" or "how" system (see Fig. 7.1A). By taking evolution into account, a different idea emerges—one that takes just a few more syllables to explain:

- In early primates, the posterior parietal cortex provided support for reaching, grasping, and manipulating objects in the fine-branch niche. As we proposed in Chapter 6, new parietal areas evolved as part of the manual-foraging system, which stored memories that mediate visuomotor transformations among various coordinate frames[99,102,103]. Figure 8.2(A) designates this relationship as visuomotor metrics.

- During anthropoid evolution, the posterior parietal cortex came to represent metrics (and relative metrics) more generally, such as location, distance, number, duration, and order information that did not necessarily link up with an automatic visuomotor transform. At the same time, these new posterior parietal representations began to interact with new, granular prefrontal areas to generate goals based on context–goal–action–outcome conjunctions[2]. Figure 8.2(B) labels this relationship as metric contexts.

An evolutionary perspective thus reconciles the monosyllabic minimalisms of "where" and "how." The properties that captured the attention of the "where" camp depend on posterior parietal interactions with the new anthropoid prefrontal areas; the properties that have most interested the "how" camp depend on posterior parietal interactions with older frontal areas, a legacy of early primates. Figure 8.2(B) highlights the anthropoid innovations, as well as the traits inherited from earlier primates (Fig. 8.2A).

Attribute features

In parallel with metric contexts sent to the dorsal and dorsolateral prefrontal cortex, the feature system provides information to the ventrolateral prefrontal cortex about the qualitative attributes of sensory contexts, such as color, visual texture, and shape. Passingham and Wise[2] review this literature in detail and propose that the ventrolateral prefrontal cortex:

> generates the goal that is appropriate to the current context and desired outcome, as evaluated in terms of current needs. The goal can be either an object, location, or action and it can be either concrete or abstract.
>
> Passingham and Wise[2] (p. 217)

Anthropoids use attribute features to generate goals in tasks involving arbitrary mapping, short-interval matching, arbitrary categorization, abstract rules, and abstract strategies.

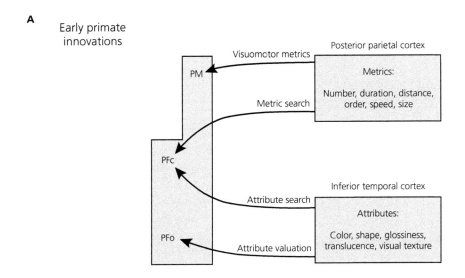

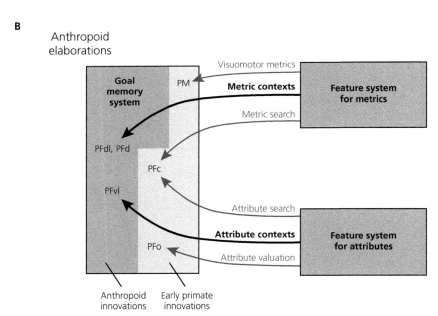

Fig. 8.2 Inputs to primate prefrontal areas. (A) Innovations of early primates. (B) Innovations of anthropoid primates (dark gray). Rostral is to the left. Abbreviations as in Fig. 8.1.

Arbitrary mapping

We have mentioned the arbitrary mapping task, also known as paired-associate learning, in previous chapters (e.g., Chapter 7, "Perception and memory"). In a typical experiment of this kind, one picture served as a goal that had to be chosen in the context of another picture. This task has also been called a visual–visual conditional association task, and it involves the arbitrary mapping of visual representations to each other.

In experiments on monkeys, cutting the uncinate fascicle impaired the learning of arbitrary visual–visual associations[104,105]. This fiber-tract lesion disconnected the inferior temporal areas from the ventrolateral prefrontal cortex, among other prefrontal areas. In another experiment, disconnecting the prefrontal cortex from the superior temporal cortex impaired a different form of paired-associate learning, in this case for arbitrary visual–auditory associations[106].

The prefrontal cortex also plays a key role in the recall of paired associates. Neurons in the temporal cortex have been found to represent such mappings, a property called pair coding[107]. After lesions of the posterior part of the corpus callosum, which connects the visual areas of the two hemispheres, visual cues represented in the right temporal cortex remained capable of generating pair coding in the left inferior temporal cortex[108]. This finding implicated commissural connections between the left and right prefrontal areas, which lie in the anterior part of the corpus callosum, as mediating this kind of recall, most likely via the ventrolateral prefrontal cortex.

Brain imaging results have also pointed to a role for the ventrolateral prefrontal cortex in representing attribute contexts. For example, in a conditional motor learning experiment, various colors and shapes instructed subjects to choose one among several actions[109,110]. The inferior temporal cortex and the ventrolateral prefrontal cortex both showed activation during the performance of this task. In a task involving two sequential attribute cues that, together, mapped arbitrarily to goals in the form of either hats or gloves, multiple-voxel similarity analysis revealed a correlation between the perirhinal cortex and the ventrolateral prefrontal cortex. More specifically, this correlation led to an ability to decode the contextual significance of the first cue[111]. These findings highlight the way that object-level representations in the perirhinal cortex contribute to the generation of goals by the ventrolateral prefrontal cortex.

Likewise, in monkey experiments, neurons in the ventrolateral and dorsolateral prefrontal cortex have been found to represent arbitrary associations, both during and after learning[83,112]. We return to this task later (see "Conditional motor learning"). Next, however, we take up the role of the ventrolateral prefrontal cortex in short-interval matching tasks.

Matching tasks

In two separate experiments, lesions of the ventrolateral prefrontal cortex in monkeys caused an impairment on the short-interval matching task for colors[113] and objects[114], and the homologue of this area has shown activation as human subjects performed analogous tasks[115,116]. In the monkey experiments, the impairment was observed even when the sample remained visible during the test phase[113], thus eliminating the need for working memory. Furthermore, increasing the delay interval had no effect once the monkeys with prefrontal cortex lesions had relearned the matching rule. These findings rule out an account of the impairment in terms of working memory and instead reflect a problem in making rule-based choices, a topic we return to later (see "Abstract rules" and "Rules and strategies"). In agreement with this interpretation, neurons in the ventrolateral prefrontal cortex encoded a rule when a sample cue served as the context for choosing a goal according to that rule[95].

Arbitrary categorization

A series of neurophysiological studies in monkeys have implicated the ventrolateral prefrontal cortex in the arbitrary categorization of stimuli based on their attribute (qualitative) features[86,91]. Likewise, in brain imaging experiments that required people to classify faces according to their attributes[117], activations occurred in both the ventrolateral and dorsolateral prefrontal cortex, especially as the task became more difficult[118,119].

The role of the prefrontal cortex in categorization remains somewhat controversial, but it shouldn't be. Critics point to the finding that a combined lesion of the ventrolateral and dorsolateral prefrontal cortex did not change the level of arousal that monkeys displayed when viewing classes of stimuli that signaled reward size or imminence[120]. This observation occurred not only for the stimuli that the monkeys had been trained on, but also for stimuli that shared features with them. However, the lesion experiment did not test *categorization* in the sense used in the neurophysiological studies[86,91]. The neurophysiology experiments required monkeys to construct *arbitrary* categories, and therefore stimuli that shared features often fell into different groupings. The monkeys could learn and unlearn such arbitrary groupings rapidly, depending on recent experience[86]. The experiment that seemed to contradict categorization instead involved *stimulus generalization*[120], a very different concept[86,121]. From an evolutionary perspective, the neurophysiological results reflect the role of the granular prefrontal cortex in categorizing visual signs of resources and selecting goals on the basis of such categories. Stimulus generalization represents a phylogenetically ancient mechanism that treats stimuli with shared features alike and does not rely on the new anthropoid parts of the prefrontal cortex, the goal system, or categorization in a strict sense.

Abstract rules

Neurophysiological studies of the monkey ventrolateral prefrontal cortex have pointed to a role in representing abstract task rules[122–124]. Such findings relate to a classic observation reported for lesions of the prefrontal cortex in humans: an impairment in switching among rules in the Wisconsin card sorting task[125]. In performing this task, the subjects need to sort cards according to one rule, such as by color, until they learn that they have made an error, at which point they should switch to a different rule. In a representative experimental design, healthy people switched to a new rule after one error, but patients with lesions of the prefrontal cortex repeated the failing rule for a mean of 12 trials[126], with similar results on a related task[127]. Such patients also switched to a new rule when they should have stuck with the current one[128]. Other tasks that depend on the prefrontal cortex have also involved shifting among different task rules[129].

In an analog of the Wisconsin card sorting task, monkeys learned matching rules based on either stimulus color or shape, which alternated in blocks of trials[50]. Lesions of the ventrolateral prefrontal cortex prevented the monkeys from relearning this task. Presumably, the need to switch between two rules blocked relearning in this case, as monkeys with ventrolateral prefrontal lesions could relearn a single, color-matching rule[113] (see "Matching tasks"). In accord with this idea, brain imaging studies have revealed activations after rule switching (and object switching[130–132]) in the ventrolateral prefrontal cortex of both humans and monkeys[133], in much the same areas that showed activation when human subjects learned about their errors on rule-switching tasks[134–136]. All these tasks involved the use of attribute contexts to generate goals.

Abstract strategies

Gaffan and his colleagues[137–139] reported several results from what they called a *strategy task*, although the task also required arbitrary categorization. On each trial, monkeys faced a choice between two stimuli, each consisting of shape and color conjunctions. The stimuli fell into two arbitrary categories. For optimal performance, the subjects had to choose a stimulus from one category for four consecutive trials, and then choose a stimulus in the other category once and only once before shifting back to the first category (Fig. 8.3A).

Lesions of the ventrolateral prefrontal cortex, but not of the orbital or dorsolateral prefrontal cortex, caused an impairment on this task (Fig. 8.3B)[138,139]. Ventrolateral prefrontal cortex lesions in macaque monkeys had only a mild effect, but crossed surgical disconnections of the prefrontal and inferior temporal cortex produced a dramatic impairment, leading to disordered choices. These results provide further support for a role of the granular prefrontal cortex in goal generation based on attribute contexts.

Summary

With their new visual traits, adaptations to diurnal foraging, and habit of moving long distances to obtain resources, relative metrics and distant qualitative attributes became especially important to evolving anthropoids. According to the proposal we presented in Chapter 7, the feature system developed new kinds of sensory representations, at levels of complexity unavailable to their ancestors—although not necessarily higher levels of complexity. These specialized representations began to serve as the contexts for generating goals once the new anthropoid prefrontal areas emerged.

Although we emphasize foraging, the same adaptations apply to social behavior. We view foraging as primary for a simple reason. The adage "you are what you eat" misses a key point: if you don't eat, you aren't. Even worse, you could be eaten along the way to eating, something our ancestors knew very well 35 million years ago or so when the goal system evolved (see Chapter 2, "Anthropoids").

In addition to using new kinds of contexts, the goal system of anthropoids reduced foraging errors by using event memories and abstract strategies.

Event memories

Passingham and Wise[2] review the results of neurophysiological and brain imaging work supporting the idea that the granular prefrontal cortex stores the memories of single

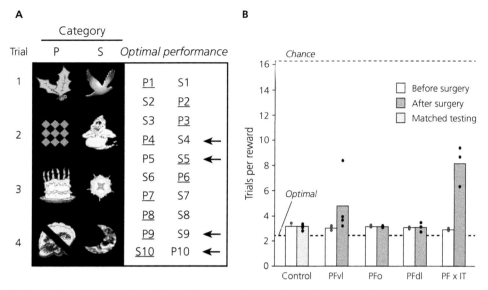

Fig. 8.3 Effect of temporal–prefrontal disconnections on the performance of a strategy task. (A) A strategy task that depended on arbitrary stimulus categorization and a shift-category rule. Monkeys needed to choose an item in the persistent (P) category at least four consecutive times in order to receive a reward (arrows). Afterward, they needed to select an item in the sporadic (S) category once and only once to obtain another reward. (B) Effects of prefrontal–inferior temporal disconnections (PF x IT) and lesions of selected parts of the prefrontal cortex. Abbreviations as in Fig. 8.1. Dashed horizontal lines indicate optimal performance (2.5 trials per reward) and chance levels of performance (random choices). Preoperative scores (unfilled bars) versus postoperative scores (gray bars). Circles, scores of individual subjects. (A) Drawings courtesy of Mark Baxter. (B) Data from Baxter et al.[138,139].

events. The most direct evidence comes from studying the effects of brain lesions, so we concentrate on those findings here.

Credit assignment

The term credit assignment applies to a problem in learning theory. Given that feedback follows some series of actions or stimuli after a time lag, how can animals attribute that outcome to the action or stimulus that (apparently) caused it?

A key line of evidence indicated that the ventrolateral prefrontal cortex contributes to this kind of credit assignment[140]. This function was initially attributed to the granular orbitofrontal cortex[141], but more recent experiments have shown that that result, along with others, depended on disrupting fiber pathways passing through or near the granular orbitofrontal cortex[142,143]. Nevertheless, for the present purpose we can consider the orbital and ventrolateral prefrontal cortex together.

In the *three-arm bandit task*[141], monkeys faced a choice among three images (Fig. 8.4A), each indicating a different reward probability. As these probabilities changed over trials,

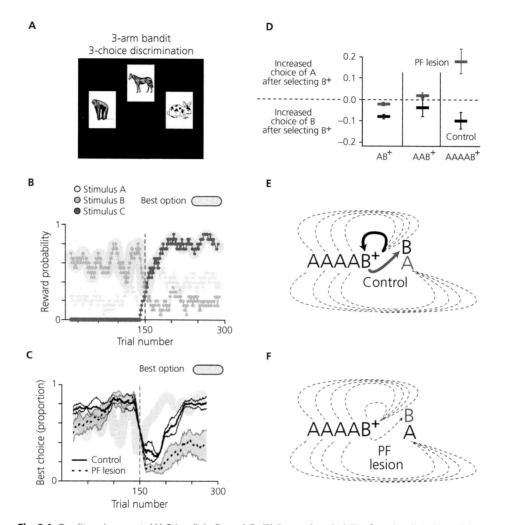

Fig. 8.4 Credit assignment. (A) Stimuli A, B, and C. (B) Reward probability for stimuli A, B, and C. The three different curves (light, medium, and dark gray) represent reward probabilities across a single test session. (Note that stimulus C has a reward probability of zero for the first half of the session.) The vertical dashed line indicates the trial when stimulus C became the best choice. (C) Performance of control monkeys and monkeys with bilateral lesions of the granular orbitofrontal cortex, but probably involving damage to fibers going to and from the ventrolateral prefrontal cortex. Thin gray and black lines denote standard error. The best option is shown as in (B). (D) After a rewarded choice of B (B+), positive values indicate an increased frequency of choosing stimulus A on the next trial and negative values correspond to an increased frequency of choosing stimulus B. Performance of control (black) and lesioned monkeys (gray). Error bars: standard error. (E) Control monkeys could link the reward that followed their choice of B to that choice (black arrow), which promoted a bias toward choosing stimulus B on the next trial (gray arrow). (F) In lesioned monkeys, only a weak link connected stimulus B with the reward on the previous trial. Abbreviation: PF, granular prefrontal cortex. From Figs. 4.6 and 4.11 in Passingham RE, Wise SP. *The Neurobiology of the Prefrontal Cortex*, © 2012, Oxford University Press. Reproduced with permission of OUP. Data in (B), (C), and (D) from Walton et al.[141].

so too might the "best choice" (Fig. 8.4B). Control monkeys quickly switched to a new "best choice," when it changed, but monkeys with lesions of the prefrontal cortex took much longer to do so (Fig. 8.4C). Control monkeys also had a strong tendency to repeat a recently rewarded choice (choice "B" in Fig. 8.4D, black bars) despite the past superiority of an alternative (choice "A"). Monkeys with lesions of the prefrontal cortex, in contrast, did not show this tendency nearly as strongly (gray bars in Fig. 8.4D), especially when they had chosen an alternative ("A") on many previous trials (depicted as AAAAB[+]). The black arrow in Fig. 8.4(E) represents the proper credit assignment in control monkeys: when a reward (+) resulted from the choice of "B", this choice–outcome (or stimulus–outcome) association should have promoted the choice of "B" on the next trial (gray arrow). The lesions in these experiments weakened or eliminated the choice–outcome (or stimulus–outcome) assignments (Fig. 8.4F), leaving previous choices of "A" to exert an undue influence on the monkeys' choices.

Most mammals behave like the lesioned monkeys, using cumulative adjustments in choice–outcome or stimulus–outcome associations to guide foraging choices (see Chapter 3). Anthropoids, in contrast, can use the memory of single events to improve their future choices, even when these conflict with the broader averages. They retain the older choice–outcome (instrumental) and stimulus–outcome (Pavlovian) mechanisms, of course. These older representational systems continue to bias choices toward those that have proved most beneficial in the past, over the long run. However, anthropoids can also use the memory of events that contradict these broad averages, and so can make better choices when ecological circumstances change rapidly.

Updating the valuation of predicted outcomes also plays a role in these choices (see Chapter 6, "Orbitofrontal–amygdala interactions"). This function depends on the granular orbitofrontal cortex[142,143] and its interactions with the amygdala (see Fig. 6.10)[144]. Taken together, two kinds of value updating contribute to foraging choices: (1) updating the likelihood that an outcome, such as a food item, will follow a given choice determines one aspect of its value; and (2) updating the valuation of these outcomes in terms of current biological needs establishes what that item is worth at any given moment. The second kind of updating extends phylogenetically old functions (see Chapter 3, "What happens in instrumental conditioning") to a set of prefrontal areas that evolved in early primates: the granular orbitofrontal cortex[140]. The visual innovations of primates play an important role in this kind of updating, especially for the visual features of outcomes. In contrast, the first kind of updating reflects something new, the ability to use single events to guide future choices. This derived trait depends on a new anthropoid area, the ventrolateral prefrontal cortex[140], and it provides an advantage over reinforcement learning alone.

Object-in-place scenes task

In Chapter 4 ("Scene memory") we described a task used to examine event memories in monkeys: the object-in-place scenes task[145,146]. Monkeys learned to choose an object-like stimulus embedded within a complex background scene (Fig. 8.5B). Although the monkeys needed to master 20 scenes concurrently, they learned the correct choice in two or three trials with a given scene, with significant one-trial learning (Fig. 8.5A, gray lines).

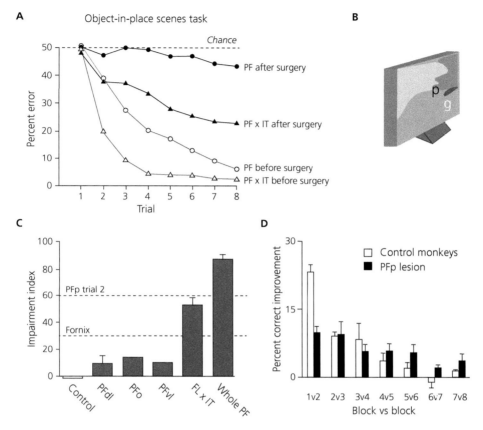

Fig. 8.5 Object-in-place scenes task. (A) Preoperative (unfilled symbols) and postoperative (black symbols) performance in two groups of monkeys: one destined to receive complete bilateral ablations of the prefrontal cortex (circles), the other to receive a crossed-disconnection lesion of prefrontal (PF) and the inferior temporal (IT) cortex (PF x IT, triangles). (B) Depiction of the video monitor that the monkeys saw, including the background (gray shapes) and goals (letters) used. (C) Performance of control monkeys (unfilled bar) and monkeys with various lesions (gray bars). Error bars: standard error. The horizontal dashed lines show the mean impairment after transection of the fornix (lower line) and for trial two after lesions of the polar prefrontal cortex (PFp). The impairment index shows the percentage of possible impairment relative to chance levels, which normalizes the scores for group differences in preoperative performance. (D) Effect of polar prefrontal cortex lesions, percent improvement for each of the first eight trials. Abbreviations as in Fig. 8.1 plus: FL, frontal lobe; PF, granular prefrontal cortex. (A), (C) Figure 8.4 in Passingham RE, Wise SP. *The Neurobiology of the Prefrontal Cortex*, © 2012, Oxford University Press. Reproduced with permission of OUP. (D) Figure 3.10 in the same source. Reproduced with permission of OUP. Data in (D) courtesy of Mark Buckley.

The inclusion of a background scene reduced errors dramatically (see Fig. 11.3A)[147]. In general, it took monkeys approximately ten trials without the backgrounds to reach the same level of performance they could attain after a single trial with the backgrounds. A scene-level context thus conferred a large learning advantage, probably by enabling the formation of unique context–goal–outcome conjunctions for each scene.

This task draws on the kinds of foraging decisions that anthropoids make in their natural habitats, in which they use signs of distant resources—signs that consist of complex visual scenes. In the laboratory, monkeys perform this task with reaching movements, so these mechanisms generalize to reachable resources as well as those attained by locomotion.

Figure 8.5(A) shows the effect of removing the granular prefrontal cortex or disconnecting it from the inferior temporal cortex. Both lesions caused a severe impairment, with bilateral lesions of the prefrontal cortex virtually abolishing the benefit provided by the background contexts. Figure 8.5(C) shows that these lesions caused a much more severe impairment than either fornix transections or lesions of various subdivisions of the granular prefrontal cortex.

Monkeys with lesions of the polar prefrontal cortex, also known as the frontal-pole cortex, had a very specific impairment on this task[148]. The second time that these monkeys saw a given scene, separated by 19 intervening scenes, they made many more errors than control monkeys did (Fig. 8.5C, top horizontal dashed line). Afterward, however, the lesioned monkeys learned at roughly the same rate as the control group (Fig. 8.5D). Similar results occurred for the first choice between two images, without background scenes. These results show that lesions of the polar prefrontal cortex specifically impair one-trial learning[148]. One-trial learning, of course, depends upon the memory of a single event and the generation of a goal based on that memory. The same lesions also impaired the learning of an abstract rule[148], a topic to which we return later (see "Abstract rules and strategies").

Conditional motor learning

Results from the conditional motor learning task resemble those from the object-in-place scenes task. In this task, monkeys learn that an arbitrary visual cue instructs a specific goal or action. We have already discussed conditional motor learning several times, and in Chapter 7 ("Perception, action, and actuality") we used results from this task to contradict the perception–action dichotomy. In a typical experiment, each of three visual cues, which differ in color and shape, instruct the subject to choose a different spatial goal (or action). Eventually, all cues, goals, and actions take on equal value, and only cue–goal (or cue–action) conjunctions predict a beneficial outcome.

Naive monkeys solve novel conditional motor problems slowly, but with experience monkeys are able to do so in just a few trials, often showing one-trial learning. Figure 8.6(A) presents learning curves before and after combined bilateral lesions of the ventrolateral and granular orbitofrontal cortex[149]. This lesion eliminated almost all of the direct interactions between the prefrontal cortex and both the inferior temporal

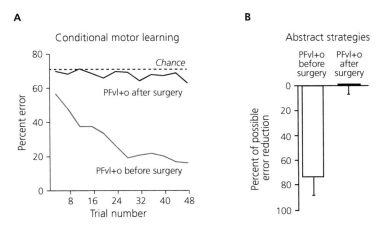

Fig. 8.6 Conditional motor learning. (A) Conditional motor learning by experienced monkeys, before (gray) and after (black) combined lesions of the ventrolateral and granular orbitofrontal cortex (PFvl+o). (B) Use of repeat–stay and change–shift strategies before (white) and after (black) the lesion. Data from Bussey et al.[149]

and perirhinal cortex, and it blocked rapid learning: not only in one or a few trials, but also within 50 trials. Given sufficient trials, monkeys with these brain lesions could solve novel problems, but they returned to the slower rates of learning typical of naive monkeys and nonprimates, such as rats[150]. Lesioned monkeys made many more errors after surgery than before, which supports the idea that the granular prefrontal cortex reduces errors.

As just mentioned, in Chapter 7 we used results from conditional motor learning experiments to refute the perception–action dichotomy (see Fig. 7.1A). The reason is simple: These experiments demonstrate that the inferior temporal cortex, which this doctrine designates as a "perception area," also plays a direct role in guiding actions. Of most relevance to the proposal in this chapter, it does so by supplying attribute contexts to the ventrolateral prefrontal cortex[151], which generates a goal or action plan based on these representations.

Temporally extended events

Many ideas about the prefrontal cortex emphasize the bridging of time gaps and integrating events over time[152]. An experimental design that tested this idea modified the standard single-pair discrimination task by introducing a visual stimulus to fill a time gap between a monkey's choice and a subsequent reward (Fig. 8.7A)[153]. This sequence created a temporally extended (or temporally complex) event. The bridging stimulus presumably helped the monkeys learn conjunctions between the choice and the outcome, and thus reduced errors. As predicted, disconnection lesions involving the inferior temporal and prefrontal cortex eliminated the advantage that the bridging event provided to control monkeys (Fig. 8.7B).

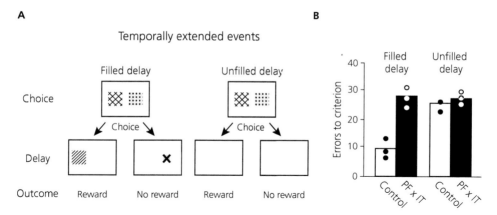

Fig. 8.7 Temporally extended events. (A) Task design. Monkeys chose between two stimuli (top row) in either a filled-delay or unfilled-delay condition. Only one choice produced a reward in each case. In the filled-delay condition, an image appeared in the place previously held by the chosen stimulus during the delay between choice and reward, and a reward followed correct choices. In the unfilled-delay condition, no image appeared after a choice, and for correct choices a reward occurred at the same time as in the filled-delay condition. (B) Errors to criterion for control monkeys and those with crossed-disconnection lesions of the prefrontal and inferior temporal cortex (PF x IT). Adapted from Figure 8.8 in Passingham RE, Wise SP. *The Neurobiology of the Prefrontal Cortex*, © 2012, Oxford University Press. Reproduced with permission of OUP. Data from Browning and Gaffan[153].

In a related experiment, monkeys needed to avoid choosing familiar stimuli in favor of novel ones[154]. Crossed-disconnection lesions of the prefrontal and inferior temporal cortex caused a severe impairment on this task, and it took these monkeys a long time to relearn the rule. Afterwards they could apply the rule normally, however. The same monkeys had a severe impairment in learning the nonmatching version of the short-interval matching task. It might seem odd that these monkeys could perform one task that used a given rule, in this case "avoid familiar stimuli," and not another task that employed the same rule. This difference also points to a role for prefrontal–temporal interactions in representing the extended temporal structure of events, such as the sample–delay–choice sequence that occurred in this task. In support of this interpretation, once the lesioned monkeys learned the matching task with 2-second delays, the introduction of lists caused an additional impairment, presumably because it disrupted the temporal structure of the task. These findings indicate that although representations of temporally extended events can reduce errors on their own (Fig. 8.7B), some behaviors require their synthesis with abstract rules. The granular prefrontal cortex plays a critical role in both aspects of error reduction, as we discuss later (see "Abstract strategies").

Summary

Their new prefrontal areas enabled evolving anthropoids to learn context–goal–action–outcome conjunctions rapidly, sometimes based on a single event. These representations reduce errors on laboratory tasks that involve assigning outcomes to choices; choosing among objects embedded in a background scene (context–goal–outcome conjunctions); choosing among actions based on arbitrary cues (context–action–outcome or context–goal–outcome conjunctions); and choosing among stimuli based on temporally extended events. In their natural habitat, faster learning and error reduction enabled our anthropoid ancestors to make more productive and less dangerous foraging choices compared with the ancestral condition. Note that it is not essential that the relevant learning takes place in just one trial; evolving anthropoids would have gained an advantage from any appreciable reduction in foraging errors.

Another way that the granular prefrontal cortex makes use of event representations is to use them for the implementation of abstract, behavior guiding strategies.

Abstract strategies

Learning set

The term learning set refers to the ability to learn faster with experience: a gradual and substantial increase in the speed of learning, usually to discriminate two stimuli. In a narrower sense, learning set refers to a specific measure of this skill, the ability to choose correctly between two novel objects—one correct, one incorrect—when seeing them for the second time (trial two). Macaque monkeys have achieved an error rate as low as about 10% on trial two, 40% or so better than chance performance.

In Chapter 7 ("The prevailing doctrine and its discontents") we called this task the single-pair task and serial discrimination learning because the subjects saw the same two stimuli trial after trial (Fig. 8.8B, left). We contrasted this version of discrimination learning with concurrent discrimination learning, also called the multiple-pair task. In this version of the task, the subjects saw a number of stimulus pairs between the presentation of any given pair (Fig. 8.8B, right).

As illustrated in Fig. 8.8(A), in the multiple-pair task control monkeys learned at a relatively slow rate (gray triangles), resembling what rats and other mammals have done on similar tasks[155]. In contrast to this slow learning, control monkeys with experience on the single-pair task developed a learning set, which reduced errors quickly (gray circles). For example, their error rate decreased by half after one trial (upward gray arrow). In contrast, on the multiple-pair task, one trial had little effect on the error rate in the time range tested (downward gray arrow), despite equivalent task experience.

The black curves in Fig. 8.8(A) show the effect of a crossed-disconnection lesion of the inferior temporal and prefrontal cortex. These lesions had little effect on learning rates for the multiple-pair task (black versus gray triangles, dashed lines) but caused a significant impairment on the single-pair task (black versus gray circles, continuous lines)[156], bringing performance into line with that for the multiple-pair task.

Murray and Gaffan[155] interpret these findings in terms of prospective coding, which refers to the ability to maintain a goal in short-term memory pending an action that achieves it. In the multiple-pair version of the task, many trials intervene before a given

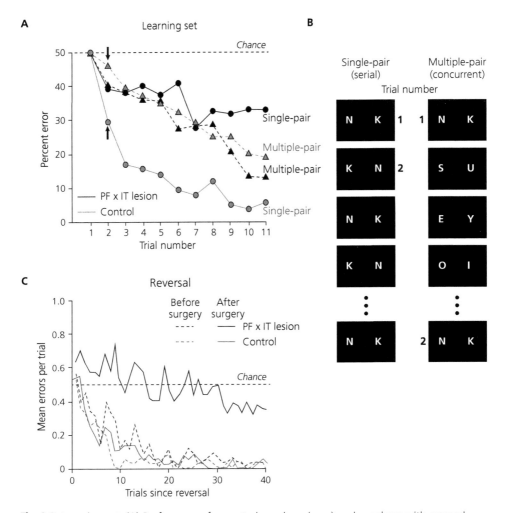

Fig. 8.8 Learning set. (A) Performance for control monkeys (gray) and monkeys with crossed disconnections of the prefrontal and inferior temporal cortex (black) on the single-pair (circles) and multiple-pair (triangles) discrimination tasks. (B) Left column: In the single-pair version of the task, the same two stimuli repeated for a series of consecutive trials. Right column: In the multiple-pair version of the task, several pairs of stimuli intervened between the first presentation of the initial pair and its second appearance. Trials one and two for a given pair are designated by numerals for both versions of the task. (C) Effect of crossed disconnections of the prefrontal and inferior temporal cortex (PF x IT lesion) on reversal performance. (A) Adapted from Figure 8.3 in Passingham RE, Wise SP. *The Neurobiology of the Prefrontal Cortex*, © 2012, Oxford University Press. Reproduced with permission of OUP. (A) Data from Browning et al.[156]. (C) Data from Wilson and Gaffan[157].

choice recurs, making it impossible to maintain a goal in prospective memory. In the single-pair task, the same two stimuli are repeated trial after trial, and so the events on one trial can be applied to the next. To succeed on trial two of this task, monkeys can use an abstract strategy called win–stay, lose–shift. If their first choice fails to produce a reward, they should avoid it on trial two and instead choose the alternative (lose–shift). If, by chance, they obtain a reward on their first choice, they should choose that object again on trial two (win–stay). In principle, monkeys could use these strategies for both the single- and multiple-pair tasks. In the multiple-pair task, however, the second trial for a given pair of stimuli takes too long to come around again.

The development of a learning set thus depends on two processes: (1) the use of a strategy to generate the goal for trial two based on the outcome of trial one; and (2) the maintenance of this goal in memory until the next trial (prospective memory). The results illustrated in Fig. 8.8(A) show that disconnecting the prefrontal cortex from the inferior temporal cortex blocked one or both of these processes, as did switching from the single-pair to the multiple-pair task. Both manipulations eliminated the learning set, although in different ways, and in both cases the learning rate of experienced monkeys reverted to the levels typical of naive monkeys and other mammals.

These findings showed that disconnecting the inferior temporal and prefrontal cortex eliminated the advantage that monkeys gained by developing a learning set, an advantage that depended on the granular prefrontal cortex. In this sense, results from the learning-set experiments resembled those illustrated in Figs. 8.3–8.7 from other tasks, all of which have demonstrated that removing the prefrontal cortex or disconnecting it from the feature system eliminated an advantage in terms of faster learning and fewer errors. In each case, this faster learning could approach the limit: one-trial learning.

The literature comparing learning sets among species remains controversial. To summarize it very briefly, many species of mammals improve their performance on discrimination tasks with experience, but not to the extent that macaque monkeys do. Claims for such performance in rodents, for example, do not stand up to critical scrutiny. Passingham and Wise[2] deal with this issue in detail, and we refer interested readers to that discussion.

Studies of discrimination-reversal tasks also indicate a prefrontally mediated advantage in terms of faster learning and fewer errors. This task required monkeys to change their choice between two objects in blocks of trials. Like a learning set, as monkeys gained experience with reversals of this kind, they switched their choices more quickly, a capacity called a reversal set. Figure 8.8(C) comes from monkeys with a reasonably strong reversal set. In these monkeys, disconnecting the prefrontal and inferior temporal cortex impaired performance[41,157], as did other lesions involving the prefrontal cortex[142,144].

In both the learning- and reversal-set experiments, a normally functioning granular prefrontal cortex reduced errors. The loss of this advantage did not result in an inability to solve the problems posed by these tasks. Instead, monkeys with lesions of the prefrontal cortex reverted to the learning rates typical of naive monkeys and other mammals, with a concomitant increase in errors. As we explained earlier (see "Event memories"), the same can be said of several other tasks.

Rules and strategies

Similar principles apply beyond win–stay and lose–shift to other rules and strategies. The concepts of a rule and a strategy are similar; both are abstractions that can be applied to novel stimuli. Rules indicate what behaviors to perform in a given context; strategies indicate what behaviors might be performed in a given context: one among two or more solutions to a problem or a partial solution to some problem.

Lesion studies in monkeys have shown that the granular prefrontal cortex uses abstract strategies to generate goals and reduce errors. In experiments employing the conditional motor learning task (see "Conditional motor learning"), monkeys used the change–shift and repeat–stay strategies. The repeat–stay strategy led to staying with the most recent goal or action when the cue repeated from the preceding trial; the change–shift strategy led to shifting from the previous choice when the cue changed from the preceding trial. For a task involving three stimuli and goals, this strategy reduced a three-choice task to a two-choice task when the cue changed from one trial to the next, and so reduced the error rate from 67% to about 50% on these trials. If applied perfectly, the repeat–stay strategy should have eliminated errors entirely when the stimulus repeated from the preceding trial. As illustrated in Fig. 8.6(B), combined lesions of the ventrolateral and granular orbitofrontal cortex completely abolished both the change–shift and repeat–stay strategies[149].

Summary

The evolution of new prefrontal areas enhanced the ability of anthropoids to generate goals based on abstract rules and strategies. According to our proposal, these behaviors depend on specialized context–goal–action–outcome conjunctions in which the goal is represented abstractly and often prospectively. As a result, anthropoids can generate goals on the basis of both concrete and abstract context–goal–action–outcome conjunctions. The former trait corresponds to an exemplar-based, list-wise approach; the latter involves abstract rules and strategies that apply to novel or rarely encountered situations. These ideas do not mean that other cortical areas in anthropoids or cortical areas in other species lack an ability to support abstract rules or strategies. Our proposal implies only that the specialized conjunctions represented in the granular prefrontal cortex of anthropoids provide an advantage in terms of faster learning and fewer errors.

Augmentation of older representational systems

The goal system of anthropoids does not work alone, of course. Animals had been learning about context, actions, and outcomes for a long time before the advent of anthropoid primates, their new prefrontal areas, or the goal system. And when the goal system emerged, the existing representational systems did not vanish. Instead of replacing the older systems, the goal system augmented their functions.

Augmentation of the manual-foraging and navigation systems

The goal system augmented the manual-foraging and navigation systems by generating abstract goals: objects in unseen or unknown locations and spatial goals in relative rather than concrete coordinates[59,158,159]. The ability to represent goals independently of the actions that achieve them provided an important advantage to evolving anthropoids.

Augmentation of the reinforcement systems

The goal system augmented the reinforcement learning systems by storing the memories of single goal-related events, thus speeding learning and reducing errors. The reinforcement systems, in contrast, update memory states without storing each event.

Put another way, the goal system increases flexibility in the time frame for averaging prior events. The reinforcement systems reflect a cumulative average over a rigid range of prior events, weighted toward more recent ones. The goal system encodes previous outcomes on a much larger variety of time-scales, representing a "reservoir" of time horizons for averaging[160,161]. Some time-scales can average events over long periods, which serve animals well in conditions of low and moderate resource volatility. At the limit, however, short time-scales can filter fast-changing outcomes in the most volatile conditions, at the level of single events. In natural foraging conditions, this translates into faster adjustments to highly volatile ecological conditions. We return to the topic of resource volatility later (see "Augmentation of the biased-competition system").

The prefrontal cortex is not unique in learning from single events, of course. Rats and other mammals can learn taste aversion in one trial, for example[162–164] (see Chapter 3, "Why Pavlovian conditioning happens") and birds learn to follow a parent based on a single exposure, a phenomenon called imprinting[165,166]. In Chapter 7 ("Rodents") we mentioned spontaneous exploration, in which rats can recognize an object and its location based on a single trial. The floor of a maze can, for example, provide a context that rats use to avoid a once-seen object and explore a novel one—not always, but about 60% of the time[167].

These examples of one-trial learning in nonprimates are perfectly compatible with the idea that a new representational system evolved in anthropoids, based on new granular prefrontal areas. The fact that some older, specialized mechanisms support one-trial learning does not negate the additional adaptive advantage of reducing the number of errors in situations outside the scope of these special-purpose mechanisms. The goal system of derived anthropoids differs from one-trial learning in other animals by integrating a broader scope of information and thereby applying fast, event-based learning to a much wider range of problems than specialized mechanisms such as taste aversion, imprinting, and spontaneous exploration.

Augmentation of the biased-competition system

The goal system also augmented the biased-competition system. It did so by extending the top-down influences that the prefrontal cortex had previously directed to the navigation and reinforcement systems (see Chapter 5, "Proposal"). In anthropoids, top-down biases from the prefrontal cortex came to involve the feature and manual-foraging systems as well. Thus, the new anthropoid prefrontal areas began to subserve what is sometimes called attentive control.

Before we discuss the role of the prefrontal cortex in attentive control, we need to address a serious problem in the literature: a tendency to rely on all-encompassing two-factor theories of behavior. These classifications invariably cause confusion because there

are more than two factors underlying behavior, just as there are more than two representational systems in the brain. So when theorists divide all behavior into two categories,
they inevitably lump unlike behaviors into a trash-can category. Table 8.1 replicates most
of Table 22.1 from Stanovich[168]. We present this table not as an endorsement of two-
factor theories of behavior but to illustrate the kinds of terms and concepts that cognitive
psychologists use to classify behaviors. In addition to the ideas that we present in Table
8.1, an active research program divides behavior into model-free and model-based reinforcement learning (see Box 4.1). This idea and some of the other dichotomies in Table
8.1 have heuristic value, especially when they wall off a particular kind of behavior for
intensive study. Their danger, and the problem inherent in Table 8.1, is the implication
that each concept in a column corresponds to all the other concepts in the same column.
For example, Table 8.1 creates the impression that all rule-based processing is conscious,
despite the obvious fact that people follow many rules, such as grammatical ones, subcon-
sciously. In Chapter 11 ("Do animals have explicit memory?") we discuss this problem in
detail.

A wealth of brain imaging data support the idea that the primate prefrontal cortex subserves the attentive control of behavior[2]. These studies have shown that the granular prefrontal cortex becomes activated when people attend to their behavior, either because of
the demanding nature of the task[3,169] or to report about their own actions[170,171]. As behaviors become automatic, the granular prefrontal cortex and its cortex–basal ganglia "loops"
become less activated, while the premotor and posterior parietal areas and their cortex–
basal ganglia "loops" become more activated[2]. Figure 8.9 illustrates this idea, incorporating some points made in Fig. 5.6.

Automatic control functions well in conditions of low to moderate resource volatility.
As explained in Chapter 3 ("Why instrumental conditioning happens"), habits are useful for exploiting resources when resource volatility is low. They have the advantage of
low computational cost and quickly executed choices. Outcome-directed behaviors, at
higher computational cost, serve animals well when resource volatility is at moderate
levels. These behaviors adapt as outcomes change, but because reinforcement learning
depends on averages over several cumulative events, it produces many errors when conditions change too rapidly for the averages to catch up. According to our proposal, attentive
control emerged as anthropoids adapted to highly volatile resources[2]. However, we have
yet to address why and when this occurred.

A regime of climatic cooling occurred about 35 million years ago, and it probably
resulted in an ecological crisis in the tropics, where anthropoids lived (and most still do).
In Chapter 2 ("Changes in brain size") we explained that the brain expansion of anthropoids probably began at about that time. Combined with a severe risk of predation and
the need to forage over large distances in dangerous daylight conditions, high volatility in necessary resources places a premium on minimizing errors. In such conditions,
top-down attentive control reduces errors by influencing which specific sensory features
will guide behavior, of the rich attribute and metric contexts available to anthropoids.
Likewise, attentive control modulates an equally rich set of visual features related to the

Table 8.1 Selected two-factor theories of behavior

Theorists	Factor 1	Factor 2
Bargh & Chartrand	Automatic processing	Conscious processing
Brainerd & Reyna	Gist processing	Analytic processing
Chaiken et al.	Heuristic processing	Systematic processing
Evans	Heuristic processing	Analytic processing
Evans & Over	Tacit thought processes	Explicit thought processes
Fodor	Modular processes	Central processes
Gawronski & Bodenhausen	Associative processes	Propositional processes
Haidr	Intuitive system	Reasoning system
Johnson-Laird	Implicit inferences	Explicit references
Kahneman & Frederick	Intuition	Reasoning
Lieberman	Reflexive system	Reflective system
Norman & Shallice	Contention scheduling	Supervisory attention system
Pollock	Quick, inflexible modules	Intellection
Posner & Snyder	Automatic activation	Conscious processing
Reber	Implicit cognition	Explicit learning
Shiffrin & Synder	Automatic processing	Controlled processing
Sloman	Associative system	Rule-based system
Smith & DeCoster	Associative processing	Rule-based processing
Strack & Deutsch	Impulsive system	Reflective system
Toates	Stimulus bound	Higher order
Wilson	Adaptive unconscious	Consciousness
Mishkin[175,176]	Habits	Memory
Squire[177]	Procedural memory	Declarative memory
Balleine & O'Doherty[178]	Habits	Goal-directed behavior

specific outcomes that should occur as a result of foraging choices. These mechanisms not only mitigate the computational bottleneck that arises from "too much information," but also ensure that most new learning is directed toward the most biologically significant features in the environment.

Earlier (see "New contexts"), we emphasized projections going from the feature system to the goal system. Top-down attentive control involves the reciprocal projection. The ventrolateral prefrontal cortex, for example, affects visual processing in the inferior temporal cortex[172], and projections from the dorsal and dorsolateral prefrontal cortex probably exert an analogous influence over the posterior parietal cortex. The key question for the present discussion is: What do goal memories have to do with attentive control? Our

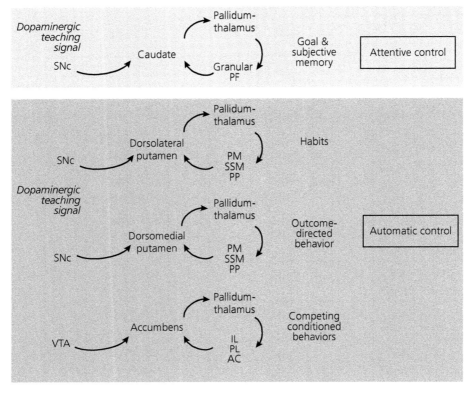

Fig. 8.9 Attentive versus automatic behavior circuits. Abbreviations: AC, anterior cingulate cortex; IL, infralimbic cortex; PF, prefrontal cortex; PL, prelimbic cortex; PM, premotor areas; PP, posterior parietal cortex; SNc, substantia nigra pars compacta; SSM, somatic sensorimotor cortex, including primary motor cortex and somatosensory areas; VTA, ventral tegmental area.

answer is that goal memories, which consist of context–goal–action–outcome conjunctions, bias temporal and parietal areas toward processing the features of contexts that are linked to goals and valuable outcomes. The same can be said for the features of predicted outcomes. For example, when foraging for blackberries the advantage goes to anthropoids that can promote glossiness detection, link the representation of glossiness to a prediction of sweetness, and bias the manual-foraging system toward grasping and manipulating berries with the feature that we call glossiness (see Fig. 6.12).

Some evidence from monkeys has provided direct support for these ideas. In one experiment, monkeys learned to distinguish among different orientations of parallel lines, which came in three different colors[173]. During testing, a separately located color cue indicated which color to use on a given trial. Lesions of the dorsolateral and ventrolateral prefrontal cortex caused a severe impairment in distinguishing different orientations of the lines with the cued color, which worsened when the color cue varied from trial-to-trial, as opposed to remaining constant for a block of trials. This finding points to a lesion-induced impairment in selecting the correct color stimulus through a top-down attentional process.

The learning theory literature makes much of the fact that all behaviors can be described in terms of stimuli, responses, and outcomes. All controlled systems can be described in terms of inputs, outputs, and feedback, of course, but this fact says nothing about their mechanisms. For our proposal to be true, evolution did not need to produce something so strange as to defy description in terms of inputs, outputs, and feedback. Instead, the goal system simply needed to provide some advantage over pre-existing representational systems. For our anthropoid ancestors, attentive control provided such advantages by promoting the learning of goal-related conjunctions on the basis of single events and by using these representations: (1) to bias sensory processing toward the stimuli associated with these goals; and (2) to bias motor processing toward actions associated with achieving these goals. The targets of these biases were discussed in Chapters 7 and 6, respectively, as the feature and manual-foraging systems.

Summary

In the ancestors of anthropoids, older representational systems made many errors when resource volatility reached high levels. Anthropoids developed a goal system, based in their new granular prefrontal areas, that provided an advantage in terms of fewer foraging errors. It did this in part by acquiring goal-related conjunctions rapidly, sometimes based on a single event, and using these memories to generate a top-down bias among competing sensory and motor representations.

Conclusions

Structure, function, advantages

Biological, anatomical, psychological, computational, and general perspectives capture the proposal advanced in this chapter in complementary ways.

In biological terms, the goal system reflects an anthropoid adaptation to a high level of resource volatility. Instincts, habits, and outcome-directed behavior work well under most ecological conditions. As a result, other animals succeed without a goal system, as did the immediate ancestors of anthropoids. A decrease in errors is always advantageous, of course, but it became a powerful selective pressure in anthropoids. As explained earlier, because of their long lives, dependence on the produce of angiosperm trees, the need to forage over long distances in daylight, predation risks, and recurrent shortfalls in necessary resources, the older representational systems made too many errors for anthropoids to thrive. At such times, the reduction of just a few foraging errors could mean the difference between life and death.

In anatomical terms, the new prefrontal areas reduce foraging errors because of three key properties: their unique pattern of extrinsic connections, which bring together high-level information about contexts, goals, actions, and outcomes in a way that other parts of the cortex cannot; their ability to integrate this information into conjunctive representations via intrinsic connections; and their relatively direct influence over premotor and posterior parietal areas that plan and specify movements[2].

In psychological terms, the goal system supports top-down attention, one-trial learning across a broad range of problems, the transfer of learned solutions to new problems (abstract strategies), arbitrary categorization, and prospective coding. It does so by processing and storing a specialized kind of neural representation, consisting of context–goal–action–outcome conjunctions, with an emphasis on visual features at high- and mid-levels of representational complexity (see Fig. 7.3).

In computational terms, the goal system uses multiple time frames for learning and alleviates both computational bottlenecks and information overload through top-down attentive control.

In general terms, the prefrontal cortex stores specialized goal representations and deploys them when current behavioral requirements exceed the capacity of more specialized cortical areas[3,4] and older representational systems[2]. Just as the perirhinal cortex represents conjunctions that identify unique objects (see Chapter 7), the new prefrontal areas of anthropoids represent conjunctions that define unique behaviors—"what to do" in a particular circumstance, including novel and rare ones.

Relation to hippocampal function

The specializations we propose for the goal system share some properties with episodic memories. Both capture single events, but they differ in crucial ways. The goal system stores particular kinds of context–goal–action–outcome conjunctions, based on its direct connections with the posterior parietal, lateral temporal, premotor, and orbitofrontal cortex[2]. The hippocampus stores related, but different, conjunctions. Not only do the outcome representations in the hippocampus have a largely different source from those in the prefrontal cortex, but the hippocampus also lacks the direct interactions with premotor areas that the prefrontal cortex has.

An important idea about the hippocampus is that it acquires information more rapidly than the neocortex, which instead learns gradually and over many experiences[174]. The invocation of one-event learning in the goal system might seem to undermine this distinction, but instead we view it as a recent adaptation, one particular to the granular prefrontal cortex. Put another way, the neocortex evolved as a slow-learning mechanism that augmented the functions of the hippocampus (and other allocortical areas), but the granular prefrontal cortex (perhaps among other neocortical areas) later adapted to fast learning.

In Chapter 11 we propose that when these two fast-learning systems—the hippocampus and the granular prefrontal cortex—work together, they generate some powerful emergent properties. But they make different contributions. The granular prefrontal cortex learns about "what happens" in relation to behavioral goals, as if every event serves as a potential principle about "how the world is." In contrast, the hippocampus learns about "what happened" at a particular time and place. The "what happens"–"what happened" distinction resembles that between semantic and episodic memory in some ways. The former corresponds to facts about a world full of goals, but these particular fact memories are often implicit and so differ from the concept of semantic memory as usually construed, which refers to explicit knowledge. We return to these topics in Chapter 11.

In Chapters 7 and 8 we have emphasized the emergence of the feature and goal systems in anthropoids; in the next chapter we consider their subsequent development during hominin evolution.

References

1. Fulton, J.F. (1949) *Physiology of the Nervous System* (Oxford University Press, New York).
2. Passingham, R.E. and Wise, S.P. (2012) *The Neurobiology of the Prefrontal Cortex* (Oxford University Press, Oxford).
3. Duncan, J. (2010) *Trends Cogn. Sci.* **14**, 172–179.
4. Gaffan, D. (2002) *Phil. Trans. R. Soc. B: Biol. Sci.* **357**, 1111–1121.
5. Shallice, T. and Burgess, P.W. (1991) *Brain* **114**, 727–741.
6. Norman, D.A. and Shallice, T. (1986) In: *Consciousness and Self-Regulation: Advances in Research and Theory*, Vol. 4 (eds. Davidson, R.J., Schwartz, G.E. and Shapiro, D.), pp. 1–18 (Plenum, New York).
7. Moscovitch, M. (1992) *J. Cogn. Neurosci.* **4**, 257–267.
8. Miller, E.K. and Cohen, J.D. (2001) *Annu. Rev. Neurosci.* **24**, 167–202.
9. Wood, J.N. and Grafman, J. (2003) *Nat. Rev. Neurosci.* **4**, 139–147.
10. Tanji, J. and Hoshi, E. (2008) *Physiol. Rev.* **88**, 37–57.
11. Roberts, A.C. and Wallis, J.D. (2000) *Cereb. Cortex* **10**, 252–262.
12. Eagle, D.M., Bari, A., and Robbins, T.W. (2008) *Psychopharmacol.* **199**, 439–456.
13. Goldman-Rakic, P.S. (1995) *Ann. NY Acad. Sci.* **769**, 71–83.
14. Fuster, J.M. (2008) *The Prefrontal Cortex* (Academic Press, New York).
15. Oates, J.F. (1987) In: *Primate Societies* (eds. Smuts, B., Cheney, D.L., Seyfarth, R.M. *et al.*), pp. 197–209 (University of Chicago Press, Chicago, IL).
16. Webster, M.J., Bachevalier, J., and Ungerleider, L.G. (1994) *Cereb. Cortex* **4**, 470–483.
17. Petrides, M. and Pandya, D.N. (2002) *Eur. J. Neurosci.* **16**, 291–310.
18. Saleem, K.S., Kondo, H., and Price, J.L. (2008) *J. Comp. Neurol.* **506**, 659–693.
19. Petrides, M. and Pandya, D.N. (1984) *J. Comp. Neurol.* **228**, 105–116.
20. Jones, E.G. and Powell, T.P. (1970) *Brain* **93**, 793–820.
21. Wallis, J.D. and Miller, E.K. (2003) *Eur. J. Neurosci.* **18**, 2069–2081.
22. Carmichael, S.T. and Price, J.L. (1996) *J. Comp. Neurol.* **371**, 179–207.
23. Barbas, H. and Pandya, D.N. (1989) *J. Comp. Neurol.* **286**, 353–375.
24. Jbabdi, S., Lehman, J.F., Haber, S.N., and Behrens, T.E. (2013) *J. Neurosci.* **33**, 3190–3201.
25. Lehman, J.F., Greenberg, B.D., McIntyre, C.C., Rasmussen, S.A. et al. (2011) *J. Neurosci.* **31**, 10392–10402.
26. Saleem, K.S., Miller, B., and Price, J.L. (2014) *J. Comp. Neurol.* **522**, 1641–1690.
27. Takahara, D., Inoue, K., Hirata, Y., Miyachi, S. et al. (2012) *Eur. J. Neurosci.* **36**, 3365–3375.
28. Lu, M.-T., Preston, J.B., and Strick, P.L. (1994) *J. Comp. Neurol.* **341**, 375–392.
29. Wang, Y., Shima, K., Isoda, M., Sawamura, H. et al. (2002) *NeuroReport* **13**, 1341–1344.

30. Dum, R.P. and Strick, P.L. (1993) In: *Neurobiology of Cingulate Cortex and Limbic Thalamus: A Comprehensive Handbook* (eds. Vogt, B.A. and Gabriel, M.), pp. 415–441 (Birkhäuser, Boston).

31. Murray, E.A. and Coulter, J.D. (1981) *J. Comp. Neurol.* **195**, 339–365.

32. He, S.-Q., Dum, R.P., and Strick, P.L. (1993) *J. Neurosci.* **13**, 952–980.

33. Luppino, G., Matelli, M., Camarda, R., and Rizzolatti, G. (1993) *J. Comp. Neurol.* **338**, 114–140.

34. Luppino, G., Rozzi, S., Calzavara, R., and Matelli, M. (2003) *Eur. J. Neurosci.* **17**, 559–578.

35. Johnson, P.B., Ferraina, S., Bianchi, L., and Caminiti, R. (1996) *Cereb. Cortex* **6**, 102–119.

36. Middleton, F.A. and Strick, P.L. (2002) *Cereb. Cortex* **12**, 926–935.

37. Alexander, G.E., DeLong, M.R., and Strick, P.L. (1986) *Annu. Rev. Neurosci.* **9**, 357–381.

38. Haber, S.N. (2003) *J. Chem. Neuroanat.* **26**, 317–330.

39. Carmichael, S.T. and Price, J.L. (1995) *J. Comp. Neurol.* **363**, 615–641.

40. Rolls, E.T. and Baylis, L.L. (1994) *J. Neurosci.* **14**, 5437–5452.

41. Wilson, C.R., Gaffan, D., Browning, P.G., and Baxter, M.G. (2010) *Trends Neurosci.* **33**, 533–540.

42. Desimone, R. and Duncan, J. (1995) *Annu. Rev. Neurosci.* **18**, 193–222.

43. Pastor-Bernier, A. and Cisek, P. (2011) *J. Neurosci.* **31**, 7083–7088.

44. Cisek, P. (2005) *Neuron* **45**, 801–814.

45. Passingham, R.E. (1985) *Behav. Neurosci.* **99**, 3–21.

46. Collins, P., Roberts, A.C., Dias, R., Everitt, B.J. et al. (1998) *J. Cogn. Neurosci.* **10**, 332–354.

47. Butters, N. and Pandya, D. (1969) *Science* **165**, 1271–1273.

48. Butters, N., Pandya, D., Stein, D., and Rosen, J. (1972) *Acta Neurobiol. Exp. (Warsz.)* **32**, 305–329.

49. Goldman, P.S., Rosvold, H.E., Vest, B., and Galkin, T.W. (1971) *J. Comp. Physiol. Psychol.* **77**, 212–220.

50. Buckley, M.J., Mansouri, F.A., Hoda, H., Mahboubi, M. et al. (2009) *Science* **325**, 52–58.

51. Passingham, R.E. (1975) *Brain Res.* **92**, 89–102.

52. Gaffan, D. and Harrison, S. (1989) *Behav. Brain Res.* **31**, 207–220.

53. Mackey, W.E., Devinsky, O., Doyle, W.K., Meager, M.R. et al. (2016) *J. Neurosci.* **36**, 2847–2856.

54. Olton, D.S., Markowska, A.L., Pang, K., Golski, S. et al. (1992) *Behav. Pharmacol.* **3**, 307–318.

55. Pochon, J.B., Levy, R., Poline, J.B., Crozier, S. et al. (2001) *Cereb. Cortex* **11**, 260–266.

56. Volle, E., Pochon, J.B., Lehericy, S., Pillon, B. et al. (2005) *Cereb. Cortex* **15**, 1064–1074.

57. Genovesio, A., Brasted, P.J., and Wise, S.P. (2006) *J. Neurosci.* **26**, 7281–7292.

58. Rainer, G., Asaad, W.F., and Miller, E.K. (1998) *Proc. Natl. Acad. Sci. USA* **95**, 15008–15013.

59. Rainer, G., Rao, S.C., and Miller, E.K. (1999) *J. Neurosci.* **19**, 5493–5505.

60. Shima, K., Isoda, M., Mushiake, H., and Tanji, J. (2007) *Nature* **445**, 315–318.

61. Averbeck, B.B., Chafee, M.V., Crowe, D.A., and Georgopoulos, A.P. (2002) *Proc. Natl. Acad. Sci. USA* **99**, 13172–13177.

62. Hoshi, E. and Tanji, J. (2004) *J. Neurophysiol.* **91**, 2707–2722.

63. Ninokura, Y., Mushiake, H., and Tanji, J. (2003) *J. Neurophysiol.* **89**, 2868–2873.

64. Yumoto, N., Lu, X., Henry, T.R., Miyachi, S. et al. (2011) *PLoS One* **6**, e19168.

65. Sakurai, Y., Takahashi, S., and Inoue, M. (2004) *Eur. J. Neurosci.* **20**, 1069–1080.

66. Berdyyeva, T.K. and Olson, C.R. (2010) *J. Neurophysiol.* **104**, 141–159.

67. Schneider, B.A. and Ghose, G.M. (2012) *PLoS Biol.* **10**, e1001413.

68. Janssen, P. and Shadlen, M.N. (2005) *Nat. Neurosci.* **8**, 234–241.

69. Leon, M.I. and Shadlen, M.N. (2003) *Neuron* **38**, 317–327.

70. Nieder, A., Freedman, D.J., and Miller, E.K. (2002) *Science* **297**, 1708–1711.

71. Ninokura, Y., Mushiake, H., and Tanji, J. (2004) *J. Neurophysiol.* **91**, 555–560.

72. Warden, M.R. and Miller, E.K. (2007) *Cereb. Cortex* **17**(Suppl. 1), i41–i50.

73. Genovesio, A., Tsujimoto, S., and Wise, S.P. (2011) *J. Neurosci.* **31**, 3968–3980.

74. Genovesio, A., Tsujimoto, S., and Wise, S.P. (2009) *Neuron* **63**, 254–266.

75. Tsujimoto, S. and Sawaguchi, T. (2005) *J. Neurophysiol.* **93**, 3687–3692.

76. Tudusciuc, O. and Nieder, A. (2009) *J. Neurophysiol.* **101**, 2984–2994.

77. Merchant, H., Crowe, D.A., Robertson, M.S., Fortes, A.F. et al. (2011) *Front Syst. Neurosci.* **5**, 2011.00069.

78. Crowe, D.A., Goodwin, S.J., Blackman, R.K., Sakellaridi, S. et al. (2013) *Nat. Neurosci.* **16**, 1484–1491.

79. Barraclough, D.J., Conroy, M.L., and Lee, D. (2004) *Nat. Neurosci.* **7**, 404–410.

80. Seo, H., Barraclough, D.J., and Lee, D. (2007) *Cereb. Cortex* **17** (Suppl. 1), i110–i117.

81. Tsujimoto, S. and Sawaguchi, T. (2004) *Cereb. Cortex* **14**, 47–55.

82. Tsujimoto, S., Genovesio, A., and Wise, S.P. (2009) *J. Neurosci.* **29**, 2569–2574.

83. Asaad, W.F., Rainer, G., and Miller, E.K. (1998) *Neuron* **21**, 1399–1407.

84. Kim, J.N. and Shadlen, M.N. (1999) *Nat. Neurosci.* **2**, 176–185.

85. Wallis, J.D. and Miller, E.K. (2003) *J. Neurophysiol.* **90**, 1790–1806.

86. Roy, J.E., Riesenhuber, M., Poggio, T., and Miller, E.K. (2010) *J. Neurosci.* **30**, 8519–8528.

87. Genovesio, A., Brasted, P.J., Mitz, A.R., and Wise, S.P. (2005) *Neuron* **47**, 307–320.

88. Rao, S.C., Rainer, G., and Miller, E.K. (1997) *Science* **276**, 821–824.

89. Miller, E.K., Erickson, C.A., and Desimone, R. (1996) *J. Neurosci.* **16**, 5154–5167.

90. Lebedev, M.A., Messinger, A., Kralik, J.D., and Wise, S.P. (2004) *PLoS Biol.* **2**, 1919–1935.

91. Freedman, D.J., Riesenhuber, M., Poggio, T., and Miller, E.K. (2002) *J. Neurophysiol.* **88**, 929–941.

92. Cohen, Y.E., Hauser, M.D., and Russ, B.E. (2006) *Biol. Lett.* **2**, 261–265.

93. Lee, D. and Seo, H. (2007) *Ann. NY Acad. Sci.* **1104**, 108–122.

94. Kennerley, S.W., Dahmubed, A.F., Lara, A.H., and Wallis, J.D. (2009) *J. Cogn. Neurosci.* **21**, 1162–1178.

95. Hoshi, E., Shima, K., and Tanji, J. (2000) *J. Neurophysiol.* **83**, 2355–2373.

96. Eiselt, A.K. and Nieder, A. (2014) *J. Cogn. Neurosci.* **26**, 1000–1012.

97. Rigotti, M., Barak, O., Warden, M.R., Wang, X.J. et al. (2013) *Nature* **497**, 585–590.

98. Ungerleider, L.G. and Mishkin, M. (1982) In: *Analysis of Visual Behavior* (eds. Ingle, J., Goodale, M.A. and Mansfield, R.J.W.), pp. 549–586 (MIT Press, Cambridge, MA).

99. Shadmehr, R. and Wise, S.P. (2005) *The Computational Neurobiology of Reaching and Pointing* (MIT Press, Cambridge, MA).

100. Kaas, J.H., Gharbawie, O.A., and Stepniewska, I. (2011) *Front. Neuroanat.* **5**, 2011.00034.

101. Milner, A.D. and Goodale, M.A. (2007) *The Visual Brain in Action* (Oxford University Press, Oxford).

102. Chang, S.W. and Snyder, L.H. (2010) *Proc. Natl. Acad. Sci. USA* **107**, 7951–7956.

103. Chang, S.W., Papadimitriou, C., and Snyder, L.H. (2009) *Neuron* **64**, 744–755.

104. Eacott, M.J. and Gaffan, D. (1992) *Eur. J. Neurosci.* **4**, 1320–1332.

105. Gutnikov, S.A., Ma, Y.Y., and Gaffan, D. (1997) *Eur. J. Neurosci.* **9**, 1524–1529.

106. Gaffan, D. and Harrison, S. (1991) *Brain* **114**, 2133–2144.

107. Sakai, K. and Miyashita, Y. (1991) *Nature* **354**, 152–155.

108. Tomita, H., Ohbayashi, M., Nakahara, K., Hasegawa, I. et al. (1999) *Nature* **401**, 699–703.

109. Toni, I., Rushworth, M.F., and Passingham, R.E. (2001) *Exp. Brain Res.* **141**, 359–369.

110. Boettiger, C.A. (2005) *J. Neurosci.* **25**, 2723–2732.

111. Libby, L., Inhoff, M.C., Love, B.C., and **Ranganath, C.** (2014) Program no. 551.14. *2014 Neuroscience Meeting Planner* (Society for Neuroscience, Washington, DC). Online.

112. Cromer, J.A., Machon, M., and **Miller, E.K.** (2011) *J. Cogn. Neurosci.* **23**, 1823–1828.

113. Rushworth, M.F., Nixon, P.D., Eacott, M.J., and **Passingham, R.E.** (1997) *J. Neurosci.* **17**, 4829–4838.

114. Kowalska, D.M., Bachevalier, J., and **Mishkin, M.** (1991) *Neuropsychologia* **29**, 583–600.

115. Rama, P. and **Courtney, S.M.** (2005) *NeuroImage* **24**, 224–234.

116. Schon, K., Tinaz, S., Somers, D.C., and **Stern, C.E.** (2008) *NeuroImage* **39**, 857–872.

117. Degutis, J. and **D'Esposito, M.** (2009) *Front. Hum. Neurosci.* **3**, 44.

118. Degutis, J. and **D'Esposito, M.** (2007) *Cogn. Affect. Behav. Neurosci.* **7**, 251–259.

119. Meyers, E.M., Freedman, D.J., Kreiman, G., **Miller, E.K.** et al. (2008) *J. Neurophysiol.* **100**, 1407–1419.

120. Minamimoto, T., Saunders, R.C., and **Richmond, B.J.** (2010) *Neuron* **66**, 501–507.

121. Buckley, M.J. and **Sigala, N.** (2010) *Neuron* **66**, 471–473.

122. White, I.M. and **Wise, S.P.** (1999) *Exp. Brain Res.* **126**, 315–335.

123. Hoshi, E., Shima, K., and **Tanji, J.** (1998) *J. Neurophysiol.* **80**, 3392–3397.

124. Wallis, J.D., Anderson, K.C., and **Miller, E.K.** (2001) *Nature* **411**, 953–956.

125. **Milner, B.** (1963) *Arch. Neurol.* **9**, 90–100.

126. Stuss, D.T., Levine, B., Alexander, M.P., **Hong, J.** et al. (2000) *Neuropsychologia* **38**, 388–402.

127. Stuss, D.T., Bisschop, S.M., Alexander, M.P., **Levine, B.** et al. (2001) *Psychol. Assess.* **13**, 230–239.

128. Barcelo, F. and **Knight, R.T.** (2002) *Neuropsychologia* **40**, 349–356.

129. Owen, A.M., Roberts, A.C., Hodges, J.R., **Summers, B.A.** et al. (1993) *Brain* **116**, 1159–1175.

130. O'Doherty, J., Critchley, H., Deichmann, R., and **Dolan, R.J.** (2003) *J. Neurosci.* **23**, 7931–7939.

131. O'Doherty, J., Kringelbach, M.L., Rolls, E.T., **Hornak, J.** et al. (2001) *Nat. Neurosci.* **4**, 95–102.

132. Cools, R., Clark, L., Owen, A.M., and **Robbins, T.W.** (2002) *J. Neurosci.* **22**, 4563–4567.

133. Nakahara, K., Hayashi, T., Konishi, S., and **Miyashita, Y.** (2002) *Science* **295**, 1532–1536.

134. Hampshire, A. and **Owen, A.M.** (2006) *Cereb. Cortex* **16**, 1679–1689.

135. Monchi, O., Petrides, M., Petre, V., **Worsley, K.** et al. (2001) *J. Neurosci.* **21**, 7733–7741.

136. Rowe, J., Hughes, L., Eckstein, D., and **Owen, A.M.** (2008) *Cereb. Cortex* **18**, 2275–2285.

137. Gaffan, D., Easton, A., and **Parker, A.** (2002) *J. Neurosci.* **22**, 7288–7296.

138. Baxter, M.G., Gaffan, D., Kyriazis, D.A., and **Mitchell, A.S.** (2008) *Eur. J. Neurosci.* **28**, 491–499.

139. Baxter, M.G., Gaffan, D., Kyriazis, D.A., and **Mitchell, A.S.** (2009) *Eur. J. Neurosci.* **29**, 2049–2059.

140. Rudebeck, P.H., Saunders, R.C., Lundgren, D., and **Murray, E.A.** (2015) Program no. 176.09. *2015 Neuroscience Meeting Planner* (Society for Neuroscience, Washington, DC). Online.

141. Walton, M.E., Behrens, T.E., Buckley, M.J., **Rudebeck, P.H.** et al. (2010) *Neuron* **65**, 927–939.

142. Rudebeck, P.H., Saunders, R.C., Prescott, A.T., **Chau, L.S.** et al. (2013) *Nat. Neurosci.* **16**, 1140–1145.

143. Rudebeck, P.H. and **Murray, E.A.** (2015) Program no. 206.10. *2015 Neuroscience Meeting Planner* (Society for Neuroscience, Washington, DC). Online.

144. Izquierdo, A., Suda, R.K., and **Murray, E.A.** (2004) *J. Neurosci.* **24**, 7540–7548.

145. **Gaffan, D.** (1992) *Eur. J. Neurosci.* **4**, 381–388.

146. **Gaffan, D.** (1994) *J. Cogn. Neurosci.* **6**, 305–320.

147. Browning, P.G., Easton, A., Buckley, M.J., and **Gaffan, D.** (2005) *Eur. J. Neurosci.* **22**, 3281–3291.

148. Boschin, E.A., Piekema, C., and **Buckley, M.J.** (2015) *Proc. Natl. Acad. Sci. USA* **112**, E1020–E1027.

149. Bussey, T.J., Wise, S.P., and Murray, E.A. (2001) *Behav. Neurosci.* **115**, 971–982.
150. Bussey, T.J., Muir, J.L., Everitt, B.J., and Robbins, T.W. (1996) *Behav. Brain Res.* **82**, 45–56.
151. Wang, M., Zhang, H., and Li, B.-M. (2000) *Eur. J. Neurosci.* **12**, 3787–3796.
152. Fuster, J.M. (2001) *Neuron* **30**, 319–333.
153. Browning, P.G. and Gaffan, D. (2008) *J. Neurosci.* **28**, 3934–3940.
154. Browning, P.G., Baxter, M.G., and Gaffan, D. (2013) *J. Neurosci.* **33**, 9667–9674.
155. Murray, E.A. and Gaffan, D. (2006) *J. Exp. Psychol. Anim. Behav. Process.* **32**, 87–90.
156. Browning, P.G., Easton, A., and Gaffan, D. (2007) *Cereb. Cortex* **17**, 859–864.
157. Wilson, C.R. and Gaffan, D. (2008) *J. Neurosci.* **28**, 5529–5538.
158. Mushiake, H., Saito, N., Sakamoto, K., Itoyama, Y. et al. (2006) *Neuron* **50**, 631–641.
159. Yamagata, T., Nakayama, Y., Tanji, J., and Hoshi, E. (2012) *J. Neurosci.* **32**, 12934–12949.
160. Bernacchia, A., Seo, H., Lee, D., and Wang, X.J. (2011) *Nat. Neurosci.* **14**, 366–372.
161. Murray, J.D., Bernacchia, A., Freedman, D.J., Romo, R. et al. (2014) *Nat. Neurosci.* **17**, 1661–1663.
162. Garcia, J., Lasiter, P.S., Bermudez-Rattoni, F., and Deems, D.A. (1985) *Ann. NY Acad. Sci.* **443**, 8–21.
163. Schwartz, M. and Teitelbaum, P. (1973) *J. Comp. Physiol. Psychol.* **87**, 384–398.
164. Rozin, P. and Kalat, J.W. (1971) *Psychol. Rev.* **78**, 459–486.
165. Horn, G. (1971) *Act. Nerv. Super. (Praha)* **13**, 119–130.
166. Horn, G., Rose, S.P., and Bateson, P.P. (1973) *Science* **181**, 506–514.
167. Eacott, M.J. and Easton, A. (2010) *Neuropsychologia* **48**, 2273–2280.
168. Stanovich, K.E. (2012) In: *The Oxford Handbook of Thinking and Reasoning* (eds. Holyoak, K.J. and Morrison, R.G.), pp. 433–455 (Oxford University Press, Oxford).
169. Rowe, J., Friston, K., Frackowiak, R., and Passingham, R.E. (2002) *NeuroImage* **17**, 988–998.
170. Lau, H.C., Rogers, R.D., Ramnani, N., and Passingham, R.E. (2004) *NeuroImage* **21**, 1407–1415.
171. Lau, H.C., Rogers, R.D., Haggard, P., and Passingham, R.E. (2004) *Science* **303**, 1208–1210.
172. Morishima, Y., Akaishi, R., Yamada, Y., Okuda, J. et al. (2009) *Nat. Neurosci.* **12**, 85–91.
173. Rossi, A.F., Pessoa, L., Desimone, R., and Ungerleider, L.G. (2009) *Exp. Brain Res.* **192**, 489–497.
174. McClelland, J.L., McNaughton, B., and O'Reilly, R. (1995) *Psychol. Rev.* **102**, 419–457.
175. Mishkin, M., Malamut, B., and Bachevalier, J. (1984) In: *Neurobiology of Learning and Memory* (eds. Lynch, G., McGaugh, J. and Weinberger, N.M.), pp. 65–77 (Guilford, New York).
176. Mishkin, M. and Petri, H. (1984) In: *Neuropsychology of Memory* (eds. Squire, L.R. and Butters, N.), pp. 287–296 (Guilford, New York).
177. Squire, L.R., Stark, C.E., and Clark, R.E. (2004) *Annu. Rev. Neurosci.* **27**, 279–306.
178. Balleine, B.W. and O'Doherty, J.P. (2010) *Neuropsychopharmacol.* **35**, 48–69.

Part IV

Hominin adaptations

In the next chapter, we begin our consideration of some evolutionary developments that occurred after the split between the ape–human lineage and other anthropoids, with an emphasis on hominin evolution. In Chapter 9 we propose that the feature and goal systems adapted to support relational reasoning and general problem solving, as well as the generalizations and categorizations of semantic memory. In Chapter 10 we discuss a new system for representing one's self and others. Then, in Chapter 11, we explore the origins of explicit memory.

Chapter 9

The goal and feature memory systems of hominins

Overview

In the lineages that produced modern apes and humans, the feature and goal memory systems adapted from a specialized role in reducing foraging errors to support broader cognitive functions. Parietal–prefrontal networks that originally represented relational metrics came to support generalized relational reasoning; temporal areas that originally represented the signs of resources came to support semantic generalizations. In addition, the prefrontal cortex adapted its top-down biasing function to memory retrieval, especially in demanding conditions. These adaptations provided advantages in meeting multiple cognitive demands.

Great moments in evolution

In a *Far Side*® cartoon by Gary Larson, "Great Moments in Evolution," three newly minted tetrapods prepare to "conquer the land," as the saying goes. The humor comes partly from the comical depiction of these creatures, but mostly from the baseball bat that one of them carries and the baseball that sits on land for them to hit (or, perhaps, swing and miss).

In addition to its humor, the cartoon makes a serious point: The adaptations of the first land vertebrates enabled the development of baseball—and football, too. It would be rank madness, of course, to claim that forelimbs evolved so that Babe Ruth could hit home runs or that hindlimbs developed to bend it like Beckham. The remedy for such fallacious teleology appeals to the concept of exaptation (see Chapter 1, "Evolution"). Tetrapod forelimbs did not evolve to support active flight, yet they developed into the engines of flight at least three times (see Box 1.1): in birds, pterosaurs, and bats (the kind that fly, not the kind that hit baseballs). In other words, forelimbs served as an exaptation for flight. The idea that a structure would emerge under one set of selective pressures and later perform others seems foreign when applied to memory and the brain, but it happens all the time in evolution.

In Chapters 7 and 8 we introduced the feature and goal memory systems of anthropoids as adaptations for reducing foraging errors; in this chapter we consider them as exaptations for multiple demand cognition and general problem solving[1], relational reasoning[2,3], and the generalized conceptual and categorical knowledge that characterizes semantic memory[4].

Evolution

As explained in Chapter 2 ("Hominins"), the ape–human lineage diverged from other catarrhines about 24–30 million years ago[5] and the last common ancestor of humans, chimpanzees, and bonobos lived somewhere around 6 million years ago. We return to the topic of human evolution, including cultural and social developments, in Chapter 11 ("Evolution"), but for the purposes of this chapter we focus on the expansion, in absolute terms, of the prefrontal, temporal, and posterior parietal cortex. Despite an aura of controversy, no one disputes the idea that these three regions of cortex expanded in absolute terms as the ape–human lineage diversified. We go into this topic in more detail in Chapter 10 ("Regional expansion"), but we preview its conclusions here because the expansion of these areas is important to the proposal in this chapter.

Experts in allometry sometimes seem to imply that because some measure of brain size falls on or near a regression line nothing really happened during evolution. Such analyses tend to downplay the importance of expansion in absolute terms, and they implicitly assume some sort of linear relationship between the amount of neural tissue and brain function. We know from computational models, however, that neural networks scale nonlinearly. Later we discuss connectionist models that learn semantic representations (see "Computational models")[6]. In general, models below a certain size failed to learn a full set of representations, and as they increased in size they reached threshold points at which generalizations emerged in addition to the representation of exemplars. In a model of writing-to-sound transformations for reading, for example, the model could not extract generalizations until it reached a certain size[7]. The proposal in this chapter suggests that something similar happened during hominin evolution.

In addition to expansion in absolute terms, the cortical areas subserving the feature and goal systems have also expanded relative to many other parts of the cortex. Not all experts agree with this conclusion, but one recent analysis showed that the prefrontal (see Fig. 2.14B, D), temporal (Fig. 9.1A), and parietal (Fig. 9.1B) cortex all expanded more

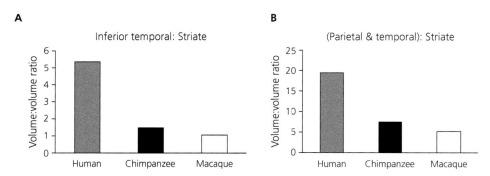

Fig. 9.1 Expansion of parietal and temporal cortex. (A) Inferior temporal cortex volume relative to the volume of primary visual (striate) cortex in three anthropoid species. (B) Temporal and parietal cortex volume, combined (as indicated by the parentheses), relative to striate cortex volume. Data from Passingham and Smaers[8].

during hominin evolution than did a reasonable reference area: the primary visual (striate) cortex[8]. Kaas[9] (p. 39), in examining this literature, also concluded that "parts of neocortex have greatly enlarged relative to the rest of neocortex, most notably prefrontal, insular, posterior parietal, and temporal cortex." Rilling and Seligman[10] (p. 527), who focused on the temporal cortex, decided that the "human temporal lobe is larger in terms of overall volume, surface area, and white matter volume than predicted for an ape with a human-sized brain."

Two studies of regional expansion are particularly important to the proposal in this chapter:

- A structural brain imaging study by Glasser et al.[11] assessed the extent of myelin-poor cortex in macaques, chimpanzees, and humans (see Plate 2C). The myelin-poor prefrontal, inferior posterior parietal, and anterior temporal regions showed dramatic expansion in the human brain, relative to these other primates. Some of the expanded areas are thought to contribute to multiple demand cognition[1] and relational reasoning[2,3] (see "Parietal–prefrontal networks").

- An analysis by Van Essen and Dierker[12] examined the differential expansion of cortical regions by using a morphing algorithm anchored to homologues in macaque and human brains (see Plate 3C). This approach revealed that the prefrontal, posterior parietal, and anterior temporal cortex expanded in human brains relative to the cortex as a whole. Of particular importance to this chapter, a comparison of Plate 3(B) and (C) demonstrates a close correspondence between some of the expanded areas and those underlying semantic memory (see "Temporal–prefrontal networks").

Proposal

Sometime after the ape–human lineage diverged from other anthropoids, parietal–prefrontal networks adapted their specialization for representing relational metrics to a more general cognitive function: relational reasoning. Likewise, parts of the temporal cortex adapted a specialization for representing the signs of resources to generalized semantic concepts and categories—at a new, hierarchically higher level. The prefrontal cortex adapted its function in top-down attentional control to the retrieval of relational and semantic memories, especially in cognitively demanding conditions, for problems that require integration over sensory modalities and cognitive domains, and when semantic memories compete within and across categories, at various levels of hierarchy.

The terms modality and domain, as used in this proposal, require some explanation because experts use them in many different ways. In this book, we use the word modality for sensory inputs such as vision and audition. In contrast, a cognitive domain corresponds to a type of knowledge, such as social or technological knowledge. The term domain can also refer to broader classes of knowledge, such as the semantic domain, as opposed to an implicit or procedural domain.

In addition to its other facets, our proposal explains the prominence of "association" cortex (Box 9.1) and helps reconcile evolutionary and traditional psychology, especially in their ongoing battle over the concept of general intelligence (Box 9.2). On the first point, the concept of "association" cortex developed because of the size and importance of the feature and goal systems in anthropoids and the expansion of the areas underlying these

> ## Box 9.1 Association cortex
>
> Taken together, the areas underlying the goal and feature memory systems make up most of the cortical territory commonly called "association cortex." Not so long ago, Eccles[141] recited the then-prevailing view that 95% of the human cerebral cortex consists of association cortex, with only a small amount devoted to sensory perception or motor control. Even at the time, neuroanatomists and neurophysiologists knew that the visual and auditory systems encompassed many of the so-called association areas. Nevertheless, the concept of "association cortex" remains influential, despite the fact that almost all neocortical areas composing the parietal, temporal, and occipital lobes can be classified as somatosensory, visual, auditory, or some combination of these sensory modalities.

system in hominins (see Plates 2C and 3C). On the second, general intelligence arose when specialized representational systems adapted to general problem solving[2]. Evolutionary and traditional psychology often seem at loggerheads, in part because they emphasize the specialized and general functions, respectively. In the next section we discuss the contribution of parietal–prefrontal networks to some of these general cognitive functions.

Parietal–prefrontal networks

In Chapter 7 ("Metrics") we proposed that the posterior parietal cortex, as part of the feature memory system, processes and stores specialized representations of relational metrics, and in Chapter 8 ("Metric features") we said that it provides this information to the prefrontal cortex for goal generation.

We also explained in Chapter 8 that the parietal–frontal networks of ancestral anthropoids built on those of early primates. The large home ranges of anthropoids led to choices among distant foraging goals and long-range paths. Many mammalian lineages faced this problem, of course, but anthropoids had to "reinvent" solutions because they descended from ancestors that foraged locally, living a life confined to the fine branches of trees (see Chapter 2, "Early primates" and Chapter 6, "Evolution"). Some of these anthropoid "reinventions" extended metric functions from their original role in planning and guiding movements (see Chapter 6, "Parietal–premotor networks") to a role in representing metric contexts more generally (see Fig. 8.2), especially for relative metrics. Examples include: the relative number of items in a patch of resources; relative distances, which correlate with estimated time and effort costs; and order information related to efficient foraging routes.

Ecology and foraging goals

Relational metrics play a central role in the foraging choices of anthropoids. One study of chimpanzees, for example, showed that they made extensive use of relative distance, number, and order[13]. They also used qualitative features, of course, but the

Box 9.2 Evolutionary psychology versus general intelligence

Psychologists have waged an ongoing battle over whether there is such a "thing" as general intelligence (*g*). Related concepts go by several names, including general problem solving, multiple demand cognition[1], the global workspace[142], domain generality[143], fluid intelligence[144], and reasoning[145]. The heritability of *g* often figures prominently in these debates. Plomin and Spinath[146], for example, conclude that *g* accounts for most of the heritable variance on intelligence tests.

An alternative view treats general problem solving as the combined influence of several traits. One recent version stressed reasoning, verbal ability, and a combination of working memory and attention[50]. Many experts who reject the concept of general intelligence emphasize that the tests used to measure *g* require not only sustained attention on a task[147], but also the motivation to perform well. (Assuming that intelligence is divided into different elements, the tasks used to measure each of them will still share some non-*g* elements, such as attention to a task. These elements could account for at least part of the correlation across diverse tasks, otherwise known as *g*, as well as its heritability.)

The concept of general intelligence has contributed to an impasse between evolutionary psychology and traditional cognitive psychology. Evolutionary psychology emphasizes specialized cognitive capacities, sometimes called modules, which arose at specific times and places as adaptations to the problems faced by particular ancestors. Many evolutionary psychologists, though not all, reject the idea that humans have a general problem-solving capacity beyond the low-level conditioning mechanisms described in Chapter 3. Traditional cognitive psychologists, on the other hand, often balk at the idea of special-purpose cognitive modules and rarely adopt an evolutionary perspective.

Our proposals reconcile these two schools of psychology in a simple way, albeit one that will probably be unsatisfying to either camp. We accept the concept from evolutionary psychology of cognitive modules as adaptations that augment ancestral capacities. During evolution, according to the principal thesis of this book, such augmentations produce the specialized representational capacities that we call memory systems. We also accept the idea that sometime after the split between the ape–human lineage and other anthropoids, some of these specialized representations adapted to broader, more general cognitive demands and thereby underlie a capacity that corresponds to general intelligence.

chimpanzees relied in large part on resource quantity, distance, and the time it took to acquire resources. They chose foraging goals according to the number of food items in a location, as well as their distance and the time it took to reach them, the time it took to manipulate the foods in order to make them consumable, and the time it took to consume a resource[13].

Chimpanzees have such impressive metric abilities that they have on occasion fooled researchers trying to study their foraging habits. One group of investigators concluded that chimpanzees "only assign value to the preferred food in a two-food mixture" (Silberberg et al.[14], p. 228)—the so-called "selective-value effect." Unfortunately, the preferred food item had a slight, uncontrolled variation in size, and their subjects simply chose the larger item[15], which illustrates the keen metric perception that anthropoids bring to the table.

Relational metric coding

Brain imaging studies in humans have implicated both the feature and goal memory systems in metric processing. Both the posterior parietal cortex (of the feature system) and the granular prefrontal cortex (of the goal system) were activated during perceptual tasks involving the number of items in a stimulus array, the proportions of lines, the size and brightness of visual stimuli, and the density of dots in a particular part of visual space[16–23]. The interaction of metrics and timing predicts collisions, for example, and so the viewing of potential collisions led to activations in parietal–prefrontal networks[24].

Lesion and stimulation studies point to the same conclusion. For example, patients with lesions of the right prefrontal cortex showed impaired processing of time intervals[25–27], and repetitive transcranial magnetic stimulation (rTMS) of the prefrontal cortex caused impairments in the perception of time intervals[28,29].

One especially important relative metric, order, applies to sequences. Parietal–prefrontal networks became activated during a transitive inference task, which depended on memories of an ordered sequence of items[30–32]. Likewise, the posterior parietal cortex showed activation when subjects maintained the order of items in working memory, and the prefrontal cortex did so when people manipulated that order mentally[33,34]. Disruptive stimulation of the posterior parietal and prefrontal cortex, by rTMS, impaired the manipulation and maintenance of order information[35,36]. In addition, lesions of the prefrontal cortex in monkeys impaired memory for the order of object choices and sequences[37]. Similar lesions also impaired the ability of humans to complete a complex sequence of assignments, such as acquiring ingredients or components in order to achieve a long-term goal[38,39]. As explained in Chapters 7 ("Metrics") and 8 ("Neurophysiology"), all of these findings have counterparts in the single-neuron activity of monkeys[40].

According to our proposal, these properties reflect the ancestral functions of anthropoid parietal–prefrontal networks. Figure 8.2(B) illustrates the idea that parietal–prefrontal developments in anthropoids augmented the visuomotor and visual search mechanisms that they inherited from early primates. Here we suggest an additional adaptation in the ape–human lineage, namely relational reasoning from relational metrics.

General problem solving

In humans, parietal–prefrontal networks appear to play a role in problem solving across a wide variety of cognitive domains. As discussed in Box 9.2, the concept of general intelligence remains controversial. Nevertheless, the tests used to assess general problem solving have had a long history. Most nonverbal varieties of such tests have required subjects to solve various puzzles, such as Raven's matrices. Figure 9.2(A) shows a typical example. To solve these problems, the subjects needed to recognize the relations among items in the columns and rows and then choose the missing piece of the puzzle. As illustrated in Fig. 9.2(A), relationships could range from simple matching to complex hierarchical relations. These puzzles test analogical reasoning and the ability to manipulate information in short-term memory[41–45].

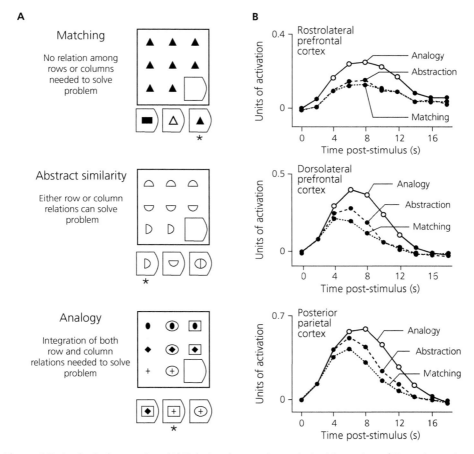

Figure 9.2 Analogical reasoning. (A) Relational reasoning task. In this version of Raven's matrix task, subjects chose from items in a menu of options, displayed below the square. The items inside the square represent stimuli that the subjects saw. For analogies (bottom), the subjects had to take into account the relationship among both rows and columns of the visual display. Asterisks mark the correct choices. (B) The time course of activations in selected parts of the posterior parietal and prefrontal cortex. Unfilled circles show significantly greater activation. Modified from Crone EA, Wendelken C, van Leijenhorst L, Honomichl RD, Christoff K, Bunge SA. Neurocognitive development of relational reasoning. *Developmental Science* 12:55–66, © 2009, Wiley-Blackwell, with permission.

Figure 9.2(B) illustrates the time course of activation in two parts of the dorsolateral prefrontal cortex: an anterior part sometimes called the rostrolateral prefrontal cortex and a more centrally located part. Along with the inferior posterior parietal cortex, both parts of the dorsolateral prefrontal cortex showed more activation for relational reasoning than for simple matching[46].

Another study involved a particularly motivated group of subjects, prospective law students, who prepared intensively for a standardized test that made extensive demands on relational reasoning, often in terms of analogical problems[47]. As Fig. 9.3(A, B) illustrates, resting state correlations among activated areas in these individuals increased selectively in a parietal–prefrontal network.

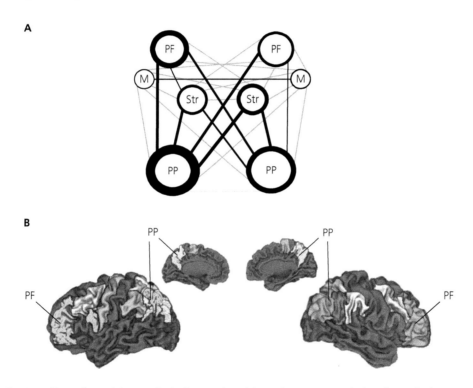

Fig. 9.3 Effect of practicing analogical reasoning. (A) Resting state correlations in cortical activations that changed after subjects studied intensively (and with a ferocious level of motivation) for the Law School Admissions Test. The diameter of each circle indicates the number of measured areas that each group included; the thickness of the lines around each circle indicates the number of changed activation correlations within a region; the thickness of the lines connecting circles corresponds to the number of connections that changed coupling between regions included in each group. (B) Brain areas that showed the changed correlations are depicted in lighter gray. Abbreviations: M, motor cortex; PF, prefrontal cortex; PP, posterior parietal cortex; Str, striatum. Reproduced from Mackey AP, Miller Singley AT, Bunge SA. Intensive reasoning training alters patterns of brain connectivity at rest. *Journal of Neuroscience* 33:4796–803, © 2013, Society for Neuroscience, with permission.

In the form of matrices and puzzles, analogical reasoning problems might seem somewhat arcane. As we explain in Chapter 11 ("Premises"), however, analogies provide much of the innovative power of human cognition. One classic example, from Thomas Henry Huxley[48], relates intellectual progress to landfill, an unlikely juxtaposition of concepts:

> … we stand on an islet in the midst of an illimitable ocean of inexplicability. Our business in every generation is to reclaim a little more land, to add something to the extent and the solidity of our possessions.

Another famous analogy comes from the history of chemistry. As the story goes, the nineteenth-century chemist Kekulé contemplated the image of a snake ingesting its own tail. According to legend, this vision inspired him to imagine how a chain of covalently linked carbon atoms could adopt a continuously linked, circular arrangement with no free ends and alternating single and double bonds: the structure of benzene. Note that a self-gnawing snake, a geometric circle, and the benzene molecule have virtually nothing in common—as sensory stimuli—except at a highly abstract relational level.

Duncan[1] synthesizes these concepts under the banner of multiple demand cognition. He suggests that parietal–prefrontal networks can integrate information from other parts of the cortex when a problem exceeds their specialized capacities. According to his idea, this network provides a cross-domain platform for generating goals under highly demanding conditions.

Because these areas have shown activation for a broad array of cognitive problems, Duncan interprets their function in terms of general intelligence[1]. Figure 9.4(A) illustrates the areas with significant activation as people performed several disparate, but demanding, tasks[1,49-51]. In support of the brain imaging results, lesions of the granular prefrontal cortex (Fig. 9.4B, left) and the posterior parietal cortex (Fig. 9.4B, right) impaired the performance of such tasks[52].

Homologues and pathways

The parietal and prefrontal components of Duncan's multiple demand system have straightforward homologues in monkeys. In Chapter 2 ("Possible new areas") we discussed activation coupling between the dorsolateral prefrontal cortex and the inferior posterior parietal cortex, which parallels cortical connections in monkeys[53,54]. These pathways appear to have changed during ape and human evolution. For example, Cloutman et al.[55], using diffusion tractography, described parietal–prefrontal pathways involving the supramarginal gyrus of the human brain, a region near the parietal–temporal junction (see Fig. 1.5). The inferior part of the supramarginal gyrus probably links auditory signals with speech production, at least in the left hemisphere, while its posterior and superior parts likely contribute to manipulating and using objects. The findings of Cloutman et al. established that the inferior supramarginal gyrus connects with the frontal cortex through an inner fascicle of fibers, whereas the superior and posterior parts connect through an outer bundle. The inner, speech-related pathway might have evolved as an elaboration of

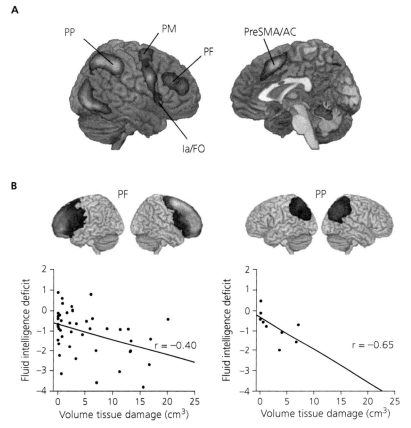

Fig. 9.4 Multiple demand cognition. (A) Activation during several problem-solving tasks that tax multiple cognitive demands. (B) Effects of brain lesions (top) on an intelligence test (bottom). Larger lesions of either the granular prefrontal cortex (left) or the posterior parietal cortex (right) led to greater impairments (more negative scores) than did smaller lesions. Abbreviations: Ia/FO, agranular insular and frontal opercular cortex; PF, dorsolateral prefrontal cortex; PM, premotor cortex; PP, posterior parietal cortex; PreSMA/AC, presupplementary motor and anterior cingulate cortex. (A) Reproduced from Fedorenko E, Duncan J, Kanwisher N. Broad domain generality in focal regions of frontal and parietal cortex. *Proceedings of the National Academy of Sciences U.S.A.* 110:16616–21, © 2013, National Academy of Sciences U.S.A., with permission. (B) From Woolgar A, Parr A, Cusack R, Thompson R, Nimmo-Smith I, Torralva T, Roca M, Antoun N, Manes F, Duncan J. Fluid intelligence loss linked to restricted regions of damage within frontal and parietal cortex. *Proceedings of the National Academy of Sciences U.S.A.* 107:14899–902, © 2010, as reproduced in Genovesio A, Wise SP, Passingham RE. Prefrontal-parietal function: from foraging to foresight. *Trends in Cognitive Sciences* 18:72–81, © 2014, Elsevier.

the visuomotor pathways inherited from the last common ancestor of humans and modern monkeys. In Chapter 2 ("Possible new areas") we mentioned an additional aspect of such remodeling and repurposing; connections between the inferior parietal and prefrontal cortex extend further anterior in humans, compared with both chimpanzees and monkeys[56]. Like the speech-related pathway described by Cloutman et al.[55], this development might also reflect an elaboration of visuomotor pathways, in this case pathways related to the manufacture and manipulation of tools[56].

The diffusion tractography studies dealt with parietal areas apart from those in Duncan's multiple demand network[1], but our proposal suggests that parietal–prefrontal relations in both cases have derived from an ancestral role involving visuomotor metrics and metric contexts.

Summary

Some time after the ape–human lineage split from other anthropoids, parietal–prefrontal networks adapted from being a specialized system for generating foraging goals based on relational metrics to a system for general relational reasoning. In modern humans, this representational system underlies analogies, metaphors, and solutions to multiple cognitive demands[1]. Parallel developments occurred in temporal–prefrontal networks, as we discuss in the next section.

Temporal–prefrontal networks

In Chapter 6 ("Temporal–orbitofrontal networks" and "Caudal prefrontal networks") we proposed that new temporal areas emerged in early primates and that they provided new prefrontal areas with information that supported search, attention, and outcome-valuation functions (see Fig. 8.2A). In Chapters 7 and 8 we proposed that, later, in anthropoids, these temporal areas: (1) elaborated into part of the feature system; (2) provided yet newer parts of the prefrontal cortex with contexts for generating goals (see Fig. 8.2B); and (3) represented the visual and acoustic signs of resources, often at a distance. According to the proposal in this chapter, after the ape–human lineage diverged from other anthropoids, these temporal areas adapted to a higher-order and more general function, namely the representation of semantic generalizations. To put it another way: Semantic memory emerged in hominins as an adaptation of anthropoid mechanisms for making foraging choices based on the signs of distant resources.

Semantic memory

The term semantic memory refers to cultural knowledge that people have about the world: the repository of facts, concepts, and categories encountered over a lifetime, including knowledge about people, places, objects, and language. Unlike episodic memories, semantic memories show context independence in that they do not include the times, sources, or circumstances of their acquisition. Some experts stretch the concept of semantic memory to cover object recognition in monkeys[57], but in this book we restrict this term to explicit semantic memories in humans. In Chapter 11 we explain why we limit the concept of semantic memory in this way.

To understand what we mean by cultural knowledge, consider the following lyric, which has perplexed generations of English-speaking people:

> Once a jolly swagman camped by a billabong,
> Under the shade of a coolibah tree,
> And he sang as he watched and waited till his billy boiled:
> "Who'll come a-waltzing Matilda, with me?"

Cultural knowledge has the ability to construct a modern intellect but can just as assuredly confound it. Later, we mention the pyramids and palm trees test of semantic memory. It is culture alone that leads researchers to choose "the pyramids and palm trees test" over "the billabongs and coolibah trees test."

Semantic memories, however, comprise more than culturally specific facts. They empower the use of cultural knowledge to make predictive inferences and draw abstract generalizations. By using their semantic memories, people can surmount the limitations of specific cognitive domains and sensory modalities to create integrative, abstract, cross-domain, and cross-modality knowledge.

Take, for example, the category "pig." Features of "pig" include a curly tail, flat snout, hooves, and four legs (except in *Animal Farm* in which pigs adopt a bipedal habit). The concept "pig" also includes the knowledge that many of them have voracious appetites, live on farms, are eaten by some people (but, for religious reasons, not by others), look upon people as their equals (according to Winston Churchill), grunt, squeal, root up the earth, and give birth to large litters of piglets. This capacious concept can also incorporate knowledge from the social domain, such as the slanderous suggestion that "pigs" take more than their fair share of something valuable.

Semantic dementia

Much of our knowledge about the neural basis of semantic memory comes from studying its breakdown in patients with a degenerative brain disease called semantic dementia: part of a spectrum of disorders known as frontotemporal dementia. The earliest reports of this disorder date from the 1890s, but recent research has raised awareness of the insights it provides for understanding semantic memory. The key observations involve the selectivity that patients exhibit in their loss of conceptual knowledge[58–60]. Furthermore, brain imaging offers the opportunity to relate the time course of semantic breakdown to the progressive anatomical deterioration that underlies the disorder[61].

Anatomy of semantic dementia

Semantic dementia results from neural degeneration, typically caused by an abnormal form of a brain protein called TDP-43. The disease results in progressive atrophy of anterior, ventral, and ventrolateral parts of the temporal lobe, including the temporal pole and the anterior fusiform gyrus, with a 50–80% loss of gray matter even at moderate stages[62]. The pathology always involves both hemispheres, but typically asymmetrically, at least early in the disease. In addition to the lateral temporal lobe, semantic dementia also affects more medial areas, including the perirhinal cortex and the amygdaloid (anterior) hippocampus[63]. First, we take up the involvement of the hippocampus, then turn to the affected neocortical areas.

Hippocampal complex

The involvement of the hippocampus in semantic dementia remains controversial, in part because the prevailing view of memory systems holds that the hippocampus subserves episodic but not semantic memory[64]. Atrophy of the hippocampus that leads to an impairment of semantic but not episodic memory seems incongruous to some experts. Nevertheless, patients in the early stages of semantic dementia show impairments of semantic memory with relatively preserved episodic memory, and they can have an overall degree of hippocampus damage similar to Alzheimer's patients, who have severe impairments of episodic memory[65].

Although patients with semantic dementia and Alzheimer's disease can have equivalent hypometabolism in and atrophy of the amygdaloid (anterior) hippocampus, Alzheimer's patients also have prominent dysfunction of the septal (posterior) hippocampus, posterior cingulate cortex, mediodorsal nucleus of the thalamus, and mammillary bodies of the hypothalamus[65], which remain largely intact in semantic dementia[66]. So the preserved episodic memory in semantic dementia might reflect the functions of these spared areas (see Chapter 10, "Medial network"). Later we propose that episodic memory arises as an emergent property from interconnected brain regions (see Chapter 11, "Modern traits"): the hippocampus and other parts of a large-scale medial network of cortical areas, including the posterior cingulate cortex. Alzheimer's disease disrupts connectivity in this network, in part because the posterior cingulate cortex degenerates along with its projections to and from the hippocampus. This degeneration might therefore underpin the earliest cognitive impairments in Alzheimer's disease, including those in episodic memory[67].

Taken together, these findings suggest that the contribution of the hippocampus to semantic memory arises from its amygdaloid (anterior) parts, a topic we return to later (see Chapter 10, "Septal versus amygdaloid hippocampus"). This idea contradicts the prevailing view of memory systems, of course, which ascribes episodic memory to the hippocampus as a whole, and assigns semantic memory to other parts of the so-called "medial temporal lobe"[64]. Instead, the hippocampus seems to contribute to both episodic and semantic memory, with specializations along its septal–amygdaloid (posterior–anterior) axis. We return to this topic in Chapter 12 ("The summation principle").

Perirhinal cortex

The perirhinal cortex is affected relatively early in semantic dementia, at least compared with the hippocampus[63,68]. Although much of the neuropathology in semantic dementia occurs in the anterior and ventrolateral parts of the temporal cortex, the early involvement of the perirhinal cortex points to some contribution of this area to semantic memory.

Lateral temporal cortex

The major focus of damage in semantic dementia occurs in the anterior, ventral, and ventrolateral temporal cortex, including the temporal pole and rostral parts of the fusiform gyrus[65,69]. According to three brain imaging methods—volume estimates, local metabolic rates, and diffusion tractography—patients with semantic dementia have significant atrophy, hypometabolism, and loss of connections in the anterior and ventral temporal lobes, with greater involvement of the left hemisphere[61].

Diffusion tractography has provided additional information about how damage to the white matter affects the broader connectivity of the anterior temporal cortex with more posterior areas, such as those for audition, language, and vision. For instance, the degeneration that occurs in the white matter seems to spare the posterior part of the inferior longitudinal fascicle, which transmits visual information between the occipital and temporal lobes. In contrast, the arcuate and uncinate fascicles, which connect temporal areas with the frontal lobe, suffer severe damage. Thus semantic dementia seems to compromise pathways between the degenerating temporal lobe and the frontal cortex, but preserves white-matter connections from the occipital cortex to the anterior temporal lobe[61]. According to one recent imaging study[70], focal atrophy in semantic dementia is confined to the anterior temporal lobe and, via fiber tracts originating there, this focal damage reduces the functionality of other cortical areas.

Summary

Patients with semantic dementia have a consistent pattern of neural damage, which selectively involves anterior and ventral parts of the temporal lobe and spares more posterior parts. Ventral and ventrolateral parts of the anterior temporal lobe suffer the most, including the temporal-pole cortex, but the damage extends medially to include the perirhinal cortex and amygdaloid (anterior) hippocampus. The degeneration affects some, but not all, of the white-matter tracts connected to these areas, with frontal–temporal interactions particularly affected.

A selective impairment

The neural degeneration in semantic dementia causes a progressive loss of conceptual and categorical knowledge, which affects all cognitive domains and sensory modalities. For example, patients cannot match the sound of an elephant to a picture of one or to the word "elephant." They also fail to associate a picture of a "masher" with a potato[71]. When these patients see two pictures of a carrot, one orange and the other green, and are asked to say which is the real one, they typically select the green carrot, increasingly so as the disease progresses[72]. Similarly, when they see two line drawings of an elephant, one with appropriately large floppy ears and one with the small ears typical of mammals, patients with semantic dementia tend to prefer the incorrect, small-eared elephant[73]. Since these patients have never seen green carrots or small-eared elephants, something other than their experience must explain their choices. The reason seems to be that as specific knowledge deteriorates, patients no longer know what carrots and elephants look like and can only recognize them as exemplars of a more general category. In these examples, a green carrot is more typical of plants and a small-eared elephant is more typical of mammals.

Memory impairments do not wax and wane in semantic dementia; once lost, patients rarely, if ever, remember the lost facts or concepts again. Consistent with this monotonic deterioration, their vocabulary narrows dramatically as the loss of conceptual knowledge progresses, which leads patients to become overly reliant upon highly familiar or super-ordinate concepts. For example, they will use the word "animal" to refer to a picture of a goat, not because they cannot retrieve the word "goat" from memory, but because their impoverished representation of goats no longer maps onto that verbal label. Instead, these patients rely on whatever general semantic knowledge remains reasonably intact and therefore usually produce a more general semantic label—in this example, "animal." The deterioration of their semantic knowledge dramatically affects the ability of patients to interpret what happens in the world. They can, for example, become frightened by a snail or confused by the daily growth of facial hair. These aberrations occur when patients lose their knowledge about snails, facial hair, and other facts about the world.

Although patients with semantic dementia have a severe impairment of semantic memory, they do not have "amnesia" in the same sense as patients like H.M. or those with some early forms of Alzheimer's disease[74]. Patients with semantic dementia can still remember their past, albeit in an impoverished fashion, and they show reasonable prospective memory[75]. Especially early in the disease, these patients often perform well on recognition memory tasks, in which they indicate whether they have previously seen particular words, scenes, or pictures. Notably, however, when items change in some way after patients first see them during a study period—a different exemplar of an item or viewing angle, for example—performance often deteriorates because they lack conceptual knowledge about the item and cannot use this knowledge to support performance on the task[76–78].

These patients also have preserved performance on tests of topographical memory, which require subjects to orient themselves in space[79], and they retain some ability to recall items from memory, as measured by reproduction of complex visual figures[80] or by the recollection of the context in which an item has occurred (source memory)[74,81,82]. These capacities probably depend on some combination of the septal hippocampal, posterior cingulate, and posterior parietal cortex. According to three lines of evidence, temporal source memory seems to be mediated by the prefrontal cortex. First, the preserved source memory in semantic dementia correlated with a composite score on tasks impaired by damage to the frontal cortex, such as the Wisconsin card sorting task and various planning tasks[74]. Second, either degenerative or focal damage to the ventromedial or orbitofrontal cortex impaired temporal source memories[83]. Third, activation occurred in the orbitofrontal cortex for semantic memory tasks involving associations of temporal (but not spatial) contexts with objects[83,84].

Patients with semantic dementia generally show good numeracy skills, such as understanding number quantity[85,86], probably due to their intact posterior parietal cortex. Likewise, these patients have fairly good skills for grasping and manipulating objects[87–89]. Even as conceptual knowledge declines, the patients remain able to play musical instruments and participate in sports such as golf and tennis, although they often lose their knowledge about the scoring systems of these games. They can apply skills to novel situations, for example by learning to retrieve objects from cylinders[90], and they can also perform well on visual problem-solving tasks, such assembling pieces of a complex jigsaw puzzle[91]. Their intact posterior parietal and premotor areas probably account for these preserved capabilities. When conceptual knowledge plays a key role in actions and object use, such as generating novel gestures and learning to use novel objects, the disabilities of these patients tend to correlate with the degree of their semantic impairment. Instead of using conceptual knowledge to guide their actions, they rely almost entirely on object affordances (see Chapter 6, "Affordances")[88].

The impressive selectivity of impairments in semantic memory relates to our proposal about episodic memory, which we advance in Chapter 11. We defer a discussion of episodic memory to that chapter, and only reiterate here what we said earlier (see "Hippocampal complex"): Explicit episodic memories depend on a large-scale network of areas that includes the hippocampus, the posterior cingulate cortex, and other medially situated areas.

Typicality and frequency

As noted earlier, semantic dementia impairs conceptual knowledge across sensory modalities and cognitive domains, and the degree of impairment correlates strongly across conceptual tasks. As the disease progresses, semantic knowledge about infrequently encountered and atypical items deteriorates first.

One example of this principle comes from a study that involved six visual and verbal tasks: delayed copy drawing, object decision, reading, spelling, lexical decision, and past-tense verb production[92]. The patients varied from mildly to severely affected; and the test items varied according to both their frequency and typicality. Four examples elucidate the concept of typicality and its various forms:

- The word "pint" has an atypical spelling-to-sound correspondence. Other words that end in "int," such as "mint" and "print," have a different and more typical pronunciation.

- The word "crypt" has an atypical spelling for a word that rhymes with "ripped."

- The past-tense of the verb "fall" is the irregular form "fell." Typical past-tense forms involve adding "–ed," as in "call–called."

- A camel is atypical among animals because it has a hump.

In all six tasks, patients with semantic dementia performed well with frequent and typical items; less well for frequent-but-atypical and for typical-but-infrequent items; and poorly for items that offer no advantages of either frequency or typicality[92]. Performance on such "disadvantaged" items in all six tasks correlated closely with an overall composite score based on standard semantic memory tasks.

Figure 9.5(A) presents data from two of the six tasks—reading words aloud and generating the past-tense form of verbs—for the patients with the more severe form of semantic dementia. Figure 9.5(B) presents an analysis of response types in the same two tasks for

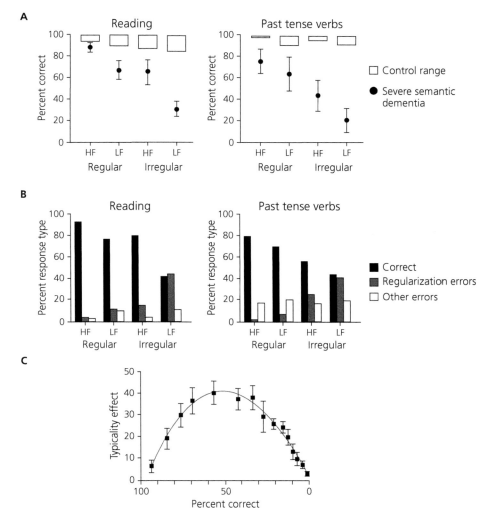

Fig. 9.5 Typicality and frequency effects in semantic dementia. (A) Two semantic memory tasks: reading single words aloud and translating the stem/present-tense forms of verbs into their past tense forms [for example, blink → blinked (regular) and think → thought (irregular)]. Abbreviations: HF, high-frequency items; LF, low-frequency items. (B) Analysis of response types for the same two tasks. Note that the scores for patients do not correspond to (A) because this plot includes both mild and severe cases. (C) The effect of concept typicality on a picture naming task. Each square indicates the size of the advantage for naming more typical versus less typical objects, at each level of performance. Error bars: 90% confidence intervals. (A, B) Adapted from Patterson K, Lambon Ralph MA, Jefferies E, Woollams A, Jones R, Hodges JR, Rogers TT. "Presemantic" cognition in semantic dementia: six deficits in search of an explanation. *Journal of Cognitive Neuroscience* 18:169–83, © 2006, reprinted by permission of The MIT Press Journals. (C) From Woollams AM, Cooper-Pye E, Hodges JR, Patterson K. Anomia: a doubly typical signature of semantic dementia. *Neuropsychologia* 46:2503–14, © 2008, Elsevier, with permission.

the entire group of patients. By far the most common errors involved excessive regularizations, such as reading "sew" to rhyme with "new" and inflecting the verb "grind" to the regular past-tense form "grinded" rather than "ground." These observations suggest that the semantic memory system plays an especially important role in processing infrequent and atypical items. Note that the tasks in this study were not overtly "semantic," in the sense that refers to meaning; few people realize that they need to retrieve the meaning of "sew" in order to read it aloud.

Figure 9.5(C) presents another demonstration, from a picture-naming task[93], of typicality effects in semantic dementia. In extremely mild cases, patients could name most objects pretty well, and in very severe cases they could scarcely name anything, so their performance differed little between typical and atypical items. At intermediate stages of disease severity, however, patients showed a significant advantage in naming high- versus low-typicality objects, reaching a peak difference of about 40%.

In a test called delayed copy-drawing, patients with semantic dementia saw several line drawings of familiar objects and studied each one. Next, they counted for 10 seconds as a distraction, after which they followed the instruction: "Draw what you were just looking at." The errors that the patients made on this task demonstrated how semantic knowledge deteriorates in this disease. Their drawings omitted the most distinctive, atypical features of items, such as the hump on a camel or the horns of a rhinoceros, while correctly including features that other members of their general category share, such as four legs and two eyes. Indeed, they began to overgeneralize such features, drawing four legs on ducks, for example[81].

These findings highlight the complex interplay between episodic retrieval and "what we know" (semantic memory). Few healthy people retain a highly faithful, literal visual image of a picture over a 10-second delay period that includes distractions. Except for the rare individual capable of eidetic imagery, people draw humps on camels because they recognize the drawing as a camel, remember that event later, and know that camels have humps. In some cases of semantic dementia, however, patients no longer know about camels, although they retain some knowledge about generic "animals," a category dominated by mammalian quadrupeds. Because generic "animals" typically lack humps and have four legs, the patients draw humpless camels and four-legged ducks. Familiar items draw on semantic representations, so what looks like an impairment in episodic retrieval—an inability to remember important aspects of a recently seen drawing—instead reflects a deeper, underlying problem with semantic memory. Novel drawings, of course, have less interaction with "what we know," and so performance suffers less.

The report illustrated in Fig. 9.5(A, B) did not include a comparison of performance with the extent of neural degeneration. A study in similar patients, however, demonstrated that the ability to read irregular (atypical) words was correlated with gray matter volume in the left anterior temporal lobe, including the temporal-pole cortex and anterior aspects of both the superior and middle temporal gyri. In contrast, the reading of nonwords was correlated with gray matter volume in the left temporal and parietal cortex[94].

Learning integrative concepts

Despite their memory losses, patients with semantic dementia can acquire new representations, although they do so differently from healthy people. In one learning experiment, both healthy subjects and patients saw a series of novel stimuli, each of which had several sensory dimensions: background color, shapes (squares and circles), number of items, and color[95]. The subjects needed to learn which of two arbitrary categories each stimulus belonged to, based solely on negative feedback when they made an incorrect choice. Although patients with semantic dementia and healthy subjects both showed some learning, the patients failed to use all four stimulus dimensions conjunctively. About half of these patients used only a single stimulus dimension to guide their learning, and as a group they used significantly fewer dimensions than healthy subjects did.

These results show that patients with semantic dementia can learn new categories, but they cannot generalize effectively across an exemplar's sensory dimensions. This learning impairment resembles the memory problems that these patients have, such as a tendency to rely on a single feature of some category rather than on a complex conjunction of features. For both learning and memory, then, semantic dementia impairs the ability to integrate representations across sensory modalities and cognitive domains[96,97].

To summarize what we have said so far: Patients with semantic dementia show a progressive and consistent loss of generalized semantic knowledge, with infrequent and atypical items suffering the most. The performance of these patients on semantic memory tests correlates with the degree of damage to the anterior temporal lobe, which supports the idea that it plays a central role in representing generalized concepts and categories. Indeed, the role of the anterior temporal lobe seems so *central* to semantic memory that it is said to function as a hub connected to specialized areas by spokes[4]. According to this wheel analogy, the "hub" lies at its metaphorical center and the "spoke" areas are arranged around its metaphorical rim.

Hub hubbub

Not all researchers accept the concept of cortical hubs. Instead, some suggest that generalized conceptual knowledge emerges from interactions among distributed, modality-specific areas without the need to invoke a hub[98]. A related view holds that conceptual knowledge emerges from interactions between the left and right temporal lobes[99], which specialize in verbal and visual knowledge, respectively. There is also emerging evidence for some degree of specialization within regions of the anterior temporal lobe. Its superior part seems, for example, to specialize in social semantic knowledge[100,101], perhaps divided between verbal and visual modalities by hemisphere. According to this idea, generalized semantic concepts depend on interhemispheric interactions of specialized areas, with impairments emerging when commissural connections deteriorate[99].

These alternative interpretations show that the work on patients with semantic dementia does not convince all experts about the existence of an anterior temporal lobe hub for semantic generalizations. Expanding the discussion to include additional evidence resolves some of these doubts. This evidence includes: (1) the properties of computational models; (2) the memory impairments suffered by patients with a particular form of encephalitis; (3) the effects of lesions of the anterior temporal lobe; (4) brain imaging results; and (5) the pattern of impairments in patients with semantic aphasia. We now take up these topics, in turn.

Computational models

The findings from semantic dementia support a model of semantic memory that depends on three elements: (1) long-term representations of semantic information, such as conceptual or categorical knowledge; (2) interactions between sensory representations and these memories; and (3) access to and selection of this knowledge for the guidance of behavior, including verbal behavior.

According to this model, domain-specific modules, exemplified by the fusiform face area and parahippocampal place area, process their specialized type of information close to where it arrives, and corticocortical connections bring this information together like spokes of a hub (Fig. 9.6B). Interactions between the hub and its "spoke" areas underlie the ability to integrate categorical and conceptually similar information, even though the items contributing to a category or concept might differ dramatically in terms of their modality- and domain-specific attributes. The category "fruit," for example, includes both grapes and bananas, which differ in color, shape, texture, and smell. Likewise, the concept of "swine" includes both boars and people prone to boorish behavior. The anterior temporal lobe hub thus represents higher-order relations among the features of the world, which facilitates inference, generalization, categorization, and problem solving, in part by applying existing knowledge to novel exemplars.

A study of resting-state activations by Pascual et al.[102] revealed some important aspects of this hub-and-spoke system. Their analysis identified four main clusters of coupled (correlated) voxels: (1) the dorsal anterior temporal lobe, which had correlated activations with auditory, somatosensory, and language networks; (2) the ventromedial temporal lobe, which was linked to visual networks; (3) the medial part of the anterior temporal lobe, which predominantly correlated with activations in the medial ring neocortex (more commonly called "limbic cortex"); and (4) the anterolateral temporal lobe, which showed coupling with both "spoke" areas of the semantic hub and a medial network of areas, thus interlinking them. The fourth cluster allows the anterolateral temporal lobe to integrate information from specialized cognitive domains and various sensory modalities, enabling the generation of domain-general representations.

In their discussion of these results, Pascual et al.[102] suggest that the anterior temporal cortex has greater complexity in humans than in other anthropoids. However, without reference to a common ancestor or quantitative support, this idea remains plausible but unsubstantiated. At first glance, their subdivisions of the anterior temporal lobe resemble the brain maps commonly accepted for monkeys. This overall similarity could, of course, mask an expansion and reorganization of the temporal cortex in humans, as mentioned earlier in this chapter (see "Evolution") and elsewhere (see Chapter 2,

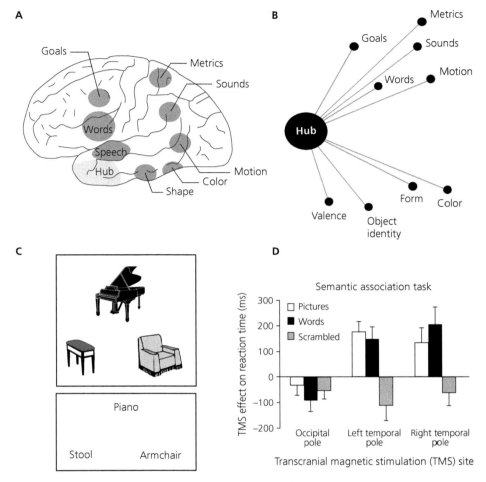

Fig. 9.6 Semantic memory. (A, B) Hub-and-spoke model of semantic memory. (C) Semantic association task with pictures (top) and words (bottom). (D) Change in reaction time induced by disruptive transcortical magnetic stimulation (TMS) of the anterior temporal cortex on pictures, words, and scrambled versions of the same stimuli. Positive values indicate slower response latencies. Error bars: standard error. From Pobric G, Jefferies E, Lambon Ralph MA (2010) Amodal semantic representations depend on both anterior temporal lobes: evidence from repetitive transcranial magnetic stimulation. *Neuropsychologia* 48:1336–42, © 2010, Elsevier, with permission.

"Possible new areas" and Chapter 10, "Regional expansion"). Independent of its comparative aspect, this study served to localize the hub of the hub-and-spoke model to the fourth cluster, the anterolateral temporal lobe, and it also suggested that the other three clusters play more specialized roles. The first one, for example, which corresponds to area TA, seems to specialize in semantic auditory representations.

Localization and comparative anatomy aside, computational models have addressed some of the uncertainties about the existence of a cross-domain hub. The behavior of these models suggests that semantic dementia occurs when the hub degenerates, leading to the loss of conceptual knowledge at specific hierarchical levels and a diminished ability to integrate information across cognitive domains. Later we consider which hierarchical levels are lost and preserved; for now we concentrate on the concept of hubs per se.

One example[103] of a connectionist, hub-and-spoke model had three layers: (1) an input layer that encoded visual features; (2) a verbal (output) layer that encoded the names of objects, categories, traits, and concepts; and (3) a middle layer that consisted of hidden units connecting the other layers. It was this middle layer that corresponded to the semantic hub. When input items shared a high degree of semantic similarity, they generated a consistent and overlapping pattern of activity. As a result, these patterns became encoded in the network's synaptic weights, and connections between the visual inputs and verbal outputs, via the hidden units, adopted an associative strength that eventually came to reflect generalized semantic concepts and categories.

These models have provided a straightforward account of the frequency and typicality effects described earlier. Frequently encountered exemplars developed stronger associative weights and typical items shared more features with other items in the same category. As a result, infrequent and atypical items had relatively fragile representations in the network. Removal of hidden units and their connections, designed to model progressive damage to the anterior temporal lobe hub in semantic dementia, therefore caused more severe impairments for these items.

Some connectionist models have included multiple input layers, simulating different sensory modalities. In these models, the modality in which an exemplar appeared had limited relevance to the abstract and categorical information encoded in the hidden layer. These models therefore predicted that impairments in the verbal and nonverbal domains should emerge together in semantic dementia, as indeed they do[103].

The same models have also accounted for the hierarchy of concepts impaired in semantic dementia. For this purpose, experts distinguish among three levels, from highest to lowest: "general," "basic," and "specific"[104]. In most circumstances, the "basic" level serves best for accessing semantic knowledge. For example, confronted with a picture of a magpie, people tend to answer the basic-level question ("Is this a bird?") faster than they will answer either the general-level question ("Is this an animal?") or the specific-level question ("Is this a magpie?"). The model networks could retrieve frequent, typical, and basic-level items relatively rapidly because they had a larger number of hidden-unit activations in common. Therefore, in addition to answering basic-level questions faster than questions at other levels, people can also decide that a robin is a bird faster than they can decide that a penguin is a bird. The reason is that robins are more common and more typical than penguins. (According to *March of the Penguins*, penguins are only "technically" birds anyway, not genuine exemplars of the concept.)

These models have suggested that items within a basic-level category, such as "bird," are represented more like other members of that category and more distinctly from items in other basic-level categories, such as "dog" or "tool." Put another way, their many shared attributes cause basic-level items to cluster more tightly in semantic feature-space, leading to stronger generalization for exemplars at the basic level than for general-level concepts. Tight clustering promotes faster decisions, and so people usually answer basic-level questions faster than general- or specific-level ones. At the general level, exemplars share fewer features, which leads to less generalization across items and slower decisions. At the specific level, generalizations provide little benefit because people need to use unique representations.

A series of experiments have provided support for these models[105]. As just mentioned, healthy subjects showed quicker and more accurate basic-level judgments, compared with both the general- and specific-level decisions. For patients with semantic dementia, however, the most accurate decisions occurred at the general level, with less successful performance at the basic level and still less at the specific level. Thus, unlike healthy subjects, patients with semantic dementia identified a kingfisher as an animal (a general-level concept) more accurately than as a bird (a basic-level concept). In the computational models, the middle (hidden) layer corresponds to the hub. With damage to this layer and its level of representation, the performance of these models resembles that of patients with semantic dementia: They, too, lose the advantage of basic-level over general-level categories.

In healthy people, the pressure to make extremely speedy decisions reversed the basic-level advantage and mimicked the pattern seen in semantic dementia. In the models, increasing the pressure to perform quickly corresponds to making decisions before the network has settled into a stable state, which leads to errors. As in semantic dementia, these errors occurred more frequently in the models for basic-level concepts than for general-level ones[103,105].

In summary, computational models support the idea that generalization and categorization underpin semantic knowledge[105]. This work also highlights the critical contribution of a hub-like network architecture and several key aspects of semantic dementia: impairments in recognizing items and concepts across cognitive domains; the loss of a basic-level advantage, especially as the disease progresses; and a larger impairment on atypical and infrequently encountered items, especially in the middle stages of the disease.

Dimming versus distorting

Another disease, *Herpes simplex virus* encephalitis (HSVE), also causes severe impairments in semantic memory, and findings in patients with this disorder seemed, at first, to conflict with the idea of a semantic hub.

People who survive HSVE often have damage to their anterior temporal lobe, so these patients should have domain-general impairments like those seen in semantic dementia. In most cases, however, HSVE patients have a more specific impairment: memory loss for animate items, with significantly better comprehension of inanimate objects[106,107]. Sometimes, they lose other "natural categories," but according to the hub-and-spoke model, none of these specialized impairments should occur. So instead of a semantic hub that generalizes information across cognitive domains, this observation suggests that the anterior temporal lobe specializes in certain domains of knowledge, such as animate objects.

A systematic comparison of impairments in HSVE and semantic dementia should, in principle, be based on performance of the same tasks. While this approach might seem obvious, it remains relatively rare. The findings from one such study clarified the contrasts and comparisons between patients with HSVE and semantic dementia. These patient groups had qualitatively different impairments, despite a similar overall level of disability[6], and they differed in three key ways:

- Patients with semantic dementia showed more anomia, an inability to recall words and names.

- Patients with semantic dementia also made more errors of omission and cross-level errors, such as substituting "animal" for "pig," whereas HSVE patients tended towards within-category errors, such as substituting "horse" for "pig."

- Patients with HSVE provided incorrect information (such as "squirrels are slimy"), while patients with semantic dementia found it difficult to generate any specific information at all.

These findings support a distinction between the "distortion" and "dimming" of semantic representations[6]. According to this idea, the acute inflammatory response in HSVE results in the "distortion" of semantic representations, whereas the progressive degeneration in semantic dementia causes the degradation or loss of these representations, or "dimming."

Connectionist models have elucidated how dimming and distortion differentially affect the semantic hub. The gradual removal of "synaptic" connections within the hidden-layer hub caused a weakening of representations across all domains, especially for less frequent and atypical items. This simulated "lesion" effect corresponds to "dimming," and it caused cross-category and cross-level errors of the kind more common in semantic dementia than in HSVE. Cross-level errors, such as using "animal" rather than "horse," result from the severe degradation or loss of basic-level representations, and the same loss accounts for anomia.

In contrast, "distorting" synaptic weights, as opposed to randomly removing "synapses," resulted in within-category ("horse" for "pig") errors like those made by HSVE patients. Distorting weights within the hidden layer resulted in less anomia and fewer cross-level errors, compared with "dimming," because the representations of basic-level categories remained relatively intact. However, distortion produced more within-category errors because it led to unreliable input–output transforms for the network as a whole.

Crucially, this study addressed a key variable that has not always been controlled in other investigations. In most tests of animate versus inanimate categories, the animate items had more in common with each other than did the inanimate items. Put another way, animate exemplars clustered more tightly in semantic space than did inanimate exemplars, and this tight clustering made semantic confusion and inappropriate substitutions more likely. To overcome this problem, inanimate categories were designed to have items that matched the tight clustering typical of animate categories. To place animate and inanimate items on an equal footing, for example, the subjects needed to name breeds of dogs and makes of cars. This manipulation abolished the category-specific impairment in HSVE, in accord with simulations in the model[6]. The distortion of weights in the hidden layer caused the model to switch its outputs incorrectly (and with poor stability) among similar concepts within a category, as HSVE patients do, for both animate and inanimate categories.

Taken together, both facets of this study—the computational simulations and the comparison of patients with HSVE and semantic dementia—supported the semantic-hub model. The category-specific semantic loss sometimes seen in HSVE[106,107], which seems to challenge that model, probably resulted from the fact that typical animate items clustered more tightly in semantic (feature) space than did inanimate ones. In experiments that controlled for this factor, the impairments in both HSVE and semantic dementia agreed with the hub-and-spoke model.

This line of research also provides a framework for understanding modality-specific impairments. One example is word deafness, a modality-specific impairment in which patients cannot understand concepts from words that they hear, but can understand visually presented concepts, such as written words or pictures[4]. Like the inability to recognize faces (prosopagnosia), word deafness results from damage to a specialized "spoke" area (Fig. 9.6B). These impairments differ from those in semantic dementia and HSVE, which results from damage to a hub that integrates specialized representations. Connectionist networks have simulated the domain- or modality-specific effects through "lesions" of the model's input or output layers.

In summary, the advantage provided by a hub, as opposed to a distributed network of specialized areas, stems from its ability to bring features together in a way that enables successful generalization across sensory modalities and cognitive domains, which people can then apply to novel, infrequent, and atypical exemplars. As is often the case for evolutionary innovations, the hub performs advantageous functions, although not necessary ones (see Chapter 1, "Homologies"). This idea accounts for some of the controversy in the literature: A hub does not seem necessary to some experts, but even so it can provide a selective advantage.

Reduced computational efficiency

Critics of the semantic hub model emphasize, quite rightly, the apparent lack of semantic memory impairments in epilepsy patients who had surgical removal of the anterior temporal lobe. They also note, equally correctly, that neither the degenerative processes underlying semantic dementia nor the infectious–inflammatory processes in HSVE cause lesions as anatomically defined as surgical ablations. Like the studies of HSVE patients, however, much of this literature has depended on relatively simple semantic tasks, rather than tests stressing the more vulnerable representations, such as those for infrequent or atypical items.

When experiments have taxed the hub's representations or have required fast responses, patients with unilateral anterior temporal lobe resections made more errors and responded more slowly than healthy subjects, in accord with the hub-and-spoke model[108]. The overall pattern of impairments resembled that in semantic dementia, albeit in much milder form. The lesser degree of impairment most likely reflected the difference between the bilateral, extensive damage in semantic dementia and HSVE in contrast to the unilateral, restricted damage in surgically lesioned patients. Removal of part of the hub did not eliminate the semantic memory system, but instead reduced the computational efficiency of the hub-and-spoke architecture as a whole[109].

One test of this idea employed disruptive, repetitive cortical stimulation (rTMS) of the anterior temporal lobe[110]. In healthy people, this disruption slowed responses on the same semantic tasks affected in semantic dementia[4,111], including semantic judgment and picture naming tasks[112]. There was no effect on equally difficult number judgments or number naming. Disruptive stimulation could also distinguish the contributions of the hub and spoke areas. Stimulation of the anterior temporal lobe in one hemisphere generated a domain-general impairment, whereas disruption of the inferior parietal lobe, a spoke area, induced a domain-specific deficit for manufactured objects[111].

Another test involved semantic associations, which semantic dementia patients performed poorly[113]. In the pyramids and palm trees test, like related tasks, subjects see an array of three pictures or words, with one at the top (Fig. 9.6C). They need to choose, as rapidly as possible, which of the two lower items "goes with" the top item. Pyramids and palm trees go together because Egypt has both. In Fig. 9.6(C), the piano and piano stool go together. In a control test, subjects see fragmented pictures or words scrambled randomly, and they need to choose the one lower item that visually matches the top item. Disruptive stimulation of either the left or right temporal lobe slowed responses during both the word and picture tasks, but not in the scrambled condition (Fig. 9.6D).

The finding that cortical disruption had the same effect for either hemisphere deserves comment, especially in view of criticisms of the hub-and-spoke model that emphasize hemispheric specialization[99]. In this experiment, healthy subjects showed a consistent impairment on verbal comprehension tasks, regardless of the hemisphere that stimulation disrupted, just as epilepsy patients do after partial lesions of either their left or right anterior temporal lobe[92]. Notwithstanding the well-known hemispheric specializations for language, these findings contradict the idea that the left and right temporal lobes play modality-specific roles in conceptual knowledge. Patients with left temporal lobe epilepsy show more anomia than patients with right temporal lobe lesions, but this symptom probably results from the greater connectivity of the left hemisphere with speech production mechanisms[114].

Brain imaging

It might seem strange that we have yet to mention brain imaging activations in semantic memory tasks. One reason relates to susceptibility artifacts[115]. These artifactual signals occur where brain tissue adjoins sinuses, which sometimes makes it difficult to interpret imaging results, especially near the temporal pole. Recent developments in imaging methods have partially mitigated this problem[116-118], and other methodological advances have included the use of novel behavioral tests and adequately demanding baseline tasks.

Semantic association tasks that involved words and pictures—variants of the pyramids and palm trees test (Fig. 9.6C)—have led to several cortical activations[119]. Healthy people showed these activations in both temporal lobes, among other areas, including the ventrolateral and orbitofrontal cortex (see Plate 3A). Within the temporal lobe, activations occurred more often in the superior temporal gyrus for the word-based task and in the fusiform gyrus for the picture-based task (see Plate 4A, B). Parts of the anterior temporal lobe had comparably high levels of activation for both the word and picture tasks (see Plate 4B, arrows), in agreement with the hub-and-spoke model.

In another brain imaging study, subjects made semantic decisions about three kinds of stimuli: audible words, environmental sounds, and pictures. Both the left and right anterior temporal lobes showed significant activation for all three kinds of stimuli, with some graded specialization of the left hemisphere for words[120]. Semantic decisions about words, pictures, and sounds led to bilateral activation of the ventral anterior temporal lobes, whereas auditory stimuli (words and environmental sounds) generated stronger activation in anterior parts of the left superior temporal gyrus. Other results were similar[121]. These findings indicate that the anterior temporal lobe hub integrates features across both sensory modalities (vision and audition) and both cognitive domains (words and pictures).

In summary, despite methodological challenges, functional brain imaging studies support the idea that the anterior temporal cortex mediates semantic representations across sensory modalities and cognitive domains, in accord with the hub-and-spoke model.

Semantic control

Left-hemisphere strokes commonly cause language impairments, such as Wernicke's and Broca's aphasia, but here we concentrate on a different stroke-induced language impairment: semantic aphasia. At first glance, this disorder resembles semantic dementia. Semantic aphasia results from damage to the left temporal–parietal junction (near and including the supramarginal gyrus), the left prefrontal cortex, or both. In apparent contradiction of the hub-and-spoke model, patients with left-hemisphere strokes that include these areas rarely have damage to the anterior temporal lobe, yet they can have prominent impairments of semantic memory.

A direct comparison of semantic aphasia and semantic dementia revealed that both groups of patients had poor verbal and nonverbal comprehension over a broad range of tasks, including those involving words, pictures, and matching sounds to either pictures or words[122]. Despite an overall similarity in their degree of impairment, the two patient groups differed in several ways:

◆ Patients with semantic dementia made more "don't know" responses and cross-level errors on naming tasks (such as "animal" instead of "pig"). They also were a more homogeneous group, with a higher correlation in their impairments across tasks.

◆ Patients with semantic aphasia produced far more implausible, unrelated, or perseverative responses, such as responding with the word "crossing" when asked to name a picture of a zebra, simply because of the unrelated concept of a "zebra crossing." Furthermore, their performance on naming and comprehension tasks improved significantly when they received an appropriate phonemic cue, such as the first sound or two of a picture's name[123]. These patients also had milder impairments on simple decision tasks, including those for words, objects, and colors, and they showed little influence of item frequency or typicality[124].

Taken together, these findings suggest that the impairment in semantic aphasia does not involve the deterioration of semantic representations per se, as occurs in semantic dementia, but instead emerges from a difficulty or abnormality in accessing this knowledge.

The same conclusion comes from a semantic judgment test, which involved a probe item and a set of potential target items[123]. This task required subjects to indicate which target item had the closest similarity in meaning with the probe. Patients with semantic aphasia performed poorly when the probe had a large semantic distance from the target. For example, when presented with the probe "broccoli" and the potential targets "lobster," "apple," and "ostrich," these patients struggled to identify the correct item: "apple," a word that, like the probe, refers to an edible plant product. In contrast, the same probe item, "broccoli," is fairly similar to the middle member of another target set: "lobster," "cauliflower," and "ostrich." In this situation, patients with semantic aphasia performed much better.

The contrasts between semantic dementia and semantic aphasia suggest that they result from different dysfunctions in semantic memory. Semantic dementia appears to involve the degradation and loss of conceptual representations, whereas in semantic aphasia these representations remain intact but with some impediment to their access and retrieval, especially for ambiguous semantic relationships. This conclusion raises an obvious question: Which brain areas control such access? A partial answer to this question is: the granular prefrontal cortex.

Given the prominent role of the anterior temporal lobe in semantic dementia, the prefrontal cortex has received less consideration in semantic memory research. The idea of a larger prefrontal–temporal network for semantic memory has found support, however, in brain imaging studies[125–128], including those mentioned earlier (see "Brain imaging", Plate 3A, B). These experiments have consistently revealed activations in the prefrontal cortex—particularly in the ventrolateral prefrontal cortex—under conditions of high semantic demand. Activations occurred there during the retrieval of demanding and nonautomatic associations, as opposed to easy and automatic ones, such as the pair tennis–ball.

In a meta-analysis of studies that contrasted highly demanding levels of attentive (semantic) control and less demanding levels[129], the ventrolateral prefrontal cortex, posterior middle temporal gyrus, dorsal angular gyrus, and cortex near the intraparietal sulcus consistently showed greater activation during more demanding tasks (red and yellow clusters in Plate 4C). These regions overlapped with the locations of lesions in semantic aphasia patients, as well as with the cortical areas that Duncan[1,130] includes in his general problem-solving, multiple demand system (see "General problem solving"). In view of their greater activation during demanding forms of semantic, phonological, and metaphor tasks (blue clusters in Place 4C, left to right), the left ventrolateral prefrontal cortex and posterior middle temporal gyrus appear to play a domain-general role.

A similar conclusion comes from disruptive stimulation of the prefrontal cortex. When subjects made semantic relatedness judgments for both strong and weak semantic associations, disruptive cortical stimulation of either the ventrolateral prefrontal cortex or the posterior middle temporal gyrus impaired demanding but not automatic decisions, inducing a 200-ms delay in making a judgment[131].

Results are also available for tasks involving semantic versus perceptual retrieval, as well as for demanding judgments about the degree of semantic relatedness versus simple feature selection. Disruptive stimulation experiments[132] have indicated that both the left ventrolateral prefrontal cortex and the posterior middle temporal gyrus contributed to semantic retrieval under these demanding conditions. Additional results showed that cortex near the intraparietal sulcus contributed to both semantic and perceptual retrieval. This finding provides further support for the idea that this part of the posterior parietal cortex contributes to a domain-general, multiple demand system.

In summary, the contrasts between semantic aphasia and semantic dementia suggest that semantic memory depends on a broadly distributed network of areas that work in concert, including the ventrolateral prefrontal, posterior parietal, middle temporal, and anterior temporal cortex. Collectively, these cortical areas enable access to both domain-specific and domain-general knowledge. Damage to the anterior temporal lobe, as occurs in semantic dementia, progressively eliminates the cross-domain representations that underlie semantic generalization and inferences. Disruption of temporal–prefrontal interactions, as occurs in semantic aphasia, impairs access to semantic knowledge, particularly in demanding conditions that require attentive (as opposed to automatic) control. The impairments in semantic aphasia correlate with those on other tests of "executive function"[122], implying that they represent a special case of a more general function.

Summary

Anterior temporal lobe hub

Some time after the ape–human lineage split from other anthropoids, part of the feature memory system came to represent generalized categories and concepts. Although there remains some controversy about hubs, as well as how they communicate with their "spoke" areas[133], converging evidence points to the anterior temporal lobe as a cortical hub for semantic memory, which integrates features across sensory modalities and cognitive domains to support semantic generalizations and inferences. Importantly, this hub is situated mainly in the lateral part of the anterior temporal lobe and therefore is not a part of the so-called "medial temporal lobe."

A semantic hub provides humans with an adaptive advantage because feature similarities provide only a partial guide to overall conceptual similarity. The membership of an item in a semantic concept and category usually has more to do with the amount of feature overlap with a "prototype" than with rigid inclusion criteria[134], a concept that goes back to Wittgenstein[96,134]. Indeed, members of a semantic category need not share any features at all[96,135]. Semantic memories augment those tied to distinct sensory modalities, cognitive domains, situations, times, and environments, thereby creating flexible, adaptable, and domain-general representations that can be applied across problems.

According to the hub-and-spoke model, experience changes the strength of associations between lower-order, domain-specific areas and cross-domain networks in the anterior temporal lobe, and this process creates a degree of representational overlap among exemplars. The strength of these associations affects the accessibility and ease of retrieval for categorical and conceptual knowledge. Greater feature overlap of an exemplar with a conceptual or categorical prototype will ease retrieval and speed responses to categorical questions. Likewise, greater overlap of one concept or category with another will increase the likelihood of further generalization. When some feature of a concept or category seems to be missing, similar representations can fill the gap, a form of inferential reasoning.

Temporal–prefrontal interactions

Like the mechanisms that establish semantic memories, their retrieval also depends on the strength of associations. In demanding situations, semantic retrieval depends on interactions between the ventrolateral prefrontal cortex and the anterior temporal hub, although other areas participate as well[129]. Demanding situations include obscure or arbitrary relations and representations widely separated in feature space, along with weak associations, often involving atypical features, and ambiguities about situational rules. Retrieving the appropriate memory requires what is commonly called "semantic control," a form of top-down biased competition.

For semantic memory, the prefrontal cortex comes to the fore when a less dominant form of a concept or category is appropriate to a given situation and a more dominant form interferes with its retrieval. For example, when people see a book they will usually retrieve the dominant concept—reading. In rare circumstances, however, a book makes a pretty good doorstop. The same goes for the competition among different hierarchical levels. Depending on the context and task rules, a picture of a "dog" might require the retrieval of representations at the general level ("animal"), the basic level ("dog"), or any of several specific levels ("terrier," "Cairn terrier," or "Toto" from *The Wizard of Oz*). A given context might require disambiguating "terrier" and "Labrador," "dog" and "puppy," and so forth. Retrieving semantic knowledge therefore requires not only a cognitive *process*, but also *knowledge* of what kind of representations to retrieve.

The distinction between process and knowledge[136] provides a link between this chapter and Chapter 8 ("Augmentation of the biased-competition system"). As part of its role in generating goals, representations in the prefrontal cortex (knowledge) produce biases (a process) among competing perceptual representations (see Chapter 7), competing motor plans (see Chapter 6), competing conditioned responses (see Chapter 5), and competing navigational frames (see Chapters 4 and 5). Semantic control emerges from analogous interactions.

As a result of degrading these interactions, certain lesions can cause semantic aphasia, in part because they block the top-down influence of the ventrolateral prefrontal cortex on the anterior temporal lobe. This blockage can occur for either of two reasons: (1) the disconnection of either direct temporal–prefrontal connections or indirect ones that are mediated by more posterior areas; or (2) the destruction of representations in the prefrontal cortex that guide semantic retrieval. The loss of rule- and context-based semantic control causes the bizarre errors and implausible responses seen in semantic aphasia. In HSVE and semantic dementia, by contrast, semantic control survives but falls on degraded ("dimmed") or distorted semantic representations. As a result, these patients make the within-level ("dog" for "pig") errors typical of HSVE or the cross-level ("animal" for "pig") errors typical of semantic dementia.

Conclusions

In Chapters 7 and 8 we discussed specialized representational systems that provided evolving anthropoids with an advantage in terms of fewer foraging errors. Here we suggest that these representations served as exaptations for more general cognitive functions. In anatomical and evolutionary terms, the posterior parietal, lateral temporal, and granular prefrontal cortex adapted their representations to support relational reasoning, semantic generalizations, and semantic control, respectively.

According to our proposal, these adaptations depended on the development of new, higher representational levels in hominins (Fig. 9.7). In Chapter 7 ("Attributes") we explained that our anthropoid ancestors developed new, primate-specific areas that represented the signs of resources at a level between low-order and object-level conjunctions (see Fig. 7.3). We think that these mid-level representations served as exaptations for semantic memory and that they did so for a simple reason: They automatically represent categories.

Figure 9.7(A) illustrates why they do so. In this heuristic sketch, the middle level (IT) represents a category ("Vis AB") of two exemplars that share features A and B. Neurons that represent the visual conjunction labeled "Vis AB" will represent all exemplars with these features: the two illustrated ("Vis ABCD" and "Vis ABEF") along with others (such as "Vis ABGH," "Vis ABD," and so forth). "Vis AB" thus corresponds to a category, as well as being appropriate for representing signs (as opposed to objects).

Figure 9.7(C) depicts several ways that higher levels of representational complexity can develop, relative to object-level representations. Even though it evolved much earlier, the hippocampus can represent higher levels because it adds spatial, temporal, and contextual dimensions to representations it receives from the perirhinal cortex (see Chapter 7)[137]. The granular prefrontal cortex adds levels by conjoining goal, strategy, outcome, and rule dimensions to information it receives from both the inferior temporal and perirhinal cortex, among other areas (see Chapter 8). According to the proposal we advance in Chapter 10, higher representational levels also develop within the granular prefrontal cortex of hominins[138,139]. And, according to the proposal presented in this chapter, something

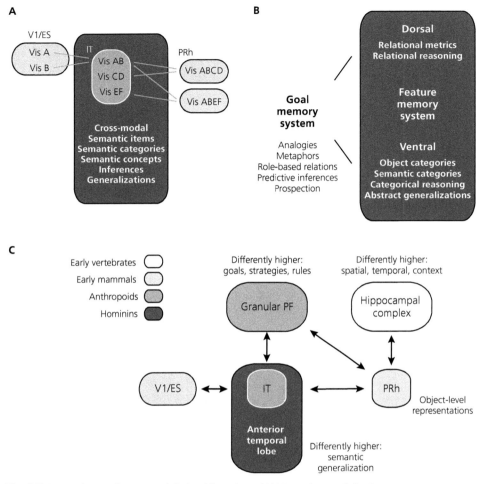

Fig. 9.7 Processing pathways and derived functions. (A) Ventral part of the feature system from Fig. 7.3. (B) Summary of goal and feature memory systems. (C) Three kinds of complex representations that build on object-level conjunctions represented in the perirhinal cortex. The key in (C) also applies to (A). The phrase "differently higher" highlights the idea that there are several processing pathways that add levels of complexity to conjunctive representations. Abbreviations: ES, extrastriate cortex; IT, inferior temporal cortex; PF, prefrontal cortex; PRh, perirhinal cortex; V1, primary visual cortex; Vis, visual features.

similar happens within the anterior temporal lobe, in which ancestrally mid-level representations support high-level concepts and categories.

Figure 9.7(B) summarizes some cognitive capacities that emerged from these developments, including cross-domain concepts and categories; productive, predictive semantic inferences; and relational, analogical reasoning. All of these traits support general problem solving and provide important advantages in demanding, novel, or rare circumstances.

Like other anthropoids, humans live long lives, and so our hominin ancestors surely benefited from remembering infrequently encountered and atypical information. Most mammals, such as rodents, "shall never see so much, nor live so long" (*King Lear, V, iii,* 345).

This chapter touches on traits that distinguish humans from other animals. About 250 years ago, Linnaeus tackled this problem in his classification of animals. According to Gould[140] (p. 251), when

> Linnaeus faced the difficult question of how to classify his own species … [h]e defined our relatives by the mundane, distinguishing characters of size, shape, and number of fingers and toes. For *Homo sapiens*, he wrote only the Socratic injunction *nosce te ipsum*—"know thyself."

In Chapter 10 we explore how our species might accomplish that feat.

References

1. Duncan, J. (2010) *Trends Cogn. Sci.* **14**, 172–179.
2. Genovesio, A., Wise, S.P., and Passingham, R.E. (2014) *Trends Cogn. Sci* **18**, 72–81.
3. Vendetti, M.S. and Bunge, S.A. (2014) *Neuron* **84**, 906–917.
4. Lambon Ralph, M.A. (2014) *Phil. Trans. R. Soc. B: Biol. Sci.* **369**, 20120392.
5. Zalmout, I.S., Sanders, W.J., Maclatchy, L.M., Gunnell, G.F. et al. (2010) *Nature* **466**, 360–364.
6. Lambon Ralph, M.A., Lowe, C., and Rogers, T.T. (2007) *Brain* **130**, 1127–1137.
7. Plaut, D.C., McClelland, J.L., Seidenberg, M.S., and Patterson, K. (1996) *Psychol. Rev.* **103**, 56–115.
8. Passingham, R.E. and Smaers, J.B. (2014) *Brain Behav. Evol.* **84**, 156–166.
9. Kaas, J.H. (2014) In: *The New Visual Neurosciences* (eds. Warner, J. and Chalupa, L.), pp. 1233–1246 (MIT Press, Cambridge, MA).
10. Rilling, J.K. and Seligman, R.A. (2002) *J. Hum. Evol.* **42**, 505–533.
11. Glasser, M.F., Goyal, M.S., Preuss, T.M., Raichle, M.E. et al. (2014) *NeuroImage* **93P2**, 165–175.
12. Van Essen, D.C. and Dierker, D.L. (2007) *Neuron* **56**, 209–225.
13. Sayers, K. and Menzel, C.R. (2012) *Anim. Behav.* **84**, 795–803.
14. Silberberg, A., Widholm, J.J., Bresler, D., Fujita, K. et al. (1998) *J. Exp. Psychol: Anim. Behav. Process.* **24**, 215–228.
15. Beran, M.J., Ratliff, C.L., and Evans, T.A. (2009) *Learn. Motiv.* **40**, 186–196.
16. Rao, S.M., Mayer, A.R., and Harrington, D.L. (2001) *Nat. Neurosci.* **4**, 317–323.
17. Dehaene, S., Piazza, M., Pinel, P., and Cohen, L. (2003) *Cogn. Neuropsychol.* **20**, 487–506.
18. Fias, W., Lammertyn, J., Reynvoet, B., Dupont, P. et al. (2003) *J. Cogn. Neurosci.* **15**, 47–56.
19. Walsh, V. (2003) *Trends Cogn. Sci.* **7**, 483–488.
20. Pinel, P., Piazza, M., Le, B.D., and Dehaene, S. (2004) *Neuron* **41**, 983–993.
21. Jacob, S.N. and Nieder, A. (2009) *Eur. J. Neurosci.* **30**, 1432–1442.
22. Bueti, D. and Walsh, V. (2009) *Phil. Trans. R. Soc. B: Biol. Sci.* **364**, 1831–1840.
23. Oliveri, M., Koch, G., Salerno, S., Torriero, S. et al. (2009) *NeuroImage* **46**, 1173–1179.
24. Assmus, A., Marshall, J.C., Ritzl, A., Noth, J. *et al.* (2003) *NeuroImage* **20** (**Suppl. 1**), S82–S88.
25. Trivino, M., Correa, A., Arnedo, M., and Lupianez, J. (2010) *Brain* **133**, 1173–1185.
26. Koch, G., Oliveri, M., Carlesimo, G.A., and Caltagirone, C. (2002) *Neurology* **59**, 1658–1659.
27. Merchant, H., Harrington, D.L., and Meck, W.H. (2013) *Annu. Rev. Neurosci.* **36**, 313–336.

28. Jones, C.R.G., Rosenkranz, K., Rothwell, J.C., and Jahanshahi, M. (2004) *Exp. Brain Res.* **158**, 366–372.

29. Koch, G., Oliveri, M., Torriero, S., and Caltagirone, C. (2003) *Neurology* **60**, 1844–1846.

30. Brzezicka, A., Sedek, G., Marchewka, A., Gola, M. et al. (2011) *Acta Neurobiol. Exp. (Wars.)* **71**, 479–495.

31. Hinton, E.C., Dymond, S., von Hecker, U., and Evans, C.J. (2010) *Neuroscience* **168**, 138–148.

32. Acuna, B.D., Eliassen, J.C., Donoghue, J.P., and Sanes, J.N. (2002) *Cereb. Cortex* **12**, 1312–1321.

33. Amiez, C. and Petrides, M. (2007) *Proc. Natl. Acad. Sci. USA* **104**, 13786–13791.

34. Champod, A.S. and Petrides, M. (2007) *Proc. Natl. Acad. Sci. USA* **104**, 14837–14842.

35. Postle, B.R., Ferrarelli, F., Hamidi, M., Feredoes, E. et al. (2006) *J. Cogn. Neurosci.* **18**, 1712–1722.

36. Koenigs, M., Barbey, A.K., Postle, B.R., and Grafman, J. (2009) *J. Neurosci.* **29**, 14980–14986.

37. Petrides, M. (1995) *J. Neurosci.* **15**, 359–375.

38. Sirigu, A., Zalla, T., Pillon, B., Grafman, J. *et al.* (1996) *Cortex* **32**, 297–310.

39. Okuda, J., Fujii, T., Ohtake, H., Tsukiura, T. et al. (2007) *Int. J. Psychophysiol.* **64**, 233–246.

40. Genovesio, A., Tsujimoto, S., and Wise, S.P. (2012) *Neuron* **74**, 656–662.

41. Volle, E., Gilbert, S.J., Benoit, R.G., and Burgess, P.W. (2010) *Cereb. Cortex* **20**, 2647–2659.

42. Bunge, S.A., Helskog, E.H., and Wendelken, C. (2009) *NeuroImage* **46**, 338–342.

43. Wendelken, C., Nakhabenko, D., Donohue, S.E., Carter, C.S. et al. (2008) *J. Cogn. Neurosci.* **20**, 682–693.

44. Christoff, K., Prabhakaran, V., Dorfman, J., Zhao, Z. et al. (2001) *NeuroImage* **14**, 1136–1149.

45. Crone, E.A., Wendelken, C., Donohue, S., van Leijenhorst, L. et al. (2006) *Proc. Natl. Acad. Sci. U.S.A.* **103**, 9315–9320.

46. Crone, E.A., Wendelken, C., van Leijenhorst, L., Honomichl, R.D. et al. (2009) *Dev. Sci.* **12**, 55–66.

47. Mackey, A.P., Miller Singley, A.T., and Bunge, S.A. (2013) *J. Neurosci.* **33**, 4796–4803.

48. Huxley, T.H. (1887, 2000) http://www.gutenberg.org/files/2089/2089-h/2089-h.htm.

49. Fedorenko, E., Duncan, J., and Kanwisher, N. (2013) *Proc. Natl. Acad. Sci. USA* **110**, 16616–16621.

50. Hampshire, A., Highfield, R.R., Parkin, B.L., and Owen, A.M. (2012) *Neuron* **76**, 1225–1237.

51. Humphreys, G.F. and Lambon Ralph, M.A. (2015) *Cereb. Cortex* **25**, 3547–3560.

52. Woolgar, A., Parr, A., Cusack, R., Thompson, R. et al. (2010) *Proc. Natl. Acad. Sci. USA* **107**, 14899–14902.

53. Neubert, F.-X., Mars, R.B., Thomas, A., Sallet, J. et al. (2014) *Neuron* **81**, 700–713.

54. Sallet, J., Mars, R.B., Noonan, M.P., Neubert, F.-X. et al. (2013) *J. Neurosci.* **33**, 12255–12274.

55. Cloutman, L.L., Binney, R.J., Morris, D.M., Parker, G.J. *et al.* (2013) *Brain Lang.* **127**, 230–240.

56. Hecht, E.E., Gutman, D.A., Bradley, B.A., Preuss, T.M. et al. (2015) *NeuroImage* **108**, 124–137.

57. Eacott, M.J., Gaffan, D., and Murray, E.A. (1994) *Eur. J. Neurosci.* **6**, 1466–1478.

58. Warrington, E.K. (1975) *Q. J. Exp. Psychol.* **27**, 635–657.

59. Snowden, J., Goulding, P., and Neary, D. (1989) *Behav. Neurol.* **2**, 167–182.

60. Hodges, J.R., Patterson, K., Oxbury, S., and Funnell, E. (1992) *Brain* **115**, 1783–1806.

61. Acosta-Cabronero, J., Patterson, K., Fryer, T.D., Hodges, J.R. et al. (2011) *Brain* **134**, 2025–2035.

62. Hodges, J.R. and Patterson, K. (2007) *Lancet Neurol.* **6**, 1004–1014.

63. Davies, R.R., Halliday, G.M., Xuereb, J.H., Kril, J.J. et al. (2009) *Neurobiol. Aging* **30**, 2043–2052.

64. Vargha-Khadem, F., Gadian, D.G., Watkins, K.E., Connelly, A. et al. (1997) *Science* **277**, 376–380.

65. Nestor, P.J., Fryer, T.D., and Hodges, J.R. (2006) *NeuroImage* **30**, 1010–1020.

66. Tan, R.H., Wong, S., Kril, J.J., Piguet, O. et al. (2014) *Brain* **137**, 2065–2076.

67. Brier, M.R., Thomas, J.B., and Ances, B.M. (2014) *Brain Connect.* **4**, 299–311.

68. Davies, R.R., Graham, K.S., Xuereb, J.H., Williams, G.B. et al. (2004) *Eur. J. Neurosci.* **20**, 2441–2446.

69. Mion, M., Patterson, K., Acosta-Cabronero, J., Pengas, G. et al. (2010) *Brain* **133**, 3256–3268.

70. Guo, C.C., Gorno-Tempini, M.L., Gesierich, B., Henry, M. et al. (2013) *Brain* **136**, 2979–2991.

71. Bozeat, S., Lambon Ralph, M.A., Patterson, K., Garrard, P. et al. (2000) *Neuropsychologia* **38**, 1207–1215.

72. Rogers, T.T., Patterson, K., and Graham, K. (2007) *Neuropsychologia* **45**, 3285–3298.

73. Rogers, T.T., Lambon Ralph, M.A., Hodges, J.R., and Patterson, K. (2004) *Cogn. Neuropsychol.* **21**, 331–352.

74. Simons, J.S., Verfaellie, M., Galton, C.J., Miller, B.L. et al. (2002) *Brain* **125**, 2523–2536.

75. Graham, K.S. and Hodges, J.R. (1997) *Neuropsychology* **11**, 77–89.

76. Ikeda, M., Patterson, K., Graham, K.S., Lambon Ralph, M.A. et al. (2006) *Neuropsychologia* **44**, 566–575.

77. Graham, K.S., Simons, J.S., Pratt, K.H., Patterson, K. et al. (2000) *Neuropsychologia* **38**, 313–324.

78. Simons, J.S., Graham, K.S., Galton, C.J., Patterson, K. et al. (2001) *Neuropsychology* **15**, 101–114.

79. Pengas, G., Patterson, K., Arnold, R.J., Bird, C.M. *et al.* (2010) *J. Alz. Dis.* **21**, 1347–1365.

80. Adlam, A.L., Patterson, K., and Hodges, J.R. (2009) *Neuropsychologia* **47**, 1344–1351.

81. Bozeat, S., Lambon Ralph, M.A., Graham, K.S., Patterson, K. et al. (2003) *Cogn. Neuropsychol.* **20**, 27–47.

82. Hoffman, P., Jefferies, E., Ehsan, S., Jones, R.W. et al. (2009) *Neuropsychologia* **47**, 747–760.

83. Duarte, A., Henson, R.N., Knight, R.T., Emery, T. et al. (2010) *J. Cogn. Neurosci.* **22**, 1819–1831.

84. Irish, M., Graham, A., Graham, K.S., Hodges, J.R. et al. (2012) *Arch. Clin. Neuropsychol.* **27**, 338–347.

85. Cappelletti, M., Butterworth, B., and Kopelman, M. (2012) *Neuropsychology* **26**, 1–19.

86. Jefferies, E., Patterson, K., Jones, R.W., Bateman, D. et al. (2004) *Neuropsychologia* **42**, 639–660.

87. Hodges, J.R., Bozeat, S., Lambon Ralph, M.A., Patterson, K. et al. (2000) *Brain* **123**, 1913–1925.

88. Bozeat, S., Lambon Ralph, M.A., Patterson, K., and Hodges, J.R. (2002) *Cogn. Affect. Behav. Neurosci.* **2**, 236–251.

89. Bozeat, S., Lambon Ralph, M.A., Patterson, K., and Hodges, J.R. (2002) *Neurocase* **8**, 127–134.

90. Hodges, J.R., Spatt, J., and Patterson, K. (1999) *Proc. Natl. Acad. Sci. USA* **96**, 9444–9448.

91. Green, H.A. and Patterson, K. (2009) *Neuropsychologia* **47**, 569–576.

92. Patterson, K., Lambon Ralph, M.A., Jefferies, E., Woollams, A. et al. (2006) *J. Cogn. Neurosci.* **18**, 169–183.

93. Woollams, A.M., Cooper-Pye, E., Hodges, J.R., and Patterson, K. (2008) *Neuropsychologia* **46**, 2503–2514.

94. Brambati, S.M., Ogar, J., Neuhaus, J., Miller, B.L. et al. (2009) *Neuropsychologia* **47**, 1893–1900.

95. Hoffman, P., Evans, G.A., and Lambon Ralph, M.A. (2014) *Cortex* **50**, 19–31.

96. Lambon Ralph, M.A., Sage, K., Jones, R.W., and Mayberry, E.J. (2010) *Proc. Natl. Acad. Sci. USA* **107**, 2717–2722.

97. Mayberry, E.J., Sage, K., and Lambon Ralph, M.A. (2011) *J. Cogn. Neurosci.* **23**, 2240–2251.

98. Martin, A. and Chao, L.L. (2001) *Curr. Opin. Neurobiol.* **11**, 194–201.

99. Gainotti, G. (2012) *Cortex* **48**, 521–529.

100. Olson, I.R., McCoy, D., Klobusicky, E., and Ross, L.A. (2013) *Soc. Cogn. Affect. Neurosci.* **8**, 123–133.

101. Zahn, R., Moll, J., Krueger, F., Huey, E.D. et al. (2007) *Proc. Natl. Acad. Sci. USA* **104**, 6430–6435.

102. Pascual, B., Masdeu, J.C., Hollenbeck, M., Makris, N. et al. (2015) *Cereb. Cortex* **25**, 680–702.

103. Rogers, T.T., Lambon Ralph, M.A., Garrard, P., Bozeat, S. et al. (2004) *Psychol. Rev.* **111**, 205–235.

104. Rosch, E., Mervis, C.B., Gray, W., Johnson, D. et al. (1976) *Cogn. Psychol.* **8**, 382–439.

105. Rogers, T.T. and Patterson, K. (2007) *J. Exp. Psychol. Gen.* **136**, 451–469.

106. Warrington, E.K. and McCarthy, R. (1983) *Brain* **106**, 859–878.

107. Warrington, E.K. and Shallice, T. (1984) *Brain* **107**, 829–854.

108. Lambon Ralph, M.A., Ehsan, S., Baker, G.A., and Rogers, T.T. (2012) *Brain* **135**, 242–258.

109. Schapiro, A.C., McClelland, J.L., Welbourne, S.R., Rogers, T.T. et al. (2013) *J. Cogn. Neurosci.* **25**, 2107–2123.

110. Lambon Ralph, M.A., Pobric, G., and Jefferies, E. (2009) *Cereb. Cortex* **19**, 832–838.

111. Pobric, G., Jefferies, E., and Lambon Ralph, M.A. (2010) *Curr. Biol.* **20**, 964–968.

112. Pobric, G., Jefferies, E., and Lambon Ralph, M.A. (2007) *Proc. Natl. Acad. Sci. USA* **104**, 20137–20141.

113. Pobric, G., Jefferies, E., and Lambon Ralph, M.A. (2010) *Neuropsychologia* **48**, 1336–1342.

114. Lambon Ralph, M.A., McClelland, J.L., Patterson, K., Galton, C.J. et al. (2001) *J. Cogn. Neurosci.* **13**, 341–356.

115. Devlin, J.T., Russell, R.P., Davis, M.H., Price, C.J. et al. (2000) *NeuroImage* **11**, 589–600.

116. Visser, M., Jefferies, E., and Lambon Ralph, M.A. (2010) *J. Cogn. Neurosci.* **22**, 1083–1094.

117. Binder, J.R., Desai, R.H., Graves, W.W., and Conant, L.L. (2009) *Cereb. Cortex* **19**, 2767–2796.

118. Halai, A.D., Welbourne, S.R., Embleton, K., and Parkes, L.M. (2014) *Hum. Brain Mapp.* **35**, 4118–4128.

119. Visser, M., Jefferies, E., Embleton, K.V., and Lambon Ralph, M.A. (2012) *J. Cogn. Neurosci.* **24**, 1766–1778.

120. Visser, M. and Lambon Ralph, M.A. (2011) *J. Cogn. Neurosci.* **23**, 3121–3131.

121. Spitsyna, G., Warren, J.E., Scott, S.K., Turkheimer, F.E. et al. (2006) *J. Neurosci.* **26**, 7328–7336.

122. Jefferies, E. and Lambon Ralph, M.A. (2006) *Brain* **129**, 2132–2147.

123. Noonan, K.A., Jefferies, E., Corbett, F., and Lambon Ralph, M.A. (2010) *J. Cogn. Neurosci.* **22**, 1597–1613.

124. Jefferies, E., Rogers, T.T., Hopper, S., and Lambon Ralph, M.A. (2010) *Neuropsychologia* **48**, 248–261.

125. Thompson-Schill, S.L., D'Esposito, M., Aguirre, G.K., and Farah, M.J. (1997) *Proc. Natl. Acad. Sci. USA* **94**, 14792–14797.

126. Wagner, A.D., Pare-Blagoev, E.J., Clark, J., and Poldrack, R.A. (2001) *Neuron* **31**, 329–338.

127. Badre, D., Poldrack, R.A., Pare-Blagoev, E.J., Insler, R.Z. et al. (2005) *Neuron* **47**, 907–918.

128. Whitney, C., Grossman, M., and Kircher, T.T. (2009) *Cereb. Cortex* **19**, 2548–2560.

129. Noonan, K.A., Jefferies, E., Visser, M., and Lambon Ralph, M.A. (2013) *J. Cogn. Neurosci.* **25**, 1824–1850.

130. Duncan, J. and Owen, A.M. (2000) *Trends Neurosci.* **23**, 475–483.

131. Whitney, C., Kirk, M., O'Sullivan, J., Lambon Ralph, M.A. et al. (2011) *Cereb. Cortex* **21**, 1066–1075.

132. Whitney, C., Kirk, M., O'Sullivan, J., Lambon Ralph, M.A. et al. (2012) *J. Cogn. Neurosci.* **24**, 133–147.

133. Binney, R.J., Parker, G.J., and Lambon Ralph, M.A. (2012) *J. Cogn. Neurosci.* **24**, 1998–2014.

134. Lakoff, G. (1987) *Women, Fire, and Dangerous Things* (University of Chicago Press, Chicago, IL).

135. Penn, D.C., Holyoak, K.J., and Povinelli, D.J. (2008) *Behav. Brain Sci.* **31**, 109–130.

136. Wood, J.N. and Grafman, J. (2003) *Nat. Rev. Neurosci.* **4**, 139–147.

137. Cowell, R.A., Bussey, T.J., and Saksida, L.M. (2010) *J. Cogn. Neurosci.* **22**, 2460–2479.

138. Lau, H. and Rosenthal, D. (2011) *Trends Cogn. Sci.* **15**, 365–373.

139. Passingham, R.E. and Wise, S.P. (2012) *The Neurobiology of the Prefrontal Cortex* (Oxford University Press, Oxford).

140. Gould, S.J. (1977) *Ever Since Darwin* (W. W. Norton, New York).

141. Eccles, J.C. (1981) *Neuroscience* **6**, 1839–1856.

142. Baars, B.J., Ramsoy, T.Z., and Laureys, S. (2003) *Trends Neurosci.* **26**, 671–675.

143. Gaffan, D. (2002) *Phil. Trans. R. Soc. B: Biol. Sci.* **357**, 1111–1121.

144. Mithen, S. (1996) *The Prehistory of the Mind* (Thames and Hudson, London).

145. Holyoak, K.J. and Morrison, R.G. (2012) *The Oxford Handbook of Thinking and Reasoning* (Oxford University Press, Oxford).

146. Plomin, R. and Spinath, F.M. (2002) *Trends Cogn. Sci.* **6**, 169–176.

147. Melnick, M.D., Harrison, B.R., Park, S., Bennetto, L. et al. (2013) *Curr. Biol.* **23**, 1013–1017.

Chapter 10

The social–subjective memory system of hominins

Overview

The granular prefrontal cortex expanded during hominin evolution, and, as it did, new and higher levels of hierarchy emerged among its specialized representations. According to our proposal, new species-specific representations of one's self and others developed in these areas as adaptations to hominin societies. As the hominin versions of these representations emerged, they began to influence older representational systems through two large-scale cortical networks. A medial network came to support perspective-taking, the recognition of situational contexts, the mental simulation of events in both the past and future, and knowledge about one's self and others gained from direct participatory experience. A lateral network came to represent social goals, norms, and concepts; categories and groups of individuals, along with their roles in society; and generalizations about one's self and others.

The horror!

> The mind of man is capable of anything—because everything is in it, all the past as well as the future.

Joseph Conrad[1] (*The Heart of Darkness*, p. 36)

In *The Heart of Darkness*, Conrad's enigmatic antihero, Kurtz, utters his famous dying words: "The horror! The horror!" We can only imagine what is going through his mind as he does so. And that is the point of this chapter: We *can* imagine what is going through his mind. Without direct evidence, without any experience of colonial Africa in the nineteenth century, and without dying ourselves, we can contemplate Kurtz's mental state as he considers the less savory aspects of "human nature." The human mind has "everything … in it, all the past as well as the future." Along with being a century-old statement about mental time travel and scenario construction, this quotation says something about memory, including the memory of fictional people like Kurtz.

In this chapter we advance the idea that evolving hominins developed new species-specific representations of self and others, which comprise the social–subjective memory system. This name draws on three meanings of the word subjective: the first emphasizes the fact that these representations pertain to the individual who has them; the second stresses an individual's traits; and the third deals with an individual's internal states. By representing our own intentions, for example, several cognitive feats become possible: we can assess and share the intentions of other people; we can develop both cooperative and competitive intentions; and we can devise social conventions[2,3]. As a result, subjective representations have a social aspect, hence the name social–subjective. "The horror," some will say, and they will have a point. But it serves our purposes well enough.

Two-chapter preview

This chapter and Chapter 11 go together in many respects, so a joint preview might be helpful. After considering the expansion of the granular prefrontal cortex during hominin evolution and presenting this chapter's proposal, we discuss some mechanisms of social cognition in anthropoid monkeys. Then we examine how new representations of one's self and others might have arisen in hominins. Several emergent properties resulted from this development, including an ability to infer the intentions of others and to generate socially appropriate goals. This chapter concludes with an examination of two large-scale cortical networks that mediate the influence of social–subjective representations over the older goal, feature, and navigation systems, including the anterior temporal lobe semantic hub (see Chapter 9, "Temporal–prefrontal networks"). Semantic memory allows people to develop generalizations about society, as well as subtle distinctions among social groups, categories of people, roles in society, personality types, individual capabilities, and social stature, all of which apply to one's self as well as others.

Then, in Chapter 11, we consider how social–subjective representations could have contributed to the emergence of explicit memory and when that might have occurred during evolution. According to the proposal we present in Chapter 11, representations of self lead to the perception of participating in events and knowing facts. Taken together, these perceptions characterize episodic and semantic memory as modern humans experience these traits.

Evolution

In Chapter 9 we discussed two evolutionary developments in hominins: generalized relational reasoning and semantic generalization. This chapter adds the idea that hominins also developed a new representational system, which underlies knowledge about one's self and others.

Social factors

Proposals about uniquely human traits inevitably incite debate, which rarely settles very much. To avoid some of the more obvious problems, we emphasize that our proposal does not imply that other species lack representations of themselves or conspecifics. We know that other species, and in particular our closest relatives, do have such representations. These species seem to infer the goals of conspecifics; distinguish among their intentions; recognize social signals from the eyes, face, and body; and engage in intentional deception, among many other social interactions[4-6]. To some extent, every animal that processes information about its own actions or motor commands possesses an element of self-representation[7]. So what we propose should be no more controversial, at least at the outset, than the claim that every member of every species represents itself and others in its own way.

Up to this point we have paid scant attention to social cognition. One reason is that primates passed through an evolutionary stage in which social interactions occurred mainly among dispersed, nocturnal animals. Early primates[8], like most modern strepsirrhines[9], probably lacked the gregarious interdependency that evolved in later primates, and especially among anthropoids[10-12]. This means that whatever neural substrates underlie social cognition in anthropoids, most of them emerged or re-emerged during primate evolution, independent of similar developments in other mammalian lineages.

Given the importance of anthropoid social systems, it should come as little surprise that the size of certain brain areas[13,14] and the total amount of neocortex[10,11,15] correlate with social complexity. Dunbar and Shultz[11], for example, conclude that the complexity of social groups, together with total brain size and longevity, have a major influence on neocortical extent. These three factors accounted for 67% of the variance in their data. The neocortex makes up so much of the primate brain that the brain size factor tells us little, which leaves social complexity and life span as the most informative covariates in their analysis.

In comparing primates with other mammals, Dunbar and Shultz stress the importance of social complexity, rather than group size per se[11,16]. Accordingly, Fig. 10.1(A) plots the percentage of the brain taken up by neocortex plotted against the mean size of social cliques for each species, rather than against mean group size. Clique size is defined as the number of individuals that interact with each other more than expected by chance; group size will often include individuals that rarely interact. The diversity of social systems among anthropoids obscures any relationship between these two variables. Nevertheless, it is clear that chimpanzees and bonobos ("X" in Fig. 10.1A) have a higher percentage of neocortex as well as larger clique sizes than do strepsirrhines (black circles). A grade shift appears to have occurred in anthropoids and again in the ape–human lineage.

Many other variables also correlate with the size of the neocortex[11], including life-history factors such as maturation rate and reproductive rate. Reproductive rate, for example, affects longevity, which in turn influences growth rate and brain size. Body size, brain size, and basal metabolic rate have a strong influence on the amount of neocortex a given species can develop. Likewise, a species must adapt its diet in order to provide sufficient energy to support large amounts of a tissue as expensive as neocortex. Some experts take such covariation as evidence against social complexity as a selective force for increases in neocortical extent[17]. The fact that other factors also affect the size of the neocortex, however, does not contradict a contribution from group complexity[16].

Figure 10.1(B) illustrates one model of how some of the key factors interact. It suggests that predation threats served as a selective pressure for larger group size, with many

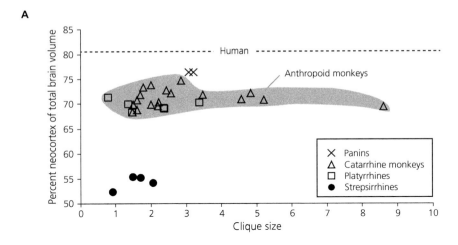

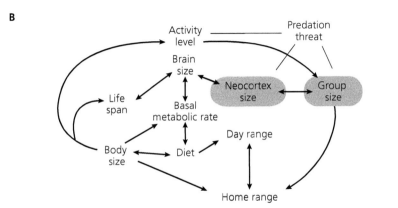

Fig. 10.1 Clique size and brain size. (A) Plot of the percentage of total brain volume taken up by neocortex, as a function of clique size. The gray shaded area shows the anthropoid range. The dashed horizontal line for humans reflects the difficulty in estimating ancestral hominin group sizes, so we do not specify an abscissa value for these data. (B) Path analysis of factors constraining the coordinated evolution of social complexity and the size of the neocortex (shaded areas). (B) Redrawn from Dunbar RIM, Shultz S. Understanding primate brain evolution. *Philosophical Transactions of the Royal Society of London B: Biological Sciences* 362:649–58, © 2007, by permission of the Royal Society. (A) Data from the same source.

interacting variables influencing the expansion of the neocortex, directly and indirectly[11]. Presumably, cognitive advantages balance the fitness costs that accompany large, energetically expensive brains[18].

Although the relative importance of social factors remains subject to debate, there is no doubt that the brain and neocortex expanded dramatically during hominin evolution. As explained in Chapter 2 ("Overall brain expansion"), early hominins had a brain roughly in the size range of modern chimpanzees, relative to body size. The encephalization quotient quantifies this statement. As the right part of Fig. 10.2(A) illustrates, this measure corresponds to the ratio of observed brain size to that predicted on the basis of body size, in this case for apes. The left part of Fig. 10.2(A) shows encephalization quotients for modern chimpanzees (gray square), modern humans (unfilled square), and extinct hominins (circles). Modern humans have encephalization quotients of well over 5 (brains of 1300–1500 cm^3 in bodies of 50–70 kg), whereas chimpanzees make do with a value of about 2 (brains of 300–400 cm^3 in bodies of 30–60 kg). Early hominins (black circles) had values a little larger than modern chimpanzees, and their descendants underwent several phases of brain expansion (Fig. 10.2A, Plate 6).

Regional expansion

Not only did the brain as a whole expand during hominin evolution, but so did the prefrontal cortex (see Chapter 9, "Evolution"). Readers familiar with the literature on cortical evolution might find this statement controversial. It is not. Modern humans have several-fold more prefrontal cortex than any other primate, a fact accepted by every expert.

If this is so, why does this literature contain so much debate? First, most studies of brain size take the absolute expansion of the prefrontal cortex for granted and so rarely emphasize this fact. Second, there are serious problems with the methods used for subdividing the cortex. In studies of the prefrontal cortex, for example, too much turns on where neuroanatomists draw its boundary with the premotor areas. Or, if they avoid this problem, these studies weaken their conclusions by lumping the primary motor, premotor, and prefrontal areas together as the frontal lobe, which obscures the contribution from prefrontal areas. Third, many of the databases used for brain-size analysis suffer from insufficient sampling, among other problems.

But the fourth and greatest reason for controversy involves allometric analysis. We touched on this topic in Chapter 9 ("Evolution"), but here we concentrate on the prefrontal cortex because it is central to the proposal in this chapter. Allometric analysis focuses on whether the prefrontal cortex expanded more than predicted by regressions based on the brains of other primates (or sometimes apes). The volume of prefrontal cortex, for example, can be plotted against the volume of the rest of the brain or the rest of the cortex. One such analysis[19,20], for example, addressed whether size estimates of the human prefrontal cortex (or various parts of it) deviated significantly from the allometric prediction for an ape or anthropoid brain scaled up to human size. The amount of human prefrontal cortex (Fig. 10.2B, unfilled circle) corresponded to that prediction. At first glance this finding seems to contradict the idea that the prefrontal cortex expanded during hominin evolution, but for reference Fig. 10.2(B) includes a vertical bar that corresponds to a five-fold difference in absolute size. Debates about allometric predictions sometimes obscure the importance of an expansion that "merely" matches an allometric prediction or is "merely" proportionate. Although the density of cells falls off in the prefrontal cortex compared with other areas, the human prefrontal cortex still has many more neurons than in any other primate[21]. In Chapter 9 ("Evolution") we explained that new representations can emerge in neural networks as they increase in absolute size.

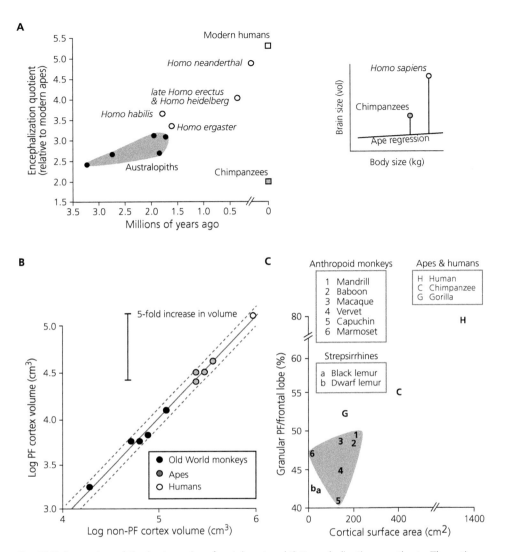

Fig. 10.2 Expansion of the brain and prefrontal cortex. (A) Encephalization quotients: The ratio of observed brain volume to the volume predicted for an ape of a given body size. Circles, fossil hominins; squares, modern species. In this figure the formal names of fossil humans, *Homo neanderthalensis* and *Homo heidelbergensis*, have been shortened to *Homo neanderthal* and *Homo heidelberg*, respectively. The gray shaded regions shows the anthropoid range. The inset to the right illustrates encephalization quotients for chimpanzees and humans, to scale. (B) Plot of prefrontal cortex size versus other cortex. (C) Granular prefrontal (PF) cortex as a percentage of the frontal lobe versus the surface area of the cortex as a whole. The gray shaded region shows the anthropoid range. (A) Adapted from Klein RG. *The Human Career*, © 2009, The University of Chicago Press. (B) Redrawn from Barton RA, Venditti C. Human frontal lobes are not relatively large. *Proceedings of the National Academy of Sciences U.S.A.* 110:9001–6, © 2013, with permission. (C) Adapted from Elston GN, Benavides-Piccione R, Elston A, Zietsch B, DeFelipe J, Manger P, Casagrande V, Kaas JH. Specializations of the granular prefrontal cortex of primates: implications for cognitive processing. *Anatomical Record Part A: Discoveries in Molecular, Cellular, and Evolutionary Biology* 288:26–35, © 2006, John Wiley & Sons.

The roughly contemporaneous expansion of several cortical regions also plagues allometric studies that focus on the prefrontal cortex. As mentioned in Chapter 9, Plates 2(C) and 3(C) show that premotor areas and major parts of both the lateral temporal and inferior parietal cortex all expanded during hominin evolution, as did the insular cortex[22]. Accordingly, the lack of selective expansion of the prefrontal cortex, relative to the brain or neocortex as a whole, might reflect the (roughly) contemporaneous expansion of several cortical regions[23].

Despite all this, two observations bring allometric analysis into perspective.

- First, the granular prefrontal cortex takes up a much greater proportion of the frontal lobe in humans than in other anthropoids, including apes[24], as shown by the data plotted on the ordinate of Fig. 10.2(C). Much more of the human frontal lobe (point H) consists of granular prefrontal cortex than in apes (points C and G), anthropoid monkeys (points 1–6), or strepsirrhines (points a and b). When the abscissa is also taken into account, the plot shows how this proportion varies as a function of cortical extent. This analysis does not contradict the plot in Fig. 10.2(B), but it helps place allometric scaling in perspective. As the volume of prefrontal cortex scaled up (Fig. 10.2B), an increasingly large proportion of the frontal lobe came to consist of granular prefrontal cortex (Fig. 10.2C).

- Second, in humans, the ratio of the prefrontal cortex to a reasonable reference area—the primary visual (striate) cortex (V1)—markedly exceeds the ratio observed for chimpanzees or anthropoid monkeys, even taking allometry into account[23]. Put another way, the volume of human prefrontal cortex exceeds that predicted for an anthropoid that has a striate cortex of the size that humans have—and dramatically so (see Fig. 2.14C, D).

Summary

We leave these debates to others because our proposal does not depend on their outcome all that much. This chapter's proposal depends on the emergence, during hominin evolution, of new and higher levels of representation of one's self and others. These innovations could have resulted from the expansion of the prefrontal cortex in absolute terms and the resulting increase in its number of neurons[21], interconnections[25–27], and other aspects of internal organization[28] or plasticity[29]. So even without taking into account allometry, the possibility of new areas, or factors such as dendritic branching, spine density, and spine number[24,25], comparative neuroanatomy provides ample support for our proposal.

Proposal

The social–subjective system specializes in representations of one's self and others, some of which developed as adaptations to hominin societies. The emergence of these representations depended on an expansion of the granular prefrontal cortex and new, higher levels of representational hierarchy that developed there. Once they evolved, species-specific social–subjective representations enabled hominins to attend to their

own intentions and perceptions and to estimate those of others. Social–subjective rep-
resentations influenced older representational systems through two large-scale cortical
networks. (1) Through interactions between social–subjective representations and an
extended hippocampal–navigation system (along with other parts of a medial network),
hominins engaged in perspective-taking; recognized situational contexts; gained knowl-
edge about themselves and others from direct participatory experience; employed men-
tal trial and error behavior and other constructive simulations of events; and established
memories of these mental activities. (2) Through interactions between social–subjective
representations and the semantic hub of the anterior temporal lobe, its associated spoke
areas, and other parts of a lateral network, hominins learned about categories of con-
specifics; concepts concerning their roles in society; generalizations about groups and
individuals, including themselves; and socially appropriate goals. Collectively, these
memories reduced foraging and social errors—or avoided them entirely.

Ancestral mechanisms

Taking into account the relative social isolation inferred for early primates, which is a characteristic of most modern strepsirrhines[8,9], some mechanisms for social cognition appear to have descended from innovations that occurred just prior to the last common ancestor of humans and monkeys or a close relative of that ancestral species. Chang et al.[30] suggest that mechanisms for nonsocial cognition became repurposed for social functions at about that time.

Three findings serve as our starting point:

- In one study, monkeys with lesions of two parts of the medial prefrontal cortex—the anterior cingulate gyrus and the prelimbic cortex—spent less time near other monkeys than control monkeys did[31].

- For cortical activations, resting-state correlations (coupling) between the anterior cingulate gyrus and the superior temporal cortex predicted the size of a monkey's social group[32].

- In another study, the size of a monkey's social group and an individual's social status correlated with gray matter volume in a group of cortical areas that included the rostral and dorsal parts of the prefrontal cortex and a middle part of the superior temporal cortex[32,33].

We have already cited evidence in humans that brain size (including the size of some areas homologous to those just mentioned) is correlated with social complexity[13,14], and later we discuss activations in prefrontal, anterior cingulate, and temporal areas during tasks that involved social cognition[34], such as making judgments about the behavioral traits and knowledge of other people.

Medial prefrontal areas also contribute to the valuation of social stimuli. These areas are well situated for mediating social emotions, rewards, and punishments, in part because they are either part of or have close connections with the ring neocortex (often called "limbic cortex")[35,36]. Striatal components of cortex–basal ganglia "loops," with their dopaminergic inputs, also contribute to valuations, as do inputs from the amygdala.

In one experiment on social valuations, monkeys had to reach near a video monitor in order to retrieve food[37]. Sometimes the monitor displayed a video clip of other monkeys showing a body part, such as a face or rump, that provided a social signal. When control monkeys viewed such video clips, they took significantly longer to retrieve the food, an indirect measure of the value they attached to socially relevant images. Monkeys with lesions of the medial prefrontal cortex did not show this social-valuation effect, indicating that they did not value social videos as much as control monkeys did. Like control monkeys, however, the lesioned monkeys increased their food-retrieval latency when reaching near an artificial snake, so the lesion effect seems to be specific to socially relevant stimuli.

Neurophysiological results also implicate the medial prefrontal cortex in social cognition. In one experiment, neurons in the anterior cingulate cortex encoded the distinction between self and others, as well as the identity of actors (agents) in conjunction with the actions they perform[38,39]. In another, pairs of monkeys performed a prisoner's dilemma task that provided different amounts of reward depending on joint choices among a small set of visual cues. In this task, anterior cingulate neurons signaled the anticipated actions of the monkey's partner[40]. An analysis of neuronal activity during the vicarious reinforcement task also revealed a role for the anterior cingulate cortex in social interactions[41,42]. In this experiment, if an actor monkey had no possibility of obtaining a reward on a given trial it could choose to either provide a reward to another monkey or ensure that no reward occurred on that trial. Neurons in the anterior cingulate cortex signaled rewards to both the actor and the partner monkey. In contrast, neurons in the granular orbitofrontal cortex encoded only what the actor monkey received[42]. Granular orbitofrontal neurons also signaled rewards in a way that reflected a social context, including social preferences and an animal's rank in the social hierarchy[43].

Other experiments have shown that two parts of the medial prefrontal cortex—the anterior cingulate gyrus and cortex in the banks of the cingulate sulcus—display distinguishable functions. Lesions of the gyral cortex decreased the interest that monkeys displayed towards images of other monkeys, such as dominant males, but lesions of the sulcal cortex did not[37]. Likewise, neurons in the gyrus signaled the impending delivery of a reward to a partner monkey, but those in the sulcus did not[42].

Homologous mechanisms do not imply, however, that nothing has changed since the common ancestor of monkeys and humans. We know that a lot has. Were it otherwise, social systems among modern anthropoids would resemble each other more closely than they do. The abscissa of Fig. 10.1(A), for example, depicts extensive diversity among the anthropoids in clique size. According to our proposal, each species—living and extinct—has (or had) social representations adapted to its particular social systems.

Social–subjective representations

Re-representation in general

If each species represents itself and conspecifics in its own way, what distinguishes hominin self-representations from those in other animals? Our suggestion relies on the concept of re-representation, as elaborated by Lau and Rosenthal[44]. Re-representation, in this sense, refers to a high-level abstraction of information represented at lower levels of a cortical-processing hierarchy. In Chapter 9 ("Computational models") we advanced a similar idea for semantic memory. There we described a model in which a high-level hub abstracts information from spoke areas that represent the sensory modalities of direct experience. This hub enables high-level re-representations that are generalized across sensory modalities and cognitive domains.

Several theorists have suggested that the human prefrontal cortex has a hierarchical organization. Their proposals often include an escalating posterior-to-anterior hierarchy that represents: (1) different time frames for establishing a context or assessing values, with a concept of *time frame* that includes temporally extended (diachronic) events[45]; (2) different event frequencies[46]; or (3) different degrees of abstraction for either behavioral contexts[47] or behavioral plans[48]. Perhaps the most general idea along these lines holds that different levels of a prefrontal hierarchy represent different degrees of relational integration, with the highest levels (relations among relations) residing in its anterior parts[44,45,49,50]. Our proposal suggests that these prefrontal hierarchies incorporate new levels of representation that emerged during hominin evolution.

Re-representations of self and others

To consider how social–subjective representations arose in hominins, we build upon three ideas about frontal hierarchies and re-representation[44], one of which comes from Graziano and Kastner[51,52]. They propose that human representations of self differ from those of other animals, including closely related primate species, because of the particular kind of social system that hominins evolved, which requires a high degree of interdependency and cooperation.

The second idea, developed by Passingham and his colleagues[53], views re-representation as an aspect of attentive control (see Chapter 8, "Augmentation of the biased-competition system"). As we explained earlier, top-down attentive control from the prefrontal cortex enhances some representations at the expense of others, either by increasing the activity of neurons preferring the favored features, by suppressing cells with opposing preferences, or both. These influences enhance the likelihood that attended features will have a selective impact on behavior. By applying these concepts to re-representational hierarchies within the medial prefrontal cortex, Passingham et al.[53] suggest that by directing attention to one's own actions and intentions, anterior parts of the medial prefrontal cortex subserve self-reflection and self-awareness.

Graziano and Kastner[51,52,54] also stress an attentional perspective. They suggest that representations of one's self arise from second-order representations of one's own attentional states, which the brain interprets as the perception of knowing, localized to one's self. According to this idea, neural networks that mediate attention to sensory stimuli also mediate attention to attentional states, which leads to the identification of our "selves" with our knowledge, location, and experiences. Their proposal builds on the idea that a network of brain regions that represents the mental states of others also underlies representations of one's self (see "Attention to others")—namely the medial prefrontal cortex, cortex near the temporal–parietal junction, cortex in the banks of the superior temporal sulcus, and the anterior temporal lobe. The concept of self results, in part, from localizing attended perceptions, intentions, and internal states to one's own body. The inference that someone else has some perception, intention, or state corresponds to an analogous attribution to that person's body. Consistent with these ideas, stimulation of cortex near the right temporal–parietal junction—an area associated with a sense of agency[55] and activated in theory of mind tasks[56]—has produced an illusion called the "out-of-body" experience[57]. This observation shows that the localization of one's self, usually centered on one's own body, can on occasion be wrong.

The third idea regarding frontal hierarchies and re-representations recognizes the need to consider both cognitive processes and knowledge when discussing cortical function, a theme that has come up repeatedly in previous chapters (see Chapter 8, "Proposal", for example). In theories of the prefrontal cortex, processes have received the most emphasis, sometimes with little consideration of the knowledge stored in the same areas[58]. If the human capacity for self-reflection stems from attention to one's own internal states, intentions, and actions[51–54], what *knowledge* guides this process?

Our general answer is that high-level re-representations[44] do. Two analogies might help explain this idea. The first draws on concepts about sensory attention. Just as a top-down bias from the prefrontal cortex to sensory areas *promotes the perception of attended stimulus features* (Fig. 10.3A), analogous interactions within the prefrontal cortex *promote the perception of attended intentions* (Fig. 10.3B), and the same idea applies to attended actions, perceptions, and other internal states. The second analogy incorporates memory into this idea by considering what happens when the prefrontal cortex directs attention to representations in sensory areas (Fig. 10.3A): *a perception results and this information can be stored in memory*. When the prefrontal cortex directs attention to representations of one's own intentions or other internal states, the same principle applies: *a perception results and this information can be stored in memory*. Two parallel examples elucidate this idea:

◆ Upon seeing a labradoodle, one might perceive certain sensory features of the dog, such as its brown, woolly coat. This information can be stored in memory, both for meeting the dog (an episodic memory) and as a generalization about labradoodles (a semantic memory).

◆ Upon attending to one's own intention to run a marathon, one might perceive certain representational features of the exercise, such as the prospect of excruciating exertion. This information can be stored in memory, both for the generation of that intention (an episodic memory) and as a generalization about running marathons (a semantic memory).

Successive re-representations of this kind can build hierarchies to a very high level, leading to second-order, third-order, and higher-order intentions. At each level, a higher-order neural network abstracts information from lower-order networks, as an emergent

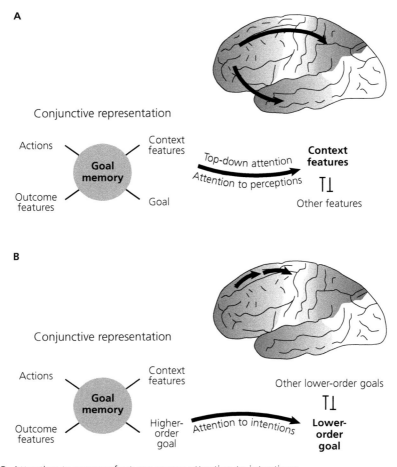

Fig. 10.3 Attention to sensory features versus attention to intentions.

property of inter-network dynamics. It is these emergent properties that provide the power that drives the development of episodic and semantic memory, as we explore in Chapter 11.

Summary

According to the proposal in this chapter, representations of one's self and others result from re-representations of attended perceptions, intentions, and other internal states. During hominin evolution, the expansion of the granular prefrontal cortex permitted these new and higher hierarchical levels to emerge (see "Regional expansion"). The re-representation of intentions plays a particularly important role in social cognition, in part because it contributes to a sense of agency and in part because it underlies inferences about the intentions of others.

Medial prefrontal cortex

Representations of one's self

Our proposal suggests that social–subjective representations initially emerged in the medial prefrontal cortex of hominins. The medial prefrontal cortex made its appearance earlier in this book, in Chapter 5, where we discussed its agranular areas and their role in regulating competing memories. In Chapter 2 ("Anthropoids") we explained that new granular prefrontal areas augmented these older, agranular prefrontal areas, and in Chapter 8 (see Fig. 8.1) we included both the granular and agranular prefrontal areas in a processing pathway for goals and actions.

Passingham et al.[53] describe something important about the medial prefrontal cortex, as reflected in a pattern of peak activations. For cortical locations distributed from posterior to anterior (Fig. 10.4A), these peaks reflected:

- attention to one's actions (peak 1);
- attention to one's intentions (peak 2);
- attention to one's internal states, such as hunger, emotions[59], and heart rate[60,61] (peaks 3, 4, and 5);
- evaluation of whether a trait applies to one's self[62,63] (peak 6);
- evaluation of one's own behavior (peak 7);
- retrieval of autobiographical events (two peaks labelled 8).

Retrieval of autobiographical events also activated the medial frontal-pole cortex[64] (Fig.10.4B, arrow) anterior to the sites labeled 8 in Fig. 10.4(A). The dorsomedial

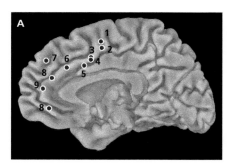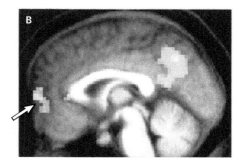

Fig. 10.4 Social–subjective activations. (A) Meta-analysis illustrating peak brain imaging loci for activations relevant to social–subjective knowledge. The numerals refer to the locations of activation peaks mentioned in the main text. (B) Activation in the medial frontal-pole cortex (arrow) and the posterior parietal cortex for the recall of real memories in contrast to imagined ones. (A) Adapted from Figure 9.7 in Passingham RE, Wise SP. *The Neurobiology of the Prefrontal Cortex*, © 2012, Oxford University Press. Reproduced with permission of OUP. (B) Modified from Hassabis D, Kumaran D, Maguire EA. Using imagination to understand the neural basis of episodic memory. *Journal of Neuroscience* 27:14365–74, © 2007, Society for Neuroscience, with permission.

prefrontal cortex and the medial frontal-pole cortex also became activated when subjects attended to their own mental states and personality traits[63,65]. Taken together, these activations point to a role for the medial prefrontal cortex in the subjective aspect of social–subjective representations. We take up the social aspect next.

Representations of others

Brain imaging studies have also revealed activations in the medial prefrontal cortex related to representing other people and making social calculations[34,66]. Reviews by Amodio and Frith[67] and by Graziano and Kastner[51,52] treat this literature in depth, so we address only selected points here.

Many brain imaging studies have indicated a close association between representations of one's self and others[51,52]. In a meta-analysis, Amodio and Frith[67] identify three parts of the medial prefrontal cortex that became activated when people related themselves to others:

◆ the presupplementary motor area for monitoring actions, whether of themselves or others;

◆ the anterior cingulate gyrus for predictions about rewards that others will receive;

◆ the ventromedial prefrontal cortex when people monitor emotions in themselves or others.

The first of these areas has a counterpart in an independently derived analysis of the medial prefrontal cortex, one based on resting-state activations and connections[68,69]. In this series of studies, four clusters of voxels corresponded to: (1) the supplementary motor area, (2) the presupplementary motor area, (3) the dorsomedial prefrontal cortex (medial area 9), and (4) the medial frontal-pole cortex (area 10) (see Plate 5C, D). The second cluster was situated dorsal to the gyral part of the anterior cingulate cortex, a region that we discussed earlier for monkeys (see "Ancestral mechanisms"). In general, the presupplementary motor area and anterior cingulate gyrus were activated when subjects monitored the actions of others, the rewards they received, or effort costs. More rostrally, activations occurred in the dorsomedial prefrontal and medial frontal-pole cortex, the third and fourth clusters, when people attended to the traits or states of others. Point 9 in Fig. 10.4(A) shows the location of one peak activation that occurred when people reflected on the thoughts and intentions of others[53], and Plate 5(A) shows some additional activation sites[68]. As mentioned earlier (see "Representations of one's self"), these areas also became activated when people attended to their own mental states and personality traits[63,65]. Stated generally, these areas seem to predict (or estimate) what other people will do, based in part on similarities or dissimilarities with one's self[70–72].

Activations also have occurred in the medial prefrontal cortex for interactions between social and subjective factors: for example when people received evaluations of their behavior from other people[73,74] and when they attended to traits attributed to them by others, called reflected self-knowledge. The medial prefrontal cortex also showed increased activation when subjects considered how to improve another person's emotional state[75], and the level of activation correlated with the degree of empathy a subject had with that individual[67].

In another brain imaging experiment, subjects learned from the experimenters whether they or another person needed to exert an effort in order to obtain some reward. In these circumstances[76]:

◆ The anterior cingulate sulcus showed activation that reflected the level of effort, regardless of who exerted it.

◆ The anterior cingulate gyrus showed activation that correlated with the net value of rewards that another person received.

◆ The nucleus accumbens showed activation that indicated the net value of rewards to one's self.

The first two findings differentiated the anterior cingulate sulcus and gyrus in a way that resembles the results mentioned earlier for monkeys (see "Ancestral mechanisms").

Another brain imaging result further underscored the interplay between social and subjective factors. In this experiment, pairs of subjects made choices for either themselves or a partner, based in part on their familiarity with their partner's preferences[77]. A large part of the medial prefrontal cortex, including the medial frontal-pole cortex, showed activation reflecting the relative value of chosen and unchosen options. When a subject made a choice based on his or her own valuations, ventral parts of the medial prefrontal cortex reflected that person's value preferences and dorsal parts signaled their partner's preferences. When the same subject made a choice based on their partner's preferences, the two regions switched roles: the ventral part signaled their partner's preferences and the dorsal part signaled their own. Ventromedial prefrontal areas therefore seem to represent the values of choices that are made, regardless of whose values they represent. In contrast, dorsomedial prefrontal areas model preferences per se.

Self-reference and memory

Representations of one's self not only contribute to social cognition and self-reflection, they also provide a memory advantage. In studies of the *self-reference effect*[78], recall improved when subjects remembered items that were relevant to themselves or were associated with self-referential judgments[79]. In these experiments, a memory enhancement occurred both for attended items and for contextual details such as sources[80].

Two sets of findings have identified the medial prefrontal cortex as playing a key role in mediating the self-reference effect. First, the level of activation there correlated with the magnitude of the memory enhancement[80]; second, lesions of the medial prefrontal cortex abolished this effect[81,82].

Similar activations have been reported for the posterior parietal cortex[80]. Specifically, when subjects actively chose an object, as opposed to passively observing another person's choice, they benefitted from the same memory enhancement as when they made self-referential judgments[83]. The medial prefrontal cortex was not significantly activated in this case, however; instead, cortex near the intraparietal sulcus was, presumably because of its relation to guiding and monitoring actions[83]. Apparently, either personal relevance or monitoring one's own actions can cause the self-reference effect, with the medial prefrontal cortex mediating the former.

Overall, this line of research leads to three conclusions: (1) processing self-referential information enhances memory; (2) the medial prefrontal cortex contributes to this effect; and (3) when people attend to self-referential information during learning, the brain areas involved in processing social–subjective information become activated, as they do later when people retrieve these memories. Accordingly, the medial prefrontal cortex appears to enhance memory retrieval when the encoding process stresses one's self or one's participation in learning. In Chapter 11, we advance the idea that a sense of participation provides the key feature that distinguishes explicit memories from memories of other kinds.

Summary

The medial prefrontal cortex represents actions, intentions, internal states, personal traits, experiences, evaluations, effort expenditure, and value preferences—both for one's self and others. Dorsal parts specialize in representing preferences that someone (one's self or a partner) has; ventral parts signal the preferences (of one's self or a partner) that guide choices[77].

These social–subjective memories provided evolving hominins with adaptive advantages in making delegated and mutual choices based, in part, on shared intentions, shared knowledge, and social conventions[2,3]. In addition to providing advantages in social cognition, reference to one's self during learning enhances recall[79].

Emergent properties

Representing mental states in others

We have mentioned the ability to read the thoughts and intentions of others. The phrase "theory of mind" usually applies to such mental activities. This term refers, in part, to an ability to estimate the knowledge, states, perceptions, and intentions of others, as well as the perception that one knows about such things[53,67,84–89]. An extensive literature deals with the distinction between simulation-based and knowledge-based assessments, and both probably contribute to a theory of mind.

Discussions of human social systems often stress the interplay between cooperation and competition, and especially shared or conflicting intentions[2]. Our hominin ancestors required considerable cooperation within their band, but this interaction entailed an element of competition as well. Individuals competed to lead the group toward the goals that they deemed beneficial, and early hominins also competed with bands of conspecifics and other hominin species. Fear and loathing, often aimed at other groups, surely goes back to early hominins[90]. Both competition and cooperation benefit from representing the mental states of others.

Competition and cooperation also depend on abstract rules that guide social choices. By way of sampling this extensive literature, we highlight two representative findings: one based on lesion effects, the other based on brain imaging. During the ultimatum game, patients with lesions of the dorsomedial prefrontal cortex made more unfair offers than control subjects did, but nevertheless knew and could explain the more socially appropriate behavior[91]. This finding indicates that the medial prefrontal cortex contributes to social choices and goals and that other areas support the knowledge of social rules. In accord with this idea, activation occurred in the dorsomedial prefrontal cortex when people chose whether to accept an unfair offer[92,93].

Perhaps the most well-known work on representing others comes from Damasio and his colleagues[94,95], who emphasize second-order representations of bodily states. They propose that understanding the thoughts, beliefs, feelings, and intentions of others begins with the representation of one's own internal state, as exemplified by autonomic signals[96]. This idea builds on the "somatic marker" hypothesis for decision making, which holds that people make choices based on autonomic and other bodily signals, "gut feelings" that the brain generates automatically based on a recognized context[97]. For assessments about other people, the key representations involve understanding or inferring how others experience their own somatic markers. People could, for example, simulate the bodily states of others, imagining themselves in the same situation in order to understand how others "feel" and what they might do. Damasio and his colleagues attribute such functions to the ventromedial prefrontal cortex, as a central component of self-representation that corresponds to self-awareness and the recognition of one's own agency. Other aspects of self-representation include introspection (metacognition and self-reflection) and representations of facts about one's self (semantic memory).

These ideas probably capture some important aspects of how people represent themselves and others, but they leave out a great deal[98,99]. The representation of internal states probably plays a more important role in empathy than in the more cognitive (and less emotional) aspects of a theory of mind, such as inferring the intentions and social knowledge of others. Furthermore, given that many internal states yield outward signs of expression, a direct sensory analysis of other people seems a more straightforward way of inferring their feelings than simulating their emotional states and markers, although all of these factors could contribute. Indeed, the ability to read emotions based on sensory signs, such as the redness of skin, might be a shared derived trait of anthropoid primates, particularly catarrhines[100,101].

In synthesizing these and related findings, Forbes and Grafman[102] emphasize the less affect-related aspects of a theory of mind. They view the capacity for a theory of mind as encompassing a broad range of social and moral knowledge, including the perceptions and goals of other people, with the medial prefrontal cortex serving as the storage site for memories of socially relevant events[103]. In support of this idea, activations occurred in the dorsomedial prefrontal and medial frontal-pole cortex when subjects told another person about social interactions and when they passed judgment about whether a sequence of events met social norms[104–106]. This kind of knowledge requires much more than "gut feelings." Furthermore, the contribution of the medial prefrontal cortex to a theory of mind is more complex than simply inferring the intentions of other people and their other internal states; it also involves the kind of person under consideration. We explain what we mean by a "kind of person" in the next section.

Goals appropriate to categories of other people

A patient with a large bilateral lesion of her medial prefrontal cortex provides some insight into theory-of-mind localization[107]. She could perform several standard tests for a theory of mind, which seems surprising given the brain imaging findings summarized earlier. Although this patient had a severe impairment in recalling autobiographical events, she could understand the intentions of others when tested with picture sequences or animations. She also recognized violations of social norms and passed a *faux pas* test that required an assessment of awkward or embarrassing social situations. Other cases have produced similar observations[95,108], which indicates that areas beyond the medial prefrontal cortex can support a theory of mind, at least as assessed with these standard tests.

Several ideas could account for these results. One appeals to distributed networks in a general sense[95], suggesting that no one region plays a necessary role in representing the mental states of other people. A more specific idea holds that some aspects of a theory of mind concern generalizations about all people, whereas others pertain to specific groups or to individuals[109]. Distinct and anatomically distributed cortical areas might specialize according to these different hierarchical levels. Yet another account stresses the generation of goals based on the inferred mental states of others, rather than a theory of mind per se[110]. The medial prefrontal cortex might specialize in the former, with other areas supporting the latter.

In an experiment that combines the last two ideas[110], subjects attempted to communicate with someone they believed to be either an adult or a child, while playing a video board game. They played the game by moving a video image with a cursor, and, as far as they knew, either a mature or immature partner in another room saw the same display and used it to achieve some goal. Control subjects transmitted information more slowly when they believed they were communicating with a child, but patients with lesions of the ventromedial prefrontal cortex did not. Furthermore, these patients failed to slow their signals after communicative failures, as control subjects did. An account in terms of goal generation agrees with the proposal we presented in Chapter 8; the prefrontal cortex generates goals based on contexts. In this case, the context included a particular category of individual—either a child or an adult—and inferences about that partner's capabilities. Patients with lesions of the ventromedial prefrontal cortex can sometimes tailor their communications to a particular audience, taking into account their gender for example[95]. The experiment summarized here, however, combined two factors; not only did the context depend on a social category (a child versus an adult), but the goal-generation process involved object-like stimuli and places on a video monitor. In Chapter 8 we explained the importance of the prefrontal cortex in generating such goals.

Illusions of otherness

People have such a strong and automatic sense of otherness that it produces a peculiar illusion. In a classic experiment, when people saw videos of animated geometric figures, such as circles or triangles, apparently interacting with each other, they attributed intentions[111] and emotions[112] to these shapes. Everyone knows, of course, that geometric forms have no such properties, but the illusion of otherness combined with apparently purposeful movement remains powerful all the same.

These illusions, like the visual ones mentioned in Chapter 7 ("Perception, action, and actuality") reflect millions of years of evolution. According to our proposals, the prefrontal cortex represents both other people (see "Representations of others") and goals (see Chapter 8), and, when these representations combine, humans automatically draw inferences about the intentions (goals) of other people. Likewise, when representations of objects and goals combine, people experience the illusion that an object has intentions. As a result, people automatically attribute intentions to just about anything that moves.

Illusions of otherness might seem maladaptive, but the attribution of intentions to inanimate objects probably did evolving hominins little harm. Indeed, attributing human-like intentions to animals might have provided advantages. Anthropomorphism, the attribution of human-like cognition to animals, lies at the heart of popular opinion about animal intelligence, not to mention the "rights" of lobsters. These ideas seem farfetched in modern times, at least to experts, but anthropomorphism probably helped early hominins deal with the animals in their midst.

Medial network

So far in this chapter we have focused on the medial prefrontal cortex, but social–subjective representations influence many other cortical areas as well. Brain imaging studies have identified a large-scale cortical network consisting mainly of medial areas: the medial prefrontal cortex, including anterior cingulate areas, along with the posterior cingulate, precuneus, medial parietal, retrosplenial, parahippocampal, subicular, and hippocampal cortex[113]. Activations have been observed in the posterior cingulate and precuneus cortex, for example, in tasks involving self-reflection[89,114,115], a theory of mind[67,88], and mentalizing about events involving one's self in both the future[116,117] and the past[118,119]. A collection of pathways called the cingulum bundle links the hippocampus and retrosplenial cortex with a broad swath of medial prefrontal cortex, especially its agranular parts[120]. These areas are often called, collectively, a default-mode network[121,122], but this name does little to capture the adaptive advantages it provided to evolving hominins or confers on people today.

As Fig. 10.5(A) illustrates, the medial network (light gray shading) includes parts of the core neocortex, medial parts of the ring neocortex, and the medial allocortex (the hippocampus). The ring neocortex evolved in early mammals, the hippocampus dates to a much earlier ancestor, and the granular prefrontal cortex emerged much later, in

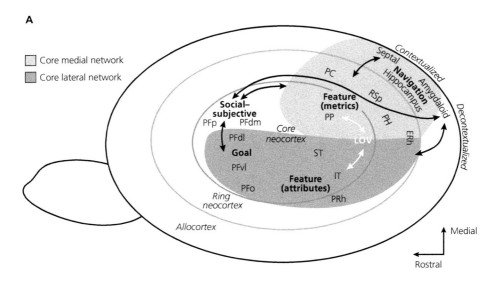

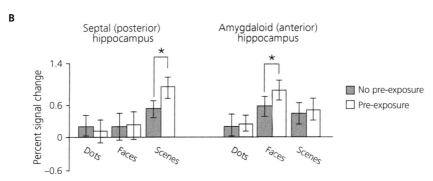

Fig. 10.5 Large-scale networks and specializations within the hippocampus. (A) Medial and lateral networks have interactions with both the social–subjective and navigation systems. The label for the amygdaloid hippocampus extends beyond the shaded area to indicate its association with the lateral network as well as the medial network. Abbreviations: ERh, entorhinal cortex; IT, inferior temporal cortex; LOV, low-order visual areas; PC, posterior cingulate cortex; PFdl, dorsolateral prefrontal cortex; PFdm, dorsomedial prefrontal cortex; PFo, granular orbitofrontal cortex; PFp, polar prefrontal (frontal-pole) cortex; PFvl, ventrolateral prefrontal cortex; PH, parahippocampal cortex; PP, posterior parietal cortex; PRh, perirhinal cortex; RSp, retrosplenial cortex; ST, superior temporal cortex. (B) Brain imaging evidence for a specialization within the hippocampus. Figure 7.8(A) illustrates the tasks, which involved perceptual learning about either dot patterns, scenes, or faces. Scene-sensitive voxels in the septal hippocampus showed selective activation for scenes (B, left) but not for faces (not illustrated). Face-sensitive voxels in the amygdaloid hippocampus showed selective activation for faces (B, right) but not scenes. (B) From Mundy ME, Downing PE, Dwyer DM, Honey RC, Graham KS. A critical role for the hippocampus and perirhinal cortex in perceptual learning of scenes and faces: complementary findings from amnesia and FMRI. *Journal of Neuroscience* 33:10490–502, © 2013, Society for Neuroscience, with permission.

anthropoids (see Chapter 2). According to our proposal, the later-evolving components of the medial network augmented the functions of the hippocampus, with the granular prefrontal cortex serving as the most recent addition.

Autobiographical memories

The medial network appears to play a central role in encoding and retrieving autobiographical memories[64,116,117,123]. In a study contrasting cortical activation during the recall of real and fictitious events, subjects were asked to remember some recent events in their lives as well as some fictional material and information about objects. Compared with object-based conditions, the retrieval of autobiographical events led to activations in the hippocampal, parahippocampal, retrosplenial, precuneus, and medial prefrontal cortex: in other words, much of the medial network. Three of these areas had higher activation for real memories than for fictional ones (Fig. 10.4B): the precuneus, posterior cingulate, and medial frontal-pole cortex. These parts of the cortex probably play some role in recalling what subjects actually experience, as opposed to what they imagine.

In a review of this literature, Schacter et al.[124] emphasize that not all of the medial network has the property just described. Some regions—and especially the hippocampus—have shown greater activation for fictional memories than for real ones. This difference might have resulted from the greater demands associated with creating fictitious memories, such as more constructive processing or a larger number of novel associations. Schacter et al. also point to specializations within the medial network. One component, more dorsally situated, appears to specialize in mentalizing generally, including imagining situations excluding one's self[123,125]. Another, which includes the posterior cingulate cortex, contributes mainly to self-referential functions, possibly functioning as a hub that integrates information from more specialized areas.

Overall, this line of research leads to three conclusions: (1) A medial network for autobiographical experiences includes the medial prefrontal, posterior cingulate, retrosplenial, and hippocampal cortex; (2) this network has both social and self-referential representations; and (3) autobiographical experience results from a constructive process that integrates information from different parts of the brain.

Constructive episodic simulation

The constructive process just mentioned goes by many names. Upon retrieving memories of past events, people often have the perception of traveling back in time, as if re-experiencing or observing the events[118]. Accordingly, the literature sometimes refers to this phenomenon as mental time travel[126].

Such mental activity need not be confined to the past, however; similar processes allow people to "play out" different approaches to problems, including strategies, routes, and sequences of actions[64,124,126–131]. This kind of cognitive activity sometimes goes by the term mental trial and error. By whatever name—mental time travel, mental trial and error, scenario construction, prospection, autobiographical simulation, social modeling, foresight, or future-thinking—the ability to imagine future events can prevent errors, in part through counterfactual thinking and learning from imaginary mistakes.

The phrase *constructive episodic simulation*[124,126,132–136] covers all of these processes. Rather than the temporal aspects of mentation—the time travel part—this label stresses the binding of disparate elements into coherent, conjunctive episodic representations. One consequence is the emergence of higher-level representations from lower-level ones. Not only does this idea apply to both actual experiences and fictitious ones, but it also applies to different kinds of fictions, such as imagining future events and revisionist histories. Indeed, people can rework previous and future events endlessly, reconstructing them in limitless varieties[137].

Two lines of evidence have indicated that the medial network underlies constructive episodic simulations, with specializations among its anterior and posterior components. First, when patients with lesions of the medial prefrontal cortex constructed narratives of future and past events they did so in the same detail as control subjects, but with significantly fewer references to themselves. Patients with lesions of the hippocampus made the same number of self-references as control subjects, but their narratives had significantly less detail[82]. So the medial prefrontal cortex seems to provide more self-referential information and the hippocampus provides more episodic detail. Second, when healthy subjects imagined events with an emphasis on their social elements, activations occurred in the dorsomedial prefrontal cortex, medial frontal-pole cortex, and posterior cingulate cortex, along with the anterior temporal lobe[138]. When they imagined the spatial aspects of such events, activations occurred in more posterior parts of the medial network, including the hippocampus. These findings support the idea that the medial prefrontal cortex contributes representations of one's self and others to the medial network.

The ability to imagine events leads to a requirement for what is sometimes called reality monitoring. Healthy people (nearly always) know whether a recollection involves a previously experienced event or a previously imagined one; and they also know the difference between having previously imagined an event and currently imagining one. In certain mental health and cognitive disorders, however, these distinctions can become distorted, with grave consequences. Along with the fitness advantages that constructive episodic simulations provided to evolving hominins, this derived trait probably produced some important vulnerabilities as well.

Situational contexts

As we explained in Chapter 2, a homologue of the hippocampus evolved in early vertebrates, and later-evolving neocortical areas augmented its function. In Chapter 4, which focused on the hippocampus, we said little about these supporting areas because early vertebrates lacked homologues of these structures. Researchers who study the human brain have no such luxury.

Augmented by neocortical areas, the hippocampus stores unique conjunctions of items, times, and places, as its homologues have throughout vertebrate history: binding in context as Ranganath and Ritchey[139] and Ritchey et al.[140] use that phrase. From this perspective, the posterior parts of the medial network—specifically the hippocampal, parahippocampal, retrosplenial, and posterior cingulate areas—function as an extended *hippocampal-navigation system*. Within this extended network, the hippocampus represents the spatial relations among various aspects of the sensory environment, emphasizing distinct situations and perspectives from one point of view or another. These specializations reflect both a legacy of the original function of the hippocampus in navigation (see Chapter 4) and the inherent nature of memories that incorporate spatial and temporal features. As a whole, the extended hippocampal–navigation network enriches and elaborates the cognitive maps that emerged *de novo* in early vertebrates. Put another way, while the hippocampus (as part of the allocortex) actively constructs new maps and updates previously learned ones, as it has throughout vertebrate history, the posterior and medial parts of the ring neocortex (see Fig. 5.1B) represent a diverse assortment of special-purpose cognitive maps. This idea implies that cognitive maps in the neocortex can control behavior without hippocampal input, especially in familiar environments.

Ranganath and Ritchey[139] and Ritchey et al.[140] suggest roles for two parts of an extended hippocampal–navigation network in humans: a posteromedial core and interacting areas. The parahippocampal, retrosplenial, and posterior cingulate cortex compose the core, which mediates the encoding and retrieval of situational models. This term refers to the gist of the spatial, temporal, and causal relationships that apply within a particular context, and it has some of the same properties as a cognitive map. The entire medial network—including the medial prefrontal cortex, the posteromedial core, and the hippocampus—constructs a model in which one's self is oriented in a particular time, place, and overall situation. Other parts of the medial network integrate information from the posteromedial core with their own kind of specialized representations, and one role of the hippocampus is to bind these complex, multidimensional representations into unique conjunctions.

The proposal in this chapter pertains to one of the specialized areas interacting with the hippocampus and the posteromedial core: the medial prefrontal cortex. We suggest that high-level re-representations of one's self and others originate in the medial prefrontal cortex and become integrated into situational models and situational perspectives. According to this idea, it is because of the derived properties of the granular prefrontal cortex in hominins that their extended hippocampal–navigation system includes species-specific re-representations of self and others. Once these re-representations emerged during evolution, the posteromedial core and hippocampus continued to do what they had long done, but with this new information. As a result, the hominin forms of situational models and cognitive maps came to include a phylogenetically novel feature—self—bound into conjunctions with the other features that characterize situational models, situational perspectives, and cognitive maps.

These ideas place the medial network in a framework broader than typical discussions of the "default-mode network." For instance, the concept of a situational context relates to perspective-taking: a comprehensive view of dynamic circumstances and one's place within those circumstances[137,141,142]. Nadel and Peterson[141] extend this idea by proposing that the medial network engages in extensive integration along a processing hierarchy. Within this hierarchy, competing representations amount to potential "interpretations" of the available information, with the best fit eventually emerging through the suppression of alternatives inconsistent with it. The prevailing "interpretation" corresponds to the most likely situational context, based on Bayesian principles that take into account biases based on prior experience. The combination of context and one's place within that context results in perspective-taking.

Support for this idea comes from patients with lesions that include the hippocampus; they have difficulty in adopting someone else's perspective[143], an idea we return to later (see "Language in amnesia").

Summary

According to our proposal, the hominin prefrontal cortex provides new, species-specific re-representations of self and others to a large-scale medial network. If we are correct, these re-representations lead to autobiographical narratives and episodic memory, topics we defer to Chapter 11. Here we stress the idea that embedding representations of one's self and others into situational models results in constructive episodic simulations, the recognition of multiple situational contexts involving one's self or one's social group, and perspective-taking, both from one's own points of view and those inferred for others.

Lateral network

In addition to the medial network, social–subjective representations also influence a large-scale lateral network, which includes various prefrontal areas (such as the ventrolateral prefrontal, granular orbitofrontal, and agranular orbital–insular cortex), along with the inferior occipital gyrus, fusiform face area, superior temporal cortex, anterior temporal lobe semantic hub, and cortex near the temporal–parietal junction[56,90,144–146]. Earlier (see "Ancestral mechanisms") we discussed evidence for an ancestral anthropoid network underlying social cognition, which includes rostral and dorsal parts of the medial prefrontal cortex (including the anterior cingulate cortex) and part of the superior temporal cortex[33].

Recent neuroanatomical findings from monkeys have revealed interconnections among many of these areas[147]. The orbital, medial, and ventrolateral prefrontal cortex, for example, all have moderate to dense interconnections with the anterior temporal lobe, including the temporal pole cortex. Notably, all parts of the medial prefrontal cortex project to the temporal pole cortex. In contrast, the dorsolateral prefrontal cortex has fewer connections with the anterior temporal lobe. The paucity of these projections might seem surprising, but it seems consistent with our proposals. As part of the goal system (see Chapter 8), the dorsolateral prefrontal cortex interacts with the posterior parietal cortex to generate goals based on metric contexts, including relational metrics, a function that is fairly distinct from those of the social–subjective system and the anterior temporal lobe semantic hub.

Granular orbitofrontal cortex

Many prefrontal areas beyond the medial ones contribute to social cognition. In one study, patients with lesions of the granular orbitofrontal cortex considered their behavior to be socially appropriate, although people observing their behavior often disagreed[148]. After they watched a video of themselves, however, the patients recognized their behavior as being socially embarrassing. Put another way, an external (video) perspective allowed these patients to apply their knowledge about social norms to themselves, but lesions of the granular orbitofrontal cortex prevented such self-awareness otherwise. In a related experiment, activations in the granular orbitofrontal cortex reflected how subjects evaluated their own traits[149]. This area also became activated when subjects made evaluative judgments about groups of people[150].

Temporal lobe

In addition to prefrontal areas, several parts of the temporal cortex and cortex near the temporal–parietal junction contribute to social cognition. Social representations in the anterior temporal lobe especially involve its superior part[151–153], area TA. Support for a social role for the temporal lobe has come from studies of paired-associate learning. Activations occurred in the superior part of the anterior temporal lobe when subjects made decisions about word pairs involving social concepts, such as honor–brave, in contrast with pairs involving animals, such as nutritious–useful[154]. In other brain imaging studies, activations in the anterior temporal lobe reflected social generalizations, including evaluative and stereotyping biases[150].

In Chapter 9 we discussed the idea of an anterior temporal lobe hub for semantic memory, and many of its concepts and categories involve the social domain. Our proposal suggests, for example, that interactions between the prefrontal cortex and the anterior temporal lobe lead to generalized social concepts and categories, including those concerning social rewards and punishments (such as exclusion and ostracism). Social concepts include the intentions of individuals, linked to what we know about them and the contribution that they can or should make to society.

In line with this idea, some patients with semantic dementia have been found to show a selective impairment in social knowledge. These patients had different degrees of impairment in word categorization for three types of material—animate items, inanimate items, and social groups[155]—and some patients performed worst on the latter. The observation that the dorsal part of the anterior temporal lobe specializes in semantic auditory functions[151–153] might account for this observation, at least in part, given the importance of audition to human social systems.

We also explained in Chapter 9 that the anterior temporal lobe hub abstracts generalized concepts and categories from lower-level representations of animate and inanimate items, and the same idea applies to social–subjective representations[151–153]. Both the semantic hub and its "spoke" areas contribute to social cognition. Inferior temporal and occipital areas represent information about faces, for example, for both individual identification and the reading of emotions, as well as postures that convey social information (body language). Collectively, these areas represent other people and groups in terms of their sensory features. More posterior (predominantly occipital) areas represent social classifications independent of evaluations, categories, and stereotypes; more anterior areas of the temporal lobe incorporate these nonsensory features into social classifications[150].

Beyond the anterior temporal lobe, the middle temporal gyrus showed activation half way along its length in a theory-of-mind experiment, as did cortex near the temporal–parietal junction[156]. These areas also became activated in semantic memory tasks[157], as illustrated in Plate 4(C).

Summary

Social–subjective knowledge extends beyond the medial prefrontal cortex to encompass other parts of the prefrontal cortex, the anterior temporal lobe semantic hub and its "spoke" areas, cortex near the temporal–parietal junction, and parts of the superior and middle temporal gyrus. The semantic memory system, as part of a large-scale lateral network of cortical areas, represents social concepts and categories of individuals, such as children versus adults, kinship relations, and social status. These categories and group representations not only contribute to perceptions and memories about society, but also to generating socially appropriate goals, such as how to act in a given social context.

Specializations of the medial and lateral networks

Episodic versus semantic memory

It is tempting to distinguish the medial and lateral networks in terms of episodic versus semantic memory functions, respectively. Granular parts of the medial prefrontal cortex have shown activation, however, as subjects classified social traits[150]. Classification reflects semantic rather than episodic memory, so the functions of the medial network must extend beyond episodic memory per se. Binder and Desai[158] argue, for example, that the posterior cingulate cortex serves as an interface between semantic and episodic memories and so is not specialized for episodic memory. In other brain imaging studies, the dorsomedial prefrontal, anterior cingulate, and retrosplenial cortex became activated in semantic memory tasks[157], which also argues against a specialization solely for episodic memories.

Instead of a simple distinction in terms of episodic versus semantic memory, some evidence supports a different division of labor: experience-near versus experience-distant knowledge. According to our proposal, the medial prefrontal cortex provides social–subjective representations to both the medial and lateral networks (Fig. 10.5A), which use them in different ways. The medial network specializes in autobiographical memory, constructive episodic simulation, perspective-taking, and situational contexts—all of which are involved in episodic memory—as well as the kinds of semantic knowledge about one's self and others that rely most directly on personal experience: experience-near knowledge.

Evidence for this idea has come from a study of amnesic patients with damage to the hippocampus. These lesions impaired both the encoding and retrieval of knowledge about personal facts, an aspect of semantic memory that relies on direct experience (experience-near knowledge)[159]. These patients had less difficulty with knowledge garnered from instruction or study (experience-distant knowledge), which probably depends on the anterior temporal lobe and other parts of the lateral network. As a result, they had a relatively preserved capacity for encoding and retrieving generalized traits associated with themselves and others, such as thoughts, beliefs, and the roles played by individuals in society[159].

Septal versus amygdaloid hippocampus

Distinctions between the medial and lateral networks might also reflect (or be reflected in) a specialization of function along the septal–amygdaloid axis of the hippocampus (see Chapter 4, "Septal versus amygdaloid hippocampus"). As illustrated in Fig. 10.5(A), both the medial and lateral networks interact with the hippocampus, but in distinct ways. In terms of the two networks, the septal (posterior) hippocampus has shown correlated resting-state activations with the medial network, including the anterior cingulate, posterior cingulate, inferior parietal, and retrosplenial cortex, along with the anterior and mediodorsal thalamus and the dorsolateral prefrontal cortex. In contrast, the amygdaloid (anterior) hippocampus has shown activations coupled with the lateral temporal cortex, including the anterior temporal lobe[160–162].

Poppenk et al.[163] link the septal hippocampus to the fine-grained analysis that underlies individuated events. In their analysis of hippocampal volume, the size of the septal hippocampus was positively correlated with better source (episodic) memory, whereas episodic memory was negatively correlated with the size of the amygdaloid hippocampus[160]. Furthermore, the ratio of septal to amygdaloid hippocampus (by volume) was correlated with the degree of explicit recollection, as opposed to familiarity judgments.

In the same vein, the septal hippocampus and medial network appear to play related roles in making fine distinctions among similar situational models, scenes, and events that have extensive feature overlap. Evidence for this idea includes activations in the septal hippocampus when people needed to detect subtle differences among scenes (Fig. 10.5B, left)[164] and when objects appeared at unexpected locations[165]. The septal hippocampus also seems to be critical for filling in scenes by extrapolating beyond scene boundaries, for example, a capacity that seems to depend on interactions among hippocampal, parahippocampal, and visual areas[166].

The amygdaloid hippocampus has different properties. It has shown activations during face recognition tasks (Fig. 10.5B, right) but not during scene recognition (Fig. 10.5B, left)[164]. It also became activated when an object appeared out of sequence[167], as opposed to when an object appeared at an unexpected location[165]. These findings support the idea that the amygdaloid hippocampus functions in large-scale integration—over large spatial territories and long time spans, incorporating affective and social information along the way.

A decrease in the volume of the amygdaloid hippocampus, relative to the septal hippo-campus, has also been reported for highly experienced London taxi drivers[168]. This find-ing probably reflects the predominance of fine-grained maps in the septal hippocampus of these experts, at the expense of coarse-grained overviews represented in the amygda-loid hippocampus. A similar shift in volume—from amygdaloid to septal hippocampus—occurs during human development[169], possibly because children and adolescents also acquire fine-grained mental maps as they mature.

In Chapter 4 ("Septal versus amygdaloid hippocampus") we mentioned brain imaging results from navigation tasks that support the idea of a transition from fine-grained to large-scale specializations along the septal–amygdaloid axis of the human hippocampus. Additionally, the integrative capacity of the amygdaloid hippocampus and its dense inter-connections with the amygdala suggest that affective information becomes integrated into its representations.

Summary

The medial and lateral network play different roles in social–subjective cognition. In broad terms, the medial network processes and underpins the emergence of autobio-graphical and other episodic memories, along with experience-near "person knowledge." The lateral network processes and stores experience-distant knowledge about social con-cepts, groups, goals, conventions, and roles in society. The septal hippocampus has a close relationship with the medial network, and it seems to specialize in situational differen-tiation and fine-grained cognitive maps; the amygdaloid hippocampus interacts closely with both the medial and lateral networks, as well as with the amygdala, and it seems to specialize in large-scale integration, incorporating affective information.

Building on their specializations, the medial and lateral networks contribute to several emergent functions, in part through their interactions with each other.

Interactions between the medial and lateral networks

Social traits and elements

One finding about interactions between the medial and lateral networks concerns a per-sonality trait called agreeableness, which applies to cooperative and empathetic individ-uals. Inferring the agreeableness of an imagined protagonist has led to activation in both the dorsomedial prefrontal cortex and the inferior temporal cortex[138], areas that also showed activation when people inferred the mental states of others[156]. These findings suggest that the assessment of personality traits, such as agreeableness, involves coopera-tive interactions between the medial and lateral networks. Personality judgments require representations of social events (a medial-network function) as well as the ability to combine this information with generalizations about social traits[138,170] (a lateral-network function).

In the same vein, an experiment in which subjects had to imagine the social elements of various situations revealed activations of the medial prefrontal and posterior cingulate areas of the medial network, along with the anterior temporal lobe of the lateral network[138]. Because this experiment isolated the spatial and social aspects of the task, it was possible to show that the social elements led to activation of the medial network—including the dorsomedial prefrontal cortex and the medial frontal-pole cortex. Coupling between the medial and lateral networks during event reconstruction probably promotes the integration of social (semantic) knowledge—including knowledge about personality traits and individual identities—into an appropriate situational context. Ritchey et al.[140] review this literature in detail, concluding that the medial network (especially its posteromedial part) functions in episodic and autobiographical memory and in social cognition, as well as in space, time, and scene perception. In their view, the lateral network (especially its anterior temporal part) specializes in semantic processing and object perception, among other functions. Crucially:

> to support the full complement of memory-guided behavior, the two systems must interact, and the hippocampal and ventromedial prefrontal cortex may serve as sites of integration between the two systems. We conclude that when considering the "connected hippocampus," inquiry should extend beyond the medial temporal lobes to include the large-scale cortical systems of which they are a part.
>
> Ritchey et al.[140] (p. 45)

Illusions of intentions

Another example of interactions between the medial and lateral networks involves the illusions about intentions discussed earlier (see "Illusions of otherness"). Such illusions have been associated with activations in both networks.

In one set of studies, people watched animations of interacting (but nonliving) "things" and later evaluated the category of an interaction[171]. Activations occurred in the several parts of the lateral network, including the dorsolateral prefrontal cortex, cortex near the temporal–parietal junction, cortex in the superior temporal sulcus, the anterior temporal lobe, and the fusiform gyrus. Importantly, activation in the superior temporal cortex showed selectivity for assessing the "intentions" of the animations, as opposed to animacy per se[172,173]. In contrast, when people made judgments about the movements of these animations through space—animacy without intentionality—posterior parietal areas became more activated. In addition to the lateral network, these experiments also revealed activation in the posterior cingulate cortex and the amygdala.

Verbal instruction and language

When subjects received verbal instructions in a brain imaging experiment, the initial activation occurred in the left ventrolateral prefrontal cortex[174], which probably reflected the retrieval of phonological representations from the temporal cortex (see Chapter 9, "Semantic control"). Temporal–prefrontal interactions pre-date language, of course, but they continued to operate after language evolved[175].

It would take a whole book to discuss the evolution of language, and, of course, many such books exist[176–180]—so we touch briefly on just three points about language, each of which involves interactions between the medial and lateral networks.

The first point relates to social goals, specifically the goal of influencing neural representations in other people. Hurford[177] suggests that early human language had a topic–comment grammar. In this simple form of language, a topic directs the listener's attention to something. After a speaker has achieved this initial goal, he or she then conveys some additional information about that topic: a comment, which establishes or modifies some representations in the listener's brain. This kind of communication depends on social–subjective representations because it requires the appreciation that a listener has perceptual representations that can be influenced. From this perspective, the impulse to direct a listener's attention to a topic involves the medial network (and its re-representations of others), with the comment usually depending on the lateral network.

The second point returns to the concept of re-representation. The relationship of language to second-, third-, and higher-order intentions is well recognized[15]. Language requires a complex interplay between one's own intentions and those of other people, often based on highly nuanced social situations. This idea highlights the social–subjective re-representations that developed in the expanding prefrontal cortex of hominins, and especially in the medial prefrontal cortex. It also points to interactions between the medial and lateral networks because much of the knowledge that people use to gauge intentions depends on concepts and categories represented in the anterior temporal lobe (see Chapter 9).

The third point involves MacNeilage's[179] frame-and-content model of the origin of speech. According to his idea, medial frontal areas provide an articulatory frame, which evolved from rhythmic social signals such as lip smacking. In contrast to theories that focus on possible gestural origins[181,182], MacNeilage's idea suggests that these socially relevant mouth, tongue, and lip movements, combined with respiratory voicing, sparked the origin of speech. Without commenting on the relative merit of gestural versus vocal origins, we note here how our proposals relate to both. MacNeilage's model suggests that the content part of the frame-and-content architecture comes from the feature and goal systems of the lateral network. The feature system represents the phonological associates of word meanings, and the goal system supports speech production. As a result, the arbitrary mapping of acoustic representations to semantic meaning mediates language reception, and similar associative processes mediate the mapping of semantic meanings to vocal outputs for expression[183]. Gestural theories of language origins also emphasize the feature and goal systems of the lateral network. Both theories are consistent with the idea that social–subjective representations in the medial network provide the impetus for communicative gestures, for either manual or vocal signaling, whereas representations in the lateral network provide much of the content.

Language in amnesia

Many experts assume that "hippocampal" amnesia spares language, in line with the idea that the hippocampus functions exclusively in memory. In Chapter 7 ("The perception–memory dichotomy") we refuted the latter idea, and here we show that the former is wrong as well. Not only is language impaired in amnesia, but the nature of the impairment highlights the interactions between social–subjective representations in the medial and lateral networks.

H.M. provides a useful starting point, as usual. Early studies suggested that he had some language impairments, such as tangential speech, which consists of straying off the topic at hand, and difficulties in describing experimental tests[184]. Most discussions of these impairments have treated them as a consequence of memory loss. An analysis by MacKay et al.[185,186], however, points to language impairments that a pure memory loss cannot explain. H.M. needed more help to discover the meaning of sentences than did control subjects, and his explanations of ambiguous sentences were less clear, concise, and effective, with more requests for clarification and elaboration. In further studies, H.M. demonstrated: (1) lexical decision impairments on low-frequency words, a pattern that became exaggerated as he aged; (2) impairments when asked to discriminate between grammatical and ungrammatical sentences, to fix sentences containing an error, and to answer questions about who did what to whom in sentences; and (3) poor performance on multiple-choice recognition of possible versus impossible sentences involving ambiguities and figurative formulations, as well as when describing the competing meanings of ambiguous sentences, phrases, and words.

Other amnesic patients also have subtle language impairments. Duff et al.[187,188] studied the linguistic behavior of patients with lesions that included the hippocampus, and their observations revealed problems in the flexible or creative use of language. In the referential communication task, for example, the subjects needed to converse with a partner in order to help them fill up a board with picture cards to match a board of their own. Although amnesic patients could establish a set of referential terms for the pictures and use them throughout the task, they showed a lack of flexibility in communicating with their partners. They failed to use language that adopted their partner's perspective, and they used culturally shared knowledge (e.g., Jerry Seinfeld's favorite cereal) less often than control subjects did[189]. And unlike healthy subjects, who quickly adopted definite referents (such as *the* windmill) when referring to the cards, amnesic patients continued to use indefinite referents (*a* windmill) throughout a session, as though they were telling their partners about the cards for the first time[190]. Definite referents signal shared knowledge, and impairment in using them suggests a problem with using social–subjective memories in support of linguistic communication.

In a follow-up experiment by Rubin et al.[191], a subject and an experimenter jointly viewed a scene containing objects, some shared in a common ground (Fig. 10.6A and B, top row) and others in a privileged ground observable by either the subject (Fig. 10.6A, bottom row) or the experimenter (Fig. 10.6B, middle row), but not both. Common

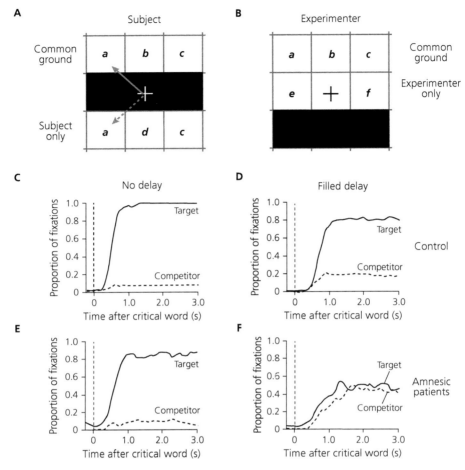

Fig. 10.6 Common-ground task. (A) Objects (a–d) seen by subjects, who could not see anything in the middle row. Each square represents a cubbyhole. (B) Objects (a–f) seen by the experimenter, who could not see anything in the bottom row. (C)–(F) Proportion of saccades made to objects in common ground (target, solid line) and to an identical object that only the subjects could see (competitor, dashed line). (C) Control subjects in the no-delay condition. (D) Control subjects in the filled-delay condition. (E) Amnesic patients in the no-delay condition. (F) Amnesic patients in the filled-delay condition. (C)–(F) Adapted from Rubin RD, Brown-Schmidt S, Duff MC, Tranel D, Cohen NJ. How do I remember that I know you know that I know? *Psychological Science* 22:1574–82, © 2011, Sage, with permission.

ground, the knowledge that we share with communication partners, helps shape the rapid and dynamic adaptation of discourse that can resolve linguistic ambiguities[192,193]. A scene in these experiments might, for example, have contained one duck in common ground and another in the subject's privileged ground. When asked to "Look at the duck," both amnesic patients and control subjects tended to look at the duck in common ground. This observation shows that these patients can distinguish between shared and private information. Even when they successfully looked at the common-ground duck, however, amnesic participants made more saccades to the privileged-ground duck than control subjects did. In the early stages of linguistic processing, therefore, the oculomotor behavior of amnesic patients reveals a subtle difficulty in establishing and maintaining common ground, which standard language tests would certainly miss.

Similar principles apply to an experiment on linguistic common ground. The subject was asked what object was located in a hidden, privileged cubbyhole that only he or she could see. The answer served to establish linguistic common ground. On a typical trial, for example, the subject was asked about a hidden compartment that contained a cactus, with another cactus located in a different, privileged cubbyhole outside this newly established common ground. Then the experimenter asked the subject to "Look at the cactus," either immediately or after a delay period of 40 seconds in which the subject related stories about the test items. Because there were two cacti in privileged cubbyholes, this command was ambiguous. In the no-delay condition, the patients (Fig. 10.6E) resolved this linguistic ambiguity much as control subjects did (Fig. 10.6C): They looked at the cactus in the linguistic common ground, the target, most of the time. After the filled delay period, however, amnesic patients showed a dramatic impairment (Fig. 10.6F), making saccades to both the competitor and target object with roughly equal frequency. Note that no one had instructed the subjects to look at the common-ground object, and they might have been entirely unaware of the basis for their choice.

The authors of this report conclude (Rubin et al.[191], p. 1474) "that declarative memory may be critical to … [the] on-line resolution of linguistic ambiguity," but we view their results differently. From our perspective, these findings provide further evidence for the perceptual functions of the hippocampus (see Chapter 7, "Humans"). Specifically, we think that the hippocampus helps resolve linguistic ambiguity by supporting perceptions about another person's knowledge, presumably based on prefrontal cortex–hippocampus interactions. This idea, in turn, suggests that the perceptual functions of the human hippocampus extend beyond a particular class of stimulus material, such as the scene stimuli discussed in Chapter 7 ("Humans"), to include information about the knowledge of others. According to this idea, impairments in both scene perception and common-ground performance result from the perspective-taking function of the hippocampus, with scene perception reflecting an ancestral role in navigation and common-ground knowledge reflecting a recently derived function related to hominin social systems.

Overall, these studies show that amnesic patients have subtle and selective language impairments that arise when their communication with partners requires either perspective-taking, resolving semantic ambiguity based on context, or establishing common ground that takes into account the knowledge of others[187]. These capacities draw on social–subjective representations, but the same ideas apply to other specialized representations as well. Studies of amnesic patients have revealed impairments in visual perception, for example, on tasks that required visual perspective-taking or resolving ambiguity among sensory features[164,194].

Conclusions

In this chapter we have ascribed the emergence of the social–subjective system to three developments in hominins:

1. Social–subjective representations adapted to the social system of each hominin species. Other species, including our closest relatives, probably have similar representations adapted to their social systems, but hominins added new and higher levels of hierarchy (re-representations) to those of their ancestors.

2. The development of new levels of hierarchy depended on the expansion of the prefrontal cortex during hominin evolution. An increase in the number of neurons and interconnections suffices to support the new representational levels that our proposal requires, without the need to invoke either new areas or any departure from allometric relationships.

3. Once new levels of social–subjective representation emerged, they became available to the navigation, feature, and goal systems via two large-scale networks: one medial, the other lateral.

The first point concerns selective factors. Perhaps, during hominin evolution, the main contribution of social–subjective re-representations involved cooperative intentions, shared action, and collective knowledge[2,3]. We do not need to assume that other primates, and especially our closest relatives, lack traits like self-reflection and self-awareness, only that the hominin form of such traits has derived properties that provided them with selective advantages.

In considering the advantages that social–subjective representations provided to evolving hominins, it is worthwhile considering how the semantic memory system might deal with them. Recall the definitions of specific-, basic-, and general-level concepts that we advanced in Chapter 9 ("Computational models"). Basic-level concepts probably provided the most important advantages to evolving hominins. General-level concepts underlie the recognition that other people resemble ourselves in an abstract sense, and specific-level representations identify individuals. These levels of representation contribute to social cognition, of course, but basic-level concepts and categories have an especially widespread social impact. They enable subtle distinctions among groups of individuals, including categories (such as kinship relations and maturity levels), roles (such as resource procurement and protection), attributes (such as personality type), capabilities (such as skills, strength, and knowledge), and hierarchy (such as leadership and dominance). This knowledge, in turn, contributes to understanding social concepts that apply to one's self or one's own group, including their roles in society. Emotional valuations apply to all of these basic-level concepts, as well as to general and specific ones.

The second point concerns the neural basis of these additional hierarchical levels. According to our proposal, new representations of self and others emerged in the granular prefrontal cortex of hominins, and especially in its medial parts.

The third point involves interactions between the new social–subjective representations and older representational systems, which are mediated by two large-scale cortical networks:

◆ A medial network distributes social–subjective representations to an extended hippocampal–navigation system (Fig. 10.5A). The medial network did not originate in hominins, but the development of higher-level re-representations of one's self and others provided the hominin version of this network with something new. In hominins, these species-specific re-representations support derived traits such as constructive episodic simulations, flexible perspective-taking that incorporates one's own points of view along with those inferred for others, the recognition of situational contexts involving one's self and others, and knowledge about the world that is drawn directly from participatory experience.

◆ A lateral network distributes social–subjective representations to the feature and goal systems, including a semantic hub in the anterior temporal lobe and language areas (Fig. 10.5A). These representations contribute to analogical, metaphorical, categorical, conceptual, and relational reasoning (see Chapter 9), as well as to the generation of goals based on these representations. They also underlie generalizations about society, groups, and individuals.

◆ Building on their specializations, interactions between these two networks contribute to social cognition in many ways, including linguistic communication that requires appreciation of a partner's perspective and intentions, establishing common ground or shared knowledge, or using context to resolve semantic ambiguity.

In *The Heart of Darkness* (Conrad[1], p. 69), Conrad has his narrator imagine Kurtz's thoughts as he utters his immortal dying words—"The horror! The horror!":

> Did he live his life again in every detail of desire, temptation, and surrender during that supreme moment of complete knowledge?

In this chapter we proposed that hominin innovations enable two aspects of this passage: the "mind reading" part, of course, but also the construction of a fictional narrative based on the author's experience and knowledge—but differing distinctly from any actual events. According to our proposals, these innovations led to something else, as well: a sense of participating in events and knowing facts. We develop this idea in Chapter 11.

References

1. **Conrad, J.** (2012) *The Heart of Darkness* (Penguin, London).
2. **Tomasello, M., Carpenter, M., Call, J., Behne, T.** et al. (2005) *Behav. Brain Sci.* **28**, 675–691.
3. **Frith, C.D.** (2012) *Phil. Trans. R. Soc. B: Biol. Sci.* **367**, 2213–2223.
4. **Rosait, A.G., Santos, L.,** and **Hare, B.** (2010) In: *Primate Neuroethology* (eds. Platt, M.L. and Ghazanfar, A.A.), pp. 117–143 (Oxford University Press, Oxford).

5. Seed, A. and Tomasello, M. (2010) *Top. Cogn. Sci.* **2**, 407–419.

6. Herrmann, E., Call, J., Hernandez-Lloreda, M.V., Hare, B. et al. (2007) *Science* **317**, 1360–1366.

7. Churchland, P.S. (2002) *Science* **296**, 308–310.

8. Müller, A.E. and Thalmann, U. (2000) *Biol. Rev. Camb. Phil. Soc.* **75**, 405–435.

9. Kappeler, P.M. (2012) In: *The Evolution of Primate Societies* (eds. Mitani, J.C., Call, J., Kappeler, P.M. *et al.*), pp. 17–41 (University of Chicago Press, Chicago, IL).

10. Dunbar, R.I.M. (2009) *Ann. Hum. Biol.* **36**, 562–572.

11. Dunbar, R.I.M. and Shultz, S. (2007) *Phil. Trans. R. Soc. B: Biol. Sci.* **362**, 649–658.

12. Shultz, S., Opie, C., and Atkinson, Q.D. (2011) *Nature* **479**, 219–222.

13. Lewis, P.A., Rezaie, R., Brown, R., Roberts, N. et al. (2011) *NeuroImage* **57**, 1624–1629.

14. Von Der, H.R., Vyas, G., and Olson, I.R. (2014) *Soc. Cogn. Affect Neurosci.* **9**, 1962–1972.

15. Dunbar, R.I.M. (2014) *Human Evolution* (Pelican-Penguin, London).

16. Pasquaretta, C., Leve, M., Claidiere, N., van de Waal, E. et al. (2014) *Sci. Rep.* **4**, 7600.

17. Charvet, C.J. and Finlay, B.L. (2012) *Prog. Brain Res.* **195**, 71–87.

18. Isler, K. and van Schaik, C.P. (2014) *Evol. Anthropol.* **23**, 65–75.

19. Barton, R.A. and Venditti, C. (2013) *Proc. Natl. Acad. Sci. USA* **110**, 9001–9006.

20. Barton, R.A. and Venditti, C. (2013) *Proc. Natl. Acad. Sci. USA* **110**, E3683–E3684.

21. Gabi, M., Neves, K., Masseron, C. et al. (2014) Program no. 446.05. *2014 Neuroscience Meeting Planner* (Society for Neuroscience, Washington, DC). Online.

22. Bauernfeind, A.L., de Sousa, A.A., Avasthi, T., Dobson, S.D. et al. (2013) *J. Hum. Evol.* **64**, 263–279.

23. Passingham, R.E. and Smaers, J.B. (2014) *Brain Behav. Evol.* **84**, 156–166.

24. Elston, G.N., Benavides-Piccione, R., Elston, A., Zietsch, B. et al. (2006) *Anat. Rec. A Discov. Mol. Cell Evol. Biol.* **288**, 26–35.

25. Elston, G.N. (2007) In: *The Evolution of Nervous Systems* (eds. Preuss, T.M. and Kaas, J.H.), pp. 191–242 (Elsevier, New York).

26. Sherwood, C.C., Holloway, R.L., Semendeferi, K., and Hof, P.R. (2005) *Nat. Neurosci.* **8**, 537–538.

27. Semendeferi, K., Teffer, K., Buxhoeveden, D.P., Park, M.S. et al. (2011) *Cereb. Cortex* **21**, 1485–1497.

28. Teffer, K. and Semendeferi, K. (2012) *Prog. Brain Res.* **195**, 191–218.

29. Krubitzer, L. and Stolzenberg, D.S. (2014) *Curr. Opin. Neurobiol.* **24**, 157–165.

30. Chang, S.W., Brent, L.J., Adams, G.K., Klein, J.T. et al. (2013) *Proc. Natl. Acad. Sci. USA* **110** (Suppl. 2), 10387–10394.

31. Hadland, K.A., Rushworth, M.F.S., Gaffan, D., and Passingham, R.E. (2003) *Neuropsychologia* **41**, 919–931.

32. Sallet, J., Mars, R.B., Noonan, M.P., Andersson, J.L. et al. (2011) *Science* **334**, 697–700.

33. Noonan, M.P., Sallet, J., Mars, R.B., Neubert, F.X. et al. (2014) *PLoS Biol.* **12**, e1001940.

34. Behrens, T.E., Hunt, L.T., and Rushworth, M.F. (2009) *Science* **324**, 1160–1164.

35. Carmichael, S.T. and Price, J.L. (1995) *J. Comp. Neurol.* **363**, 615–641.

36. Haber, S.N. and Knutson, B. (2010) *Neuropsychopharmacol.* **35**, 4–26.

37. Rudebeck, P.H., Buckley, M.J., Walton, M.E., and Rushworth, M.F.S. (2006) *Science* **313**, 1310–1312.

38. Yoshida, K., Saito, N., Iriki, A., and Isoda, M. (2011) *Curr. Biol.* **21**, 249–253.

39. Yoshida, K., Saito, N., Iriki, A., and Isoda, M. (2012) *Nat. Neurosci.* **15**, 1307–1312.

40. Haroush, K. and Williams, Z.M. (2015) *Cell* **160**, 1233–1245.

41. Chang, S.W., Winecoff, A.A., and Platt, M.L. (2011) *Front. Neurosci.* **5**, 27.

42. Chang, S.W., Gariepy, J.F., and Platt, M.L. (2013) *Nat. Neurosci.* **16**, 243–250.

43. Azzi, J.C., Sirigu, A., and Duhamel, J.R. (2012) *Proc. Natl. Acad. Sci. USA* **109**, 2126–2131.

44. Lau, H. and Rosenthal, D. (2011) *Trends Cogn. Sci.* **15**, 365–373.

45. Summerfield, C. and Koechlin, E. (2009) In: *The Cognitive Neurosciences* (ed. Gazzaniga, M.S.), pp. 1019–1030 (MIT Press, Cambridge, MA).

46. Krueger, F., Moll, J., Zahn, R., Heinecke, A. et al. (2007) *Cereb. Cortex* **17**, 2346–2353.

47. Badre, D. (2008) *Trends Cogn. Sci.* **12**, 193–200.

48. Botvinick, M.M. (2008) *Trends Cogn. Sci.* **12**, 201–208.

49. Bunge, S.A., Helskog, E.H., and Wendelken, C. (2009) *NeuroImage* **46**, 338–342.

50. Koechlin, E. and Summerfield, C. (2007) *Trends Cogn. Sci.* **11**, 229–235.

51. Graziano, M.S. and Kastner, S. (2011) *Cogn. Neurosci.* **2**, 125–127.

52. Graziano, M.S. and Kastner, S. (2011) *Cogn. Neurosci.* **2**, 98–113.

53. Passingham, R.E., Bengtsson, S.L., and Lau, H.C. (2010) *Trends Cogn. Sci.* **14**, 16–21.

54. Kelly, Y.T., Webb, T.W., Meier, J.D., Arcaro, M.J. et al. (2014) *Proc. Natl. Acad. Sci. USA* **111**, 5012–5017.

55. Nahab, F.B., Kundu, P., Gallea, C., Kakareka, J. et al. (2011) *Cereb. Cortex* **21**, 48–55.

56. Saxe, R. and Powell, L.J. (2006) *Psychol. Sci.* **17**, 692–699.

57. Blanke, O., Ortigue, S., Landis, T., and Seeck, M. (2002) *Nature* **419**, 269–270.

58. Wood, J.N. and Grafman, J. (2003) *Nat. Rev. Neurosci.* **4**, 139–147.

59. Luo, Q., Mitchell, D., Jones, M., Mondillo, K. et al. (2007) *NeuroImage* **38**, 631–639.

60. Siep, N., Roefs, A., Roebroeck, A., Havermans, R. et al. (2009) *Behav. Brain Res.* 149–158.

61. Critchley, H.D., Wiens, S., Rotstein, P., Ohman, A. et al. (2004) *Nat. Neurosci.* **7**, 189–195.

62. Ochsner, K.N., Ray, R.D., Cooper, J.C., Robertson, E.R. et al. (2004) *NeuroImage* **23**, 483–499.

63. Ochsner, K.N., Beer, J.S., Robertson, E.R., Cooper, J.C. et al. (2005) *NeuroImage* **28**, 797–814.

64. Hassabis, D. and Maguire, E.A. (2009) *Phil. Trans. R. Soc. B: Biol. Sci.* **364**, 1263–1271.

65. Gilbert, S.J., Spengler, S., Simons, J.S., Steele, J.D. et al. (2006) *J. Cogn. Neurosci.* **18**, 932–948.

66. Harris, L.T. and Fiske, S.T. (2007) *Soc. Cogn. Affect. Neurosci.* **2**, 45–51.

67. Amodio, D.M. and Frith, C.D. (2006) *Nat. Rev. Neurosci.* **7**, 268–277.

68. Sallet, J., Mars, R.B., Noonan, M.P., Neubert, F.-X. et al. (2013) *J. Neurosci.* **33**, 12255–12274.

69. Beckmann, M., Johansen-Berg, H., and Rushworth, M.F. (2009) *J. Neurosci.* **29**, 1175–1190.

70. Frith, C.D. and Frith, U. (2006) *Brain Res.* **1079**, 36–46.

71. Mitchell, J.P., Macrae, C.N., and Banaji, M.R. (2006) *Neuron* **50**, 655–663.

72. Ramnani, N. and Miall, R.C. (2004) *Nat. Neurosci.* **7**, 85–90.

73. Somerville, L.H., Kelley, W.M., and Heatherton, T.F. (2010) *Cereb. Cortex* **20**, 3005–3013.

74. Moran, J.M., Macrae, C.N., Heatherton, T.F., Wyland, C.L. et al. (2006) *J. Cogn. Neurosci.* **18**, 1586–1594.

75. Reniers, R.L., Vollm, B.A., Elliott, R., and Corcoran, R. (2014) *Soc. Neurosci.* **9**, 50–62.

76. Apps, M.A. and Ramnani, N. (2014) *J. Neurosci.* **34**, 6190–6200.

77. Nicolle, A., Klein-Flugge, M.C., Hunt, L.T., Vlaev, I. et al. (2012) *Neuron* **75**, 1114–1121.

78. Symons, C.S. and Johnson, B.T. (1997) *Psychol. Bull.* **121**, 371–394.

79. Leshikar, E.D., Dulas, M.R., and Duarte, A. (2015) *Neuropsychol. Dev. Cogn. B Aging Neuropsychol. Cogn.* **22**, 388–412.

80. Leshikar, E.D. and Duarte, A. (2012) *Soc. Neurosci.* **7**, 126–145.

81. Philippi, C.L., Duff, M.C., Denburg, N.L., Tranel, D. et al. (2012) *J. Cogn. Neurosci.* **24**, 475–481.

82. Kurczek, J., Wechsler, E., Ahuaja, S., Jensen, U. et al. (2015) *Neuropsychologia* **73**, 116–126.

83. Powell, L.J., Macrae, C.N., Cloutier, J., Metcalfe, J. et al. (2010) *J. Cogn. Neurosci.* **22**, 2186–2197.

84. Happe, F., Malhi, G.S., and Checkley, S. (2001) *Neuropsychologia* **39**, 83–90.

85. Shallice, T. (2001) *Brain* **124**, 247–248.

86. Stuss, D.T., Gallup, G.G., and Alexander, M.P. (2001) *Brain* **124**, 279–286.

87. Rowe, A.D., Bullock, P.R., Polkey, C.E., and Morris, R.G. (2001) *Brain* **124**, 600–616.

88. Kumaran, D. and Maguire, E.A. (2005) *J. Neurosci.* **25**, 7254–7259.

89. Johnson, S.C., Baxter, L.C., Wilder, L.S., Pipe, J.G. et al. (2002) *Brain* **125**, 1808–1814.

90. Amodio, D.M. (2014) *Nat. Rev. Neurosci.* **15**, 670–682.

91. Krajbich, I., Adolphs, R., Tranel, D., Denburg, N.L. et al. (2009) *J. Neurosci.* **29**, 2188–2192.

92. Sanfey, A.G., Rilling, J.K., Aronson, J.A., Nystrom, L.E. et al. (2003) *Science* **300**, 1755–1758.

93. Gabay, A.S., Radua, J., Kempton, M.J., and Mehta, M.A. (2014) *Neurosci. Biobehav. Rev.* **47**, 549–558.

94. Damasio, A.R. (1994) *Descartes' Error: Emotion, Reason, and the Human Brain* (Avon, New York).

95. Philippi, C.L., Feinstein, J.S., Khalsa, S.S., Damasio, A. et al. (2012) *PLoS One* **7**, e38413.

96. Singer, T., Seymour, B., O'Doherty, J., Kaube, H. et al. (2004) *Science* **303**, 1157–1162.

97. Bechara, A. and Damasio, A.R. (2005) *Games Econ. Behav.* **52**, 336–372.

98. Dunn, B.D. (2006) *Neurosci. Biobehav. Rev.* **30**, 239–271.

99. Apperly, I.A. (2008) *Cognition* **107**, 266–283.

100. Changizi, M.A. (2009) *The Visual Revolution* (Benbella, Dallas, TX).

101. Khan, S.A., Levine, W.J., Dobson, S.D., and Kralik, J.D. (2011) *Psychol. Sci.* **22**, 1001–1003.

102. Forbes, C.E. and Grafman, J. (2010) *Annu. Rev. Neurosci.* **33**, 299–324.

103. Krueger, F., Barbey, A.K., and Grafman, J. (2009) *Trends Cogn. Sci.* **13**, 103–109.

104. Dreher, J.C., Koechlin, E., Tierney, M., and Grafman, J. (2008) *PLoS One.* **3**, e3227.

105. Goel, V., Grafman, J., Tajik, J., Gana, S. et al. (1997) *Brain* **120**, 1805–1822.

106. Sirigu, A., Zalla, T., Pillon, B., Grafman, J. et al. (1996) *Cortex* **32**, 297–310.

107. Bird, C.M., Castelli, F., Malik, O., Frith, U. et al. (2004) *Brain* **127**, 914–928.

108. Leopold, A., Krueger, F., Dal, M.O., Pardini, M. et al. (2012) *Soc. Cogn. Affect. Neurosci.* **7**, 871–880.

109. Welborn, B.L. and Lieberman, M.D. (2015) *J. Cogn. Neurosci.* **27**, 1–12.

110. Stolk, A., D'Imperio, D., di Pellegrino, G., and Toni, I. (2015) *Curr. Biol.* **25**, 1–6.

111. Heider, F. and Simmel, M. (1944) *Am. J. Psychol* .**57**, 243–259.

112. Klein, A.M., Zwickel, J., Prinz, W., and Frith, U. (2009) *Q. J. Exp. Psychol.* **62**, 1189–1197.

113. Andrews-Hanna, J.R., Reidler, J.S., Sepulcre, J., Poulin, R. et al. (2010) *Neuron* **65**, 550–562.

114. Conway, M.A. and Pleydell-Pearce, C.W. (2000) *Psychol. Rev.* **107**, 261–288.

115. Whitfield-Gabrieli, S., Moran, J.M., Nieto-Castanon, A., Triantafyllou, C. et al. (2011) *NeuroImage* **55**, 225–232.

116. Addis, D.R., Moscovitch, M., and McAndrews, M.P. (2007) *Brain* **130**, 2327–2342.

117. Hassabis, D., Kumaran, D., and Maguire, E.A. (2007) *J. Neurosci.* **27**, 14365–14374.

118. Tulving, E. (2002) *Annu. Rev. Psychol.* **53**, 1–25.

119. Wheeler, M.A., Stuss, D.T., and Tulving, E. (1997) *Psychol. Bull.* **121**, 331–354.

120. Heilbronner, S.R. and Haber, S.N. (2014) *J. Neurosci.* **34**, 10041–10054.

121. Raichle, M.E. and Snyder, A.Z. (2007) *NeuroImage* **37**, 1083–1090.

122. Raichle, M.E., MacLeod, A.M., Snyder, A.Z., Powers, W.J. et al. (2001) *Proc. Natl. Acad. Sci. USA* **98**, 676–682.

123. Andrews-Hanna, J.R., Saxe, R., and Yarkoni, T. (2014) *NeuroImage* **91**, 324–335.

124. Schacter, D.L., Addis, D.R., Hassabis, D., Martin, V.C. et al. (2012) *Neuron* **76**, 677–694.

125. Andrews-Hanna, J.R., Smallwood, J., and Spreng, R.N. (2014) *Ann. NY Acad. Sci.* **1316**, 29–52.

126. Suddendorf, T., Addis, D.R., and Corballis, M.C. (2009) *Phil. Trans. R. Soc. B: Biol. Sci.* **364**, 1317–1324.

127. Buckner, R.L. and Krienen, F.M. (2013) *Trends Cogn. Sci.* **17**, 648–665.

128. Passingham, R.E. and Wise, S.P. (2012) *The Neurobiology of the Prefrontal Cortex* (Oxford University Press, Oxford).

129. McLelland, V.C., Devitt, A.L., Schacter, D.L., and Addis, D.R. (2015) *Memory* **23**, 1255–1263.

130. Gaesser, B., Spreng, R.N., McLelland, V.C., Addis, D.R. et al. (2013) *Hippocampus* **23**, 1150–1161.

131. Prebble, S.C., Addis, D.R., and Tippett, L.J. (2013) *Psychol. Bull.* **139**, 815–840.

132. Suddendorf, T. and Redshaw, J. (2013) *Ann. NY Acad. Sci.* **1296**, 135–153.

133. Suddendorf, T. (2013) *Trends Cogn. Sci.* **17**, 151–152.

134. Suddendorf, T. and Corballis, M.C. (2007) *Behav. Brain Sci.* **30**, 299–313.

135. Suddendorf, T. and Corballis, M.C. (2010) *Behav. Brain Res.* **215**, 292–298.

136. Suddendorf, T. and Busby, J. (2003) *Trends Cogn. Sci.* **7**, 391–396.

137. Buckner, R.L. and Carroll, D.C. (2007) *Trends Cogn. Sci.* **11**, 49–57.

138. Hassabis, D., Spreng, R.N., Rusu, A.A., Robbins, C.A. et al. (2014) *Cereb. Cortex* **24**, 1979–1987.

139. Ranganath, C. and Ritchey, M. (2012) *Nat. Rev. Neurosci.* **13**, 713–726.

140. Ritchey, M., Libby, L.A., and Ranganath, C. (2015) *Prog. Brain Res,* **219**, 45–64.

141. Nadel, L. and Peterson, M.A. (2013) *J. Exp. Psychol. Gen.* **142**, 1242–1254.

142. Buckner, R.L. (2010) *Annu. Rev. Psychol.* **61**, 27–28.

143. Beadle, J.N., Tranel, D., Cohen, N.J., and Duff, M.C. (2013) *Front. Psychol.* **4**, 69.

144. Frith, C.D. and Frith, U. (2007) *Curr. Biol.* **17**, R724–R732.

145. Blakemore, S.J. (2008) *Nat. Rev. Neurosci.* **9**, 267–277.

146. Saxe, R. and Kanwisher, N. (2003) *NeuroImage* **19**, 1835–1842.

147. Mohedano-Moriano, A., Muñoz, M., Sanz-Arigita, E., Pro-Sistiaga, P. et al. (2015) *J. Comp. Neurol.* **523**, 2570–2598.

148. Beer, J.S., John, O.P., Scabini, D., and Knight, R.T. (2006) *J. Cogn. Neurosci.* **18**, 871–879.

149. Beer, J.S. and Hughes, B.L. (2010) *NeuroImage* **49**, 2671–2679.

150. Gilbert, S.J., Swencionis, J.K., and Amodio, D.M. (2012) *Neuropsychologia* **50**, 3600–3611.

151. Simmons, W.K., Reddish, M., Bellgowan, P.S., and Martin, A. (2010) *Cereb. Cortex* **20**, 813–825.

152. Ross, L.A. and Olson, I.R. (2010) *NeuroImage* **49**, 3452–3462.

153. Olson, I.R., McCoy, D., Klobusicky, E., and Ross, L.A. (2013) *Soc. Cogn. Affect. Neurosci.* **8**, 123–133.

154. Zahn, R., Moll, J., Krueger, F., Huey, E.D. et al. (2007) *Proc. Natl. Acad. Sci. USA* **104**, 6430–6435.

155. Rumiati, R.I., Carnaghi, A., Improta, E., Diez, A.L. et al. (2014) *Cogn. Neurosci.* **5**, 85–96.

156. Mars, R.B., Sallet, J., Schuffelgen, U., Jbabdi, S. et al. (2012) *Cereb. Cortex* **22**, 1894–1903.

157. Wirth, M., Jann, K., Dierks, T., Federspiel, A. et al. (2011) *NeuroImage* **54**, 3057–3066.

158. Binder, J.R. and Desai, R.H. (2011) *Trends Cogn. Sci.* **15**, 527–536.

159. Grilli, M.D. and Verfaellie, M. (2014) *Neuropsychologia* **61**, 56–64.

160. Poppenk, J. and Moscovitch, M. (2011) *Neuron* **72**, 931–937.

161. La, J.R., Landeau, B., Perrotin, A., Bejanin, A. et al. (2014) *Neuron* **81**, 1417–1428.

162. Ritchey, M., Yonelinas, A.P., and Ranganath, C. (2014) *J. Cogn. Neurosci.* **26**, 1085–1099.

163. Poppenk, J., Evensmoen, H.R., Moscovitch, M., and Nadel, L. (2013) *Trends Cogn. Sci.* **17**, 230–240.

164. Mundy, M.E., Downing, P.E., Dwyer, D.M., Honey, R.C. et al. (2013) *J. Neurosci.* **33**, 10490–10502.

165. Kumaran, D. and Maguire, E.A. (2007) *J. Neurosci.* **27**, 8517–8524.

166. Chadwick, M.J., Mullally, S.L., and Maguire, E.A. (2013) *Cortex* **49**, 2067–2079.

167. Kumaran, D. and Maguire, E.A. (2006) *PLoS Biol.* **4**, e424.

168. Woollett, K., Spiers, H.J., and Maguire, E.A. (2009) *Phil. Trans. R. Soc. B: Biol. Sci.* **364**, 1407–1416.

169. Gogtay, N., Nugent, T.F., Herman, D.H., Ordonez, A. et al. (2006) *Hippocampus* **16**, 664–672.

170. Freeman, J.B. and Ambady, N. (2011) *Psychol. Rev.* **118**, 247–279.

171. Tavares, P., Lawrence, A.D., and Barnard, P.J. (2008) *Cereb. Cortex* **18**, 1876–1885.

172. Saxe, R., Xiao, D.K., Kovacs, G., Perrett, D.I. et al. (2004) *Neuropsychologia* **42**, 1435–1446.

173. Tavares, P., Barnard, P.J., and Lawrence, A.D. (2011) *Soc. Cogn. Affect. Neurosci.* **6**, 98–108.

174. Hartstra, E., Waszak, F., and Brass, M. (2012) *NeuroImage* **63**, 1143–1153.

175. Hickok, G. and Poeppel, D. (2000) *Trends Cogn. Sci.* **4**, 131–138.

176. Hurford, J.R. (2007) *The Origins of Meaning* (Oxford University Press, Oxford).

177. Hurford, J.R. (2012) *The Origins of Grammar* (Oxford University Press, Oxford).

178. Fitch, W.T. (2010) *The Evolution of Language* (Cambridge University Press, Cambridge UK).

179. MacNeilage, P.F. (2008) *The Origin of Speech* (Oxford University Press, Oxford).

180. Burling, R. (2005) *The Talking Ape* (Oxford University Press, Oxford).

181. Rizzolatti, G. and Arbib, M.A. (1998) *Trends Neurosci.* **21**, 188–194.

182. Sterelny, K. (2012) *Phil. Trans. R. Soc. B: Biol. Sci.* **367**, 2141–2151.

183. Murray, E.A., Brasted, P.J., and Wise, S.P. (2002) In: *The Neurobiology of Leaning and Memory* (eds. Squire, L.R. and Schacter, D.), pp. 339–348 (Guilford, New York).

184. Sidman, M., Stoddard, L.T., and Mohr, J.P. (1968) *Neuropsychologia* **6**, 245–254.

185. MacKay, D.G., Stewart, R., and Burke, D.M. (1998) *J. Cogn. Neurosci.* **10**, 377–394.

186. James, L.E. and MacKay, D.G. (2001) *Psychol. Sci.* **12**, 485–492.

187. Duff, M.C. and Brown-Schmidt, S. (2012) *Front. Hum. Neurosci.* **6**, 69.

188. Duff, M.C., Hengst, J., Tranel, D., and Cohen, N.J. (2006) *Nat. Neurosci.* **9**, 140–146.

189. Duff, M.C., Hengst, J., Tranel, D., and Cohen, N.J. (2008) *Brain Lang.* **106**, 41–54.

190. Duff, M.C., Gupta, R., Hengst, J.A., Tranel, D. et al. (2011) *Psychol. Sci.* **22**, 666–673.

191. Rubin, R.D., Brown-Schmidt, S., Duff, M.C., Tranel, D. et al. (2011) *Psychol. Sci.* **22**, 1574–1582.

192. Hanna, J.E., Tanenhaus, M.K., and Trueswell, J.C. (2003) *J. Mem. Lang.* **49**, 43–61.

193. Brown-Schmidt, S. (2012) *Lang. Cogn. Process.* **27**, 62–89.

194. Lee, A.C., Buckley, M.J., Pegman, S.J., Spiers, H. et al. (2005) *Hippocampus* **15**, 782–797.

Chapter 11

The origin of explicit memory in hominins

Overview

Most accounts of memory assume that rodents, monkeys, and humans have a homologous neural system for explicit memory. If so, then it must have developed fairly early in mammalian evolution, if not beforehand. Alternatively, we propose: (1) that explicit memory is a derived hominin trait; (2) that it emerges from interactions among several representational systems; (3) that these systems evolved at different times in response to a variety of selective pressures, one in early vertebrates and others later, including one in hominins; (4) that high-order, hominin-specific re-representations of self contribute to both the perception of participating in ongoing, attended events and the perception of knowing attended facts; (5) that these self-representations become a dimension of conjunctive representations that correspond to explicit memories; and (6) that when people retrieve representations with this dimension they re-experience the sense of participating in events and of knowing facts that characterizes explicit memory.

Lions, popes, and people

> What makes the Hottentot so hot?
> What puts the "ape" in apricot?
> What have they got that I ain't got?
>
> The Cowardly Lion in *The Wizard of Oz*[1]

We propose a two-word answer to the Cowardly Lion's last question—explicit memory. It takes courage to say so because his enquiry epitomizes an age-old dilemma: What separates "man from beast"? People have pondered this question as long as people have existed, with some concluding that neurobiology cannot contribute very much to answering it. A statement on evolution by Pope John Paul II[2] says as much. "The sciences," it asserts, "can discover at the experimental level a series of very valuable signs indicating what is specific to the human being." But, by papal pronouncement, neurobiology can go only so far; it can never grasp "the experience of … self-awareness and self-reflection" that instead "falls within the competence of philosophical analysis …."

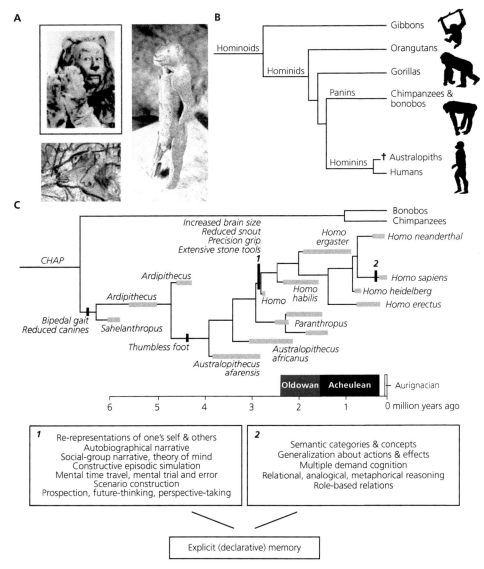

Fig. 11.1 Hominin evolution. (A) The Cowardly Lion (upper left), the Lion Man of Hohlenstein (right), and a lion drawing in the Chauvet cave (lower left). (B) The ape–human lineage. (C) A conjectural cladogram of the panin–hominin lineage. We present a color version of this figure in Plate 6. The sets of traits labelled with the numerals 1 and 2 are listed in the large boxes at the bottom. Together, their interactions produce the experience of participating and knowing that characterizes explicit (declarative) memory. The thick parts of the cladogram lines indicate the range of fossil specimens for the species in question. Abbreviation: CHAP, chimpanzee–human ancestral population. As in Fig. 10.2, the formal names of fossil humans, *Homo neanderthalensis* and *Homo heidelbergensis*, have been shortened to *Homo neanderthal* and *Homo heidelberg*, respectively. (A, upper left) From http://www.artfire.com/ext/shop/product_view/Vintage-Poster-Place/9747001/. (A, lower left) From http://www.bradshawfoundation.com/chauvet/. (A, right) Scanned from *Archaeology* magazine.

The pontiff has a point. A full understanding of "what is specific to the human being" would require the identification of cognitive traits that emerged at various times after the panin–hominin split, in a variety of extinct hominin species (Fig. 11.1C, Plate 6). For neural processes, that is a hard nut to crack. With due deference to this problem, we think that the Cowardly Lion's questions suggest a way forward: not his specific questions so much as the fact that he asked any questions at all. We just used the word "fact," but of course it is not a fact that the Cowardly Lion asked these questions; it is a fiction. As a rule, lions neither pose questions nor obsess about their inadequacies. The Cowardly Lion represents a person with leonine traits, a concept that springs from the human capacity for metaphor. Could otiose questions from a beastly metaphor contribute to understanding the origin of explicit memory? We think that they might.

The reason is that people have generated such metaphors for a long time. Like the Cowardly Lion, the Lion Man of Hohlenstein combines traits of humans and lions (Fig. 11.1A). Someone carved it from a mammoth's tusk 30,000 to 35,000 years ago, and it remains one of the oldest examples of a part human, part animal figurine: a three-dimensional metaphor. The Lion Man arose from the *Aurignacian* culture: the same people who created flutes for music, drew lions in the Chauvet cave (Fig. 11.1A), and carved a female figurine 35,000 years ago[3]. Later, we list some additional artifacts produced by these anatomically modern humans, who buried their dead in elaborate graves and created items for personal ornamentation (see "Evolution"). Ceremonial burials demonstrate the ability to imagine a far-off future (constructive episodic simulation, as explained in Chapter 10); figurative art, music, and ornamentation accompany symbolic communication. Both capacities are hallmarks of explicit memory. Therefore it is obvious that these people had a modern form of memory, with all its implications. The literature is chockfull of claims about human capacities that other animals lack, each matched to counterclaims debunking the idea. By carving the Lion Man and drawing lions, our Aurignacian ancestors revealed a cognitive gap between humans and other animals that no reasonable person can deny.

Clearly, we've got something that they ain't got, and this chapter proposes that this "something" is a derived trait called explicit memory. Instead of trying to solve the problem of "what is specific to the human being" writ large, we explore a smaller, more tractable question: How might explicit memory have emerged from an ancestral condition that—for all of its cognitive power—lacked this trait?

Evolution

The Lion Man of Hohlenstein and the Chauvet cave drawings resulted from an acceleration in human innovation, which occurred fairly recently by evolutionary standards. Klein[4] (p. 742), summarizes the innovations of behaviorally and anatomically modern hominins, as follows:

- Substantial growth in the diversity and standardization of artifact types.
- Rapid increase in the rate of artifactual change through time and in the degree of artifact diversity through space.

- First routine shaping of bone, ivory, shell, and related materials into formal artifacts ("points," "awls," "needles," "pins," etc.).

- Earliest appearance of incontrovertible art and personal ornamentation.

- Oldest undeniable evidence for spatial organization of camp floors, including elaborate hearths and the oldest indisputable structural "ruins."

- Oldest evidence for the transport of large quantities of highly desirable stone raw materials over scores and even hundreds of kilometers.

- Earliest secure evidence for ceremony or ritual, expressed both in art and in elaborate graves.

- First evidence for human ability to live in the coldest ... parts of Eurasia.

- First evidence for human population densities approaching those of historic hunter–gatherers in similar environments.

- First evidence for fishing and for other significant advances in the human ability to extract energy from nature.

Some of these points remain controversial. Arguments persist about how much Neanderthals resembled modern humans in some of the traits just listed[5]. For example, a Neanderthal necklace made from eagle talons dates to about 100,000 years ago[6]. Experts also differ about how suddenly and recently cultural creativity accelerated, with some favoring a gradual accumulation of new capacities from about 200,000 years ago[7] or even more gradually from about 500,000 years ago. Others view the time course as more compressed: a "creative explosion" that occurred as recently as 50,000 years ago[4]. Without denying that many important developments occurred earlier, we accept expert opinion holding that something important happened in human evolution either about 50,000 years ago as Klein[4] would have it or about 100,000 years ago as Sterelny[8] suggests. We do not need to choose between these opinions or the earlier dates because, as they bear on our proposal, they are all relatively recent. Archeologists who favor gradualism dislike the phrase "creative explosion," but it seems to capture what happened fairly well, at least when viewed against the time-scale of vertebrate, mammalian, and primate evolution.

The more important question for our purposes is: How did human inventiveness accelerate? Sterelny[9] (p. 2) suggests that:

> There are two broad approaches to explaining behavioral modernity. One focuses on the social world of Paleolithic hominins, with the idea that behavioral modernity is a response to increasing social complexity .... An alternative centers on ... a genetic change that led to a change in the intrinsic cognitive capacity ... [producing] upgrades to language; to theory of mind; or to working memory.

A speculative depiction of hominin evolution, which incorporates both of these approaches, appears in Fig. 11.1(C) and Plate 6. Any neuroscientist who reproduces these figures or uses them in public risks being hooted down by experts in human evolution, with considerable justification. These cladograms render, in concrete form, relationships that remain poorly established—to say the least. Nevertheless, these illustrations have two virtues: They are specific and they facilitate a comparison of brain expansion (see

Fig. 10.2A) and hominin evolution (Fig. 11.1C) on the same time-scale. Plate 6 does so on the same page, with a matching color code. According to these plots, the hominin brain reached its modern size relative to body mass 200,000 to 600,000 years ago[10,11], which implies that any changes after that time involved some aspect of neural organization, broadly construed, rather than further changes in relative brain size. Such changes could underlie the second approach to which Sterelny refers.

Figure 11.1(C) and Plate 6 also mark some key traits that emerged during hominin evolution. The first developments involved bipedal locomotion and reduced canine teeth. The emergence of bipedal gait in australopiths, 5–7 million years ago, accompanied a life spent more at ground level than in the ancestral condition, probably in response to selective pressures involving deforestation. Their dental changes, likewise, point to increasing reliance on the tougher foods found at ground level. According to Klein[4] (p. 275) "australopiths were essentially bipedal apes, who still spent considerable time feeding, sleeping, or avoiding predation in trees." Their most impressive adaptations occurred from the waist down.

The first evidence for the use of tools to butcher meat and extract marrow dates to about 3.4 million years ago[12,13], pre-dating the earliest known *Homo* specimens by about 600,000 years[14]. The *Oldowan* tradition of simple flake tools corresponds roughly with the appearance of *Homo habilis* about 2.5 million years ago. These hominins developed a suite of adaptations that included the increased use and manufacture of stone tools, an increased reliance on meat as a source of calories, and larger brains. Figure 10.2(A) and Plate 6 illustrate the encephalization quotients of *Homo habilis* in relation to australopiths and modern chimpanzees.

The more complex, bifacial hand axes of the *Acheulean* tool kit roughly correlate with the appearance of *Homo ergaster*, whose descendants or close relatives probably included *Homo erectus* and *Homo heidelbergensis*, who we call the Heidelberg people for short. As illustrated in Fig. 11.1(C), the transition from Oldowan to Acheulean artifacts occurred about 1.6 million years ago, and a transition from an older Acheulean tradition to a newer one might have occurred around 600,000 years ago, when the Heidelberg people appear in the record. (Box 11.1 presents a brain imaging finding related to the observation of tool-making skills.)

Unambiguous evidence for controlled fire dates from about 1 million years ago[15]. The details remain sketchy, but the decreased degree of sexual dimorphism in *Homo ergaster, Homo erectus,* and the Heidelberg people suggests that they had already adopted a new social system. A high level of sexual dimorphism often points to operational specializations between males and females in a species. In hominins, the declining morphological differences between the sexes probably indicates a more egalitarian society. According to Klein[4] (p. 735), the "decreased dimorphism in [*Homo*] *ergaster* may ... mark the beginnings of a distinctively human pattern of sharing and cooperation between the sexes, prefiguring the social organization of historic hunter–gatherers." Figure 10.2(A) shows encephalization quotients for these species, which exceed the australopith range.

Box 11.1 Imitation and tools

People learn, in part, by imitating others. Although copying an observed behavior provides an advantage in performing the same behavior later, inferring the imitated person's intentions—and then imitating their actions—is a much more powerful way to achieve goals.

When subjects watched an expert knapper making a complex Acheulean stone tool compared with a simple Oldowan one, greater activation occurred in the ventrolateral prefrontal cortex for the more complex tool[128]. Both novices and expert knappers showed this effect, but experts differed from the novices in a key way: They also had activations in the dorsomedial prefrontal cortex. It seems likely that this medial prefrontal activation had something to do with experts reading the intentions of other experts, something the novices could not do.

Along the same lines, Frith[129] suggests that a fitness advantage arises from shared intentions and joint actions, and he proposes that these are uniquely human traits. In Chapter 10, we pointed to various kinds of mental simulations, including mental trial and error behavior, as a way to reduce the large number of errors involved in learning[130]. Imitation, especially when combined with inferences about intentions, provides another way to reduce errors.

Until about 50,000 to 100,000 years ago, hominin artifacts and anatomy changed more or less in concert[4]. Afterwards, behavioral, cultural, and tool-making innovations accelerated rapidly without additional anatomical changes, at least for crude measures such as brain size.

In summary, according to many experts an acceleration in cultural innovation occurred:

◆ more than 4.5 million years after the transition to a bipedal gait and reduced canines that indicated a shift in living conditions and diet;

◆ long after the Oldowan tool-making tradition and a major phase of brain expansion about 2.5 million years ago (Fig. 10.2A);

◆ long after the shift to more sophisticated Acheulean tools, which occurred about 1.6 million years ago;

◆ long after the reduced sexual dimorphism that points to a new social system, also about 1.6 million years ago, which might have included cooperation in foraging;

◆ long after the size of the hominin brain stabilized 200,000 to 600,000 years ago.

This evolutionary sequence constrains ideas about the evolution of memory systems. Changes in sexual dimorphism suggest that the social developments central to our proposal in Chapter 10 occurred, or at least began, much earlier than the acceleration in cultural innovation that characterized the "creative explosion."

Although many uncertainties remain, modern humans probably evolved in Africa from a founding population of approximately 10,000 interbreeding individuals, whose descendants later migrated throughout the world and replaced other hominin species that had preceded them[4,16]. An origin outside Africa remains possible, but wherever they arose these people produced cave art, carved the Lion Man of Hohlenstein, and one of their descendants—much, much later—created the Cowardly Lion (Fig. 11.1A).

Definitions

As with many aspects of biology, such as the definition of life, a formal definition of explicit memory remains illusive. As Medawar and Medawar[17] (p. 66) explain:

> In certain formal contexts—mathematical logic, for example, in which a definition is a rule for substituting one symbol for one or more others—definitions are crucially important, but in … biology their importance is highly exaggerated. It is simply not true that no discourse is possible unless all technical terms are precisely defined; if that were so, there would be no biology. A principal purpose of definition is to bring peace of mind. Sometimes, though, it is too dearly bought: a "definition," as the word itself connotes, has a quality of finality that is often unjustified and misleading and may have the effect of confining the mind instead of liberating it.

Nevertheless, we need to explain what we mean by explicit memory. For the purposes of this book, explicit memories are characterized by a subjective perception of participating in events or knowing facts. We know that some definitions of explicit memory invoke conscious recollection[18] (see Chapter 12, "The monkey model"), but it is conceivable, at least, that the human sense of participating and knowing could have arisen without conscious recollection. Accordingly, we set aside the concepts of phenomenal awareness and consciousness in order to explore a narrower and potentially separate topic: the emergence of explicit memory during hominin evolution.

Terminology is always a problem in such discussions, so we need to be clear about ours. In this book, explicit memory, declarative memory, explicit knowledge, and declarative knowledge all mean the same thing.

Premises

Discussions of cognitive capacities that might separate "man from beast" often focus on "one big thing." The development of language, politics, economic traditions, cultural transmission, social systems, tool use, a theory of mind, mental time travel, prospection, self-awareness, a certain kind of agency, metacognition, and high-order relational reasoning, among other cognitive capacities, have all had adherents as that "one big thing," and some still do. Gross[19] traces the history of these efforts, including one emphasizing an obscure ventricular ridge called the hippocampus minor, which, as it turns out, has nothing to do with the hippocampus. Instead of "one big thing," we propose that a combination of several evolutionary developments—several "sizable things"—led to the emergence of explicit memory.

The proposal in this chapter depends, in part, on three ideas discussed in Chapters 9 and 10:

1. In hominins, parietal–prefrontal networks adapted from representing relational metrics to a new, more general function: support for relational reasoning of the sort that

solves analogical problems and underpins multiple demand cognition (see Chapter 9, "Parietal–prefrontal networks").

2. The lateral temporal cortex, and especially the anterior temporal lobe, also adapted to a new, more general function in hominins. From its origins in representing the signs of resources, it came to represent the generalized concepts and categories of semantic memory (see Chapter 9, "Temporal–prefrontal networks").

3. The granular prefrontal cortex developed high-level, species-specific re-representations of self and others as an adaptation to the interdependent and cooperative social systems of hominins (see Chapter 10).

In addition to these three premises, the discussion in this chapter adopts some of the concepts and terms that Penn et al.[20] use, and so we introduce them here. These investigators contrast human and animal cognition and argue that in humans:

> mental representations are *compositional*—that is, complex mental representations are formed by combining discrete representational states into more complex structures … in a combinatorial fashion …. [But they] are compositional … in a specific fashion: … formed by *concatenation*, thereby retaining the identity of the original constituents, rather than by some other conjunctive mechanism that sacrifices the integrity of the original constituents.
>
> Penn et al.[20] (pp. 124–125, italics in original)

This idea sheds some light on the origin of the anterior temporal lobe hub. In Chapter 2 we explained that the perirhinal cortex evolved in early mammals and that most inferior temporal areas emerged much later, in primates. A key aspect of conjunctive representations in the perirhinal cortex is that they "sacrifice the integrity" of mid- and low-level conjunctions in order to represent objects at a specific level, disambiguating unique object identities (see Chapter 7, "Attributes" and "The perception–memory dichotomy"). When primates developed the inferior temporal cortex, this innovation initiated a long series of adaptations that preserved the mid-level conjunctions. In hominins, these conjunctions developed the additional and higher hierarchical levels that underlie semantic concepts and categories (see Chapter 9, "Temporal–prefrontal networks").

A particularly important aspect of semantic memory is that its generalized representations are not necessarily tied to sensory features. As we said in Chapter 9 ("Anterior temporal lobe hub") "members of a semantic category need not share any features at all"[21]. Penn et al. argue that unlike animals:

> A human subject is perfectly capable of reasoning about a *role-based category* such as "lovers" or "mothers" or "tools" without there being any set of perceptual features that all lovers, mothers, or tools have in common.
>
> Penn et al.[20] (p. 125, italics ours)

This idea emphasizes the role that semantic items and categories appear to play in the world, which relates to cause-and-effect knowledge, agency, and analogies among items and categories that seem to have similar effects on the world. Penn et al.[20] (p. 125, italics ours) particularly emphasize "the ubiquitous human capacity to find *analogical* correspondences between perceptually disparate relations ...—one of the hallmarks of the human mind and a prominent feature of abstract causal reasoning and [a theory of mind]." For example, consider the concept of a "mother ship," which issues forth alien-filled vessels to conquer the world. The relationship between this kind of "mother" and other kinds depends on shared roles and relations, not shared perceptual features. At one level, the semantic concept of "mother" is an analogy for anything that seems to have the role of emitting smaller things somewhat like itself.

Concepts and categories, like object representations, depend on conjunctive representations. Although the discussion of conjunctions in Chapter 7 focused on concrete features such as colors, shapes, metrics, and so forth, an *abstraction* can also serve as a dimension that enters into conjunctive representations. For example, the roles played by an object, concept, or category—the effects it seems to have on the world—can enter into conjunctions. So, too, can representations of one's self and one's role in the world (action–effect knowledge, also known as agency).

To illustrate this point, Fig. 11.2 depicts various conjunctive representations. Certain conjunctions allow people to differentiate glossy, sweet berries from dull, bitter ones or,

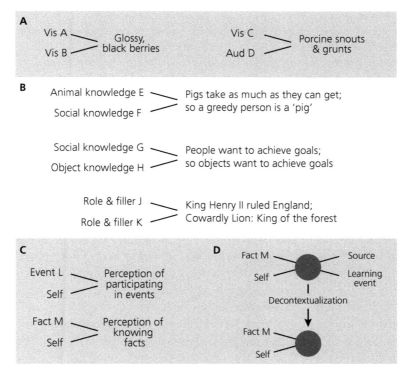

Fig. 11.2 Representational conjunctions. (A)–(C) A feature-conjunction view of role-based relations, semantic concepts and categories, metaphors, and explicit memories. (D) Decontextualization as a process.

through pattern completion, to recognize a pig from either its grunt or its snout (Fig. 11.2A). Semantic representations in the anterior temporal lobe underlie some additional capacities (see Chapter 9, "Temporal–prefrontal networks"); they contribute to analogical and meta-phorical conjunctions, which can include role-based relations (Fig. 11.2B).

We have already mentioned a contribution of the anterior temporal lobe to the role-based use of objects. In Chapter 9 ("A selective impairment") we pointed out that although semantic dementia spares motor skills, and although tool use depends primarily on parietal–prefrontal networks, when patients need to employ conceptual knowledge to use a new tool, they have impairments that correspond with their performance on tests of semantic memory[22]. This obser-vation suggests the existence of conjunctive representations that include an object's sensory fea-tures, affordances, and the role that the object plays in a world of actions, causes, and effects.

With this background, and having established the three premises listed earlier, we can now state our proposal on the origin of explicit memory.

Proposal

Explicit memory evolved in hominins after their new, species-specific re-representations of self developed in the granular prefrontal cortex and began to interact with older rep-resentational systems. These interactions have two consequences: (1) people perceive themselves as participating in ongoing, attended events and knowing attended facts, and (2) representations of self become embedded into the memories of attended facts and events. Upon retrieval of these memories, people perceive themselves as knowing facts (semantic memory) and re-experiencing events as a participant or observer (epi-sodic memory): the hallmarks of explicit memory. Not only do actual events and facts have these properties, but imagined events and fictions have them as well.

Decontextualization

According to this proposal, when humans attend to events or facts, their hominin-spe-cific re-representations of *self* automatically enter into higher-order representations that underlie both episodic and semantic memories (Fig. 11.2C). In the terms used by Penn et al.[20], these representations are compositional, concatenated conjunctions. At first, they not only include the facts of semantic memory but also the source of this knowledge and the events linked to learning. For semantic memories, this knowledge becomes *decon-textualized*, which means that the conjunctions lose their source- and event-specific fea-tures. According to our proposal, the self-representation feature remains concatenated with the items, concepts, and categories of semantic memory (Fig. 11.2D). In Chapter 9 ("Computational models") we outlined a model in which the representations in a seman-tic hub correspond to abstractions gleaned from modality- and domain-specific represen-tations in "spoke" areas. The concept of decontextualization presented here extends this idea to abstractions derived from the representations of events.

At first glance, it might seem like a proper decontextualization process should eliminate the self-representation feature as well as features reflecting sources and events, but "ineffi-ciencies" of this sort occur commonly in evolution. The self-representation feature might remain concatenated in semantic memories (Fig. 11.2D) simply because its persistence provided an adaptive advantage to evolving hominins. A feature indicating that a fact had once been attended to, with a sense of participating in the learning event, might have been beneficial in its own right. For example, we know that self-referential attention improves memory (see Chapter 10, "Self-reference and memory"). A self-representation feature might also have contributed to communicating facts to other people, a topic we return to later (see "Language").

Contributing representational systems

According to our proposal, four representational systems contribute to explicit memory:

- The social–subjective system, which contributes high-level, hominin-specific re-representations of self that distinguish explicit memories from memories of other kinds (see Chapter 10, "Social–subjective representations" and "Medial frontal cortex").
- The extended hippocampal–navigation system, which integrates spatial, temporal, and object representations that underlie perspective-taking and situational models (see Chapter 10, "A medial network").
- The feature system, which represents attributes, metrics, objects, semantic concepts and categories, and relations among relations (see Chapters 7 and 9).
- The goal system, which represents behaviors, strategies, and the effects of behavior on the world (see Chapters 8 and 9).

Together, these interacting representational systems enable the acquisition and later retrieval of explicit memories. However, each of them evolved at a different time in relation to selective pressures in the distant past. Furthermore, none of them evolved in a teleological pursuit of explicit memory; they provided advantages to some ancestral species in their time and place. According to our proposals, the cognitive innovation that we call explicit memory evolved from interactions among representational systems that had emerged much earlier:

- The navigation system evolved early in vertebrate history as these distant ancestors adopted a mobile, predatory life (see Chapters 2 and 4).
- The feature and goal systems emerged in anthropoids as they came to depend on highly volatile resources distributed over a large home range and on the signs of resources at a distance (see Chapters 2, 7, and 8).
- The social–subjective system developed as an adaptation to hominin social systems (see Chapter 10).

Excluded systems

Other representational systems contribute very little, if anything, to explicit memory. For example, when we reach to and grasp an object we usually have explicit knowledge about that goal and the fact that we are reaching to it, but the memories that transform the object's location from visual coordinates into the requisite joint-angle changes and forces remain a mystery (see Chapter 6). Likewise, responses based on reinforcement learning often become apparent in retrospect, but their genesis does not (see Chapter 3 and, later in this chapter, "Choices based on predicted outcomes" and "Conditioned responses"). The same can be said for an implicit "sense of direction" mediated by the navigation system (see Chapter 4) and biases among competing memories (see Chapter 5), competing sensory representations (see Chapter 7), and competing goals (see Chapter 8).

Precedents

Our proposal has many precedents, of course. We have already emphasized the debt owed to Penn et al.[20]. The link between the hippocampus, navigation, and explicit memory resembles ideas advanced from different perspectives by both Raby and Clayton[23] and Buzsáki and Moser[24]. The latter link the hippocampus and associated structures with both cross-domain memory and place cells in an attempt to reconcile two seemingly contradictory views about the function of the hippocampus: explicit memory and spatial processing. They propose that both functions derive from the neural mechanisms of navigation and that "navigation in real and mental space are fundamentally the same" (Buzsáki and Moser[24], p. 130). Raby and Clayton[23], recognizing the lack of evidence that animals engage in mental time travel or have genuine episodic memory, generalize the concept to include other forms of foresight, prospection, or future-thinking. They propose that semantic memory evolved as a mechanism for learning facts about the physical world and that episodic memory evolved for social functions, in order to establish an awareness of both one's self and others. In several writings, Buckner and his colleagues[25-27] explore similar ideas, emphasizing the importance of prospection and self-representation and attempting to place these ideas in an evolutionary context. In Chapter 10 we discussed the contributions of Tulving, Suddendorf, Moscovitch, Addis, Schacter, Maguire, and their many colleagues, who discuss mental time travel, constructive episodic simulation, scenario construction, and episodic memory[28-35]. In Chapter 10 we also introduced the ideas of Graziano and Kastner[36], who propose that human cognition developed when hominins recognized themselves in others and localized re-representations of their goals and attentional states to their own body. Passingham et al.[37] and Lau and Rosenthal[38] explain the concept of re-representation and the emergence of new and higher hierarchical levels during human evolution[39]. Ideas about attention that include a decision to engage with perceptual representations[40] also agree with and precede our proposal. The works cited here, of course, only scratch the surface of a voluminous literature. Our proposal contributes to this tradition by placing explicit memory in a concrete evolutionary context and by emphasizing the importance of species-specific re-representations of self.

Exaptations

Some readers might assume that a cognitive capacity as sophisticated as explicit memory must depend on newly evolved structures. However, evolution often adapts old structures to new functions. We provided several examples in Chapters 1 and 2: wings are forelimbs with new functions; inner-ear ossicles are jaw bones with new functions; and renal glomeruli are capillaries with new functions. In Chapter 9 ("Great moments in evolution") we discussed this phenomenon, known as exaptation, more generally. The proposal in this chapter invokes exaptation by suggesting that episodic memory emerged from cortical areas common to all anthropoids: granular prefrontal, posterior parietal, and lateral temporal cortex, along with an extended hippocampal–navigation system.

Critics might object that, while it is all well and good to invoke exaptation, emergent properties, and interacting representational systems, we should state more concretely what produced explicit memory, as well as how and when it emerged. We now attempt to meet this challenge.

The origin of explicit memory

Modern traits

Episodic and semantic memory

According to our proposal, explicit memories result from interactions among representational systems able to generate, via their interactions, the subjective experience of explicit memory. Only humans have this trait because explicit memory requires the high-level, species-specific re-representations of self that developed during hominin evolution (see Chapter 10).

The species specificity of these representations merits further comment. In Chapter 10 we emphasized the existence of many types of self-representation, each adapted to the social systems of a given species. There we proposed that as the prefrontal cortex expanded during hominin evolution, new and higher levels of re-representation developed. These re-representations supported the second-, third-, and higher-order intentions thought to play an essential role in language, among other social functions. More generally, they led to the human capacity for representing one's own attentional states and perceptual judgments, as well as intentions.

Our proposal posits that re-representations of self in the hominin prefrontal cortex interact with the extended hippocampal–navigation system, which gives rise to the perception of participating in—and having participated in—the events of one's life. Crucially, retrieval of these memories leads to the recollection of these events as if observing or re-experiencing them[35]. Accordingly, these memories underlie the construction of an autobiographical narrative.

In contrast to episodic memories, which are by definition explicit, *implicit* event memories merely reflect a record of experiences tied to a particular time, place, and context. A simple example illustrates this point: No one would claim that a video recorder has episodic memory or explicit knowledge, despite the fact that it establishes and retains a record of events. Later we suggest that the same goes for animals (see "Do animals have explicit memory?"). Like other implicit memories, implicit event memories lack concatenated re-representations of one's self. As a result, when implicit event memories are retrieved no sense of participation comes along with recall. Explicit event memories, according to our proposal, *do* have concatenated re-representations of self as one of their features, and so these representations produce the perception of participating in events—both as they occur and upon retrieval (Fig. 11.2C, top).

Hominin re-representations of self also underlie semantic memories (see Chapter 9, "Semantic memory"). In parallel with the distinction between explicit and implicit event memories, the difference between semantic memories, which are by definition explicit, and *implicit* fact memories involves the presence or absence of concatenated re-representations of self. According to our proposal, implicit fact memories do not have them and semantic memories do (Fig. 11.2C, bottom). These representations of self produce the perception of knowing factual and cultural knowledge. Because facts that we can write or talk about are necessarily explicit, the concept of implicit factual knowledge is inherently foreign. Yet many human behaviors depend on facts about the world that are implicit. Examples include the trajectories of falling objects, the affordances of objects, the structures of speech and grammar, and the illusion described in Box 11.2.

Contrast with the prevailing view

Obviously, the ideas about explicit memory espoused here contrast with the prevailing view of memory systems, which designates a group of four cortical areas—the hippocampal, entorhinal, perirhinal, and parahippocampal cortex—as the brain "center" for explicit (declarative) memory. Proponents of the prevailing view rarely use the term "center," presumably because it has gone out of fashion, but that is the underlying concept all the same. As support for the idea of a single memory center, these experts point to what

---

Box 11.2 Implicit fact knowledge

The concept of implicit fact knowledge is counterintuitive, but a simple example involves the perception of moving objects. People perceive small, attended objects as moving against stationary backgrounds, even when the opposite is true. The background frame captures perception, which reflects a broad statistical regularity about the relative movement of objects and background scenes in the everyday world. Our hominin ancestors surely saw the sun as moving across a stationary sky, and it took modern humans a long time to understand this illusion.

In the laboratory, a perceptual phenomenon that goes by terms such as induced motion or the Duncker illusion reveals this kind of implicit fact-knowledge. When a large background actually moves, but a small, attended object remains still, people perceive the situation the other way around. Subjects perceive the object as moving. If both the object and background jump at the same time in the same direction, but the background jumps farther, people perceive the attended object as moving in a direction opposite to what actually occurs[131]. People seem to "know," implicitly, that large background scenes are stationary—even when this is wrong—and monkeys know the same thing[132].

they describe as a "global" anterograde amnesia that supposedly follows the removal or dysfunction of the four "memory" areas (see Chapter 1, "What happened to Henry?"). However, we explained in Chapter 7 ("The perception–memory dichotomy") that lesions of these areas do not cause global amnesia. Instead, each cortical area has its own specialized representations, which support both perception and memory. Also contrary to the prevailing view, explicit memory depends on many cortical areas in addition to the four it designates as the "medial temporal lobe" memory center (see "Contributing representational systems").

Disconnection

We still need to explain why the lesions in H.M. and other amnesic patients cause such devastating impairments. Unfortunately, this explanation requires a great deal of anatomical detail. Readers who would rather avoid such intricacies might skip to the next section (see "Summary"). According to our proposal, amnesia-inducing lesions disconnect high-order, prefrontal, social–subjective representations from other key representational systems, specifically from:

- the hippocampal–navigation system, a part of the medial network (see Chapter 10, "Medial network");
- the anterior temporal lobe semantic hub and its "spoke" areas, components of the lateral network (see Chapter 10, "Lateral network").

These disconnections occur in different ways for the medial and lateral networks. For the medial network, the disconnections in amnesic patients are mostly caused by damage to the cortical gray matter; lesions disrupt interactions between the prefrontal cortex and posteromedial parts of the medial network, although damage to the fornix and fimbria contribute as well. For the lateral network, the disconnections are mostly caused by damage to white matter; lesions disrupt interactions between the prefrontal cortex and anterior temporal areas. Of course, the medial and lateral networks have extensive interactions with each other (see Fig. 10.5)[41], which are also disrupted in these patients. Note, however, that none of these disruptions has anything more than a tangential relationship with the "medial temporal lobe" as usually construed.

Networks described as medial and lateral might seem distant from each other. In primate brains, however, both come together near a narrow passage called the temporal stem, a part of the subcortical white matter that lies near the amygdala and the amygdaloid (anterior) hippocampus (see Chapter 2, "Distortions of the medial cortex").

The crucial issue concerns the location and extent of damage to the white matter. Even without direct evidence, we know that H.M.'s surgeons must have cut many fiber tracts connecting his remaining cortical areas with both the thalamus and the prefrontal cortex. White matter tracts can suffer considerable functional disruption without damage that is obvious enough to merit comment in a postmortem or structural imaging (MRI) analysis. Indeed, critics of the prevailing view have long accounted for much of H.M.'s impairment in terms of damage to pathways traversing the temporal stem, rather than as a result of the cortical areas removed by his neurosurgeons[42,43].

Damage to white matter in the temporal stem and to other fiber tracts near the amygdala disrupts many connections between the temporal and prefrontal cortex, both directly and indirectly via the thalamus. Obviously, lesions of the hippocampus and entorhinal cortex, as occurred in H.M., will block interactions between the prefrontal cortex and these areas and thus disrupt the function of the medial network (see Chapter 12, "H.M.'s ablation" and Box 12.2). Less obviously, lesions that include the amygdala, which also occurred in H.M., will cause many additional disconnections, including those cutting off the perirhinal cortex and parts of the inferior temporal cortex from both the thalamus and other cortical areas (see Chapter 12, "Falsification of the first model" and Fig. 12.2D). These disconnections affect the function of the lateral network.

The autopsy results on H.M. confirm the suspected white matter damage[44]. The authors of this postmortem description did not focus on the temporal stem, but their presentation reveals enough to demonstrate extensive white matter damage there. Nissl-stained sections at the level of the amygdala indicate that virtually nothing of H.M.'s white matter remained between the gray matter lesion site and the nearby callosal sulcus. This observation means that his neurosurgeons cut most or all of the fiber tracts lateral to the amygdala and the amygdaloid (anterior) hippocampus. Figure 2h in the autopsy report[44] illustrates this part of the lesion, and a recent paper revisits the extent of H.M.'s fiber-tract damage[45]. By comparing the structural brain images acquired from H.M. in 1993 to tractography reconstructions of white matter pathways in healthy individuals, it was possible to detect significant damage to H.M.'s right uncinate fascicle, which runs between the frontal and temporal cortex and contributes to the temporal-stem pathway. This white matter damage adds to what the autopsy shows.

Despite the fact that the autopsy report excludes H.M.'s fimbria from its discussion, the published Nissl-stained sections reveal that it is smaller and more densely stained than in an intact brain (Figs. 2k and 2l versus Fig. 2q in Annese et al.[44]). These features usually indicate a damaged pathway. Accordingly, H.M.'s surgery probably damaged many of the fibers running through the fimbria and entering the fornix, which connects the entorhinal, perirhinal, and subicular cortex with the thalamus[46], among other structures. Consistent with this conclusion, the mammillary bodies, which receive projections from the hippocampal complex via the fornix, are shrunken in H.M.'s histological material[44].

Fiber-tracing experiments in monkeys can explore homologous pathways and the damage done to them by surgery like H.M.'s. In these experiments, surgical removal of the amygdala in combination with the hippocampus severely damages axonal pathways that either originate or terminate in the prefrontal cortex[47].

Part of the reason for these disconnections involves the temporal stem, as in the case of H.M. Many fibers to and from the anterior temporal lobe and inferior temporal cortex run through the stem, where they make up part of a fiber bundle located next to the amygdala[48]. To reach the prefrontal cortex, fibers from the anterior temporal, entorhinal, and perirhinal cortex contribute to a medial part of the uncinate fascicle. This fiber bundle coalesces near the rostral and dorsal part of the amygdala before entering the frontal lobe to merge with the remainder of the uncinate fascicle. Axons from the prefrontal cortex run in the opposite direction.

Because of their proximity to the temporal stem, combined lesions of the amygdala and hippocampus do extensive damage to the medial uncinate fascicle[47]. These lesions cut many of the connections between the medial prefrontal cortex and the anterior temporal, perirhinal, and superior temporal cortex. The disconnected prefrontal areas include agranular areas 25 (infralimbic cortex), 32 (prelimbic cortex), and 24 (anterior cingulate cortex), along with area 14 of the orbitofrontal cortex. H.M.'s lesion probably produced similarly widespread disconnections of the anterior and superior temporal lobe from the prefrontal cortex.

These inadvertent disconnections not only involve direct projections between the prefrontal and temporal cortex, but also information relayed via the thalamus. To reach the thalamus, fibers to and from the temporal cortex enter the ventral amygdalofugal and ventrostriatal pathways, both of which gather near the lateral and dorsal amygdala, somewhat like the uncinate fascicle. Aspiration lesions of the amygdala substantially reduce the number of cells projecting from inferior temporal cortex (area TE) to the mediodorsal nucleus of the thalamus, specifically its medial magnocellular part[48]. This disconnection can occur either by disrupting white matter in the temporal stem or by damaging the amygdalofugal or ventrostriatal pathways. The disconnected part of the thalamus has reciprocal connections with the granular orbitofrontal and agranular orbital–insular cortex[49,50], so lesions of the amygdala would eliminate many thalamic routes between the inferior temporal and prefrontal cortex. As we explain in Chapter 12 ("H.M.'s ablation" and Box 12.2), H.M.'s ablation included most of the amygdala, so thalamically mediated connections between the temporal and prefrontal cortex would have been severely damaged, in addition to the amygdalothalamic inputs that also influence the prefrontal cortex[51].

Summary

H.M.'s neurosurgeons intended to remove the hippocampus, the amygdala, and most of the entorhinal cortex. Although they removed less of the hippocampus than originally estimated[52], they did extensive damage to fiber pathways in the region of the temporal stem. Their removal of the amygdaloid (anterior) hippocampus and most of the entorhinal cortex[53,54] eliminated prefrontal connections with these parts of the hippocampal–navigation system, of course. In addition, along with removing the amygdala, they inadvertently severed pathways connecting the prefrontal cortex with several remaining parts of the temporal cortex, including the ventroanterior temporal, superior temporal, inferior temporal, and perirhinal cortex. These areas include the anterior temporal lobe semantic hub, a number of its "spoke" areas, and other parts of the feature system. The neurosurgeons also interrupted connections between the hippocampal–navigation system (see Chapter 10, "Medial network") and the anterior temporal lobe hub (see Chapter 10, "Lateral network").

As a result of these disconnections, interactions among the representational systems that contribute to explicit memory formation suffered a severe disruption in H.M. (see "Contributing representational systems"). According to our proposal, new explicit memories require prefrontal re-representations of self to interact with these systems in order to form new conjunctive representations that include the "self" dimension. So it is clear why H.M.'s lesion had such a devastating impact on his ability to establish new explicit memories; only highly indirect pathways remained available for forming the requisite conjunctions.

In contrast, for memories established before H.M.'s surgery, his species-specific re-representations of self had already been incorporated into stored representations (Fig. 11.2C). Despite the abnormalities related to his epilepsy, when H.M. learned something in his presurgical life, his social–subjective system provided its representations to both the medial and lateral networks. So during the retrieval of these presurgical memories, H.M. experienced the perception of knowing and participating that underlies explicit memory. This account explains his relatively preserved retrograde memories, and the same principles apply to other amnesic patients.

Along with the dysfunction caused by damaged white matter in H.M. (and other amnesic patients), it is instructive to consider the specializations of white matter tracts in healthy people[55]. A recent study found that microstructural variation in the inferior longitudinal fascicle correlated with performance accuracy on the odd-stimulus-out task for *faces* (see Chapter 7, "Humans"). This kind of structural variation, detected by diffusion tractography, mainly reflects individual differences in myelination and axon density. In contrast to the inferior longitudinal fasciculus, which connects occipital visual areas with the perirhinal cortex (among other areas), microstructural variation in the fornix correlated with performance on the odd-stimulus-out task for *scenes*. In parallel, brain imaging activations in the perirhinal cortex correlated with performance accuracy on the face task, whereas activations in the hippocampus did so for the scene task. The microstructural variation in the two fiber tracts also correlated with cortical activation levels in a task- and region-specific manner. These findings extend the discussion of specialized representations in the perirhinal and hippocampal cortex to specific white matter tracts associated with these areas (see Chapter 7, "Humans").

In summary, H.M.'s disconnections degraded interactions among the prefrontal cortex, the medial network, and the lateral network, which blocked the establishment of new episodic and semantic memories. As we mentioned in Chapter 10 ("Episodic versus semantic memory"), it is tempting to link prefrontal–medial network interactions to episodic memory and prefrontal–lateral network interactions to semantic memory. At a very rough level this idea has some value. However, we do not mean to imply a rigid specialization of this kind. Along with their role in episodic memory, the hippocampus and rest of the medial network make an important contribution to semantic memory (see also Chapters 9, "Hippocampal complex", 12, "The summation principle", and 13, "H.M.'s amnesia"). Nevertheless, in order to incorporate re-representations of self into all kinds of semantic memories, regardless of where they are stored, social–subjective representations in the prefrontal cortex need to interact—or at least have interacted in the past—with both the medial and lateral networks. The combined white- and gray matter damage in H.M. blocked all of the routes mediating these interactions, and therefore he could not establish either new semantic memories or new episodic memories.

Ancestry

If we are correct, then the evolutionary developments discussed in Chapters 9 and 10 led to explicit memory, but we have said little so far about how this trait relates to language.

Language

We assume that language emerged as an adaptation to hominin social systems[20,56]. As discussed in Chapter 10 ("Language"), even protolanguage in a topic–comment form[57] presupposes that other people have attention to direct and representations to influence. For example, Dunbar[58] concludes that language requires three levels of intentional re-representation (third-order intentions) and that yet higher-order levels evolved as language matured. Of course, once language evolved it came to dominate explicit memory, as the terms semantic and declarative illustrate.

No one knows when language evolved, but genetic studies provide some hints, many of them involving the so-called "language gene" *FoxP2*. According to Dunbar[58], one analysis points to events about 2.5 million years ago, when a gene related to the jaw musculature underwent modification. However, this change could reflect dietary developments rather than communicative ones. An early study of the *FoxP2* gene yielded an estimate for its origin at about 60,000 years ago, which corresponds roughly with the emergence of fully modern humans. But a more recent analysis led to a different conclusion, with an estimate of this gene's origin at 400,000 to 800,000 years ago in an ancestor common to modern humans and Neanderthals[59]. (The morphology of the hyoid bone, which supports tongue and larynx movements[60], has also suggested a language capacity in Neanderthals[5].) Finally, an intron that affects expression of the *FoxP2* gene changed and was selected for (fixed) in modern humans[61].

Regardless of its origins, the era of exaggerated claims about the *FoxP2* gene seems to be nearly over, at long last. It is not a specific "language gene," as celebrated in popular science. For example, in one famous family a mutation in the *FoxP2* gene affected both speech and other aspects of orofacial coordination[62]. Brain imaging results in these individuals pointed to structural and activation abnormalities in the dorsal striatum, which expresses this gene. These striatal defects appear to affect coordinated movement sequences generally, not just those for speech. However, the speech impairments are particularly severe, which could reflect any of several factors: a greater requirement for coordination; the fact that the effectors used for speech have more degrees of freedom than other effectors; or the need to integrate auditory feedback into precisely timed articulatory gestures[62]. The latter possibility agrees with the idea that the fundamental function of the basal ganglia involves the use of feedback to adjust ongoing behavior (see Chapter 12, "If not habits, what?").

Studies of the vocal tract in hominins suggest that some kind of voiced articulation might have evolved about 800,000 years ago, and a related opinion points to the roughly contemporaneous development of larger passageways for motor innervation of the tongue and mouth[58]. Yet another estimate concentrates on developments about 500,000 years ago, when the ear canal changed in a way that might help people decode language by improving transmission in the 2–4 kHz range, which conveys key speech elements[60]. None of these estimates constrain our understanding of memory systems very much, except to suggest that language, or at least some form of protolanguage, preceded the acceleration in cultural innovation that occurred sometime around 50,000 to 100,000 years ago (see "Evolution").

If not language, what?

If the development of language did not lead directly to the "creative explosion," what did? Mithen[63] proposes a useful metaphor that places ideas about cognitive modules in an evolutionary context, drawing heavily on the evolutionary psychology of Cosmides and Tooby[64]. He suggests that the ancestral condition corresponded to a medieval "cathedral" containing several "chapels," walled off from each other. Each "chapel" symbolizes a specialized cognitive domain. Mithen emphasizes knowledge about society (the social domain), objects and affordances (the tools and technology domain), and biology (the plant and animal domains). For evolving hominins, plants and animals served as resources or threats; technological knowledge supported their exploitation of resources with a manufactured tool kit; and social knowledge maintained cooperation and a division of labor. Chapter 9 ("Temporal–prefrontal networks") discussed these kinds of knowledge in terms of semantic concepts and categories.

However, the mere existence of these specialized forms of knowledge cannot account for the "creative explosion" because they were all in place long beforehand. For example, hominins have made extensive use of manufactured stone tools, lived in cooperative social groups, and exploited meat for energy for more than a million years, and perhaps twice that long. Developments that occurred 1 to 2 million years ago—or 500,000 to 800,000 years ago as Dunbar[58] estimates for language—have little likelihood of accounting for cultural developments that took place 50,000 to 100,000 years ago. According to Mithen, it was not the existence of social, biological, and technical knowledge that engendered the "creative explosion." Instead, dramatic cultural advances depended on new interactions among these specialized cognitive domains.

In terms of Mithen's "cathedral" metaphor, the "walls" that once separated the "chapels" represent barriers between specialized cognitive domains. Generalization among these domains awaited neural developments that breached these "walls." This idea resembles both Rozin's[65] proposal that general intelligence stems from access to multiple cognitive domains and the concept of a global workspace. Once the breach occurred, a new level of generalization empowered the human proficiency with analogies, metaphors, and relations among relations previously unimaginable (literally). Innumerable innovations flowed from the generalizations that hominins could then abstract from specialized knowledge, a concept that we call *explosive generalization*.

We suggest that "explosive generalization" was mediated in large part by the anterior temporal lobe semantic hub, which breached the "walls" of Mithen's metaphorical "chapels" at some point during hominin evolution.

In terms of timing, it seems plausible that new levels of hierarchy formed in the granular prefrontal cortex first, which led to new, high-level re-representations of self (see Chapter 10, "Social–subjective representations"). Later, new levels of hierarchy formed in the anterior temporal lobe (see Chapter 9, "Temporal–prefrontal networks") and in parietal–prefrontal networks (see Chapter 9, "Parietal–prefrontal networks"), resulting in "explosive generalization." In Fig. 11.1(C) and Plate 6, we group these developments as trait sets 1 and 2, respectively.

We think that both sets of derived traits depended on cortical expansion in absolute terms (see Chapter 10, "Evolution"), although organizational[66] and genetic[67] changes probably accompanied that expansion. For example, a comparison of the genomes of modern humans and chimpanzees revealed changes in genes that promote synaptic plasticity. In adulthood, human brains appear to have an enhanced capacity for anatomical adaptation[66,67], which could reflect an extension into later life of developmental gene expression that is usually confined to young animals[68]. The very lengthy developmental trajectories of human cortex also support this view[69,70]. Furthermore, after the split between Neanderthals and modern humans, several genes seem to have developed more activity in the latter[71]. Compared with the genome as a whole, these genes have almost twice the likelihood of being associated with behavioral disorders such as autism and schizophrenia[71]. This finding leads to two conjectures that can be expressed in terms of our proposals: (1) autism might result from aberrations of the hominin-specific social–subjective system; and (2) schizophrenia might result from constructive episodic simulations divorced from social–subjective representations. For example, a difficulty in linking re-representations of self with the products of mental simulations might lead to the perception that they arose from external sources. Perhaps the derived cognitive traits of modern humans depend disproportionately on the more active genes just mentioned[71], which seem to be particularly vulnerable to disruption. These ideas are speculative, of course, but liabilities often accompany adaptive advantages in evolution.

We can, likewise, only speculate about the ecological and social forces that favored explicit memory. Traditional thinking has focused on hunting, scavenging for meat, and the level of social cooperation needed for such activities. However, Sayers and Lovejoy[72] challenge these assumptions, emphasizing the high costs of obtaining and processing resources compared with their benefits. They argue against hunting and long-range scavenging as factors driving the cognitive adaptations of australopiths and other early hominins. For bipedal animals, traveling long distances has a particularly high cost. Travel time, processing time, carrying capacity, and other cost factors all figure into the final tally. Instead of hunting and scavenging for meat, Sayers and Lovejoy suggest that an extreme form of ecological generalism drove cognitive developments in hominins. Shifting to a highly varied diet required a broad range of knowledge, especially about volatile, atypical, rarely encountered, and diverse botanical resources. Infrequently encountered and atypical concepts would have become essential, as would the social structures that promoted this way of life[58,73]. In Chapter 9 we discussed the role of the anterior temporal lobe hub in representing infrequent and atypical items.

Sterelny[8] emphasizes social factors, proposing that modern cognition evolved in response to an economic crisis that advantaged foragers who came to rely on intermediaries in a social group, as opposed to the direct reciprocation of material and nutritional goods between two individuals. In addition, this reciprocation sometimes needed to occur in the far distant future. Social–subjective representations and constructive episodic simulation, respectively, must have played crucial roles in such economic arrangements.

Sayers and Lovejoy[72] (p. 347) suggest that early hunter–gatherers, who relied on long-distance hunting and scavenging as well as on multiple-party economic exchanges[8], did not emerge until relatively late in hominin evolution, once "social cooperation and cohesion, along with … major advancements in communication and tool-making skills" became "sufficient to overcome the inherent disadvantages" of bipedal locomotion. If so, then perhaps the most recent suite of developments that enabled the "creative explosion"—labeled 2 in Fig. 11.1(C) and Plate 6—occurred about 50,000 to 100,000 years ago or a little before that.

Do animals have explicit memory?

Because we propose that explicit memory evolved during hominin evolution, we need to address the extensive literature implying that nonhuman animals have this form of memory. If we are correct, then animals lack explicit memory as defined in our proposal, despite a widespread assumption to the contrary. Although animals certainly remember events and facts, our proposal implies they do not experience a sense of participating in events or knowing facts. If their knowledge is not explicit, it must by definition be implicit—and our proposal suggests that all knowledge in nonhuman animals corresponds to what in humans would be called implicit memory or implicit knowledge.

The impediment to knowing whether animals have explicit memory, of course, is that they can only express their knowledge through performance, a topic that we revisit in Chapter 12 ("The monkey model"). In our opinion, the performance measures that experts advance for explicit memory in animals are subject to alternative interpretations. In each instance, we believe that the attribution of explicit memory to animals reflects unverified (and often unverifiable) assumptions, bolstered by the use of proxy terms that avoid the words explicit and declarative. Some proxy terms rely on classifying memories. In these cases, exemplified by the concepts of goal- or outcome-directed behavior and "episodic-like" memory, the conclusion that animals have explicit memory depends on the assumption that the proxy classification corresponds exclusively to explicit memory and that there are no forms of implicit memory lurking within the same class of memories. In "Choices based on predicted outcomes", "Episodic memory", and "Episodic-like memory" we show how these classifications can include implicit memories. In "One-trial associative learning", "Conditioned responses", "Receiver operating characteristic analysis", and "Report-based approach" we discuss attributes thought to characterize explicit memory in animals, again showing that implicit memories can have the same attributes.

Choices based on predicted outcomes

According to Balleine and O'Doherty[74], all behavior, including all human behavior, falls into one of two categories: habits or goal-directed behavior. To be fair, they and other like-minded theorists often accept additional categories such as Pavlovian learning and a separate episodic memory system, but habits and goal-directed behavior receive the lion's share of attention. By a goal, learning theorists usually mean reward or reinforcement or some other unconditioned stimulus (see Chapter 3). Because we recognize other kinds of goals in this book, such as objects or places that serve as the targets of action, we use the phrase outcome-directed behavior instead of goal-directed behavior.

To accept the idea that all human cognition can be classified as either habitual or outcome-directed, one has to believe that instrumentally conditioned responses belong in the same category of behavior as contemplating the aesthetics of the Mona Lisa and its place in cultural history. As explained in Chapter 8 ("Augmentation of the biased-competition system"), behavioral dichotomies create trash-can categories, and so they inevitably lead to absurdities of this kind. In a better world, they would elicit little more than a wry smile.

In essence, the dichotomy between habits and outcome-directed behaviors classifies all human behavior into habits versus "everything else," with the unstated implication that the category "everything else" might correspond to explicit memory. The same goes for the habit–memory dichotomy, which attempts to equate the nonhabit category with explicit memory. We explain the deficiencies of this idea in detail in Chapter 12 ("The habit–memory dichotomy").

The problem with both of these dichotomies, like other two-factor theories of human behavior (see Table 8.1), is their implication about explicit memory. In this case, the problem is that outcome-directed behavior can be either implicit or explicit. Explicit outcome-directed behavior is obvious in humans, but it takes an experiment to show that people make outcome-directed choices implicitly.

Johnsrude et al.[75,76] report the results of such an experiment. In one version of their task, subjects had to count the number of red stimuli that appeared along with some black ones. Whenever a red stimulus appeared, so did a visual pattern, and subjects sometimes obtained candy or raisins shortly thereafter. These rewards followed each visual pattern at a variable probability, ranging from 0.1–0.9. When the subjects were asked about these probabilities, they could not report anything about them. Nevertheless, specific testing showed that the subjects established memories of the association between visual patterns and values. When subjects chose between two patterns, they usually chose the one associated with the higher value. Not only did the subjects fail to report the reward likelihoods, but they concocted spurious reasons for their choices, saying, for example, that the pattern "looked like a nerve cell" (Johnsrude et al.[75], p. 258). The results of Johnsrude et al.[75,76] show that people can acquire stimulus–outcome (pattern–value) memories implicitly and use these memories to make choices.

Stimulus–outcome (S–O) memories result from Pavlovian learning, by defini-tion, which does not necessarily involve behavioral choices. However, the findings of Johnsrude et al. enable us to conclude that choice behavior can be based on implicit knowledge—including choices based on predicted outcomes. We recognize that critics will say that the study of Johnsrude et al. did not demonstrate outcome-directed behavior in a rigorous way because they did not use widely accepted assays of such behavior, such as reinforcer devaluation (see Chapter 3, "What happens in instrumental conditioning"). We expect that future studies will confirm our interpretation of these results, but in the meantime we content ourselves with the demonstration that people sometimes make choices that depend on their implicit knowledge about predicted outcomes, even if that does not correspond to a more restricted sense of the term outcome-directed behavior. The existence of *implicit* outcome-directed behavior in humans is important because it undermines any interpretation of outcome-directed behavior in animals as evidence for explicit memory.

In a related experiment, fasting subjects faced a choice between high-calorie and low-calorie yoghurt drinks, which had either a red or a blue label[77] (otherwise, the drinks had the same sensory features). After 2 weeks of experiencing both types of yoghurt drink in the red- or blue-labeled cups, the subjects then chose freely between cups of the two col-ors. Most subjects (58% versus 42%) chose the high-calorie option. Although a 16% bias might not seem all that impressive, note that the information the subjects used to make these choices depended on a delayed and vague visceral effect. As in the experiment of Johnsrude et al., the subjects in this experiment knew nothing about the basis for their choices and reported the color–calorie association no more accurately than expected by chance, with equal confidence when right or wrong. This experiment provides further support for the idea that people can learn stimulus–outcome (color–caloric value) asso-ciations implicitly and use these memories to make choices.

A third example involves conditioned place preferences and aversions. In this experi-ment, subjects could explore either of two "houses" using a virtual reality display[78]. They did so by moving an avatar from the "street" into the interior of each house, at which time they saw realistic internal scenes. As the subjects explored the houses, they heard a sound clip generated by a laboratory worker pretending to set up a future experi-ment. The subjects heard consonant (pleasant) music while they explored one house as opposed to static noise for the other house. In later testing without the sound clips, the subjects could choose to spend time in either house, and they showed a strong tendency to dwell in the house previously associated with the pleasant sounds. In fact, they spent 84% of their time in that house. In a separate experiment, which examined conditioned place aversions, the subjects first explored houses associated with either the static noise or with dissonant (unpleasant) music. In that experiment, subjects avoided the house associated with unpleasant sounds, spending 96% of their time in the other one. When the subjects were later asked about their choices, they denied that either the music or the static noise had influenced them in any way. Their behavior—choosing which of two houses to explore—seemed on the surface to depend on explicit knowledge, but it did not.

Accordingly, conditioned place preferences and aversions provide no evidence for explicit memory in animals.

Several additional studies involving a combination of instrumental and Pavlovian conditioning offer examples of how subjects make choices without being able to report the basis for their choice. Examples include the Iowa gambling task[79], a probability-based weather prediction task[80,81], and others that Johnsrude et al.[75] cite, but perhaps the most interesting is an experiment by Wegner[82]. His subjects had *some* influence over the movements of a cursor as it traversed images of various objects, but only *some*. In fact, the ultimate destination of the cursor remained under the control of the investigator throughout the experiment. When the subjects heard the name of an object just before the cursor stopped over it, this acoustic stimulus tricked them into concluding that they had just chosen that object. They evidently generated an explicit, retrospective account about why the cursor stopped where it did, wrongly attributing that choice to themselves. Their behavior appeared—both to observers and to the subjects themselves—to reflect explicit choices, but this cannot be true for the simple reason that the subjects did not make any choice at all.

Episodic memory

The object-in-place scenes task[83], which requires monkeys to learn and choose the correct object-like stimulus embedded in a complex background scene (Fig. 11.3A, inset), was explained in Chapters 4 ("Scene memory") and 8 ("Object-in-place scenes task"). We discuss these results again here because of the idea that this task measures episodic memory—a form of explicit memory.

The presence of a background scene dramatically improves the ability of monkeys to remember which stimulus to choose. Monkeys can remember the correct choice after just one or two trials, each separated by 19 intervening trials that involve different choice stimuli and background scenes (Fig. 11.3A, unfilled circles). Without the background scenes, monkeys learn much more slowly (Fig. 11.3A, gray triangles). It typically takes monkeys ten or more trials without the background scenes to reach the level that they attain after just one trial with the scenes. The relevance to episodic memory, and therefore to explicit memory, comes in part from this one-trial learning, which by definition involves the capture of a single event. We return to one-trial learning later (see "One-trial associative learning"), but for now we concentrate on the neural substrates of this kind of memory.

The idea that this task measures explicit, episodic memory appears to gain support from the finding that fornix transections impair object-in-place scene learning in both monkeys[83] (Fig. 11.3A) and humans (Fig. 11.3B)[84]. Lesions of the mammillary bodies and anterior thalamic nuclei in monkeys also cause impairments on this task, of about the same magnitude[83,85,86].

Given the link between these brain structures and episodic memory[87], findings from this task have led some experts to conclude that monkeys have episodic memories. The

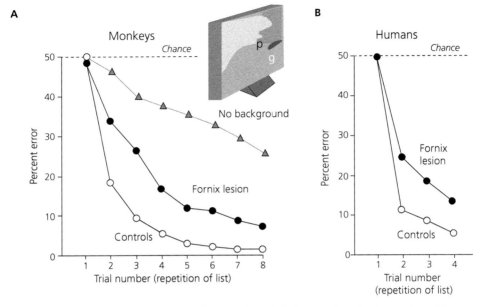

Fig. 11.3 Object-in-place scenes task. (A) Effect of fornix lesions on learning in monkeys. The inset shows an example scene. Learning curves for control monkeys with (unfilled circles) and without (gray triangles) the background scenes. Fornix transections (black circles) impaired learning mildly. (B) Effect of fornix lesions on learning in humans. (A) Adapted from Gaffan D. Against memory systems. *Philosophical Transactions of the Royal Society of London B Biological Sciences* 357:1111–21, © 2002, Royal Society.

evidence, however, does not necessarily support that conclusion. The problem arises from classifying these memories as episodic, with that term's inherent implication about explicit memory. If there are implicit forms of scene memory, then neither the scene learning in monkeys nor the similarity between the effects of fornix lesions in humans and monkeys demonstrates explicit memory in monkeys. These findings could instead reflect the contribution of specialized representations that underlie implicit forms of scene memory in both monkeys and humans, which probably depend on homologous neural substrates.

Episodic-like memory

This book neglects birds because, despite their fascinating behavior, no birds are numbered among our ancestors (see Box 2.1). Nevertheless, an influential literature suggests the existence of explicit memory in scrub jays and other corvids. Experiments have demonstrated that these birds have memories of where and when they cached food, as well as what kind of foods they cached[88,89]. The classification of these "what–where–when" memories as episodic implies that these animals have explicit memory.

Given the demonstration of this capacity in an avian species, the difficulty of demonstrating something similar in mammals has come as a surprise to some. A number of attempts to demonstrate "what–where–when" memories in rats or monkeys have failed[90,91]. This difficulty would indeed be surprising on the assumption that "what–where–when" memories are homologous in humans and scrub jays. But their last common ancestor, a relatively early amniote, lived around 320 million years ago[92] (see Fig. 1.5). If this creature had episodic memory, then this trait appeared much earlier than seems reasonable, in an animal implausibly associated with explicit (declarative) knowledge. The idea that the lineages leading to rats and monkeys later lost this powerful trait is even less plausible. More likely, "what–where–when" memories reflect convergent evolution among food-caching species—analogous, not homologous functions.

The deeper problem, however, lies in the assumption that event memories correspond to episodic memories. Notably, humans can have "what–where–when" memories without episodic memories of these events, and people can remember events without explicit knowledge of what, where, and when they occurred[93,94]. Earlier we referred to these memories as implicit event knowledge (see "Episodic and semantic memory"). The existence of implicit "what–where–when" memories undermines the assumption that event memories are explicit in animals. The creation of yet another proxy term, "episodic-like" memory[95], changes nothing of substance, unless this is understood to reflect analogies and not homologies. Analogous behaviors that evolved in parallel probably differ in many properties (see Box 1.1) and therefore tell us relatively little about episodic memory in humans.

One-trial associative learning

Like the object-in-place scenes task, the conditional motor learning task is relevant to episodic memory because monkeys show one-trial learning, an attribute of explicit memory. In a typical version, an object-like visual stimulus signals monkeys to choose one goal and different stimuli signal other goals. The basic pattern of spared and impaired memory resembles human amnesia fairly closely.

After extensive experience with solving similar problems, monkeys often remember what to do for novel stimuli based on one trial. Lesions of the fornix[96,97] and lesions that include the hippocampus, along with the subiculum and entorhinal cortex[98], cause a sizable impairment in new learning (Fig. 11.4A) and prevent one-trial learning entirely (Fig. 11.4B). Recent evidence indicates that inactivation of the entorhinal cortex, alone, causes this impairment[99]. And although lesions of the fornix profoundly disrupt one-trial learning, they have no effect on the recall of familiar stimulus–goal associations (Fig. 11.4C), a pattern resembling the relatively severe impairment in establishing new memories in human amnesia, combined with better retrograde memory. Monkeys with hippocampus lesions also continue to employ abstract strategies that require an intact short-term memory[100], which corresponds to the relatively intact short-term memory and strategic planning seen in human amnesia.

Despite these similarities, one-trial conditional motor learning does not demonstrate that monkeys have explicit memory. First, there is no way of excluding the possibility of implicit one-trial learning. Second, the impairment in monkeys pales in comparison with that of H.M. and similar patients. Monkeys with these lesions make more errors, but

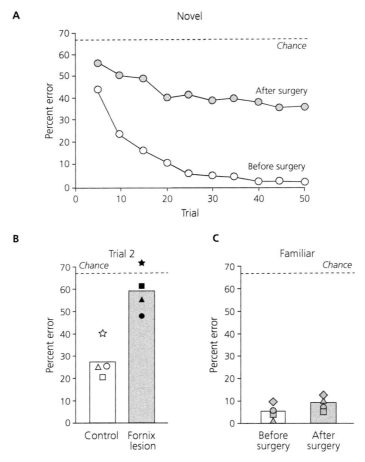

Fig. 11.4 Conditional motor learning. (A) Learning of novel mappings between visual signs and goals (or actions). Average learning curves for monkeys before lesions (unfilled circles) and after aspiration lesions of the hippocampus and the caudal entorhinal cortex (gray circles). (B) Effects of fornix lesion on one-trial learning. Scores on trial two with no prior errors and one or more intervening trials. Control monkeys, unfilled bar; monkeys with fornix transections, gray bar. Symbols: individual subjects. (C) Recall of familiar mappings for control monkeys (unfilled bar) and monkeys with hippocampus lesions (gray bar). Data in (A) and (C) from Murray and Wise[98]. Data in (B) from Brasted et al.[97].

given a sufficient number of trials they eventually solve every problem[96,97]. Accordingly, the comparison with human amnesia breaks down at this level of detail.

Conditioned responses

In Chapter 3 we discussed fear conditioning, which includes learning to make defensive responses. It is common to refer to these responses as "fear," although no evidence supports the impression that animals experience the subjective emotional experience that humans report as fear[101]. A trait called "fear" should not be considered homologous among humans and animals unless it shares the subjective, affective features so central to fear in humans. The associated defensive and autonomic responses are likely to be homologous, however.

The use of the same word, "fear," for both conditioned responses and the subjective experience of human emotions makes it is easy to assume that animals experience what humans do. The same problem also applies to all conditioned responses, including all varieties of reinforcement learning. To put it another way, Pavlovian or instrumentally conditioned responses do not serve as evidence for explicit memory in animals. Indeed, the prevailing view of memory systems usually treats them as implicit, an opinion we endorse.

Receiver operating characteristic analysis

Many studies of the hippocampus emphasize a role in explicit recollection, as contrasted with familiarity judgments[102–104]. These studies take advantage of an analytical method from signal detection theory called the receiver operating characteristic (ROC). The ROC measures a trade-off between sensitivity and selectivity. At high sensitivity, receivers detect a signal reliably (hits), but at the risk of accepting something other than that signal (false alarms). At low sensitivity, receivers often fail to detect a valid signal (misses), but reliably reject inputs other than the signal (correct rejections). In practice, this analysis involves plotting hits as a function of false alarms, resulting in an ROC curve. At the highest level of sensitivity (but lowest selectivity), the probability of a hit and a false alarm converges at one: the right extreme of the ROC curve (Fig. 11.5, left). The left extreme of the curve corresponds to the lowest level of sensitivity: The probability of a false alarm decreases to zero, but so does the ability to detect a valid signal (a hit). The left half of the ROC curve, therefore, represents a regime with low sensitivity and high selectivity.

As shown in Fig. 11.5(A), the ROC curve had an asymmetrical shape when this analysis was applied to word recognition in human subjects. In this task, subjects reported confidence judgments for the recognition of previously seen word pairs (versus rearranged pairs). The asymmetry of the ROC curve resulted from the detection of valid memories with relatively high reliability at low sensitivity levels, which shifted the left part of the curve upward[104].

Fortin et al.[105] also observed an asymmetric ROC curve in rats, based on an olfactory version of the short-interval matching task (Fig. 11.5B). This task used a nonmatching rule and, when a nonmatch occurred, rats could obtain food by digging into a test cup; otherwise they could get food from a standard cup at the back of their test cage. The experimenters biased the rats toward hits and false alarms by adjusting the amount of food in the standard cup and by increasing the cost of choosing the test cup by making it taller. Monkeys also had asymmetric ROC curves on a similar task[106].

The similarity between animals and humans extended to subjects with memory impairments. Both amnesic patients with damage said to be confined to the hippocampus and rats with hippocampus lesions had symmetrical ROC curves (Fig. 11.5A, B, gray circles)[105]. A separate analysis estimated recognition due to familiarity judgments (Fig. 11.5, right).

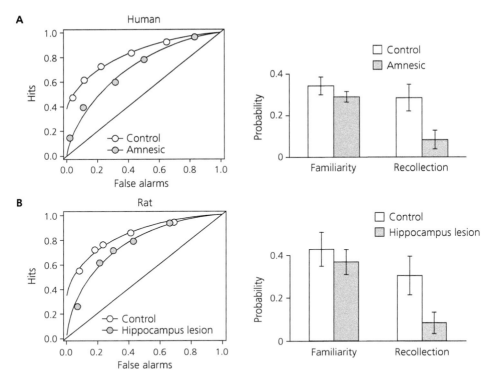

Fig. 11.5 Receiver operating characteristic (ROC) curves. (A) Data from humans. Left: ROC curves. Right: Familiarity versus recollection components. Control subjects, unfilled circles and bars; amnesic patients, gray circles and bars. (B) Data from rats. Left: ROC curves. Right: Familiarity versus recollection components. Control rats, unfilled circles and bars; rats with hippocampus lesions, gray circles and bars. (A) Reprinted from Yonelinas AP, Kroll NE, Quamme JR, Lazzara MM, Sauve MJ, Widaman KF, Knight RT. Effects of extensive temporal lobe damage or mild hypoxia on recollection and familiarity. *Nature Neuroscience* 5:1236–41, © 2002, by permission from Macmillan Publishers Ltd. (B) Reprinted from Fortin NJ, Wright SP, Eichenbaum H. Recollection-like memory retrieval in rats is dependent on the hippocampus. *Nature* 431:188–91, © 2004, by permission from Macmillan Publishers Ltd.

According to Fortin et al.[105], two conclusions can be drawn from these studies: (1) in healthy people and control rats, an asymmetry in the ROC curves results from explicit recollection; and (2) in humans and rats with damage to the hippocampus, the ROC curves revert to a symmetrical form that reflects relatively intact familiarity judgments, as opposed to explicit recollection.

We do not dispute the findings that led to these conclusions, but a problem arises when an attribute of these curves, asymmetry, serves as a proxy for explicit memory. This interpretation depends on the assumption that only explicit memory can lead to this attribute. If some other function of the hippocampus can generate such asymmetry, then these observations do not demonstrate explicit memory in either rats or monkeys.

In monkeys, for example, recency memory could serve as this other function. A recency strategy would improve task performance at low sensitivity levels (the left part of the ROC curve) because it provides information in addition to stimulus identity. Because fornix lesions have been shown to impair recency judgments for an ordered sequence of stimuli in monkeys[107], we can account for the asymmetry in ROC curves without invoking explicit memory.

Report-based approach

Animals can be said to "report" about their memories through their actions. In one such experiment, a modified short-interval matching task, monkeys saw a sample stimulus and then two additional stimuli[108]. The choice of one of these two stimuli led to a matching test, which yielded a preferred outcome if the subject performed the task correctly. The choice of the other stimulus, a "no-test" option, produced a less preferred outcome. Choices of the less-desired reward were taken as a "report" that the monkey did not remember the sample, and vice versa for choices leading to the matching test. In other words, the assumption in these experiments was that monkeys can report on the contents of their working memory, as the terms metamemory and memory awareness indicate. On the surface, the monkeys' behavior on control, catch trials seemed to support this view. On these trials, the "no-test" choice was the best the monkey could do because no sample stimulus had appeared. Indeed, the monkeys reliably chose the "no-test" stimulus on catch trials. Furthermore, as the memory period was lengthened, the monkeys chose the "no-test" option more frequently, as expected for forgetting the sample and knowing so explicitly.

These results, however, do not provide any evidence for explicit memory in monkeys because a simple conditioning account can explain them. As discussed earlier, conditioned responses can depend on implicit memory in humans, so we can assume the same for monkeys. Through experience, the monkeys in this experiment probably learned to choose the lower-value, but reliable, pay-off whenever this choice—the "no-test" option—could be predicted to yield a better net return, on average, taking delay and effort costs into account. Monkeys have counterintuitive value-discounting functions[109], which this experiment did not control for. As a result, its findings fail to provide convincing evidence for metamemory, memory awareness, or explicit memory in monkeys.

In a related experiment, called the tubes test, monkeys had to choose among four opaque tubes, one of which contained food[110]. On some trials (called overtly baited trials), the monkeys could observe an experimenter putting food into a tube, but on other trials (covertly baited trials) they could not. Later, the monkeys could select one tube by lifting it, which caused any food in the tube to slide out. The monkeys could select only one tube per trial, but they were allowed the opportunity to look down any of the tubes before making a selection. The result was that the monkeys examined the contents of the tubes more frequently on covertly baited trials than on overtly baited ones. On the surface this behavior seems to be a "report": not only that the monkeys lack any knowledge of the food's location on covertly baited trials, but also that they have explicit knowledge about the contents of their working memory. Pigeons and rats can also perform tasks of this kind[90,111,112].

Like the matching task, the tubes test fails to provide any evidence for explicit memory in monkeys. On the overtly baited trials, the monkeys simply moved toward the tube that they had seen baited earlier during a trial. This behavior requires a short-term memory of the food's location, which some experts call working memory. This sense of the term working memory, however, does not imply that these memories are explicit. On the covertly baited trials, the monkeys necessarily resorted to exploratory foraging in order to find the hidden food items; so naturally they looked into the tubes before making their choice. These observations do not demonstrate that the monkeys have explicit memory; they simply show that monkeys make foraging choices based on the remembered locations of food when they can and otherwise explore likely food locations.

Other proxy terms for explicit memory, such as contextual[113], associational[114], relational[115,116], and serial or temporal-order[117] memory, suffer from the same conceptual problems. In humans, explicit memories often have these attributes, but so do some forms of implicit memory. As explained in several previous chapters, and especially in Chapter 7 ("The perception–memory dichotomy"), the pattern of preserved and impaired performance reflects specialized representations that have no fealty to concepts such as perception, implicit memory, or explicit memory.

Prefrontal cortex–hippocampus connections

The proposal on explicit memory in this chapter emphasizes interactions between the prefrontal cortex and older representational systems, among which the extended hippocampal–navigation system figures prominently. Some readers might find this emphasis puzzling because of Fig. 11.6(A), which remains highly influential. This anatomical summary situates the perirhinal cortex and the parahippocampal cortex as gateways to both the hippocampus and entorhinal cortex, and so we call it the gateway doctrine. Figure 11.6(A) suggests that inputs from the prefrontal cortex to the hippocampus and entorhinal cortex need to pass through these gateways, and it reduces more direct prefrontal cortex inputs to the catch-all box labeled "other."

The anatomical summary in Fig. 11.6(A) has remained virtually unchanged for two decades[118,119], but it creates a number of misleading impressions. Aggleton[120] reviews the literature in detail, so we touch on only two points here.

First, contrary to the gateway doctrine, a variety of prefrontal areas have direct connections with the subiculum (Fig. 11.7A) and hippocampus (Fig. 11.7B), as well as with the entorhinal cortex (Fig. 11.6B)[53,121-124]. Interactions between the prefrontal cortex and the hippocampus, therefore, do not require the mediation of either the perirhinal or the parahippocampal cortex. Figure 11.6(C) summarizes some of the connections that bypass these postulated "gatekeepers."

Second, the entorhinal cortex has connections with most of the ring neocortex, not just the two ring areas that the gateway doctrine emphasizes. These areas include the

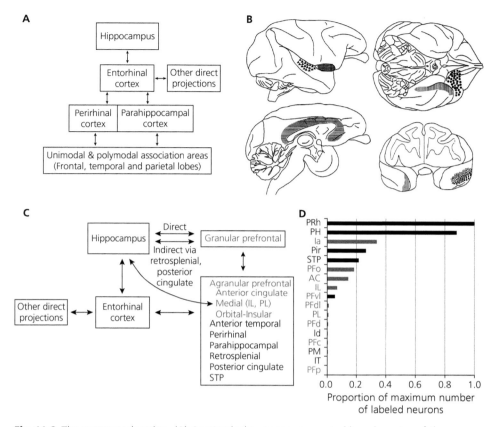

Fig. 11.6 The gateway doctrine. (A) Anatomical summary promoted by advocates of the prevailing view of memory systems. (B) Areas projecting to the entorhinal cortex. Each fi l type shows a region with such connections, including parts of the superior temporal cortex (triangles), the agranular insular cortex (cross-hatch), the temporal pole (vertical hatch), the cingulate and retrosplenial cortex (horizontal hatch), the orbitofrontal cortex (filled circles), the rostral superior temporal cortex (unfilled circles), and the rostral inferior temporal cortex (squares). (C) Summary of connections. (D) Relative number of retrogradely labeled neurons after injections of tracer into various parts of the monkey entorhinal cortex. The plot shows the maximum for any single injection site, as a proportion of the number of labeled cells in the perirhinal cortex. Abbreviations: AC, anterior cingulate cortex; Ia, agranular insular cortex; Id, dysgranular insular cortex; IL, infralimbic cortex; IT, inferior temporal cortex (excluding PRh); PFc, caudal prefrontal cortex; PFd, dorsal prefrontal cortex; PFdl, dorsolateral prefrontal cortex; PFo, granular orbitofrontal cortex; PFp, polar prefrontal cortex; PFvl, ventrolateral prefrontal cortex; PH, parahippocampal cortex; Pir, piriform cortex; PL, prelimbic cortex; PM, premotor cortex; PRh, perirhinal cortex; STP, superior temporal polysensory area. Parts of the prefrontal cortex appear in gray type. (A) Redrawn from Zola-Morgan S, Squire LR, Alvarez-Royo P, Clower RP. Independence of memory functions and emotional behavior: separate contributions of the hippocampal formation and the amygdala. *Hippocampus* 1:207–20, © 1991, John Wiley & Sons, with permission. (B) Reproduced from Mohedano-Moriano A, Pró-Sistiaga P, Arroyo-Jiménez MM, Artacho-Pérula E, Insausti AM, Marcos P, Cebada-Sánchez S, Martínez-Ruiz J, Muñoz M, Blaizot X, Martínez-Marcos A, Amaral DG, Insausti R. Topographical and laminar distribution of cortical input to the monkey entorhinal cortex. *Journal of Anatomy* 211:250–60, © 2007, John Wiley & Sons, with permission. (D) Data from Insausti et al.[122].

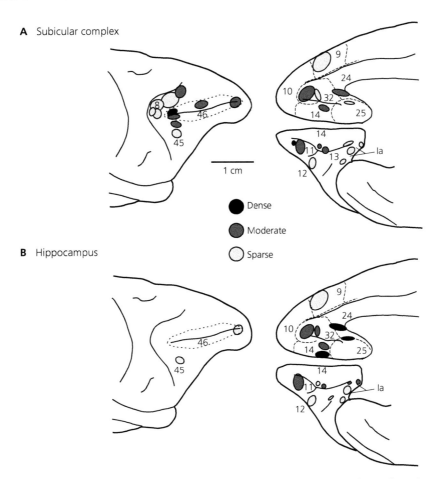

Fig. 11.7 Prefrontal–hippocampal connections. Direct connections between the prefrontal cortex and either the subiculum (A) or the hippocampus (B). Gray levels at the various tracer injection sites indicate the density of retrogradely labeled cells in the hippocampal complex. The numerals corresponds to cortical areas (see Fig. 1.4). From Murray EA, Wise SP. Why is there a special issue on perirhinal cortex in a journal called *Hippocampus*? The perirhinal cortex in historical perspective. *Hippocampus* 22:1941–51, © 2012, reproduced with permission from John Wiley & Sons. Based on drawings in Barbas and Blatt[53].

infralimbic, prelimbic, orbital–insular, anterior cingulate, posterior cingulate, and retrosplenial cortex, among others (Fig. 11.6B). Figure 11.6(D) shows that although the two "gateway" areas have the largest number of cells projecting to the entorhinal cortex, many other areas contribute such inputs as well.

Taking these two points together, and using neuroanatomical findings in macaque monkeys as a proxy for connections in humans, we conclude that the granular prefrontal cortex has several routes for interacting with the extended hippocampal–navigation system. According to the proposal that we advanced earlier in this chapter, these connections help to establish and retrieve explicit memories. As we summarize in Fig. 11.6(C), granular prefrontal areas not only have direct connections with the hippocampus, but also connect to it indirectly via the retrosplenial[125] and posterior cingulate cortex, as well as via agranular prefrontal areas. Figure 11.6(C) still leaves out a great deal, but—in contrast to Fig. 11.6(A)—our less-filtered anatomical summary provides ample support for the proposal presented in this chapter. Specifically, our proposal requires the granular prefrontal cortex to provide re-representations of self to both the extended hippocampal–navigation system and to other aspects of the large-scale medial network discussed in Chapter 10, as well as to the lateral network discussed in the same chapter.

Conclusions

We know for sure that explicit memory originated in one of our ancestors. With equal certainty, we know that some of our ancestors lacked this trait. For example, early animals did not have a brain at all, so it would be preposterous to suggest that they had "precursors" of explicit memory in any meaningful sense. In Chapter 1 ("Why ask 'why'?") we expressed the same thought differently:

◆ The kinds of memory that H.M. lost did not exist in all of his ancestors.

◆ Yet in some of them it did.

That is not a proposal; it is an obvious fact.

We state the obvious because it frames the key question: In which of our ancestors did explicit memory first emerge? In other words, which ancestors combined their cognitive capacities in a way that first produced a perception of participating in remembered and imagined events (episodic memory) and knowing facts (semantic memory)?

In answering these questions, we have come the view that, of extant animals, only humans have explicit memory. Obviously, this idea differs dramatically from the belief that a "precursor" of episodic memory evolved in a common ancestor of birds and mammals[126]. It also conflicts with the commonly accepted assumption that rodents, humans, and monkeys have a homologous explicit (declarative) memory system (see "Do animals have explicit memory?"). Instead of "ancient ancestry," we propose that explicit memory arose relatively recently, in hominins, as an emergent property of the derived traits discussed in Chapters 9 and 10 and their interactions. The proposal in Chapter 10 discussed some of these hominin traits:

◆ The elaboration of new and higher hierarchical levels of re-representation in the prefrontal cortex empowered attention to and perception of one's own intentions, perceptions, actions, traits, and internal states. This development, in turn, produced new, higher-level, species-specific re-representations of self in hominins, which allowed the localization of intentions, perceptions, and attentional states to one's self and others. The selective pressures for these developments probably involved the gregariously interdependent social systems adopted by evolving hominins (see Chapter 10, "Social–subjective representations").

◆ Once the hominin form of self-representation arose in the prefrontal cortex, it could become a dimension of representations processed and stored by the hippocampus and the rest of the extended hippocampal–navigation system (Fig. 11.2C). According to our proposal, this species-specific self-representational dimension produces the perception of participating in ongoing, attended events. Later, when memories with this dimension are retrieved, humans re-experience the remembered events as participants—the characteristic quality of episodic memory.

In Chapter 9 we discussed some additional hominin traits:

◆ The elaboration of new and higher hierarchical levels of representation in the anterior temporal lobe produced "explosive generalization" across cognitive domains (see Chapter 9, "Temporal–prefrontal networks"). Comparable adaptations in parietal–prefrontal networks enabled high-order relational reasoning and multiple demand cognition (see Chapter 9, "Parietal–prefrontal networks").

◆ After these developments occurred, interactions between the prefrontal cortex and the anterior temporal lobe could embed species-specific representations of self into the kinds of memories that the semantic hub and its "spoke" areas store: attentively acquired facts, concepts, categories, and generalizations (Fig. 11.2C). According to our proposal, this species-specific self-representational dimension produces the perception of knowing facts as they are encountered. Later, when memories with this dimension are retrieved, humans experience the sense of knowing that characterizes semantic memory.

Figure 11.1(C) and Plate 6 take a stab at placing these developments in an evolutionary context. In this scenario, the derived traits discussed in Chapter 10 developed first (marked by the numeral 1). As just mentioned, these innovations led to interactions between hominin representations of self and the extended hippocampal–navigation system. The latter continued doing what it had long done, but its new inputs led to several emergent properties, including an autobiographical narrative covering an individual's life span. A related capacity also emerged at about this time, which goes by many names: constructive episodic simulation, mental time travel, mental trial and error, scenario construction, prospection, foresight, and future-thinking. As a result, autobiographical narratives could extend into the distant past and the far future, including revisionist histories and imaginary possibilities. We regard these capacities as derived traits in humans, but they reflect conserved specializations of the hippocampal–navigation system.

Later, the innovations discussed in Chapter 9 contributed to a dramatic acceleration in cultural innovation (marked by the numeral 2 in Fig. 11.1C and Plate 6). This suite of derived traits included a semantic hub in the anterior temporal lobe, which enabled the capacity for "explosive generalization" that led to far-reaching analogical and metaphorical reasoning, as well as the establishment of highly abstract and generalized concepts and categories. Developments in parietal–prefrontal networks added knowledge about relations among relations, including action–effect and cause-and-effect relations that underlie concepts about agency.

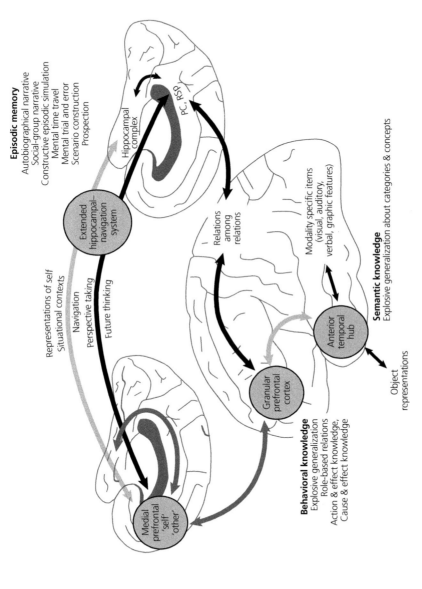

Fig. 11.8 Participating and knowing. Summary of interactions among representational systems, including two cortical hubs, one in the anterior temporal lobe, the other in the granular prefrontal cortex. Abbreviations: PC, posterior cingulate cortex; RSp, retrosplenial cortex.

The following labels appear within the figure:

Episodic memory
Autobiographical narrative
Social-group narrative
Constructive episodic simulation
Mental time travel
Mental trial and error
Scenario construction
Prospection

Hippocampal complex

PC, RSp

Extended hippocampal–navigation system

Representations of self
Situational contexts
Navigation
Perspective taking
Future thinking

Relations among relations

Modality specific items
(visual, auditory, verbal, graphic features)

Semantic knowledge
Explosive generalization about categories & concepts

Anterior temporal hub

Object representations

Granular prefrontal cortex

Behavioral knowledge
Explosive generalization
Role-based relations
Action & effect knowledge
Cause & effect knowledge

Medial prefrontal 'self' 'other'

Many theorists point to "explosive generalization" as a key characteristic of human cognition, although in different terms. For example, Mithen[63] emphasizes the ability to use language outside the social domain and to apply role-based, cause-and-effect knowledge about tools to animals and social groups. Penn et al.[20] emphasize analogies among different cognitive domains. They propose that human cognition differs from that of other animals in three main ways: (1) it allows the application of solutions gained for one cognitive domain to others, resulting in highly abstract problem-solving strategies; (2) it empowers the representation of role-based relations, divorced from their perceptual features; and (3) it enables the arbitrary symbolic associations of speech and language. We do not know when "explosive generalization" developed, but it might have been as recently as 100,000 years ago, after which our ancestors began to bury members of their social group in elaborate graves and draw animals on the walls of caves (see "Evolution").

Despite its power, "explosive generalization" cannot account for explicit memory on its own, at least not as modern humans experience this trait. However, interactions among the derived traits discussed in Chapters 9 and 10 might do so, especially because the prefrontal cortex and the anterior temporal lobe provide inputs to each other. These reciprocal connections enable a particularly powerful form of representational recursion, which can integrate both social–subjective knowledge and episodic memories with semantic concepts and categories (Fig. 11.8). The anterior temporal lobe can draw on inputs from the granular prefrontal cortex to develop semantic generalizations that are enriched by representations of one's self and others, including one's own perceptions, strategies, intentions, and emotional states; the prefrontal cortex can draw on inputs from the anterior temporal lobe to enhance its goal and social–subjective representations with the cultural constructs collected over a lifetime. After the self-representational dimension becomes established in memories stored by the anterior temporal lobe hub and its "spoke" areas, they can provide the medial network with what it needs to establish new explicit memories, even in the absence of a contribution from the prefrontal cortex (see Chapter 13, "Episodic memory").

According to the scenario depicted in Fig. 11.1(C) and Plate 6, human cognition adopted its modern character only after all these developments fell into place: first explicit memory, then "explosive generalization." At that point, a combination of the two fueled a "quantum advance in the human ability to innovate …." (Klein and Edgar[127], p. 272). Once it did, modern humans increased their population, expanded their range, displaced other hominins, and conjured up the Cowardly Lion.

References

1. **Fleming, V.** (director) (1939) Metro-Goldwyn-Mayer.
2. **Pope John Paul II** (1996) *L'Osservatore Romano.* http://www.ewtn.com/library/papaldoc/jp961022.htm.
3. **Conard, N.J.** (2009) *Nature* **459**, 248–252.
4. **Klein, R.G.** (2009) *The Human Career* (University of Chicago Press, Chicago, IL).
5. **Dediu, D.** and **Levinson, S.C.** (2013) *Front. Psychol.* **4**, 397.

6. Radovcic, D., Srsen, A.O., Radovcic, J., and Frayer, D.W. (2015) *PLoS One* **10**, e0119802.

7. Lind, J., Lindenfors, P., Ghirlanda, S., Liden, K. et al. (2013) *Sci. Rep.* **3**, 1785.

8. Sterelny, K. (2014) *Biol. Theory* **9**, 65–77.

9. Sterelny, K. (2011) *Phil. Trans. R. Soc. B: Biol. Sci.* **366**, 809–822.

10. Bookstein, F., Schafer, K., Prossinger, H., Seidler, H. et al. (1999) *Anat. Rec.* **257**, 217–224.

11. Conroy, G.C., Weber, G.W., Seidler, H., Recheis, W. et al. (2000) *Am. J. Phys. Anthropol.* **113**, 111–118.

12. McPherron, S.P., Alemseged, Z., Marean, C.W., Wynn, J.G. et al. (2010) *Nature* **466**, 857–860.

13. Harmand, S., Lewis, J.E., Feibel, C.S., Lepre, C.J. et al. (2015) *Nature* **521**, 310–315.

14. Villmoare, B., Kimbel, W.H., Seyoum, C., Campisano, C.J. et al. (2015) *Science* **347**, 1352–1355.

15. Berna, F., Goldberg, P., Horwitz, L.K., Brink, J. et al. (2012) *Proc. Natl. Acad. Sci. USA* **109**, E1215–E1220.

16. Mellars, P. (2006) *Proc. Natl. Acad. Sci. USA* **103**, 9381–9386.

17. Medawar, P.B. and Medawar, J.S. (1983) *Aristotle to Zoos. A Philosophical Dictionary of Biology* (Harvard University Press, Cambridge, MA).

18. Clark, R.E., Manns, J.R., and Squire, L.R. (2002) *Trends Cogn. Sci.* **6**, 524–531.

19. Gross, C.G. (1998) *Brain, Vision, Memory* (MIT Press, Cambridge, MA).

20. Penn, D.C., Holyoak, K.J., and Povinelli, D.J. (2008) *Behav. Brain Sci.* **31**, 109–130.

21. Lambon Ralph, M.A., Sage, K., Jones, R.W., and Mayberry, E.J. (2010) *Proc. Natl. Acad. Sci. USA* **107**, 2717–2722.

22. Bozeat, S., Lambon Ralph, M.A., Patterson, K., and Hodges, J.R. (2002) *Cogn. Affect. Behav. Neurosci.* **2**, 236–251.

23. Raby, C.R. and Clayton, N.S. (2009) *Behav. Process.* **80**, 314–324.

24. Buzsáki, G. and Moser, E.I. (2013) *Nat. Neurosci.* **16**, 130–138.

25. Buckner, R.L. and Krienen, F.M. (2013) *Trends Cogn. Sci.* **17**, 648–665.

26. Buckner, R.L. (2010) *Annu. Rev. Psychol.* **61**, 27–28.

27. Buckner, R.L. and Carroll, D.C. (2007) *Trends Cogn. Sci.* **11**, 49–57.

28. Poppenk, J. and Moscovitch, M. (2011) *Neuron* **72**, 931–937.

29. Addis, D.R., Moscovitch, M., and McAndrews, M.P. (2007) *Brain* **130**, 2327–2342.

30. Suddendorf, T., Addis, D.R., and Corballis, M.C. (2009) *Phil. Trans. R. Soc. B: Biol. Sci.* **364**, 1317–1324.

31. Tulving, E. (2002) *Annu. Rev. Psychol.* **53**, 1–25.

32. Wheeler, M.A., Stuss, D.T., and Tulving, E. (1997) *Psychol. Bull.* **121**, 331–354.

33. Schacter, D.L., Addis, D.R., Hassabis, D., Martin, V.C. et al. (2012) *Neuron* **76**, 677–694.

34. Conway, M.A. and Pleydell-Pearce, C.W. (2000) *Psychol. Rev.* **107**, 261–288.

35. Hassabis, D., Kumaran, D., and Maguire, E.A. (2007) *J. Neurosci.* **27**, 14365–14374.

36. Graziano, M.S. and Kastner, S. (2011) *Cogn. Neurosci.* **2**, 98–113.

37. Passingham, R.E., Bengtsson, S.L., and Lau, H.C. (2010) *Trends Cogn. Sci.* **14**, 16–21.

38. Lau, H. and Rosenthal, D. (2011) *Trends Cogn. Sci.* **15**, 365–373.

39. Vendetti, M.S. and Bunge, S.A. (2014) *Neuron* **84**, 906–917.

40. Kiani, R. and Shadlen, M.N. (2009) *Science* **324**, 759–764.

41. Ritchey, M., Libby, L.A., and Ranganath, C. (2015) *Prog. Brain Res.* **219**, 45–64.

42. Horel, J.A. (1978) *Brain* **101**, 403–445.

43. Gaffan, D. (2001) *Behav. Brain Res.* **127**, 5–11.

44. Annese, J., Schenker-Ahmed, N.M., Bartsch, H., Maechler, P. et al. (2014) *Nat. Commun.* **5**, 3122.

45. Thiebaut de Schotten, M., Dell'Acqua, F., Ratiu, P., Leslie, A. et al. (2015) *Cereb. Cortex* **25**, 4812–4827.

46. Saunders, R.C., Mishkin, M., and Aggleton, J.P. (2005) *Exp. Brain Res.* **167**, 1–16.

47. Muñoz, M., Mishkin, M., and Saunders, R.C. (2009) *Cereb. Cortex* **19**, 2114–2130.

48. Goulet, S., Dore, F.Y., and Murray, E.A. (1998) *Exp. Brain Res.* **119**, 131–140.

49. Ray, J.P. and Price, J.L. (1992) *J. Comp. Neurol.* **323**, 167–197.

50. Ray, J.P. and Price, J.L. (1993) *J. Comp. Neurol.* **337**, 1–31.

51. Timbie, C. and Barbas, H. (2015) *J. Neurosci.* **35**, 11976–11987.

52. Corkin, S., Amaral, D.G., Gonzalez, R.G., Johnson. K.A. et al. (1997) *J. Neurosci.* **17**, 3964–3979.

53. Barbas, H. and Blatt, G.J. (1995) *Hippocampus* **5**, 511–533.

54. Cavada, C., Company, T., Tejedor, J., Cruz-Rizzolo, R.J. et al. (2000) *Cereb. Cortex* **10**, 220–242.

55. Hodgetts, C.J., Postans, M., Shine, J.P., Jones, D.K. et al. (2015) *eLife* 10.7554/eLife.07902.

56. Burling, R. (2005) *The Talking Ape* (Oxford University Press, Oxford).

57. Hurford, J.R. (2012) *The Origins of Grammar* (Oxford University Press, Oxford).

58. Dunbar, R. (2014) *Human Evolution* (Pelican-Penguin, London).

59. Krause, J., Lalueza-Fox, C., Orlando, L., Enard, W. et al. (2007) *Curr. Biol.* **17**, 1908–1912.

60. Martinez, I., Arsuaga, J.L., Quam, R., Carretero, J.M. et al. (2008) *J. Hum. Evol.* **54**, 118–124.

61. Maricic, T., Gunther, V., Georgiev, O., Gehre, S. et al. (2013) *Mol. Biol. Evol.* **30**, 844–852.

62. Watkins, K. (2011) *Prog. Brain Res.* **189**, 225–238.

63. Mithen, S. (1996) *The Prehistory of the Mind* (Thames and Hudson, London).

64. Cosmides, L. and Tooby, J. (2013) *Annu. Rev. Psychol.* **64**, 201–229.

65. Rozin, P. (1976) *Prog. Psych. Physiol. Psych.* **6**, 245–280.

66. Krubitzer, L. and Stolzenberg, D.S. (2014) *Curr. Opin. Neurobiol.* **24**, 157–165.

67. Preuss, T.M. (2012) *Proc. Natl. Acad. Sci. USA* **109 (Suppl. 1)**, 10709–10716.

68. Somel, M., Franz, H., Yan, Z., Lorenc, A. et al. (2009) *Proc. Natl. Acad. Sci. USA* **106**, 5743–5748.

69. Shaw, P., Kabani, N.J., Lerch, J.P., Eckstrand, K. et al. (2008) *J. Neurosci.* **28**, 3586–3594.

70. Gogtay, N., Giedd, J.N., Lusk, L., Hayashi, K.M. et al. (2004) *Proc. Natl. Acad. Sci. USA* **101**, 8174–8179.

71. Gokhman, D., Lavi, E., Prufer, K., Fraga, M.F. et al. (2014) *Science* **344**, 523–527.

72. Sayers, K. and Lovejoy, C.O. (2014) *Q. Rev. Biol.* **89**, 319–357.

73. Dunbar, R.I.M. (2009) *Ann. Hum. Biol.* **36**, 562–572.

74. Balleine, B.W. and O'Doherty, J.P. (2010) *Neuropsychopharmacol.* **35**, 48–69.

75. Johnsrude, I.S., Owen, A.M., and Zhao, W.V. (1999) *Lean. Motiv.* **30**, 250–264.

76. Johnsrude, I.S., Owen, A.M., White, N.M., Zhao, W.V. et al. (2000) *J. Neurosci.* **20**, 2649–2656.

77. Zandstra, E.H. and El-Deredy, W. (2011) *Appetite* **57**, 45–49.

78. Molet, M., Billiet, G., and Bardo, M.T. (2013) *Behav. Proc.* **92**, 31–35.

79. Bechara, A., Damasio, H., Tranel, D., and Damasio, A.R. (1997) *Science* **275**, 1293–1295.

80. Knowlton, B.J., Squire, L.R., and Gluck, M.A. (1994) *Learn. Mem.* **1**, 106–120.

81. Knowlton, B.J., Mangels, J.A., and Squire, L.R. (1996) *Science* **273**, 1399–1402.

82. Wegner, D.M. (2002) *The Illusion of Conscious Will* (MIT Press, Cambridge, MA).

83. Gaffan, D. (1994) *J. Cogn. Neurosci.* **6**, 305–320.

84. Aggleton, J.P., McMackin, D., Carpenter, K., Hornak, J. et al. (2000) *Brain* **123**, 800–815.

85. Parker, A. and Gaffan, D. (1997) *J. Cog. Neurosci.* **9**, 512–521.

86. Parker, A. and Gaffan, D. (1997) *Neuropsychologia* **35**, 1093–1102.

87. Vann, S.D., Tsivilis, D., Denby, C.E., Quamme, J.R. et al. (2009) *Proc. Natl. Acad. Sci. USA* **106**, 5442–5447.

88. Clayton, N.S. and Dickinson, A. (1998) *Nature* **395**, 272–274.

89. Clayton, N.S. and Dickinson, A. (1999) *J. Exp. Psychol. Anim. Behav. Process.* **25**, 82–91.

90. Hampton, R.R. and Schwartz, B.L. (2004) *Curr. Opin. Neurobiol.* **14**, 192–197.

91. Hampton, R.R., Hampstead, B.M., and Murray, E.A. (2005) *Learn. Motiv.* **36**, 245–259.

92. Phillips, M.J., Bennett, T.H., and Lee, M.S. (2009) *Proc. Natl. Acad. Sci. USA* **106**, 17089–17094.

93. Suddendorf, T. and Corballis, M.C. (2007) *Behav. Brain Sci.* **30**, 335–345.

94. Suddendorf, T. and Corballis, M.C. (2007) *Behav. Brain Sci.* **30**, 299–313.

95. Clayton, N.S., Bussey, T.J., Emery, N.J., and Dickinson, A. (2003) *Trends Cogn. Sci.* **7**, 436–437.

96. Brasted, P.J., Bussey, T.J., Murray, E.A., and Wise, S.P. (2003) *Brain* **126**, 1202–1223.

97. Brasted, P.J., Bussey, T.J., Murray, E.A., and Wise, S.P. (2005) *Behav. Neurosci.* **119**, 662–676.

98. Murray, E.A. and Wise, S.P. (1996) *Behav. Neurosci.* **110**, 1261–1270.

99. Yang, T., Bavley, R.L., Fomalont, K., Blomstrom, K.J. et al. (2014) *Hippocampus* **24**, 1102–1111.

100. Wise, S.P. and Murray, E.A. (1999) *Hippocampus* **9**, 101–117.

101. LeDoux, J.E. (2013) *Trends Cogn. Sci.* **17**, 155–156.

102. Aggleton, J.P. and Brown, M.W. (2005) *Q. J. Exp. Psychol. B* **58**, 218–233.

103. Diana, R.A., Yonelinas, A.P., and Ranganath, C. (2007) *Trends Cogn. Sci.* **11**, 379–386.

104. Eichenbaum, H., Yonelinas, A.P., and Ranganath, C. (2007) *Annu. Rev. Neurosci.* **30**, 123–152.

105. Fortin, N.J., Wright, S.P., and Eichenbaum, H. (2004) *Nature* **431**, 188–191.

106. Guderian, S., Brigham, D., and Mishkin, M. (2011) *Proc. Natl. Acad. Sci. USA* **108**, 19425–19430.

107. Charles, D.P., Gaffan, D., and Buckley, M.J. (2004) *J. Neurosci.* **24**, 2037–2044.

108. Hampton, R.R. (2001) *Proc. Natl. Acad. Sci. USA* **98**, 5359–5362.

109. Kralik, J.D. and Sampson, W.W. (2012) *Behav. Process.* **89**, 197–202.

110. Hampton, R.R., Zivin, A., and Murray, E.A. (2004) *Anim. Cogn.* **7**, 239–246.

111. Sutton, J.E. and Shettleworth, S.J. (2008) *J. Exp. Psychol. Anim. Behav. Process.* **34**, 266–282.

112. Roberts, W.A., Feeney, M.C., McMillan, N., MacPherson, K. et al. (2009) *J. Exp. Psychol. Anim. Behav. Process.* **35**, 129–142.

113. Gaffan, D., Parker, A., and Easton, A. (2001) *Neuropsychologia* **39**, 51–70.

114. Eichenbaum, H. and Bunsey, M. (1995) *Curr. Dir. Psychol. Sci.* **4**, 19–23.

115. Cohen, N.J., Poldrack, R.A., and Eichenbaum, H. (1997) *Memory* **5**, 131–178.

116. Eichenbaum, H. and Cohen, N.J. (2014) *Neuron* **83**, 764–770.

117. Kesner, R.P., Gilbert, P.E., and Barua, L.A. (2002) *Behav. Neurosci.* **116**, 286–290.

118. Zola-Morgan, S., Squire, L.R., Alvarez-Royo, P., and Clower, R.P. (1991) *Hippocampus* **1**, 207–220.

119. Wixted, J.T. and Squire, L.R. (2011) *Trends Cogn. Sci.* **15**, 210–217.

120. Aggleton, J.P. (2011) *Neurosci. Biobehav. Rev.* **36**, 1579–1596.

121. Muñoz, M. and Insausti, R. (2005) *Eur. J. Neurosci.* **22**, 1368–1388.

122. Insausti, R., Amaral, D.G., and Cowan, W.M. (1987) *J. Comp. Neurol.* **264**, 356–395.

123. Mohedano-Moriano, A., Pró-Sistiaga, P., Arroyo-Jiménez, M.M., Artacho-Pérula, E. et al. (2007) *J. Anat.* **211**, 250–260.

124. Aggleton, J.P., Wright, N.F., Rosene, D.L., and Saunders, R.C. (2015) *Cereb. Cortex* **25**, 4351–4373.

125. Morris, R., Pandya, D.N., and Petrides, M. (1999) *J. Comp. Neurol.* **407**, 183–192.

126. Allen, T.A. and Fortin, N.J. (2013) *Proc. Natl. Acad. Sci. USA* **110** (Suppl. 2), 10379–10386.

127. Klein, R.G. and Edgar, B. (2002) *The Dawn of Human Culture* (John Wiley & Sons, New York).

128. Stout, D., Passingham, R., Frith, C., Apel, J. et al. (2011) *Eur. J. Neurosci.* **33**, 1328–1338.

129. Frith, C.D. (2012) *Phil. Trans. R. Soc. B: Biol. Sci.* **367**, 2213–2223.

130. Passingham, R.E. and Wise, S.P. (2012) *The Neurobiology of the Prefrontal Cortex.* (Oxford University Press, Oxford).

131. Wong, E. and Mack, A. (1981) *Acta Psychol.* **48**, 123–131.

132. Lebedev, M.A., Douglass, D.K., Moody, S.L., and Wise, S.P. (2001) *J. Neurophysiol.* **85**, 1395–1411.

Part V

Deconstructing and reconstructing memory systems

In the first 11 chapters of this book (Parts I–IV) we traced the evolution of ideas about memory systems (Chapter 1), of the vertebrate brain (Chapter 2), and of multiple, interacting representational systems (Chapters 3–11). We have also explored how an evolutionary perspective can contribute to a new view of memory, one that emphasizes specialized neural representations and the advantages that they provided to specific ancestors in the distant past. Part IV brought to an end our series of proposals but left a key question unanswered: If the prevailing view of memory is so unsatisfactory, how did it arise and come to dominate the field? In Chapter 12 we answer this question by explaining how a reluctance to incorporate evolution, or doing so inadequately, has fostered some of the prevailing view's most significant flaws. In Chapter 13 we present a chapter-by-chapter summary, consider some tests of our proposals, revisit H.M.'s amnesia one last time, and offer some concluding remarks.

Deconstructing amnesia

Overview

The proposals presented in Parts II–IV bear scant resemblance to the prevailing view of memory systems, which came to prominence in the 1980s. Since that time, its four principal tenets have dominated the field: (1) Four cortical areas—the hippocampal, entorhinal, parahippocampal, and perirhinal cortex—function cooperatively in the service of explicit memory; (2) these areas function collectively to support episodic and semantic memory; (3) "memory areas" lack perceptual functions; and (4) the basal ganglia, as a whole, subserves habits and other implicit memories—but not explicit memory. Compelling evidence contradicts all of these ideas. In this chapter we explain how research on monkeys and a particular choice made in the 1980s produced the prevailing view. We also explain how neglect or misunderstanding of evolution—and an outdated attitude toward animal models—contributed to its contradictions.

The road not taken

The themes of this chapter bring to mind the famous and often-quoted poem by Robert Frost—*The Road Not Taken*[1]. A traveler faces a fork in the road, considers the situation, and chooses the path that seems less trodden. Although the two roads do not differ all that much, the choice will influence affairs for a long time to come.

Something similar happened in memory research. In Chapter 2 we pointed out that the prevailing view of explicit memory treats a diverse mixture of allocortical and neocortical areas as a single functional entity—the "medial temporal lobe memory system"—despite the fact that these structures evolved at very different times in response to distinct selective pressures. The prevailing view also ignores the contributions of the basal ganglia to explicit memory, despite the fact that some cortex–basal ganglia "loops" include the same "medial temporal lobe" areas said to subserve explicit memory, including the hippocampus (see Plate 1).

These problems provide ample signs that something is amiss in world of memory research, but we appreciate that few neuroscientists will find such arguments persuasive on their own. Accordingly, in this chapter we address two questions:

- ◆ If there is no such thing as a "medial temporal lobe memory system," then how did this idea develop?

- If we dismiss the idea of a "medial temporal lobe memory system," in general, does this apply to all four of its principal tenets: (1) that four cortical areas contribute similarly to explicit memory, to the exclusion of other cortical areas (see "The equipotentiality principle"); (2) that its four "memory areas" specialize in either episodic or semantic memory, thereby summing to explicit memory (see "The summation principle"); (3) that "memory areas" lack perceptual functions (see "The perception–memory dichotomy"); and (4) that the basal ganglia, being a "habit system," lacks a role in explicit memory (see "The habit–memory dichotomy")?

In answering the first question, we explain why and when the field took the path that it did. History shows that, at a particular juncture in the 1980s, memory researchers faced a fork in the road. The pioneers of the field felt, no doubt, that the path they picked was the right one, as the traveler in *The Road Not Taken*[1] first supposes. In retrospect, however, the alternative might have prevented a long detour.

In the beginning of memory systems research in the 1950s and 1960s, most experts thought that amnesia—defined as an impairment in explicit memory—resulted from damage to the hippocampus. If this idea had prevailed in the interim, memory researchers might have reached the proposal in Chapter 11 on explicit memory, or something like it, much sooner. Instead, in the late 1970s and 1980s, memory research changed course abruptly; it shifted from a focus on the hippocampus to include three nearby cortical areas said to share an explicit-memory function with the hippocampus. This diversion had several unfortunate consequences: (1) it deflected attention from the representational specializations of those four cortical areas, including the hippocampus; (2) it hindered an appreciation of how other areas—such as the granular prefrontal cortex and the anterior temporal lobe—contribute to explicit memory; (3) it de-emphasized hippocampus–prefrontal and hippocampus–anterior temporal lobe interactions; and (4) it obscured the special status and role of the medial allocortex, known in mammals as the hippocampus.

In the first part of this chapter ("The Road Taken") we explain that experiments on monkeys triggered this momentous shift in ideas about memory, which was then applied to humans and other animals. Contrary to the proposal in Chapter 11, these experiments depended on the assumption that monkeys and humans share a homologous explicit memory system. A deeper appreciation of evolutionary relationships among monkeys, humans, and other animals—and a more sophisticated approach to animal models (Box 12.1)—might have prevented some of the problems that ensued.

The road taken

H.M.'s ablation

The history of memory systems research began with H.M., of course (see Chapter 1, "What happened to Henry?"). Books and articles too numerous to mention tell his story, culminating in Corkin's[2] recent reminiscences, but here we emphasize just one point. The early discussions of H.M.'s case, in the 1950s and 1960s, emphasized the loss of hippocampal function as the cause of his amnesia. An influential 1957 paper by Scoville and

Box 12.1 Animal models in perspective

Many comparative and evolutionary biologists cringe when the talk turns to animal models[113]. Animal research can provide important insights, often based on methods that can never be applied to humans, but we appreciate the uneasiness of these experts.

For monkey models of explicit memory, not only must advocates of the prevailing view assume (like it or not) that monkeys have a human-like experience of participating in events and knowing facts, but they need to extend this assumption to an extinct species that lived dozens of millions of years ago—the last common ancestor of monkeys and humans. When rodents are included, the relevant common ancestors lived many tens of millions of years before that. Advocates of the prevailing view of memory rarely articulate either assumption, but the animal models of human amnesia become incoherent without them.

To examine whether these assumptions can withstand critical scrutiny, consider two examples of monkey models, which we touched upon in Chapters 1 and 2:

1. Trichromacy (full-color vision) emerged in Old World anthropoids (catarrhines), and modern Old World monkeys, apes, and humans share this trait by inheritance. Consequently, Old World monkeys serve as pretty good models of human color vision, although not perfect ones[113].

2. For other traits, monkeys make miserable models. Chapter 1 ("Precursors of the past") used vocal communication as an example. Social behavior, including vocal communication, shows tremendous diversity among modern primate species. No one knows which species resemble the last common ancestor of humans and monkeys in this regard, and it is likely that none of them do so very closely.

To evaluate a monkey model of human amnesia, we need to know whether it more closely resembles the terrific model of human trichromacy or the terrible model of human language. More generally, after millions of years of independent evolution, we need to recognize both the similarities inherited from our last common ancestor and the differences that have emerged in the interim. As explained in this chapter, a failure to embrace this principle plagued early work on animal models of human memory—and afflicts it still.

Milner[3], for example, had the title "Loss of recent memory after bilateral hippocampal lesions." Another early paper, from 1959, had a similar title: "The memory defect in bilateral hippocampal lesions"[4].

These pioneering researchers knew full well that H.M.'s neurosurgeons had removed many brain structures in addition to the hippocampus, but they had good reasons—based on a linked set of observations—to focus on the hippocampus[3-5]:

- Severe amnesia did not follow bilateral lesions of the anterior temporal lobe, including the anterior aspect of the structures removed in H.M.

- Severe amnesia did not follow unilateral lesions of the structures removed in H.M.

◆ Severe amnesia did occur when unilateral lesions of the sort made in H.M. happened to combine with pre-existing pathology of the hippocampus in the opposite hemisphere.

Collectively, these observations supported the idea that bilateral removal of the hippocampus had caused H.M.'s amnesia.

This conclusion depends, of course, on the assumption that the actual lesion in H.M. corresponded reasonably well with the planned one. H.M.'s neurosurgeon intended to remove the amygdala, the hippocampus, and the cortex ventral to these two structures[3]. Figure 12.1 shows a drawing of the proposed ablation, depicted on one hemisphere, along

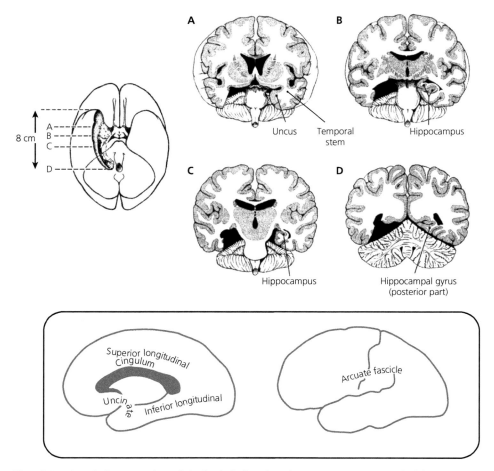

Fig. 12.1 H.M.'s lesion. Drawing of the brain lesion that the neurosurgeon intended for H.M. Top, left: Ventral view of a brain showing the levels of sections in the frontal plane depicted in (A–D). The neurosurgeon made lesions in both hemispheres, but the drawings in (A–D) show one hemisphere intact to display the structures removed. The drawings at the bottom show the approximate locations of some key fiber fascicles. Top: Reproduced from Scoville WB, Milner B. Loss of recent memory after bilateral hippocampal lesions. *Journal of Neurology, Neurosurgery and Psychiatry* 20:11–21, © 1957, with permission from BMJ Publishing Group Ltd.

Box 12.2 Refinements in understanding H.M.'s lesion

In addition to neurosurgical notes, we now have H.M.'s autopsy results[114], along with a structural brain imaging study conducted about a decade before his death[115] and some additional fiber-tract analysis[116]. The intended lesion, the brain imaging, and the autopsy results differ in some ways, but the basic picture remains reasonably consistent.

According to the imaging study[115], H.M.'s neurosurgeon made a fairly symmetrical lesion. The cortical areas that he removed extended from the temporal pole through the medial part of the anterior temporal lobe and the largest part of the amygdala. The lesion included the entorhinal cortex and the amygdaloid (anterior) half of the hippocampal complex. The surgery left the septal (posterior) hippocampus in place, but it underwent considerable atrophy. Portions of the perirhinal cortex also sustained direct damage.

The postmortem findings[114] indicated that H.M.'s parahippocampal cortex was more intact than the structural imaging had suggested, with somewhat more of the septal (posterior) hippocampus spared as well. Only a small medial corner of the entorhinal cortex remained, along with medial parts of the amygdala.

In addition to this gray matter damage, cortical and thalamic disconnections likely accompanied the intended lesion, which resulted from cutting fiber tracts. A recent paper examined the extent of H.M.'s fiber-tract damage[116] by contrasting tractography reconstructions of control subjects with data from H.M.'s structural imaging scans. This analysis shows that, in the right hemisphere at least, H.M.'s uncinate fascicle had sustained significant damage. In Chapter 11 ("Disconnection") we detailed additional disconnections that the postmortem analysis revealed[114].

with the rough location of some key fiber fascicles. When the initial ideas about memory systems developed, researchers had nothing to go on apart from these drawings and the associated description. Now, of course, we know more (Box 12.2), especially about involvement of white matter and fiber tracts (see Chapter 11, "Disconnection"). But at the time, the idea that damage to the hippocampus caused profound amnesia seemed perfectly reasonable.

Other cases

Additional evidence, from postmortem analysis of other amnesic patients[6–8] also pointed to hippocampus lesions as a cause of amnesia. We focus here on five patients, which the literature calls R.B., G.D., L.M., W.H., and E.P. For clarity of exposition, we call them Patients 1–5, respectively. Patients 1–3 had lesions said to be confined to the hippocampus; Patient 4 had lesions of the hippocampus and entorhinal cortex; and Patient 5 had yet more extensive lesions, including the structures involved in Patient 4's lesion, along with the amygdala, perirhinal cortex, and parts of the parahippocampal, fusiform, lateral temporal, parietal, and insular cortex. Patients 1–3 had a clinically significant anterograde amnesia[6,7]; Patient 4 had more severe anterograde amnesia; and Patient 5 resembled H.M., both in the extent of his brain damage and in the greater degree of impairment[8].

The finding that Patients 1–3 had significant amnesia with damage supposedly confined to the hippocampus provides some support for the proposal we presented in Chapter 11. The postmortem analyses did not convince all experts, however, in part because of the possibility of unreported (or unseen) brain damage and in part because the amnesia in Patients 4 and 5 was more severe than in Patients 1–3.

In the 1950s and 1960s, these reports had yet to appear, but in that era such observations would surely have been taken as support for the concept of "hippocampal amnesia." The finding that Patients 1–3 had a significant amnesia opens the possibility of hippocampus–prefrontal interactions as a key contributor to episodic memory and points to three-way interactions among the hippocampus, prefrontal cortex, and anterior temporal lobe as a substrate for semantic memory (see Fig. 11.8).

When the case reports for Patients 1–5 appeared, however, the more severe amnesia in Patients 4 and 5 was interpreted in terms of a "medial temporal lobe memory system," in which the hippocampus is merely one among four cortical areas that make a comparable contribution to explicit memory. As we explained in Chapter 7 ("The perception–memory dichotomy") and take up again later in this chapter (see "The equipotentiality principle" and "The summation principle"), we interpret these findings differently. H.M., Patient 4, and Patient 5 had a greater impairment because of the specific, additional disconnections caused by their larger lesions (see also Chapter 11, "Disconnection").

These divergent interpretations highlight the uncertainty about which aspect of H.M.'s lesion caused his impairment in explicit memory, and the same doubts apply to other amnesic patients as well. At first glance, a monkey model of human amnesia should have been able to resolve any doubts about the neural substrates of explicit memory. In Chapter 11 ("Do animals have explicit memory?") we discussed several problems with the assumption that monkeys have explicit memory, but little of this was recognized as the prevailing view took shape. At the time, it seemed as though a monkey model merely required a task that measured explicit memory, combined with selective brain lesions. Monkeys have obvious homologues of each cortical area removed from H.M., so nothing but time and effort appeared to stand in the way of confirming the "hippocampus theory" of explicit memory. A fundamental problem, however, loomed over the entire enterprise.

The monkey model

The monkey model of human amnesia faced a major difficulty from the start: how to measure explicit (declarative) memory in monkeys. The prevailing view is expressed by Squire and his colleagues (Clark et al.[9], p. 524, italics ours):

> the fundamental distinction is between the capacity for conscious recollection of facts and events … and nondeclarative memory, which supports skill and habit learning and other forms of memory that are *expressed through performance* rather than recollection.

This quotation refers to human memory, but, as discussed in Chapter 11, it has direct implications for monkey research. Monkeys, obviously, express all of their memories through performance, and so these definitions imply that they lack explicit memory. Yet the prevailing view of memory systems depends on precisely the opposite assumption. In Chapter 11 ("Do animals have explicit memory?") we explained why we doubt claims of explicit memory in monkeys and other animals, arguments that many experts will no doubt reject. Regardless, when an entire field of research depends upon an unverified (and perhaps unverifiable) assumption—that animals have explicit memory—it has a problem worth keeping in mind.

We now review, in some detail, a series of monkey experiments that shifted the field's original focus from the hippocampus to the "medial temporal lobe." Readers with only a passing interest in this history might skip to the summary of this section, which presents our key conclusions.

First attempts

When neuropsychologists began work on a monkey model of human amnesia in the 1960s, they assumed that monkeys have the same kinds of memory as people do. They soon learned, however, that monkeys differ from humans in surprising ways.

The early attempts at modeling H.M.'s amnesia assumed that one memory test would serve as well as any other. Accordingly, for the most part they used discrimination tasks. These tasks have long been the mainstay of animal psychology, in part because of their simplicity and the fact that any animal can perform them. Subjects usually choose between two stimuli, and the correct choice yields a reward. Discrimination tasks have two serious drawbacks, however: (1) subjects can perform these tasks in several different ways; and (2) although people can use explicit memory to perform discrimination tasks, they do not always need to do so.

The neuropsychologists of the 1960s considered discrimination tasks to be generic memory tests. Although they do test certain kinds of memory, human subjects can perform these tasks in many ways:

1. They can learn the association between a stimulus and a reward. This form of stimulus–outcome learning corresponds to Pavlovian memory, as we discussed in Chapter 3. Having learned this association, subjects can then choose high-value stimuli, a behavior called Pavlovian approach or sign tracking.

2. They can learn stimulus–response–outcome associations (see Chapter 3).

3. They can treat the two stimuli as a single, compound stimulus and use conditional motor learning to solve the problem. For stimuli A and B, the compound conditional cues are A–B and B–A: the first component to the left; the second to the right. The compound stimulus A–B instructs a movement to the left (stimulus A), and B–A instructs a movement to the right (stimulus A again).

4. They can learn what "response" to make upon seeing the correct stimulus, without reference to predicted outcomes: a stimulus–response association or habit.

5. They can explicitly recall which of the two stimuli should be chosen.

6. They can implicitly learn an abstract rule that depends on the previous trial. If they chose stimulus A on the previous trial and received positive feedback, subjects can

employ a win–stay strategy to choose stimulus A again on the next trial. If they chose stimulus B on the previous trial and received negative feedback, they can use a lose–shift strategy to choose stimulus A on the next trial.

7. They can explicitly learn such an abstract rule.

Once the discrimination task is viewed as a problem that a subject needs to solve, it becomes obvious that it has many solutions. In this context, the failure of the early attempts to model human amnesia with the discrimination task should come as no surprise. If a brain lesion prevents one solution to the problem, subjects will solve it another way.

In the 1960s, however, the failure of these experiments came as an enormous surprise. Monkeys with lesions of the hippocampus performed perfectly well on the discrimination learning task—both in acquisition and retention—and on an early version of the short-interval matching task[10–13]. As a consequence, several experts invoked "species differences" to account for the failure of their experiments—after the fact. Applied so vaguely, this idea explains nothing. It certainly could not mask the fact that the early researchers in the field did not understand why their experiments had failed. Frustration peaked in the early 1970s, as neuropsychologists grappled with the absence of the predicted results on memory tests while trying to understand the impairments that hippocampus lesions caused on other tasks[14]. None of this work produced much progress.

Then, after decades of failure, when it seemed as though no lesion would ever affect performance on any memory task that monkeys could actually perform, finally, and at long last, one did.

First successes

In the first success, Gaffan[15] cut the fornix and used the short-interval matching task to demonstrate a memory impairment. To increase the demand on memory, he presented a series of sample stimuli, called a *list*, for testing at various intervals, and, in a separate procedure, lengthened the memory delay period. Figure 12.2(C) shows that the lesioned monkeys performed the task poorly in the most demanding conditions. For a list of ten objects, control monkeys performed correctly 85% of the time, but monkeys with fornix transections could manage only a little above chance level, performing correctly 55% of the time. After such prolonged frustration, neuropsychologists of the 1970s understandably interpreted Gaffan's result in terms of H.M.'s amnesia. This attitude seemed to gain support from the slightly subpar performance of H.M. on a similar task[16].

Advocates of the prevailing view often refer to short-interval matching procedures as "object recognition" or "visual recognition" tasks, but in Chapter 1 ("Task names") we warned about the danger of such names. Like discrimination problems, the matching task presents a problem amenable to several solutions. For the matching rule, subjects see a sample then, after a delay period, need to chose it over a foil. Subjects can choose the sample because:

1. they have an explicit recollection of the item or explicitly rehearse it in short-term memory;

2. they judge it to be the most familiar stimulus;

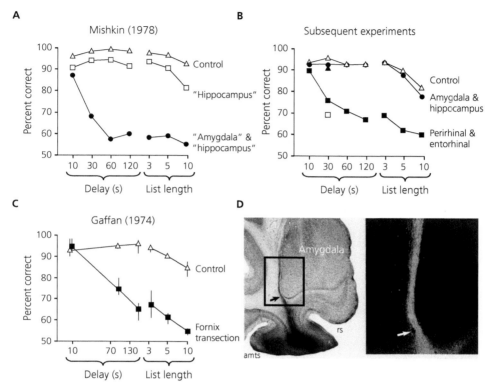

Fig. 12.2 Performance of monkeys on the short-interval matching task. (A) Percent correct at various delays with a single sample (delays) and with a variable number of samples (list length). (B) Results that falsified the "amygdala plus hippocampus" model of amnesia. The unfilled square shows the result of excitotoxic lesions of the perirhinal and entorhinal cortex, combined; the filled triangle shows the control data for that experiment. (C) Effect of fornix transection. Vertical lines through each data point show the range of scores for the animals in a group. (D) Anterograde labeling of efferent fibers from the perirhinal cortex. Left: Nissl-stained section through the amygdala. The box corresponds to the region shown in dark-field illumination to the right. The arrow points to a blood vessel common to both photomicrographs. Right: The labeled axons appear white. Medial is to the right, dorsal is up. (A), (B) From Murray EA, Wise SP. Why is there a special issue on perirhinal cortex in a journal called *Hippocampus*? The perirhinal cortex in historical perspective. *Hippocampus* 22:1941–51, © 2012, reproduced with permission from John Wiley & Sons. (C) Redrawn from Gaffan D. Recognition impaired and association intact in the memory of monkeys after transection of the fornix. *Journal of Comparative and Physiological Psychology* 86:1100–9, © 1974, American Psychological Association. (D) Reproduced from Murray EA. Medial temporal lobe structures contributing to recognition memory: the amygdaloid complex versus the rhinal cortex. In *The Amygdala: Neurobiological Aspects of Emotion, Memory, and Mental Dysfunction*, pp. 453–70, © 1993, CCC Republication.

3. they judge it to be the stimulus encountered most recently.

For the nonmatching rule, subjects simply avoid the sample in favor of the alternative, using the same solutions. In the jargon of the field, these two rules are usually called delayed matching-to-sample and delayed nonmatching-to-sample, respectively. The phrase short-interval matching covers both.

The prevailing view of memory systems typically assumes the first possibility, but human subjects can perform the task using either familiarity or recency strategies, without explicit recall. Furthermore, the short-interval matching task typically requires memories to persist for only a few minutes or less, and H.M. could remember most items very well over such short intervals. Taken together, its inappropriate time-scale and the fact that people can perform the task without explicit memory make this task an unlikely assay for explicit memory in monkeys, as memory researchers have pointed out from time to time[17,18].

Despite these limitations, the short-interval matching task provided researchers with a way to measure *some* form of memory in monkeys and, after refining the task to employ different stimuli on each trial, Mishkin used it to generate the first monkey model of human amnesia. In a brief but highly influential article[19], he concluded that combined lesions of the "amygdala plus hippocampus" produced a severe impairment in explicit memory. We place this description of the lesion in quotation marks because, as we explain later, it is highly inaccurate.

In Mishkin's experiment, monkeys with the so-called "amygdala plus hippocampus" lesion performed the task normally at delays of 10 seconds or so (Fig. 12.2A), which eliminated any account of the impairment in terms of sensory processing or stimulus discrimination. The same observation also showed that the lesioned monkeys could remember and apply the task rule. With longer memory intervals, however, monkeys with this lesion performed the task poorly (Fig. 12.2A, black circles). Importantly, animals said to have either bilateral "hippocampus" lesions alone (Fig. 12.2A, squares) or bilateral "amygdala" lesions alone (not illustrated) performed quite well. For example, in the most demanding conditions monkeys with the so-called "hippocampus" lesions (Fig. 12.2A, squares) made some errors, but their performance did not differ very much from that of control monkeys (Fig. 12.2A, triangles). Monkeys with the combined "amygdala plus hippocampus" lesion had a severe impairment and could not perform appreciably better than chance level at delay intervals of 1 minute, even with just one sample item (Fig. 12.2A).

Mishkin's model of amnesia led to the idea that H.M.'s impairment in explicit memory resulted from damage to more than the hippocampus. Indeed, this idea was appealing to some experts precisely because of the close correspondence between H.M.'s brain damage and the so-called "amygdala plus hippocampus" lesion. At a stroke, these results seemed to rule out species differences of any importance[20].

The inclusion of the "amygdala" in Mishkin's model contradicted earlier ideas about the cause of H.M.'s amnesia, which focused on the hippocampus alone. We have already mentioned the impairments that followed Gaffan's fornix transections[15] (Fig. 12.2C), which appeared to support the idea of "hippocampal amnesia." Furthermore, in contrast to the results illustrated in Fig. 12.2(A), other investigators reported an impairment on the short-interval matching task after hippocampus lesions (see "Hippocampus lesions: effect or no effect?").

So at this point in the history of the field, one set of findings focused on the hippocampus—in accord with ideas about H.M.'s amnesia from the 1950s and 1960s—but another suggested that the model needed an additional structure, specifically the amygdala. A series of subsequent studies in the mid-1980s attempted to reconcile these two ideas. At first, they seemed to do so in favor of the "amygdala plus hippocampus" model[21-26]. Whenever a lesion disrupted the function of both the hippocampus and the amygdala, it produced an impairment on short-interval matching tasks. The impairment also extended across different sensory modalities and so seemed to be "global," in this limited sense of the word. In these studies, lesions that spared either the hippocampus or the amygdala caused only mild impairments, if any. The concept of a "medial temporal lobe memory system" emerged from this line of research, but only after a dramatic overhaul.

Falsification of the first model

From the start, some experts had serious doubts about the "amygdala plus hippocampus" model of human amnesia. In Chapter 11 ("Disconnection") we mentioned the temporal stem. Horel[27], for example, suspected that the surgery in H.M. had damaged fiber tracts in that part of the temporal white matter. Unfortunately, although one monkey experiment that tested this idea yielded an impairment on the short-interval matching task[28], a lesion of the temporal stem placed more posteriorly had no effect[24]. As a consequence, proponents of the "amygdala plus hippocampus" model continued to champion ideas that discounted impairments caused by inadvertent damage to fiber tracts. They also tended to neglect the damage to nearby cortical areas that accompanied the intended lesions. As it turned out, these two problems proved to be related: Together, inadvertent damage to fiber tracts and damage to adjacent areas caused the impairment that Mishkin[19] had observed. The amygdala had nothing to do with it.

The key to understanding this conclusion comes from a detailed consideration of anthropoid neuroanatomy. Both the perirhinal and entorhinal cortex lie mainly ventral to the amygdala and the amygdaloid (anterior) hippocampus in monkeys, as they do in humans. When Mishkin[19] made aspiration lesions of the amygdala and hippocampus, he removed the rostral part of the entorhinal cortex to gain access to the amygdala and the caudal part of the entorhinal cortex to reach the hippocampus. Therefore, in experiments based on the "amygdala plus hippocampus" model, only the combined lesion removed the entire entorhinal cortex.

The combined "amygdala plus hippocampus" lesion also compromised the entire perirhinal cortex, but for more complicated reasons. First, Mishkin probably did some direct damage to the rostral perirhinal cortex in order to gain access to the amygdala. Second, and more importantly, his lesions had the unintended effect of cutting axons going to and from the perirhinal cortex. As explained in Chapter 11 ("Disconnection"), many of these connections run through fiber tracts adjacent to the amygdala (Fig. 12.2D). In aggregate, these pathways have a sheet-like architecture that extends from near the amygdala into more caudal aspects of the temporal lobe, so only the combined "amygdala plus hippocampus" lesion severed both the rostral and caudal components of these fiber tracts. As a result, Mishkin inadvertently disconnected the entire perirhinal cortex from the thalamus and most other cortical areas.

It is clear, therefore, that the combined lesion in monkeys did much more than remove the "amygdala plus hippocampus," and subsequent experiments showed that damage to the perirhinal and entorhinal cortex—not the amygdala–hippocampus combination—had caused the impairment.

In the first of these studies, lesions of the entorhinal and perirhinal cortex were added to a removal of the amygdala. This three-component, combined lesion caused a severe impairment on the short-interval matching task[29]. As a historical matter, this result—reported in the mid-1980s—appeared to push proponents of the prevailing view toward including the perirhinal cortex as a component of their "medial temporal lobe memory system." Yet, despite the assumption that the hippocampus is part of this "system," the combined amygdala–entorhinal–perirhinal lesion caused a severe impairment without any direct damage to either the hippocampus or the fornix.

To complement the addition of entorhinal–perirhinal lesions to a removal of the amygdala, the same experimenters intended to add entorhinal–perirhinal lesions to a removal of the hippocampus[29]. An anatomical analysis confirmed that they removed the entire hippocampus in four of six subjects. The fact that these four monkeys achieved a score of 89% correct, on average, ruled out a contribution of the hippocampus to the short-interval matching task—at least for the version used in this experiment. Contrary to the experimenters' intentions, however, they left about half of the perirhinal cortex intact[30]. The relatively good performance of this group of monkeys provided the first clue that the perirhinal cortex plays a particularly important role in the performance of short-interval matching tasks.

Figure 12.2(B) illustrates the results that finally ruled out the "amygdala plus hippocampus" model of human amnesia. In the key experiment, combined aspiration lesions of the entorhinal and perirhinal cortex caused a severe impairment on the short-interval matching task[31], and a detailed histological analysis confirmed that the lesion had spared both the amygdala and hippocampus. In a follow-up study, excitotoxic lesions of the perirhinal and entorhinal cortex—which spared fiber tracts through and near these areas as well as leaving the amygdala and hippocampus intact—also caused a severe impairment, even at a 30-second delay with just one sample item (Fig. 12.2B, unfilled square)[32,33].

Combined, excitotoxic lesions of the amygdala and the hippocampus complemented this work. These lesions left the perirhinal and entorhinal cortex intact[34], and Fig. 12.2(B) shows that they had little, if any, effect on task performance.

These results not only overturned Mishkin's "amygdala plus hippocampus" model, but they also showed that the hippocampus is not necessary for successful performance of the short-interval matching task per se. Although some advocates of the prevailing view continue to emphasize the effects of hippocampus lesions on certain versions of this task, no results contradict two conclusions:

1. Monkeys that have had their hippocampus completely removed, bilaterally, can perform some versions of the short-interval matching task as well as control monkeys. This result demonstrates that the hippocampus is not necessary for performing short-interval matching tasks per se.

2. Lesions confined to the perirhinal and entorhinal cortex, which leave the hippocampus completely intact, cause a severe impairment on this task[35]. This finding shows that an intact hippocampus is not sufficient to support good matching-task performance.

We return to the first point later when we explore why hippocampus lesions *do* affect performance on some various versions of the matching task (see "Hippocampus lesions: effect or no effect?").

In summary, by the late 1990s, it had become clear that the first monkey model of human amnesia—the "amygdala plus hippocampus" model—was wrong. It foundered for several reasons, some of which continue to plague the field. First, it depended on the unwarranted assumption that the short-interval matching task measures explicit memory; second, the damage done to the perirhinal and entorhinal cortex—some of it inadvertent and none of it emphasized at the time—had caused the impairment; and third, partly for this reason, the choice of stimulus material mattered more than anyone realized in the 1980s and early 1990s.

Why did the stimulus material matter so much? We explained in Chapter 7 ("The perception–memory dichotomy") that the perirhinal cortex functions as a component of the feature system and that it represents feature conjunctions at the level of natural objects. We can therefore understand the contribution of the monkey perirhinal cortex in terms of a specialization for object representations. So when memory tests use objects or other stimuli with object-level feature overlap, impairments will follow perirhinal cortex lesions or combined lesions of the perirhinal and entorhinal cortex. Box 12.3 addresses the relative contributions of these two cortical areas.

Fork in the road

The failure of the first monkey model led to a fork in the road. One path offered an opportunity to revise the model by dispensing with the amygdala and substituting the cortical areas necessary for performing the short-interval matching task. That is essentially what happened in the 1980s. The other path, "the road not taken," would have involved discarding both the task and the cortical areas that came along with it.

Readers might wonder about a third option: Why not simply switch to better tests of explicit memory? An early proposal suggested a battery of three explicit-memory tasks for monkeys, in addition to the short-interval matching task: two varieties of visual discrimination learning and the spatial delayed response task[26]. Unfortunately—and quite aside from the issues about explicit memory in animals discussed earlier (see Chapter 11, "Do animals have explicit memory?")—the three additional tests all fell by the wayside. Briefly, the impairments observed on discriminations tasks depended on the stimulus

Box 12.3 Entorhinal versus perirhinal cortex

Combined lesions of the perirhinal and entorhinal cortex account for the impairment on most versions of the short-interval matching task, but which area contributes the most? Figure 12.3(B) summarizes results pointing to the perirhinal cortex as the answer to this question. After perirhinal cortex lesions that left 96% of the entorhinal cortex intact (Fig. 12.3B, filled circles), monkeys performed the task poorly in the most demanding conditions. In contrast, after lesions of the entorhinal cortex that left about half of the perirhinal cortex intact, monkeys performed fairly well (Fig. 12.3B, unfilled circles), in agreement with another report[117]. Taken together, these findings suggest a more important role for the perirhinal cortex than for the entorhinal cortex in performing the short-interval matching task with objects or other object-like stimuli.

However, combined lesions of the entorhinal and perirhinal cortex (Fig. 12.3B, filled squares) caused a more severe impairment than did perirhinal cortex lesions alone (Fig. 12.3B, filled circles), despite the fact that these groups had roughly the same amount of damage to the perirhinal cortex (leaving only 12–15% of this area intact). Therefore it seems likely that the entorhinal cortex makes some contribution to performance of the short-interval matching task, especially when the perirhinal cortex is functionally compromised.

material used (see Chapter 7, "The perception–memory dichotomy")[36–40], and lesions of the so-called "memory areas" had no effect on performance on the spatial delayed response task[12,41,42]. As a result, the dominant monkey model of human amnesia came to depend almost entirely on the short-interval matching task.

Summary

The monkey model of human amnesia has always included a task and a lesion:

- The model began with a battery of tasks thought to measure explicit memory in monkeys, but eventually only the short-interval matching task remained. Most versions of this task use objects or other object-like stimuli, with a strong emphasis on vision.
- The lesion began as a combination of the "amygdala plus hippocampus." After experimental evidence ruled out that model, three cortical areas—the perirhinal, entorhinal, and parahippocampal cortex—quietly replaced the amygdala.

Although the "amygdala plus hippocampus" model failed utterly (Fig. 12.2B), somehow this fact did not trigger a serious reconsideration of its two core features: (1) the assumption that short-interval matching tasks measure explicit memory; and (2) the idea that the lesion needs to include a combination of diverse structures in the so-called "medial temporal lobe." By the mid- to late 1980s, the short-interval matching task had become entrenched as a test of explicit memory in animals. So instead of eliminating the task from the model, its advocates simply replaced a (largely) subcortical structure, the amygdala, with nearby cortical areas—and the prevailing view of memory systems morphed into something like its present form.

That choice, made in the 1980s, has influenced the path followed ever since. Research on the neural substrates of explicit memory began to concentrate on a conceptual construct called the "medial temporal lobe" and lost its initial focus on the hippocampus. *The Road Not Taken*[1] tells a similar tale. Choices, once made, can be difficult to change. The traveler in Frost's poem, to his credit, appreciated that he would probably never revisit his initial choice. In contrast, memory researchers can still return to the road not taken in the 1980s.

What would that entail? First, the field would need to abandon the current practice of patching the prevailing view as contradictions emerge. Second, it would discard the object-based, short-interval matching task as a canonical test for explicit memory. Third, the cortical areas that came along with this task would depart the so-called "medial temporal lobe memory system" and return to their rightful place among the evolutionary innovations of early mammals.

By revisiting the choice made three decades ago, memory researchers can also reconsider species differences in a more principled way, embracing both diversity and evolutionary principles. This point is especially important because underlying the frustrations, falsifications, failures, and false starts, monkey models of amnesia have depended on the denial or dismissal of diversity. Monkey memory does not match human memory all that well, but neither does it differ completely. Exploring the "road not taken" in the 1980s would require treating a monkey model realistically: not terribly terrific, but not terrifically terrible either (Box 12.1). The "amygdala plus hippocampus" model vanished in the face of contradictory evidence, and its replacement conflicts with a great deal of evidence as well. Nevertheless, monkey models can still provide important insights into human memory provided that experimenters take evolution into account and recognize certain limitations. The value of any such model depends on the exact memory tests used, of course, but above all on an appreciation of experimental results in the context of how each species adapted to its way of life. These principles apply to all animal models, of course, not just to those involving monkeys—a topic we revisit in Chapter 13 ("Only humans have explicit memory").

The remainder of this chapter attempts to clear some of the obstacles that continue to hamper travel along "the road not taken." Although it comes in many varieties, the prevailing view of memory systems usually has four principal tenets, which we call the equipotentiality principle, the summation principle, the perception–memory dichotomy, and the habit–memory dichotomy. We now take up these topics in turn.

The equipotentiality principle

The equipotentiality principle holds that each component of the "medial temporal lobe memory system" functions in a similar, cooperative way—as a unitary system. As one authoritative source expresses its key prediction: "The severity of memory impairment increases as additional components of the medial temporal lobe memory system are damaged" (Zola-Morgan et al.[43], p. 493). To be fair, this tenet does not rule out area-by-area specializations entirely; the perirhinal cortex, for example, could still have an object-related specialization in addition to its role in explicit memory. Furthermore, the prevailing view does not necessarily demand precisely equal contributions. But to have any coherence, it must predict an additive effect as more components of the so-called "medial temporal lobe memory system" are added to a lesion.

Experts in human memory have dispensed, by and large, with the equipotentiality principle. In Chapter 7 ("Humans") we explained that both the perirhinal and hippocampal cortex represent specialized kinds of information in humans, as other cortical areas do. In monkey research, however, the equipotentiality principle remains highly influential.

Falsification

This chapter has already presented some of the evidence that rules out the equipotentiality principle. Figure 12.2(B) shows that lesions of the perirhinal and entorhinal cortex caused almost the entire impairment on one version of the short-interval matching task, and Fig. 12.3(A, B) presents similar results. The equipotentiality principle predicts that damage to additional "memory areas" should have worsened the impairment, but it did not. When a removal of the hippocampus was added to lesions of the perirhinal and entorhinal cortex (Fig. 12.3A, circles), the monkeys actually performed better than after combined lesions of the perirhinal and entorhinal cortex that left the hippocampus intact (Fig. 12.3A, squares). The finding, alone, falsifies the equipotentiality principle.

The experiment just mentioned involved adding a hippocampus lesion to a removal of nearby cortical areas. The complementary approach is to add lesions of nearby cortical areas to a removal of the hippocampus. The equipotentiality principle predicts that adding a perirhinal cortex lesion to a hippocampus lesion should increase the degree of impairment. An influential paper by Zola-Morgan et al.[44] reported this result, but its conclusions were unconvincing for two reasons. First, their so-called "hippocampus" lesion included the entorhinal cortex, hence the quotation marks. These investigators actually made a hippocampus plus entorhinal cortex lesion. As we explained earlier, the perirhinal and entorhinal cortex mediate performance of the short-interval matching task, at least as tested with the usual stimulus material. Accordingly, the addition of the perirhinal cortex to a hippocampus plus entorhinal cortex lesion inadvertently completed the perirhinal–entorhinal lesion. A similar problem plagues another paper from the same laboratory[45]. Monkeys with lesions of the hippocampus plus the entorhinal cortex performed the short-interval matching task normally at delays of less than 30 seconds, probably because the perirhinal cortex remained intact. However, these monkeys had mild impairments for 1- and 10-minute delays, which probably resulted from damage to the entorhinal cortex.

Because of these findings, and because complete lesions of the hippocampus (Fig. 12.2A) often have no effect on short-interval matching performance, we can reject the equipotentiality principle.

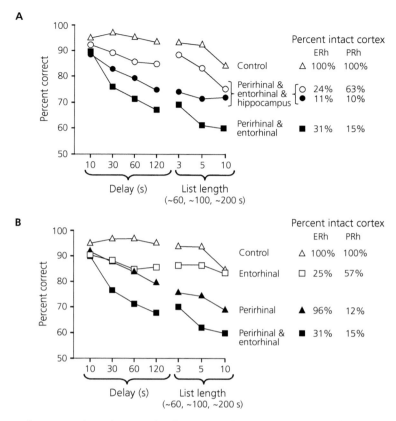

Fig. 12.3 Performance of monkeys on the short-interval matching task. (A) Effect of adding a hippocampus lesion to a lesion of the perirhinal and entorhinal cortex. Format as in Fig. 12.2. The key shows the proportion of the latter two cortical areas that remained intact, based on a histological analysis (means across hemispheres and subjects). There were two groups of monkeys with combined lesions of the perirhinal cortex, the entorhinal cortex, and the hippocampus. In one of these groups, more of the perirhinal cortex remained intact (unfilled circles) than in the other (filled circles). Although for clarity this plot does not give ranges or variances, the key differences apparent in these plots are statistically significant. (B) Effect of aspiration lesions intended to remove the perirhinal cortex, the entorhinal cortex, or both. (A) Based on data from Meunier M, Hadfield W, Bachevalier J, Murray EA. Effects of rhinal cortex lesions combined with hippocampectomy on visual recognition memory in rhesus monkeys. *Journal of Neurophysiology* 75:1190–1205, © 1996, American Physiological Society. (B) From Meunier M, Bachevalier J, Mishkin M, Murray EA. Effects on visual recognition of combined and separate ablations of the entorhinal and perirhinal cortex in rhesus monkeys. *Journal of Neuroscience* 13:5418–32, © 1993, Society for Neuroscience, with permission.

Hippocampus lesions: effect or no effect?

As Fig. 12.2(C) shows, lesions of the hippocampus or the fornix do sometimes cause impairments on the performance of short-interval matching tasks[15,46,47], an inconsistency that reflects the relatively unconstrained nature of this task. As explained in Chapter 7 ("The perception–memory dichotomy"), the contribution of a cortical area to the short-interval matching task, like other tasks, depends on the relationship between its specialized representations and the stimulus material used in a given experiment. Results also depend on the various strategies available to subjects, such as the familiarity or recency strategy, neither of which requires the explicit recall or rehearsal of the sample items (see "First successes"). In addition, the number of stimuli used for testing (set size) affects the results, among other technical factors. With intermediate and small set sizes, stimuli reappear repeatedly, which impedes familiarity judgments because all the stimuli become familiar. With trial-unique stimuli, the stimulus items are never familiar, at least at the start of a trial.

An interaction between set size and strategy probably explains a great deal of the controversy about the effects of hippocampus lesions. Experiments involving intermediate set sizes have tended to report impairments on short-interval matching tasks[46,47]. Gaffan's[15] original study on the effects of fornix transections, for example, used an intermediate set size—60 objects at a time, 300 in total—and he observed a clear impairment (Fig. 12.2C). Many technical factors might have contributed to this result, but a subsequent experiment points to one plausible account. Monkeys with fornix lesions had an impairment in remembering the temporal sequence of stimuli, a judgment that depended on recency memory[48]. So the impairments that have been observed on matching tasks after hippocampus or fornix lesions probably resulted from disrupting a recency strategy: an account consistent with the idea that the hippocampus incorporates temporal context into conjunctive representations[49,50]. Experiments using small and intermediate set sizes promoted a recency strategy because they precluded a familiarity strategy. Put another way, because all the test items were familiar, relative recency became a better solution to the problem that the monkeys faced. This interpretation does not imply that the hippocampus specializes in recency detection, of course, only that its specialized representations help animals implement such a strategy.

In contrast to experiments employing small and intermediate set sizes, those that used trial-unique stimuli have tended to produce negative results on short-interval matching tasks. In four separate investigations, fornix transections[51] caused only a mild impairment and selective hippocampus lesions did not cause any impairment at all[34,52,53]. These results probably reflected the fact that successful task performance could depend on familiarity judgments. At the time of the choice, the sample had some familiarity but the alternative did not. In accord with this account, fornix transections had no effect on a version of the matching task that used highly familiar samples and novel foils[48].

As a historical matter, the chronology of these findings had a major influence on the field. Researchers discovered the large and consistent effect caused by lesions of the perirhinal and entorhinal cortex long after the mild and inconsistent impairments that sometimes followed lesions of the hippocampus or fornix. Had the former been reported first, little controversy concerning the effects of hippocampus lesions would have ensued, and animal researchers might have developed more skepticism about using the matching task as an assay for explicit memory. The remaining uncertainty involves the relatively minor question of whether the hippocampus contributes to some versions of the short-interval matching task. It does, but only in a way that reflects the specialized representations of the hippocampus, not the equipotentiality principle. Advocates of the prevailing view sometimes claim that technical factors account for the lack of an impairment after selective hippocampus lesions, such as whether the initial training took place before or after the lesion or whether the lesions were made in one surgical procedure or two[54], but these accounts have been ruled out[52,53].

Parahippocampal cortex

So far, we have said relatively little about the parahippocampal cortex. This area is less well studied than the other so-called "memory areas" of the prevailing view, hence the paucity of data. One report showed that complete lesions of the parahippocampal cortex did not cause any impairment on the short-interval matching task[53]. This finding contradicts the equipotentiality principle, of course, as does the finding that combined lesions of the hippocampus and parahippocampal cortex had little or no effect on performance of this task[22].

Additional tests

As summarized in Chapter 7 ("The perception–memory dichotomy"), lesions of the perirhinal cortex were responsible for dramatic impairments on discrimination tasks that used stimulus material with high levels of feature ambiguity. Lesions of the hippocampus, however, either caused no impairment or facilitated performance on these tasks[55] (see Fig. 7.5C). Such findings strongly contradict the idea that the perirhinal cortex and the hippocampus perform cooperative functions, as the equipotentiality principle maintains.

Summary

The monkey model of human amnesia has led some proponents of the prevailing view to embrace the equipotentiality principle. However, a broad range of experimental findings contradict this idea. Instead of a common function, each cortical area included in the so-called "medial temporal lobe memory system" has specialized representations for specialized functions. We know more about the specializations of the hippocampus and the perirhinal cortex than the other two so-called "memory areas," but in summary:

◆ The hippocampus contributes to scene memory and perception, as its homologues have since the origin of vertebrates (see Chapters 2 and 4), and observations in humans support this conclusion (see Chapter 7, "Humans"). This specialization reflects the ancestral role of the hippocampus homologue in navigation (see Chapter 4).

- The perirhinal cortex represents feature conjunctions at the level of natural objects (see Chapter 7, "The perception–memory dichotomy"), as it has since the advent of mammals.

- The entorhinal cortex plays a role in linking object-like stimuli to spatial goals[56], as well as serving as an intermediary between the perirhinal cortex and the hippocampus[49] (see Fig. 9.7C) and mediating interactions between the prefrontal cortex and the extended hippocampal–navigation system (see Chapter 11, "Prefrontal–hippocampus connections").

- The parahippocampal cortex represents conjunctions of objects and their locations[57], which supports perspective-, place-, or scene-based rules[53] (see Chapter 10, "A medial network"). In support of this idea, lesions of the parahippocampal cortex showed that it contributes, along with the hippocampus, to scene memory. These lesions caused impairments in discriminating among complex scenes in monkeys[58], in accord with the finding that this area became activated when either humans or monkeys viewed such scenes[59].

The summation principle

Even if each component of the "medial temporal lobe memory system" has specialized functions, perhaps they combine to produce all of the varieties of explicit memory. According to one version of this idea, the hippocampus subserves episodic memory and other parts of the "medial temporal lobe" underlie semantic memory[60,61]. Together, episodic and semantic memory add up to explicit (declarative) memory, so we call this idea the summation principle. Another theme in the literature divides functions in a different way, suggesting that the hippocampus mediates explicit recollection and the remainder of the "medial temporal lobe" subserves familiarity judgments: a two-process or dual-channel model[62].

We reject the summation principle, but only a particular piece of it. As explained in Chapter 9 ("Temporal–prefrontal networks"), many parts of the temporal lobe contribute to semantic memory, and the same areas probably contribute to familiarity judgments as well. The anterior temporal lobe semantic hub and most of its domain-specific "spoke" areas lie outside the so-called "medial temporal lobe." But one "spoke" area, the perirhinal cortex, is usually included. We reject the concept of a "medial temporal lobe memory system," but we do not dispute the idea that the specialized representations of the perirhinal cortex contribute to semantic memory or that these representations can underlie familiarity judgments. Likewise, in Chapters 10 and 11 we summarized a small selection of the evidence in favor of the idea that the hippocampus makes a central contribution to episodic memory. So we do not dispute that piece of the summation principle either. In fact, this idea plays a crucial role in the proposal that we advanced in Chapter 11 on episodic memory. Accordingly, we concentrate here on just one part of the summation principle: the exclusion of the hippocampus from a role in semantic memory.

The key question for our purposes therefore becomes: Do lesions of the hippocampus spare semantic memory? Some reports have claimed that they do[60,61]. Children with damage to the hippocampus, according to these reports, were said to have severe impairments in episodic memory with nearly normal semantic memory. Structural brain imaging in these patients suggested that the hippocampus, alone among the four "memory areas" of the prevailing view, had a smaller than normal volume.

However, other studies have led to a different conclusion. They showed that adult patients with hippocampus lesions have impairments in semantic memory[63,64], especially for new and rapid semantic learning[63,65,66]. It is well known, for example, that people can permanently acquire knowledge about the meaning of a novel word after just one exposure. Patients with hippocampus lesions seem to have a specific impairment in fast semantic learning, sometimes known as fast mapping.

Critics might argue: (1) that the children in these studies had more selective hippocampus lesions than the adult subjects did or (2) that children acquire semantic information over long time-scales, which the laboratory studies could not replicate. Neither objection holds much sway, however. On the first point, the neuroanatomical analysis performed on the children was about the same as for the adults, which is to say very approximate at best. There was no indication that the lesions in adult patients extended farther into the temporal neocortex than did the lesions in the children. On the second point, the problem in hippocampal amnesia lies in fast semantic learning, not in learning over long time-frames. Adult patients with hippocampus lesions can eventually acquire new semantic information, although only slowly and through repeated exposure[63,65].

Compared to hippocampal amnesia, patients with semantic dementia have the opposite pattern of impairments. In two related studies, these patients learned rapidly upon initial exposure to new semantic items (e.g., vocabulary referring to familiar concepts)[67,68]. Unfortunately, they could only maintain these memories by repeatedly practicing and rehearsing them, with little sustained gain in semantic knowledge. In addition, patients with semantic dementia showed little generalization across concepts, except in the milder stages of the disease and when learning involved extensive variety[69,70]. These findings suggest a specialization of the areas most affected in semantic dementia for slow semantic learning and semantic generalizations, in contrast to a specialization of the hippocampus for fast semantic learning.

In summary, we can reject the summation principle on the basis of several studies[63–66]. The hippocampus has a role in both episodic and semantic memory, especially for rapidly learned semantic representations and those based on direct, participatory experience (see Chapter 10, "Episodic versus semantic memory"). Its specialization in rapid acquisition also accounts for the distinction between recollection and familiarity judgments. Furthermore, these conclusions agree with a distinction between the functions of the hippocampus and those of most neocortical areas in terms of learning rate[71]. According to this idea, the hippocampus acquires information rapidly, but with limited capacity. Most of the neocortex learns slowly, providing both additional long-term storage capacity and a diversity of specialized representations. From this perspective, the neocortex can be viewed as augmenting the functions of ancestral, allocortical areas such as the hippocampus.

The perception–memory dichotomy

In Chapter 7 we dealt with the perception–memory dichotomy in detail (Box 12.4). This tenet of the prevailing doctrine arose from a straightforward observation: H.M., like other amnesic patients, had little difficulty with perception in his daily life and in most standard clinical tests of perception. From this observation, advocates of the prevailing view propose separate neural substrates for perception and memory, with the perirhinal cortex being a "memory area," along with the other parts of the so-called "medial temporal lobe." In turn, they classify the inferior temporal cortex as a "perception area" devoid of memory functions (see Fig. 7.1B).

In Chapter 7 ("The perception–memory dichotomy") we explained the problems with this idea and offered an alternative view, one based on ideas about feature conjunctions and the disambiguation of feature overlap[72].

In the absence of an evolutionary perspective, the perception–memory dichotomy might seem plausible. But once brain evolution is taken into account, it makes little sense. In place of the perception–memory doctrine, we propose that particular selective pressures led to the perirhinal and inferior temporal cortex representing feature conjunctions at the levels that they do—for both perception and memory. The inferior temporal cortex encodes and stores the visual *signs* of resources. In the laboratory, experimenters call these signs *cues*, and they are used by animals to perform tasks. Ancestral anthropoids, however, used them to improve foraging choices at a distance. High-acuity, trichromatic vision—enhanced by exquisite distance information provided by stereopsis—delivered these sensory signs to the brains of the large, long-lived, far-ranging, diurnal foragers that anthropoids became (see Chapter 2, "Anthropoids"). The perirhinal cortex, in contrast, encodes and stores feature conjunctions at the level of objects that early mammals encountered while foraging. Evolutionary developments separated by so much time

---

Box 12.4 Sources cited in support of the prevailing view

This chapter does not deal with all of the evidence cited by proponents of the prevailing view. Another set of issues was discussed in Chapter 7 ("The perception–memory dichotomy" and "Conclusions"). Proponents of the prevailing view of memory systems deny that the hippocampus and perirhinal cortex, or other parts of the so-called "medial temporal lobe memory system," play any role in perception[107–109,118,119]. Their reports on human subjects, likewise, regularly claim intact perception in amnesic patients[110–112]. A parallel literature in rats gainsays findings that support a role for the perirhinal cortex[120,121] or the hippocampus[121] in perception. We refute these arguments in Chapter 7.

usually reflect different selective pressures, none of which suggest a specialization in terms of perception versus memory.

In summary, cortical areas specialize in different kinds of representations, not in psychological processes like perception or memory[72,73].

The habit–memory dichotomy

The final tenet of the prevailing view holds that the basal ganglia, as a whole, subserves habits[74-76]. In learning theory, habits—also called S–R associations—are characterized by slow acquisition, high stability, poor transfer, and, most importantly, a lack of sensitivity to predicted outcomes (see Chapter 3, "What happens in instrumental conditioning"). In cognitive psychology, habits are identified by low sensitivity to a competing (dual) task that attracts attention. (In biology, the term has a completely different meaning, which we avoid in this chapter.) Combined with the doctrine that the "medial temporal lobe" subserves explicit memory, the idea that the basal ganglia subserves habits gives rise to what we call the habit–memory dichotomy.

Evolution

In Chapter 2 ("Outdated concepts") we summarized some ideas about brain evolution that influenced the development of the habit–memory dichotomy. Early proponents relied on ideas advanced by MacLean, who believed that the basal ganglia evolved as part of a "reptilian" brain. He also claimed that the hippocampus and other limbic structures evolved later, in "primitive" mammals, and that "higher" cortical areas emerged yet later, in "advanced" mammals. Accordingly, an early formulation of the habit–memory dichotomy[74] suggested that habits and the basal ganglia go together, in part, because they both evolved before mammals, as "primitive" traits in vertebrates "lower" on the "phyletic scale" than mammals (see Mishkin et al.[74], p. 73). The same authors also proposed that explicit memory came along with limbic structures, including the hippocampus, in mammals.

Unfortunately, these ideas relied on the biology of a bygone era, long gone even as the habit–memory dichotomy developed in the 1980s. There is no "phyletic scale" on which species rank from "primitive" to "advanced." The notion of reptilian structures inside mammalian heads is nonsense. More specifically, we explained in Chapter 2 ("Early vertebrates") that the basal ganglia did not evolve before homologues of the hippocampus, as these early versions of the habit–memory dichotomy assumed[74]. Both structures arose early in the history of vertebrates. According to the proposal in Chapter 11, explicit memory does indeed depend on recent evolutionary developments, but not on the emergence of the hippocampus or its homologues in mammals, "primitive" or otherwise. As for habits, some parts of the basal ganglia mediate habits, but other parts have different functions.

Rodents

Results from experiments on rodents directly contradict the habit–memory dichotomy. They have demonstrated that a dorsomedial part of the rodent striatum subserves outcome-directed behavior (otherwise known as goal-directed behavior), whereas only a dorsolateral part of the striatum underlies habits[77,78].

In a decisive experiment, rats learned to press a lever for sucrose under a reinforcement schedule that promoted habit formation[77]. Later, half of the rats developed a taste aversion to sucrose because the experimenters paired its ingestion with lithium chloride injections, which induced nausea or malaise. This procedure devalued the sucrose outcome. Later, all the rats pressed the lever under extinction conditions (which means that they could no longer get any sucrose). Control rats continued to press the lever at a typical extinction rate, about 60% of the end-of-training rate, including rats that had undergone the outcome-devaluation procedure (Fig. 12.4A). As expected, this behavior reflected a stimulus–response habit, which was characterized by an insensitivity to predicted outcomes. In contrast, rats with lesions of the dorsolateral striatum pressed the lever much less often after the outcome-devaluation procedure (Fig. 12.4B). Despite having a previously established lever-pressing habit, the lesioned rats showed a strong sensitivity to the predicted outcome. Dorsolateral striatal lesions therefore had two related effects: they impaired the performance of habits and they restored sensitivity to predicted outcomes.

In an experiment that yielded a complementary result, rats performed a task that should have promoted the learning of stimulus–response–outcome associations (outcome-directed behaviors)[78]. The experimenters then tested whether their subjects actually performed an outcome-directed behavior by using the devaluation procedure. In control rats, as expected, the rate of lever pressing decreased for devalued outcomes (Fig. 12.4C, gray bar) and increased for nondevalued outcomes (unfilled bar) relative to the end-of-training rate (circles, dashed horizontal line). Lesions of the dorsomedial striatum blocked this devaluation effect, thus demonstrating that they disrupted outcome-directed behavior (Fig. 12.4D and E). Because lesions that preceded training decreased the rate of lever pressing (Fig. 12.4D, circles) compared with control rats (Fig. 12.4C, circles), in another experiment the rats received their lesions after training. This procedure produced similar results (Fig. 12.4E); the lesioned rats continued to press the lever at the end-of-training rate, with little sensitivity to predicted outcomes.

Taken together, these experiments show that the dorsomedial and dorsolateral striatum perform different functions. The dorsolateral striatum underlies habits, but the dorsomedial striatum contributes to outcome-directed behavior. These findings contradict the habit–memory dichotomy, which holds that the basal ganglia, as a whole, subserves habits. Although these data come from rodents, we know of no reason to suppose that any other mammal differs in this respect, a sentiment captured in Fig. 5.6(B).

A common misunderstanding in comparative neuroanatomy is worth mentioning here. It is tempting to equate the dorsomedial (outcome-directed) part of the rodent striatum with the head of the caudate nucleus of primates[79]. But as we explained in Chapter 2, most of the head of caudate nucleus emerged during the evolution of primates, like the granular prefrontal areas that project to it. So the "outcome-directed" part of the rodent basal ganglia is not homologous to the head of the caudate nucleus in primates. Instead, this part of the rodent striatum is homologous (mostly) with a dorsomedial part of the putamen,

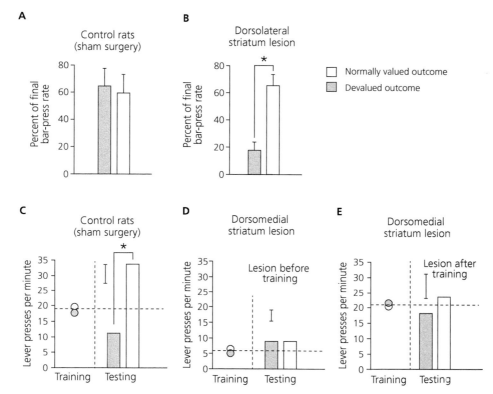

Fig. 12.4 Habits versus outcome-directed behavior. (A) The performance of control rats for (B). Rats were over-trained before being tested using a devaluation procedure. (B) The effect of lesions of the dorsolateral striatum. (C) Performance of control rats for (D), (E). The circles show lever pressing rates at the end of training but before the devaluation procedure. Dashed horizontal line: end-of-training response rate, across groups. The error bars in (C–E) show a measure of variance: the within-subject standard error of the difference of the means. (D) The effect of lesions of the dorsomedial striatum before training. (E) The effect of lesions of the dorsomedial striatum made after training. Asterisks indicate significant differences. (A), (B) Adapted from Yin HH, Knowlton BJ, Balleine BW. Lesions of dorsolateral striatum preserve outcome expectancy but disrupt habit formation in instrumental learning. *European Journal of Neuroscience* 19:181–9, © 2004, John Wiley & Sons. (C)–(E) From Yin HH, Ostlund SB, Knowlton BJ, Balleine BW. The role of the dorsomedial striatum in instrumental conditioning. *The European Journal of Neuroscience* 22:513–23. © 2005, John Wiley & Sons.

which functions in "loops" that include motor and somatosensory areas[80] (see Chapter 2, "Rings, loops, and memories"). Figure 5.6(B) illustrates these relations. This concept is especially important because the emergence of new prefrontal areas in early primates and in anthropoids (see Fig. 8.2) led to derived functions—not only for these new areas of cortex but also for their cortex–basal ganglia "loops." These derived functions extended the role of the basal ganglia beyond habits and outcome-directed behavior to include the cognitive traits that emerged during primate evolution (see Chapter 8, "Augmentation of older representational systems"), including those that arose during hominin evolution (see Chapters 9–11).

Proponents of the habit–memory dichotomy often cite a different rodent experiment[81]. In this task, rats navigated through a plus maze that had one arm blocked (Fig. 12.5A, B; see also Fig. 5.7A). In an example series of trials, rats started at the south end of the maze (with its north arm blocked) and learned that only the west arm had food. After the rats had learned this layout, they were placed at the north end of the maze (with its south arm blocked). Early in training, most rats used a place rule (e.g., go west, young rat; Fig. 12.5A). After extensive experience, however, most rats switched to a "response" rule (e.g., turn left; Fig. 12.5B).

Figure 12.5(C, D) contrasts behavior before and after brain lesions. Early in training, lesions of the dorsolateral striatum had no effect (Fig. 12.5C, left), but hippocampus lesions caused rats to use the "response" rule more than usual (Fig. 12.5C, gray bar) and the place rule less (hatched bar). In contrast, after extensive training, hippocampus lesions had no effect (Fig. 12.5D, right), but lesions of the dorsolateral striatum caused rats to use the place rule more than usual for that stage of training (Fig. 12.5D, hatched bar).

Advocates of the prevailing view see these results as support for the habit–memory dichotomy, but this interpretation depends entirely on two unverified assumptions:

◆ Behavior early in training and implementation of the place rule reflected the use of explicit memory, a function of the hippocampus.

◆ Behavior late in training and implementation of the "response" rule reflected the use of stimulus–response habits, a function of the basal ganglia.

These experiments provide important results, but we disagree with the way that some experts interpret them. In Chapter 11 ("Do animals have explicit memory?") we explained the problems with the assumption that rodents have explicit memory. As for habits, it is fine to say that stimulus–response habits produce insensitivity to predicted outcomes and their current value, but over-training has other effects as well. It allows animals to act quickly in response to some stimuli while neglecting others, in order to mitigate computational overload (see Chapter 3, "Why instrumental conditioning happens").

In this context, we can understand that the experiment illustrated in Fig. 12.4 addresses a distinction pertinent to the reinforcement systems—outcome-directed behavior versus habits (see Chapter 3). In contrast, the results depicted in Fig. 12.5 deal with a distinction relevant to the navigation system—intrinsic versus extrinsic guidance frames (see Chapter 4). Our interpretation of the plus-maze experiment (Fig. 12.5) draws on the proposal we presented in Chapter 4 and avoids any unverified assumptions about the existence of explicit memory in rats:

◆ Behavior early in training and implementation of the place rule reflected the use of an extrinsic frame of reference and extramaze visual cues.

◆ Behavior late in training and implementation of the "response" rule reflected the use of an intrinsic frame of reference and learned motor programs (the sequence and timing of movements required to obtain food).

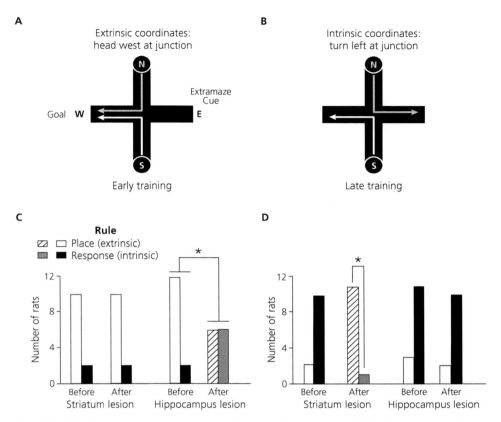

Fig. 12.5 Shift from extrinsic to intrinsic coordinates with experience. (A) During training, rats began running the maze at the place labeled S (south). In this example, the spatial goal was the end of the west arm, and an example extramaze cue is illustrated. In order to probe the coordinate frame used by each subject, the experimenters placed the rat at the place labeled N (north) after training (probe trials). White arrows represent training trials; gray arrows show probe trials. Performance on the probe trials indicated the use of extrinsic coordinates (a place rule) early in training. (B) The gray arrow illustrates the spontaneous use of intrinsic coordinates (a "response" rule) late in training. (C) Performance of two groups of rats early in training, before and after lesions of either the dorsolateral striatum or the hippocampus. The asterisk indicates a significant effect of the lesion. (D) Performance of two groups of rats late in training. Hatched and gray bars in (C) and (D) emphasize the significant behavioral effects of the lesions. (A) Figure 3.6 (top) in Passingham RE, Wise SP. *The Neurobiology of the Prefrontal Cortex*, © 2012, Oxford University Press. Reproduced with permission of OUP. (B) Adapted from Packard MG, McGaugh JL. Inactivation of hippocampus or caudate nucleus with lidocaine differentially affects expression of place and response learning. *Neurobiology of Learning and Memory* 65:65–72, © 1996, Elsevier, with permission.

Put another way, with experience rats shift from using extrinsic navigation to running motor programs: a straightforward interpretation of these results that appeals, if nothing else, to common sense. The hippocampus subserved the place rule in these experiments because it guides navigation in an extrinsic frame of reference (see Chapter 4);

the dorsolateral striatum subserved the "response" rule because it guides navigation in an intrinsic frame of reference, in part by using proprioceptive feedback to adjust motor programs. We return to this idea later (see "If not habits, what?").

Despite these arguments, advocates of the habit–memory dichotomy maintain that both habits and intrinsic guidance are stimulus–response (S–R) behaviors that depend on the basal ganglia. In another rat experiment[82], lesions of the striatum caused an impairment on a win–stay version of the eight-arm radial arm maze, which proponents of the habit–memory dichotomy take as evidence for a role in stimulus–response memories. But the use of various foraging strategies, such as win–stay[82], or a shift from extrinsic to intrinsic guidance (Fig. 12.5) says nothing about either explicit memory or habits, except for one coincidence. As mentioned earlier, extensive experience (over-training) leads both to habits (neglect of predicted outcomes) and intrinsic guidance (neglect of extramaze cues). This combination manifests itself in many ways as animals adjust their foraging strategies based on prior experience and changing circumstances, but provides no support for the habit–memory dichotomy. Notwithstanding the many experiments that have produced results weakly consistent with this doctrine, the findings illustrated in Fig. 12.4 have conclusively ruled it out (Box 12.5).

Monkeys

Proponents of the prevailing view also cite some experimental results from monkeys as support for the habit–memory dichotomy. According to one of these experiments[83], lesions of the tail of the caudate nucleus were said to impair performance on a habit task but not on an explicit-memory task. Lesions of the "amygdala plus hippocampus" were said to produce the opposite results[38], thus completing a double dissociation of function.

In this experiment, the multiple-pair (concurrent) discrimination task—discussed in Chapter 7 ("The prevailing doctrine and its discontents") and illustrated in Fig. 8.8(B,

---

Box 12.5 Meta-analysis and falsification

In an era of brain research dominated by functional brain imaging and the meta-analyses that synthesize these results, it might seem strange that we rely so much on a single set of studies to reject a habit function for the basal ganglia as a whole.

As discussed in Chapter 1 ("Other methods"), brain imaging methods cannot rule out functional contributions for a brain structure. The lack of a significant activation in some area in some experimental contrast provides hints, but such findings can never provide a definitive refutation of any claim about that area's function. In contrast, if some behavior survives the lesion of that structure, then we can conclude that the lesioned area is not necessary for that behavior—at least within limits imposed by adaptations in remaining structures. Accordingly, a single lesion study can sometimes provide definitive evidence, especially in falsifying a theory, such as the one positing a habit function for the basal ganglia as a whole.

right)—was assumed to assess habits. (Set aside, for the time being, the fact that proponents of the prevailing view sometimes interpret this testing procedure as a "perception
task," for reasons explained in Box 7.1.) Monkeys with tail-of-the-caudate lesions learned
the task to the same, 90% correct criterion as control monkeys, but made many more
errors along the way. The authors interpreted this increase in errors to criterion as an
impairment in habits. The same monkeys performed normally on a short-interval matching task, so their [explicit] memory was said to be intact.

In a related experiment[84], monkeys with combined lesions of the hippocampus and the
tail of the caudate nucleus had impairments on the multiple-pair discrimination task, but
monkeys with lesions confined to the hippocampus did not. This finding also seemed to
support the idea that the caudate nucleus is part of a "habit system."

We reject these conclusions because they follow from faulty assumptions. First, short-
interval matching performance does not measure explicit memory. As explained earlier
(see "Falsification of the first model"), impairments on this task result not from the loss
of some global, explicit memory function mediated by a "medial temporal lobe memory
system," but instead from damage to the perirhinal and entorhinal cortex and the loss of
their specialized representations. This idea explains the impairment that follows so-called
"amygdala plus hippocampus" lesions without invoking either explicit memory in monkeys or the habit–memory dichotomy.

Second, the multiple-pair discrimination task is not a specific test of habits. Not only did
H.M. perform this task very poorly, despite his supposedly intact "habit system"[85], but the
choices that monkeys make on the multiple-pair task are sensitive to outcome valuations[86],
which contradicts the assumption that this task measures habits. Instead of impairing habits in these experiments[83,84], lesions of the tail of the caudate nucleus disrupted the function
of cortex–basal ganglia "loops" involving the inferior temporal cortex. In Chapter 7 ("The
prevailing doctrine and its discontents") we discussed experiments in which lesions of the
inferior temporal cortex caused an impairment on the multiple-pair task. Lesions of its
projection targets in the striatum, the tail of the caudate nucleus and the posterior limit of
the putamen, would be expected to have the same effect. This idea accounts for the effects
of tail-of-the-caudate lesions without appealing to the habit–memory dichotomy.

Other findings from monkeys have directly contradicted the habit–memory dichotomy. In the detour task, monkeys needed to reach around a transparent barrier in order
to obtain a visible piece of food. Without the barrier, the monkeys performed the habit,
acquired over a lifetime, of reaching directly for the food. Monkeys treated with MPTP had
a severe dysfunction of the basal ganglia because this neurotoxin destroyed its dopaminergic inputs. Nevertheless, the monkeys continued to reach directly for a visible target even
with the barrier present, and so they hit the barrier[87]. They therefore had an abnormally
persistent habit, not the habit impairment predicted by the habit–memory dichotomy.

Humans

Like other aspects of the prevailing view, arguments in support of the habit–memory
dichotomy come from clinical observations as well as from animal experiments. The most

influential of these findings come from probabilistic classification tasks. In one such task, subjects learned to construct categories of stimuli based on informative but inconclusive feedback. They believed that they were learning to predict the "weather," and so this task is sometimes called the weather prediction task. In accord with the habit–memory dichotomy, patients with basal ganglia disease had an impairment on this task, but amnesic patients did not, at least not in early trials[75,88]. Furthermore, brain imaging studies showed that as control subjects learned this task, activation occurred in the striatum. Proponents of the prevailing view refer to this test as a "habit task" because they see it as gradual stimulus–response learning in the absence of awareness.

An alternative interpretation of the same results focuses on a different aspect of the task—the prediction and processing of feedback. Tests of patients with Huntington's disease or Parkinson's disease have revealed impairments in various skills requiring the integration of feedback with ongoing behavior, such as mirror reading[89], maintaining contact with a moving target[90], solving puzzles like the Tower of Hanoi task[91], and learning sequences of movements[92,93]. In similar studies, amnesic patients learned and performed such skills normally, as H.M. did[94–96]. Although some experts cite these results as support for the habit–memory dichotomy, these impairments, along with others, can be reinterpreted in terms of a problem with using feedback efficiently. Brain imaging studies have revealed that activation in the striatum during feedback-based learning exceeds that during feedback-free learning, and clinical testing has shown that Parkinson's disease impairs the former but not the latter[97,98]. These findings suggest that the basal ganglia integrates feedback with ongoing behavior, an idea we explain later (see "If not habits, what?"). Here we focus on just one well-documented observation.

We mentioned in Chapter 6 ("Autopilot control") that as Huntington's disease progresses, especially in the early stages of the disease and in asymptomatic gene carriers, most damage occurs in the dorsal striatum. In a reaching task, both asymptomatic and symptomatic gene carriers had impairments in correcting ongoing movements based on feedback. Their movements started normally but became irregular and inefficient (jerky) from the time that the earliest feedback arrived, about 300 ms after the movement started, until the end of the movement[99,100]. This finding indicates that, for reaching movements at least, the basal ganglia uses feedback to adjust movements as they unfold. Because these findings were based on a rigorous psychophysical analysis, we regard them as more solid and reliable than the results cited by proponents of the habit–memory dichotomy, which can be interpreted in terms of either habits or feedback processing.

Summary

We reject the habit–memory dichotomy on two grounds. First, results from rats convincingly contradict the idea that the basal ganglia, as a whole, subserves habits[77,101,102]. Restriction of the dichotomy to the dorsal basal ganglia[103] does nothing to salvage it because these studies contrast the function of two parts of the dorsal striatum and demonstrate that only a part of the rodent basal ganglia has anything to do with habits. In primates, even less of the basal ganglia has this function, when viewed as a proportion of the total volume of the basal ganglia.

Second, each part of the cortex sends projections to the striatum (see Chapter 2, "Rings and loops"). The hippocampus, for example, has its striatal territory just as other cortical areas have theirs. This understanding undermines the habit–memory dichotomy fundamentally. It makes no sense to contrast the memory functions of something called "the medial temporal lobe" and the basal ganglia because all cortical areas (including the hippocampus and all of the other components of the so-called "medial temporal lobe") function in cooperation with the basal ganglia (see Fig. 2.3 and Plate 1).

If not habits, what?

So if the basal ganglia, as a whole, does not subserve habits, what does it do? One idea is that the basal ganglia functions as part of a forward model[104]. This term refers to a neural computation that predicts the feedback signals that should arrive in the brain as actions unfold, based on motor command signals and taking into account neural delays (see Chapter 6 and Fig. 6.7). The concept of a forward model accounts for all of the impairments caused by basal ganglia disease (see "Humans") because they all involve feedback processing. For reaching movements, this computation allows the brain to compensate for neural noise, faulty estimates about the mass or momentum of a grasped object, or external forces that can generate errors in reaching. When feedback deviates sufficiently from predictions, an adjusted motor command can compensate for the error. In more general terms, a forward model uses motor commands to generate predictions about feedback. In the example just given, the feedback involves proprioceptive and visual signals (see Chapter 6), but another form of feedback consists of behavioral outcomes, such as food availability or effort costs (see Chapter 3).

According to this idea, the basal ganglia predicts feedback in order to adjust ongoing behavior. By predicting feedback, the basal ganglia can contribute not only to skills and motor behavior, such as reaching movements, but also to cognitive functions such as planning, changing plans (switching), generating a series of plans (sequences), and constructing various types (categories) of plans. The product of the basal ganglia goes by many names: decisions, choices, schedules, sequences, priorities, adjustments, adaptations, and control policies, among others. Collectively, they take into account the current sensory context, predicted biological costs and benefits, other kinds of predicted feedback (such as proprioceptive and visual signals), and constraints on behavior (such as risks and dangers). The actual feedback can either match expectations or deviate from predictions, leading to an adjustment in ongoing behavior.

These ideas explain why so much of the basal ganglia has nothing to do with habits. In primates, for example, "prefrontal" parts of the striatum help the prefrontal cortex do what it does: generate goals based on a current context and up to date biological needs (see Chapter 8)[105]. Just as cortex–basal ganglia "loops" involving the prefrontal cortex support the goal system, "loops" that include the premotor, primary motor, somatosensory, and posterior parietal cortex support the manual-foraging system. As Chapter 6 explained, these representations transform extrinsic, visual coordinates into joint-angle changes and muscle forces, among similar functions. Calling these sophisticated computations "habits" contributes little to understanding them, although they, like habits, involve automatic (as opposed to attentive) behaviors.

Conclusions

The road less traveled by

Advocates of the prevailing view sometimes treat its chief tenets as facts established by rigorous research in the distant past. This chapter reveals a very different history. Forgetting its frail foundation, supporters of a "medial temporal lobe memory system" and a "striatal habit system" frequently focus on a flood of weakly consistent findings and demand disproof to dislodge these doctrines[106-112]. In a field like memory research, disproof is not a realistic standard. Rather than disproving the dominant doctrines, Chapters 1–11 explored the "road not taken" in the 1980s. That road, we submit, leads not only to a better understanding of memory systems, but also of their history and of the ancestral species in which they emerged.

The "road taken" by the field of memory research depended in large part on a monkey model of human amnesia that took shape in the late 1970s and 1980s. This model relied on the short-interval matching task, which has three crucial shortcomings: It measures memory on an inappropriate time-scale; it does not require explicit memory; and its results depend on both the stimulus material used and stimulus set size, among other factors. The first version of the model claimed that combined damage to the amygdala and hippocampus causes amnesia. When subsequent experiments showed that these results arose from inadvertent and incidental brain damage, advocates of the prevailing view retained the task and replaced the amygdala with three nearby cortical areas: the perirhinal, entorhinal, and parahippocampal cortex. As a result, theories of explicit memory began to place less emphasis on the hippocampus and more on these nearby areas.

Taken to its logical conclusion, the finding that short-interval matching tasks depend on the perirhinal and entorhinal cortex in monkeys—and not to any significant extent on the hippocampus—would exclude the hippocampus from the "medial temporal lobe memory system" in monkeys. Of course, we do not accept this conclusion because we reject both the assumption that these tasks measure explicit memory and the concept of a "medial temporal lobe memory system."

In contrast to the prevailing view, our approach to understanding explicit memory aligns reasonably well with ideas about "hippocampal amnesia" dating to the 1950s (see "H.M.'s ablation"). According to the proposal that we presented in Chapter 11, interactions of the extended hippocampal–navigation system with both the granular prefrontal cortex and the anterior temporal lobe subserve explicit memory in humans, including both its episodic and semantic varieties (see Fig. 11.8).

Evolution

Neglect or misunderstanding of evolution has led to many shortcomings of the prevailing view:

◆ The equipotentiality principle ignores the idea that the hippocampal, entorhinal, perirhinal, and parahippocampal cortex have different evolutionary histories, which involved distinct selective pressures faced by diverse ancestral species distributed over hundreds of millions of years. According to our proposals, these selective factors produced the distinct and specialized representations housed in all four of these cortical areas.

◆ The summation principle neglects the idea that the neocortex evolved in mammals, long after the hippocampal homologue, which evolved in early vertebrates. According to our proposals, posteromedial parts of the mammalian ring neocortex augmented the function of the medial allocortex (the hippocampus in mammals), which was inherited from ancestral amniotes (see Chapter 2, "Early amniotes"). From this perspective, the summation principle appears to posit that the neocortical components of the "medial temporal lobe" added semantic memory to a pre-existing episodic memory system, which seems exceedingly unlikely.

◆ The perception–memory dichotomy fails to consider the perirhinal and inferior temporal cortex in the context of the ancestral species in which these areas first emerged. Our proposals relate the specialized representations in both areas to the foraging problems faced by these ancestors in their time and place: The perirhinal cortex supported the perception and memory of objects encountered by early mammals; the inferior temporal cortex supported the perception and memory of signs used by anthropoids to locate distant resources.

◆ The habit–memory dichotomy stems, in part, from serious misconceptions about brain evolution and about evolution in general. Furthermore, this doctrine neglects two important ideas that depend on an evolutionary perspective: (1) new cortex–basal ganglia "loops" emerged during evolution; and (2) the hippocampus contributes to its own cortex–basal ganglia "loops." As illustrated in Fig. 2.3 and Plate 1, our proposals incorporate this archetypal telencephalic architecture into the evolutionary accretion model of memory.

Outdated ideas about evolution have led some memory researchers down the wrong road from time to time (see "The habit–memory dichotomy"), but neglect of evolution has been a much more pervasive impediment to progress. When the broad scope of vertebrate evolution—and especially brain evolution—is considered in sufficient detail, it provides a key insight: Representational systems exist in modern brains because they provided a specific set of advantages to a particular ancestral species. By traveling the "road not taken" in the 1980s, memory researchers can someday assimilate anatomy, ancestors, and adaptations into accounts of amnesia.

References

1. Frost, R. (1920) *Mountain Interval* (Henry Holt, Bartleby.com/119, New York).
2. Corkin, S. (2013) *Permanent Present Tense* (Basic Books, New York).
3. Scoville, W.B. and Milner, B. (1957) *J. Neurol. Neurosurg. Psychiatr.* **20**, 11–21.
4. Milner, B. (1959) *Psychiatr. Res. Rep. Am. Psychiatr. Assoc.* **11**, 43–58.
5. Penfield, W. and Mathieson, G. (1974) *Arch. Neurol.* **31**, 145–154.
6. Zola-Morgan, S., Squire, L.R., and Amaral, D.G. (1986) *J. Neurosci.* **6**, 2950–2967.
7. Rempel-Clower, N., Zola, S., Squire, L., and Amaral, D. (1996) *J. Neurosci.* **16**, 5233–5255.
8. Stefanacci, L., Buffalo, E.A., Schmolck, H., and Squire, L.R. (2000) *J. Neurosci.* **20**, 7024–7036.
9. Clark, R.E., Manns, J.R., and Squire, L.R. (2002) *Trends Cogn. Sci.* **6**, 524–531.
10. Correll, R.E. and Scoville, W.B. (1965) *J. Comp. Physiol. Psychol.* **60**, 175–181.
11. Correll, R.E. and Scoville, W.B. (1965) *J. Comp. Physiol. Psychol.* **60**, 360–367.
12. Correll, R.E. and Scoville, W.B. (1967) *Exp. Brain Res.* **4**, 85–96.
13. Orbach, J., Milner, B., and Rasmussen, T. (1960) *Arch. Neurol.* **3**, 230–251.
14. Izquierdo, I. (1975) *Prog. Neurobiol.* **5**, 37–75.
15. Gaffan, D. (1974) *J. Comp. Physiol. Psychol.* **86**, 1100–1109.
16. Sidman, M., Stoddard, L.T., and Mohr, J.P. (1968) *Neuropsychologia* **6**, 245–254.
17. Mandler, G. (1980) *Psychol. Rev.* **87**, 252–271.
18. Aggleton, J.P. and Brown, M.W. (1999) *Behav. Brain Sci.* **22**, 425.
19. Mishkin, M. (1978) *Nature* **273**, 297–298.
20. Mishkin, M. (1982) *Phil. Trans. R. Soc. Lond. B, Biol. Sci.* **298**, 83–95.
21. Bachevalier, J., Parkinson, J.K., and Mishkin, M. (1985) *Exp. Brain Res.* **57**, 554–561.
22. Murray, E.A. and Mishkin, M. (1984) *J. Neurosci.* **4**, 2565–2580.
23. Saunders, R.C., Murray, E.A., and Mishkin, M. (1984) *Neuropsychologia* **22**, 785–796.
24. Zola-Morgan, S., Squire, L.R., and Mishkin, M. (1982) *Science* **218**, 1337–1339.
25. Zola-Morgan, S. and Squire, L.R. (1984) *J. Neurosci.* **4**, 1072–1085.
26. Zola-Morgan, S. and Squire, L.R. (1985) *Behav. Neurosci.* **99**, 22–34.
27. Horel, J.A. (1978) *Brain* **101**, 403–445.
28. Cirillo, R.A., Horel, J.A., and George, P.J. (1989) *Behav. Brain Res.* **34**, 55–69.
29. Murray, E.A. and Mishkin, M. (1986) *J. Neurosci.* **6**, 1991–2003.
30. Meunier, M., Hadfield, W., Bachevalier, J., and Murray, E.A. (1996) *J. Neurophysiol.* **75**, 1190–1205.
31. Meunier, M., Bachevalier, J., Mishkin, M., and Murray, E.A. (1993) *J. Neurosci.* **13**, 5418–5432.
32. Malkova, L., Bachevalier, J., Mishkin, M., and Saunders, R.C. (2001) *NeuroReport* **12**, 1913–1917.
33. Baxter, M.G. and Murray, E.A. (2001) *Eur. J. Neurosci.* **13**, 1228–1238.
34. Murray, E.A. and Mishkin, M. (1998) *J. Neurosci.* **18**, 6568–6582.
35. Baxter, M.G. and Murray, E.A. (2001) *Hippocampus* **11**, 201–203.
36. Buffalo, E.A., Stefanacci, L., Squire, L., and Zola, S.M. (1998) *Behav. Neurosci.* **112**, 3–14.
37. Gaffan, D. and Murray, E.A. (1992) *Behav. Neurosci.* **106**, 30–38.
38. Malamut, B.L., Saunders, R.C., and Mishkin, M. (1984) *Behav. Neurosci.* **98**, 759–769.
39. Phillips, R.R., Malamut, B.L., Bachevalier, J., and Mishkin, M. (1988) *Behav. Brain Res.* **27**, 99–107.
40. Bussey, T.J. and Saksida, L.M. (2007) *Hippocampus* **17**, 898–908.
41. Murray, E.A. and Mishkin, M. (1986) *J. Neurosci.* **6**, 1991–2003.
42. Waxler, M. and Rosvold, H.E. (1970) *Neuropsychologia* **8**, 137–146.

43. Zola-Morgan, S., Squire, L.R., and Ramus, S.J. (1994) *Hippocampus* 4, 483–495.

44. Zola-Morgan, S., Squire, L.R., Clower, R.P., and Rempel, N.L. (1993) *J. Neurosci.* 13, 251–265.

45. Alvarez, P., Zola-Morgan, S., and Squire, L.R. (1994) *Proc. Natl. Acad. Sci. USA* 91, 5637–5641.

46. Beason-Held, L.L., Rosene, D.L., Killiany, R.J., and Moss, M.B. (1999) *Hippocampus* 9, 562–574.

47. Zola, S.M., Squire, L.R., Teng, E., Stefanacci, L. et al. (2000) *J. Neurosci.* 20, 451–463.

48. Charles, D.P., Gaffan, D., and Buckley, M.J. (2004) *J. Neurosci.* 24, 2037–2044.

49. Cowell, R.A., Bussey, T.J., and Saksida, L.M. (2010) *Hippocampus* 20, 1245–1262.

50. Cowell, R.A., Bussey, T.J., and Saksida, L.M. (2006) *J. Neurosci.* 26, 12186–12197.

51. Bachevalier, J., Saunders, R.C., and Mishkin, M. (1985) *Exp. Brain Res.* 57, 547–553.

52. Buckmaster, C.A., Eichenbaum, H., Amaral, D.G., and Rapp, P.R. (1999) *Soc. Neurosci. Abstr.* 25, 88.

53. Nemanic, S., Alvarado, M.C., and Bachevalier, J. (2004) *J. Neurosci.* 24, 2013–2026.

54. Zola, S.M. and Squire, L.R. (2001) *Hippocampus* 11, 92–98.

55. Saksida, L.M., Bussey, T.J., Buckmaster, C.A., and Murray, E.A. (2007) *Cereb. Cortex* 17, 108–115.

56. Yang, T., Bavley, R.L., Fomalont, K., Blomstrom, K.J. et al. (2014) *Hippocampus* 24, 1102–1111.

57. Malkova, L. and Mishkin, M. (2003) *J. Neurosci.* 23, 1956–1965.

58. Bachevalier, J. and Nemanic, S. (2008) *Hippocampus* 18, 64–80.

59. Nasr, S., Liu, N., Devaney, K.J., Yue, X. et al. (2011) *J. Neurosci.* 31, 13771–13785.

60. Vargha-Khadem, F., Gadian, D.G., Watkins, K.E., Connelly, A. et al. (1997) *Science* 277, 376–380.

61. Vargha-Khadem, F., Gadian, D.G., and Mishkin, M. (2001) *Phil. Trans. R. Soc. B: Biol. Sci.* 356, 1435–1440.

62. Tsivilis, D., Vann, S.D., Denby, C., Roberts, N. et al. (2008) *Nat. Neurosci.* 11, 834–842.

63. Holdstock, J.S., Mayes, A.R., Isaac, C.L., Gong, Q. et al. (2002) *Neuropsychologia* 40, 748–768.

64. Kapur, N. (1994) *Cogn. Neuropsychol.* 11, 661–670.

65. Gardiner, J.M., Brandt, K.R., Baddeley, A.D., Vargha-Khadem, F. et al. (2008) *Neuropsychologia* 46, 2865–2868.

66. Manns, J.R., Hopkins, R.O., and Squire, L.R. (2003) *Neuron* 38, 127–133.

67. Graham, K.S., Patterson, K., Pratt, K.H., and Hodges, J.R. (1999) *Neuropsychology* 13, 359–380.

68. Dewar, B.K., Patterson, K., Wilson, B.A., and Graham, K.S. (2009) *Neuropsychol. Rehabil.* 19, 383–421.

69. Mayberry, E.J., Sage, K., Ehsan, S., and Lambon Ralph, M.A. (2011) *Neuropsychologia* 49, 3591–3598.

70. Hoffman, P., Clarke, N., Jones, R.W., and Noonan, K.A. (2015) *Neuropsychologia* 76, 240–253.

71. McClelland, J.L., McNaughton, B., and O'Reilly, R. (1995) *Psychol. Rev.* 102, 419–457.

72. Saksida, L.M. and Bussey, T.J. (2010) *Neuropsychologia* 48, 2370–2384.

73. Graham, K.S., Barense, M.D., and Lee, A.C. (2010) *Neuropsychologia* 48, 831–853.

74. Mishkin, M., Malamut, B., and Bachevalier, J. (1984) In: *Neurobiology of Learning and Memory* (eds. Lynch, G., McGaugh, J. and Weinberger, N.M.), pp. 65–77 (Guilford, New York).

75. Knowlton, B.J., Mangels, J.A., and Squire, L.R. (1996) *Science* 273, 1399–1402.

76. Broadbent, N.J., Squire, L.R., and Clark, R.E. (2007) *Learn. Mem.* 14, 145–151.

77. Yin, H.H., Knowlton, B.J., and Balleine, B.W. (2004) *Eur. J. Neurosci.* 19, 181–189.

78. Yin, H.H., Ostlund, S.B., Knowlton, B.J., and Balleine, B.W. (2005) *Eur. J. Neurosci.* 22, 513–523.

79. Balleine, B.W. and O'Doherty, J.P. (2010) *Neuropsychopharmacol.* 35, 48–69.

80. Wise, S.P. (2008) *Trends Neurosci.* 31, 599–608.

81. Packard, M.G. and McGaugh, J.L. (1996) *Neurobiol. Learn. Mem.* 65, 65–72.

82. McDonald, R.J. and White, N.M. (1993) *Behav. Neurosci.* **107**, 3–22.

83. Fernandez-Ruiz, J., Wang, J., Aigner, T.G., and Mishkin, M. (2001) *Proc. Natl. Acad. Sci. USA* **98**, 4196–4201.

84. Teng, E., Stefanacci, L., Squire, L.R., and Zola, S.M. (2000) *J. Neurosci.* **20**, 3853–3863.

85. Hood, K.L., Postle, B.R., and Corkin, S. (1999) *Neuropsychologia* **37**, 1375–1386.

86. Malkova, L., Gaffan, D., and Murray, E.A. (1997) *J. Neurosci.* **17**, 6011–6020.

87. Taylor, J.R., Roth, R.H., Sladek, J.R., and Redmond, D.E. (1990) *Behav. Neurosci.* **104**, 564–576.

88. Knowlton, B.J., Squire, L.R., and Gluck, M.A. (1994) *Learn. Mem.* **1**, 106–120.

89. Martone, M., Butters, N., Payne, M., Becker, J.T. *et al.* (1984) *Arch. Neurol.* **41**, 965–970.

90. Heindel, W.C., Butters, N., and Salmon, D.P. (1988) *Behav. Neurosci.* **102**, 141–147.

91. Saint-Cyr, J.A., Taylor, A.E., and Lang, A.E. (1988) *Brain* **111**, 941–959.

92. Knopman, D. and Nissen, M.J. (1991) *Neuropsychologia* **29**, 245–254.

93. Willingham, D.B., Nissen, M.J., and Bullemer, P. (1989) *J. Exp. Psychol. Learn. Mem. Cogn.* **15**, 1047–1060.

94. Squire, L.R., Knowlton, B., and Musen, G. (1993) *Annu. Rev. Psychol.* **44**, 453–495.

95. Sherry, D.F. and Schacter, D.L. (1987) *Psychol. Rev.* **94**, 439–454.

96. Schacter, D.L. and Tulving, E. (1994) In: *Memory Systems 1994* (eds. Schacter, D.L. and Tulving, E.), pp. 1–38 (MIT Press, Cambridge, MA).

97. Aron, A.R., Watkins, L., Sahakian, B.J., Monsell, S. *et al.* (2003) *J. Cogn. Neurosci.* **15**, 629–642.

98. Poldrack, R.A., Desmond, J.E., Glover, G.H., and Gabrieli, J.D. (1998) *Cereb. Cortex* **8**, 1–10.

99. Smith, M.A., Brandt, J., and Shadmehr, R. (2000) *Nature* **403**, 544–549.

100. Smith, M.A. and Shadmehr, R. (2005) *J. Neurophysiol.* **93**, 2809–2821.

101. Yin, H.H. (2005) *Eur. J. Neurosci.* **22**, 513–523.

102. Yin, H.H., Knowlton, B.J., and Balleine, B.W. (2006) *Behav. Brain Res.* **166**, 189–196.

103. Packard, M.G. and Knowlton, B.J. (2002) *Annu. Rev. Neurosci.* **25:563–593**, 563–593.

104. Aron, A.R., Wise, S.P., and Poldrack, R.A. (2009) In: *Encyclopedia of Neuroscience* (ed. Squire, L.R.), pp. 1069–1077 (Academic Press, Oxford).

105. Passingham, R.E. and Wise, S.P. (2012) *The Neurobiology of the Prefrontal Cortex* (Oxford University Press, Oxford).

106. Mishkin, M., Suzuki, W.A., Gadian, D.G., and Vargha-Khadem, F. (1997) *Phil. Trans. R. Soc. B: Biol. Sci.* **352**, 1461–1467.

107. Squire, L.R., Wixted, J.T., and Clark, R.E. (2007) *Nat. Rev. Neurosci.* **8**, 872–883.

108. Suzuki, W.A. (2009) *Neuron* **61**, 657–666.

109. Stark, C.E.L. and Squire, L.R. (2000) *Learn. Mem.* **7**, 273–278.

110. Levy, D.A., Shrager, Y., and Squire, L.R. (2005) *Learn. Mem.* **12**, 61–66.

111. Shrager, Y., Gold, J.J., Hopkins, R.O., and Squire, L.R. (2006) *J. Neurosci.* **26**, 2235–2240.

112. Kim, S., Jeneson, A., van der Horst, A.S., Frascino, J.C. et al. (2011) *J. Neurosci.* **31**, 2624–2629.

113. Preuss, T.M. and Robert, J.S. (2014) In: *The Cognitive Neurosciences* (eds, Gazzaniga, M.S. and Mangun, G.R.), pp. 59–66 (MIT Press, Cambridge, MA).

114. Annese, J., Schenker-Ahmed, N.M., Bartsch, H., Maechler, P. et al. (2014) *Nat. Commun.* **5**, 3122.

115. Corkin, S., Amaral, D.G., Gonzalez, R.G. et al. (1997) *J. Neurosci.* **17**, 3964–3979.

116. Thiebaut de Schotten, M., Dell'Acqua, F., Ratiu, P., Leslie, A. et al. (2015) *Cereb. Cortex* **25**, 4812–4827.

117. Leonard, B.W., Amaral, D.G., Squire, L.R., and Zola-Morgan, S. (1995) *J. Neurosci.* **15**, 5637–5659.

118. Suzuki, W.A. (2010) *Trends Cogn. Sci.* **14**, 195–200.

119. Squire, L.R., Shrager, Y., and Levy, D.A. (2006) *Learn. Mem.* **13**, 106–107.

120. Clark, R.E., Reinagel, P., Broadbent, N.J., Flister, E.D. et al. (2011) *Neuron* **70**, 132–140.

121. Hales, J.B., Broadbent, N.J., Velu, P.D., Squire, L.R. et al. (2015) *Learn. Mem.* **22**, 83–91.

Chapter 13

Reconstructing memory's past

Anybody can have a brain. That's a very mediocre commodity. Every pusillanimous creature that crawls on the earth or slinks through slimy seas has a brain!

The Wizard in *The Wizard of Oz*[1]

In *The Wizard of Oz*, the Scarecrow wants a brain and the Cowardly Lion craves courage, but according to the Great and Powerful Oz, all they need is a diploma and a medal, respectively. Even if we pay no attention to the man behind the curtain, we know that the Wizard's way will never work. Diplomas and medals validate memories, and without such memories they signify nothing. H.M. deserved both degrees and medals for his contributions to memory research[2], but what good would they have done him? Such mementos would have seemed to him like awards to someone else.

We opened this book with H.M., and we return to him later, after a chapter-by-chapter summary and a few thoughts about testing our proposals.

Summary

Part I

In Chapter 1 we provided an introduction and some background material. Among its themes: (1) memory seems to come in distinct systems because novel forms of representation arose at various times and augmented existing forms; (2) the functions of these systems extend beyond the selective factors that led to their development; and (3) representational systems perform many functions in addition to memory. Table 1.2 lists our proposals, and Table 1.3 contrasts them with the prevailing view of memory systems.

We outlined a version of vertebrate brain evolution in Chapter 2, and Fig. 13.1 illustrates its main conclusions: (1) the telencephalon, which evolved in early vertebrates, included homologues of the hippocampus and basal ganglia; (2) the neocortex evolved in early mammals; (3) early primates evolved the first granular prefrontal areas, along with new parts of the premotor, posterior parietal, and temporal cortex; (4) additional parts of the granular prefrontal cortex emerged during anthropoid evolution, as the posterior parietal and lateral temporal cortex became more elaborate; and (5) the prefrontal, posterior parietal, and lateral temporal cortex expanded dramatically during hominin evolution.

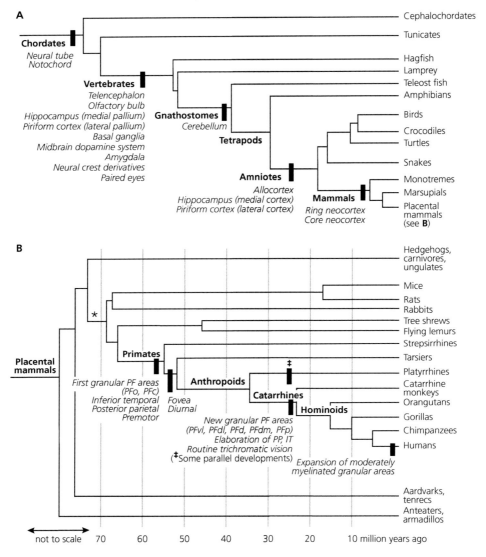

Fig. 13.1 Summary cladogram. (A) Chordates. (B) Placental mammals. The asterisk denotes the last common ancestor of rodents and primates. The derived traits of selected lineages appear beneath the black bars.

Part II

In Chapter 3 we presented a brief sketch of reinforcement learning, which evolved early in the history of animals. Despite surface similarities, reinforcement learning depends on several diverse and neurophysiologically unrelated mechanisms, as demonstrated by the finding that sea anemones, which have no central nervous system, can establish Pavlovian memories. The fact that both the cerebellum and the telencephalon can subserve Pavlovian learning, independent of each other, supports the same conclusion, as does the wide variety of protostomes and vertebrates that show both Pavlovian and instrumental learning, despite sharing few, if any, homologous brain structures. As new memory systems emerged during evolution (see Chapters 4–10), reinforcement learning persisted in modified forms, but it cannot account for derived aspects of human cognition such as analogical, metaphorical, or relational reasoning, abstract problem-solving strategies, constructive episodic simulation, mental time travel, scenario construction, mental trial and error, autobiographical narratives, language, a theory of mind, or explicit (declarative) memory.

According to Chapter 4, a navigation system emerged during the major evolutionary transition that produced stem vertebrates. These animals adapted to a life of predatory foraging, based in part on vision and olfaction, and among their many derived traits was a homologue of the hippocampus. According to our proposal, the hippocampal homologue of early vertebrates housed a new representational system, sometimes called a cognitive map, which enabled these animals to reach goals via various routes, including novel ones. These map-like representations incorporated locations, objects, and odors, as well as the sequences in which they should be encountered during a journey, including their timing. Once these specialized representations developed, they became available for other cognitive functions.

In Chapter 5 we proposed that a biased-competition system arose in the agranular prefrontal cortex of early mammals and that it regulates competition among and within other representational systems. According to Chapter 5, the biases that these areas generate depends on their representations of the contexts in which one kind of behavior should prevail over others and the successes that such biases have promoted in the past. Examples of competing representations include outcome-directed behaviors versus habits, Pavlovian versus instrumental behaviors, navigation via extrinsic versus intrinsic coordinates, newer and fragile memories versus older and sturdy ones, and current versus obsolete contexts for guiding foraging.

Part III

In Chapter 6 we examined the manual-foraging system, which emerged in early primates as these animals adapted to a life confined to the fine branches of trees and shrubs. Their derived traits included grasping hands and feet, forward-facing eyes, and a hindlimb-dominated mode of locomotion that freed their hands for specialized functions. A suite of new cortical areas emerged in these animals, including several premotor and posterior parietal areas. These areas stored memories—in the form of visuomotor transforms—about how to reach toward, grasp, and manipulate objects. In addition, two parts of the granular prefrontal cortex also emerged in early primates: one guided the search for and attention to items dispersed among the fine branches; the other updated the valuation of items and actions in accord with current biological needs. New inferior temporal areas augmented visual processing by representing new kinds of feature conjunctions. Taken together, these developments provided advantages in finding, keeping track of, evaluating, and obtaining items in a cluttered and mechanically unstable environment.

According to Chapter 7, as anthropoids evolved from small, local foragers into large, far-ranging animals, new and elaborated temporal and posterior parietal areas came to support a feature system. This name refers to two particular classes of features, which we call attributes and metrics. The temporal cortex came to represent conjunctions of attributes such as color, shape, and visual texture, along with analogous acoustic features; the posterior parietal cortex represented metrics such as number, order, duration, and distance. The feature system provided anthropoids with advantages in identifying the signs of distant resources, including mid-level visual conjunctions simpler than whole objects but more complex than elemental features and low-order conjunctions. Along with its new and elaborated areas, the feature system incorporated older sensory areas, such as the perirhinal cortex, which continued to represent feature conjunctions at the level of objects, as it had since the advent of mammals. The feature system augmented the navigation system for the perception and memory of objects, signs, and scenes.

In Chapter 8 we discussed the goal system and the several new granular prefrontal areas that evolved in anthropoids. Unlike the reinforcement learning systems (see Chapter 3), which learn cumulatively and discard event information, the goal system stores representations of single, goal-related events. By generating goals based on the memory of goal-related events and abstract behavioral strategies, anthropoids could decrease their frequency of dangerous foraging choices. During shortfalls in resources—in the face of fierce competition and a serious risk of predation—any reduction in foraging errors would have provided an important selective advantage[3].

Part IV

According to Chapter 9, the feature and goal systems underwent important changes after the ape–human lineage diverged from other anthropoids. From their origins in generating foraging goals based on relational metrics, prefrontal–posterior parietal networks came to support relational reasoning more generally[4]; from their origins in identifying the signs of resources, parts of the lateral temporal lobe came to represent generalized concepts and categories. These developments led to semantic memory, analogical reasoning, and multiple demand cognition, among other cognitive capacities.

We introduced the social–subjective system in Chapter 10. According to the proposal in that chapter, species-specific re-representations of self and others emerged in the expanding prefrontal cortex of hominins as adaptations to their particular social systems. As these new re-representations evolved, they could influence older representational systems. A large-scale medial network—encompassing the medial prefrontal cortex and the hippocampus, among other posteromedial areas—came to support perspective-taking, the recognition of situational contexts, and constructive episodic simulations (scenario construction, mental time travel, and mental trial and error). A lateral network—including the lateral prefrontal cortex, the superior temporal cortex, and the anterior temporal lobe, among other areas—came to represent social goals and concepts, categories of individuals along with their roles in society, and generalizations about one's self and others.

In Chapter 11 we explored the origin of explicit memory, proposing that episodic memory developed in hominins when their new, species-specific re-representations of self became integrated into conjunctive representations of events (see Figs. 11.2C and 13.2A). Upon retrieval of these memories, ancestral hominins re-experienced events as if observing or participating in them. Similarly, hominins began to acquire factual, cultural, and conceptual knowledge as part of attended, participatory experience, and re-representations of self became an integral part of these memories as well (see Figs. 11.2C and 13.2A). As ancestral hominins acquired such knowledge, the self-representation feature generated the perception of knowing these facts and generalizations. Likewise, upon retrieval, this representational dimension produced the sense of knowing that characterizes semantic memories.

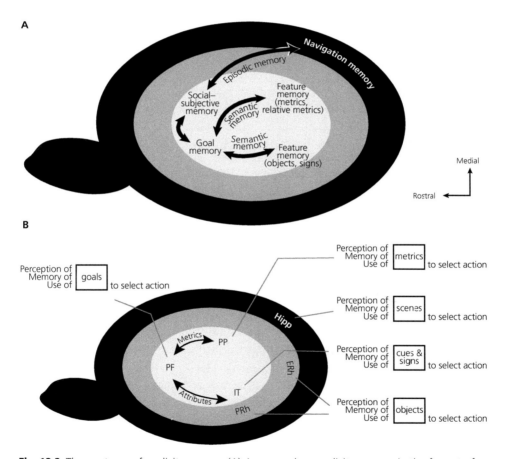

Fig. 13.2 The anatomy of explicit memory. (A) A proposal on explicit memory, in the format of Fig. 2.1. (B) Cortical areas specialize in representations, not memory or perception. Abbreviations: ERh, entorhinal cortex; Hipp, hippocampus; IT, inferior temporal cortex; PF, prefrontal cortex; PP, posterior parietal cortex; PRh, perirhinal cortex.

Part V

Taken together, Parts I–IV showed how an evolutionary perspective can provide a conceptual framework for understanding how distinct representational systems interact and generate a sense of participating in our past, present, and future—both as individuals and as members of society. In Part V we returned to the history of research on memory systems, a topic that we introduced in Chapter 1. According to Chapter 12, a series of experiments in monkeys led to the two concepts that have dominated the field of memory research for three decades: a "medial temporal lobe memory system" and a basal ganglia (or striatal) "habit system." Neglect or misunderstanding of evolution, and especially brain evolution, contributed to the many shortcomings of these doctrines.

In this chapter we conclude by considering some possible tests of the evolutionary accretion model, revisiting the famous patient H.M., summarizing our main conclusions, and indulging in some concluding commentary.

Tests

To have scientific value, our proposals must be testable in some way, like any other hypothesis or theory. Evolutionary theories present special difficulties in this regard because they depend on information about extinct species or about a diverse selection of modern species.

Each species has its own set of representational systems

The first test concerns the overarching theme of this book: New representational systems emerged as evolutionary adaptations to new ways of life. We predict that when comparative research has identified the representational systems in a sufficient diversity of vertebrates, their distribution will demonstrate that each lineage developed a unique set of such systems, adding to or subtracting from each one's ancestral state. That information will be a long time coming, however, and it will require considerable research on species that have received little attention from laboratory researchers to date.

The hippocampus specializes in navigational representations

Our proposal depends upon the idea that the mammalian hippocampus performs a navigational function that has been conserved among vertebrates. If future experiments overturn this idea, our proposal would perish. A comparative analysis might someday show, for example, that some other structure in the vertebrate brain subserves navigation.

Our proposal does not, however, imply that hippocampal function is confined to navigation. Indeed, in Chapter 4 we explained that the hippocampus adopted additional functions based on the specialized representations used for navigation and that, as new representational systems evolved and provided the hippocampus with novel kinds of information, its functions expanded further. The proposal we presented in Chapter 11 depends on this idea.

So our prediction is that the hippocampus of modern vertebrates performs a mixture of conserved and derived functions. In Chapter 10 ("Situational contexts") we discussed the idea of perspective-taking for scenes as one example of a derived function. Another involves the perception of someone else's knowledge, which people can use as contextual information for alleviating semantic ambiguities and establishing semantic common-ground (see Chapter 10, "Language in amnesia").

The granular prefrontal cortex evolved in primates

The proposals presented in Chapters 6, 8, 10, and 11 depend on several unorthodox (and, in some circles, unpopular) ideas: that the first granular prefrontal areas evolved in primates; that other such areas evolved in anthropoid primates; and that these areas became elaborated during hominin evolution. The refutation of these ideas would invalidate our proposals. (Readers who reject them probably reached that conclusion early in Chapter 1, anyway). We explained in Chapter 2, in brief form, some of the arguments that support our view of cortical evolution. It should be easy to show that we are wrong, if that is the case. If the several granular prefrontal areas in anthropoids have homologues in murine rodents, for example, then rodent researchers should be able to support this conclusion by citing a constellation of diagnostic properties that distinguish the granular prefrontal cortex from all other cortical areas. Neither vague allusions to amalgams nor a list of similarities will do, but the standards of comparative neurobiology can be met if a homologue of the granular prefrontal cortex exists in murine rodents and other nonprimate mammals.

Small violations could be accommodated. Perhaps the polar prefrontal cortex first appeared in early primates and did not await the upward grade shift in brain size that occurred in anthropoids (see Chapter 2, "Anthropoids"). If so, then the amendments to our proposal would not shake it too much. Along the same lines, rodents and primates diverged tens of millions of years ago, which has allowed ample time for the properties of homologous areas to change. Accordingly, the demonstration of differences between homologous cortical areas in primates and rodents would not weaken our proposal appreciably, absent a comprehensive phylogenetic analysis.

Multiple demand cognition depends on elaborated anthropoid areas

Our proposal also depends on current ideas about cross-domain, multiple demand processing in the granular prefrontal and posterior parietal cortex (see Chapter 9, "Parietal–prefrontal networks") and similar ideas about a semantic hub in the anterior temporal lobe (see Chapter 9, "Temporal–prefrontal networks"). It would contradict important aspects of our proposal, therefore, if, as some experts currently believe, there is no semantic hub and no such thing as multiple demand cognition.

It would not, however, contradict our proposal if additional cortical hubs came to light. According to one idea, the interactions between the prefrontal cortex and the anterior temporal lobe are paralleled by hub-like interactions between the prefrontal and postero-medial cortex[5], an idea we explored in Chapter 10 ("Situational contexts").

Humans have a species-specific form of self-representation

Because re-representations of one's self and others are central to our ideas about explicit memory, we expect that a comprehensive assessment of the kinds and levels of social–subjective representations across primates would be helpful in either confirming or over-turning the proposals we presented in Chapters 10 and 11.

Prefrontal–hippocampal interactions are crucial to explicit memory

The proposal in Chapter 11 on explicit memory relies on reasonably direct connections between the hippocampus and the prefrontal cortex (see Fig. 11.6, excluding part A, and Fig. 11.7). If future work undermines the neuroanatomical findings that we rely upon, that would argue against our ideas. Some experts, for example, believe that these connections are less extensive than our reading of the literature suggests.

Only humans have explicit memory

The idea that explicit (declarative) memory is a derived hominin trait is sure to generate some resistance, to put it mildly. If explicit memory can be demonstrated in rodents or monkeys, for example, then we must be wrong. We know that many experts believe that this trait has already been demonstrated in animals, but we explained in Chapter 11 ("Do animals have explicit memory?") why we disagree. Exploration of these issues will require a validated nonverbal assay for explicit memory.

The idea that animal researchers cannot study explicit memory—because their subjects do not have this trait—might seem, at first glance, to undermine the study of animal memory. It shouldn't. If we are correct, then animal experiments can-not examine explicit memory directly, but they *can* explore exaptations for explicit memory. We recognize that this idea might not be particularly satisfying, either for funding agencies or for popular accounts of memory. That is unfortunate, but as Darwin[6] (p. 147) put it so gracefully, "there is grandeur in this view of life." Memory researchers can magnify that grandeur in a way that scientists in other fields can never hope to match. Rather than viewing other species as "models" of ourselves, we can strive to appreciate each species in its own right, in relation to the lives that its individuals lead—to quote Darwin[6] (p. 147) again—in "endless forms most beautiful and most wonderful."

Methodological advances for testing our proposals

Currently, the disruption of cortical activity by rTMS cannot test our proposals because it mostly affects the surface of the brain. In the future, however, it might become possible to inactivate deep brain structures temporarily and selectively in humans. We imagine a method analogous to optogenetic manipulations, in which neurons might be filled with an otherwise innocuous molecular agent that selectively inactivates them only when con-verging beams of energy (like x-rays) sum in a precisely delineated area to exceed a thresh-old. This imaginary method would allow investigators to selectively and simultaneously inactivate structures such as the hippocampus and prefrontal cortex before, during, and after an attempt to acquire new episodic memories, for example. Another new approach might involve the study of functional dissociations among white matter pathways that align with distinct representational systems[7]. Given that much of our interpretation of H.M.'s amnesia relates to disconnections, methods that reversibly inactivate selected fiber tracts would enable several tests our proposals.

H.M.'s amnesia

Future tests aside, some readers will wonder whether our proposals can even account for current knowledge about human amnesia. To address this issue, we return to the famous case of H.M. In Chapter 1 we described his impairment in traditional terms—an anterograde amnesia for long-term semantic and episodic memories, supposedly global in scope.

Episodic memory

According to our proposals, the establishment of new episodic memories requires re-representations of one's self to interact with the extended hippocampal–navigation system. In Chapter 10 ("Medial network") we explored this network in detail. Removal of H.M.'s amygdaloid (anterior) hippocampus and entorhinal cortex cut many of the connections between his hippocampus and prefrontal cortex, especially for the medial prefrontal cortex. These aspects of H.M.'s lesion probably eliminated the contribution of the medial network to establishing new episodic memories.

The idea that prefrontal–hippocampal interactions underlie the acquisition of episodic memories raises two related questions: (1) why don't bilateral lesions of the prefrontal cortex cause amnesia; and (2) how did H.M.'s lesion cause severe anterograde amnesia even though his entire prefrontal cortex and some of his hippocampus remained intact?

On the first question, we proposed in Chapter 10 ("Medial prefrontal cortex") that species-specific self-representations originate in the medial prefrontal cortex. During childhood, however, representations of self become distributed elsewhere in the cortex, such as the lateral prefrontal cortex, the cortex of the temporal–parietal junction, the superior temporal cortex, and the anterior temporal lobe semantic memory system (see Chapter 10, "Lateral network"). For example, as people mature they develop concepts and generalizations about themselves that probably draw on representations in the medial prefrontal cortex but reside in the lateral network—the anterior temporal lobe in this case. These representations are probably sufficient to generate a sense of participation in events, even in the absence of a contribution from more direct prefrontal–hippocampal interactions.

This idea also helps answer the second question. H.M.'s lesion eliminated indirect pathways for establishing episodic memories as well as relatively direct ones, so it did not matter (for this purpose) that his prefrontal cortex and some of his hippocampus remained intact. According to our proposals, H.M.'s lesion disrupted fiber tracts in his anterior temporal stem and other parts of his temporal white matter (see Chapter 11, "Disconnection" and Chapter 12, "H.M.'s ablation"). These lesions not only disrupted prefrontal–temporal interactions, but also those between self-representations in his lateral network and what remained of his extended hippocampal–navigation system. In less affected patients, these pathways can support the establishment of new episodic memories.

H.M.'s impairment in episodic memory was anterograde because his intact cortex retained the self-representation features that had been incorporated into episodic memories established before his surgery, as illustrated in Fig. 11.2(C). A great deal of attention has been devoted to the extent of retrograde amnesia in H.M. and other amnesic patients, and they do have some difficulties in this regard[8–10]. For example, H.M. struggled to recollect his presurgical life in detail[2]. However, his impairment in the recall of past events paled in comparison with his devastating incapacity to remember events that occurred after his surgery, and so it is reasonable to emphasize his anterograde amnesia.

Although H.M. had many intact retrograde memories, like everyone else he failed to remember events from his early childhood. Young children have excellent memories, but adults (and even adolescents) recollect very few, if any, episodic memories about their early childhood. This universal phenomenon is called neonatal amnesia, and it probably results from the immaturity of the prefrontal cortex, the hippocampus, or both[11,12]. In terms of our proposals, the immaturity of these structures prevents the encoding of episodic memories in a form typical of adults or adolescents. As childhood progresses and self-representations become widely distributed in the cortex, the semantic memory system develops progressively more complex generalizations and concepts about one's self. Accordingly, the nature of self-representation changes, and the simpler, early forms no longer evoke the sense of having participated in a recalled event.

Semantic memory

In addition to his impairment in episodic memory, H.M. had a severe inability to establish and recall new semantic memories[13]. Other amnesic patients also have impairments in semantic learning, but they can acquire new knowledge much better than H.M. could, albeit slowly, and these memories can persist[14,15].

According to our proposals, H.M.'s semantic memory impairment was more severe than that of typical amnesic patients because of the more extensive fiber-tract damage in his case (see Chapter 11, "Disconnection" and Chapter 12, "H.M.'s ablation"). As a result, his anterior temporal lobe had more difficulty integrating self-representations into new semantic memories. Removal of his amygdaloid (anterior) hippocampus caused additional impairments, especially for rapidly acquired semantic memories (see Chapter 9, "Hippocampal complex" and Chapter 12, "The summation principle").

In less-affected patients, both prefrontal–temporal routes and other "spoke"-to-hub pathways supply self-representations to the semantic memory system in a way that can bypass the medial network (see Chapter 10, "Medial network"), including the hippocampus. As a result, self-representations can enter into their new semantic memories, although only slowly and with repeated exposure (see Chapter 12, "The summation principle").

Short-term memory

H.M.'s relatively preserved capacity for short-term memory depended on his intact sensory and prefrontal areas, as did his ability to attend to sensory information. This does not imply that H.M. had an entirely normal short-term memory, however. Recent research has demonstrated impairments in amnesic individuals for certain kinds of short-term memory, in particular for tasks that require a flexible, viewpoint-independent representation of a spatial environment[16]. These observations highlight the representational specializations of the hippocampus and the fact that its functions cut across process-related concepts like perception and memory.

Perception

In Chapter 7 we dismissed the perception–memory dichotomy on empirical grounds. The fact remains, however, that H.M.'s amnesia was not accompanied by pervasive perceptual impairments. H.M.'s intact prefrontal and posterior parietal cortex probably accounted for much of his preserved perceptual and perceptual-learning ability, along with whatever temporal areas remained both intact and connected with other parts of the cortex. From the study of other amnesic patients, we know that they have preserved or impaired perceptual learning depending on the stimulus material used for testing[17]. Again, representational specializations explain these results; process-based concepts do not.

Skill memory

H.M.'s preserved motor skill learning resulted from his intact manual–foraging system (see Chapter 6), and he also had fairly normal language skills. Upon closer examination, however, H.M. had some intriguing language impairments, including problems in answering questions about agents and subjects in sentences, in dealing with sentences that included ambiguities and figurative phrases, and in describing the competing meanings of ambiguous language (see Chapter 10, "Language in amnesia"). As in other amnesic patients, these impairments probably reflected the disruption of interactions between H.M.'s social–subjective and hippocampal–navigation systems, which led to problems with perspective-taking, identifying with communication partners, and using context to resolve ambiguities.

Conclusions

The prevailing view of memory systems consists of several related tenets: (1) four cortical areas—the parahippocampal, perirhinal, entorhinal, and hippocampal cortex—compose a "medial temporal lobe" system for explicit (declarative) memory; (2) the basal ganglia, as a whole, subserves habits; (3) the four so-called "memory areas" lack perceptual functions; and (4) monkeys, humans, and rodents share explicit memory by virtue of inheritance from a common ancestor.

The proposals presented in this book, which we call the evolutionary accretion model, differ from these tenets in every respect (see Table 1.3):

1. All cortical areas store memories based on their specialized representations (Fig. 13.2B). Accordingly, several areas outside the so-called "medial temporal lobe" contribute to explicit memory, including the prefrontal cortex and the anterior temporal lobe.

2. The basal ganglia supports each representational system as a component of cortex–basal ganglia "loops" (see Fig. 2.3B and Plate 1B)—an archetypal telencephalic architecture that evolved early in the history of vertebrates. This concept explains why only a part of the basal ganglia has anything to do with habits.

3. Many cortical areas function in both perception and memory, including those that the prevailing view classifies as parts of the so-called "medial temporal lobe" (Fig. 13.2B).

4. Modern humans have inherited several representational systems, each of which evolved in the distant past as a specific ancestor adapted to a new way of life (Fig. 13.3). Explicit memory does not arise from any one of these systems. Instead, this uniquely human trait depends on interactions between species-specific re-representations of self and other representational systems, including a navigation system that evolved early in the history of vertebrates (Fig. 13.2A). A sense of experiencing events and knowing facts results from these interactions.

When—sometime during hominin evolution—episodic and semantic memories combined with "explosive generalization" across cognitive domains (see Fig. 11.8), our ancestors developed rich autobiographical narratives, a repository of conceptual knowledge, and the capacity for cultural innovation that characterizes modern humans (see Fig. 11.1C and Plate 6).

Epigraphs and endings

We conclude with comments on two epigraphs, the one that began this chapter and the one for the book as a whole. In the former, the Wizard of Oz calls the brain a "very mediocre commodity" because "every ... creature that crawls on the earth or slinks through slimy seas" has one. Even wizards are sometimes wrong. Anemones slink through seas every now and then, entirely without a brain. And simply "having" a brain doesn't explain very much. Many of the lineages depicted in Figs. 13.1 and 13.3 have developed their own brains, and they all deserve attention. Given the relentlessly promoted "language" capacities of parrots[18], monkeys[19], chimpanzees[20], and orangutans[21,22], perhaps they will tell us all about it someday. And by orangutans, here, we mean the orange-haired apes who live in earthly jungles, not the guardians of scientific orthodoxy on the *Planet of the Apes*[23].

In the epigraph for this book, a chimpanzee on that planet, Dr. Zira, explains evolution to a human astronaut. Apes and humans, she says, "evolved from a point in common but in different directions, the former gradually developing to the stage of rational thought,

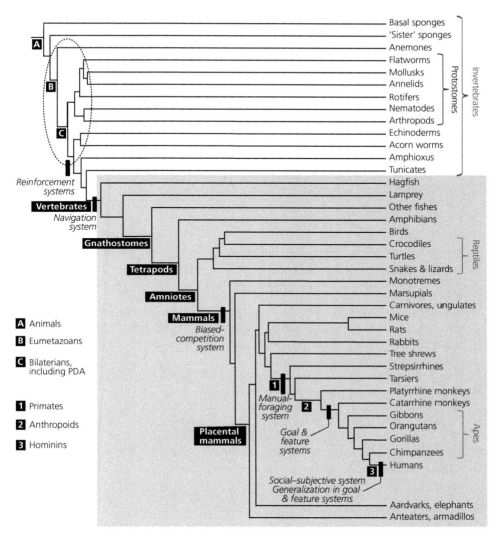

Fig. 13.3 Cladogram of animals. Background shading marks the vertebrates. Vertical black bars indicate the lineage in which each memory system first appeared.

the others stagnating in their animal state" (Boulle[23], p. 127). Readers of the novel eventually learn that Dr. Zira harbors some serious misconceptions about primate evolution on her planet. Not only do its humans have "rational thought," but neither apes nor humans are likely to "stagnate" very much on any planet.

As an up-and-coming chimpanzee at the mercy of old-school orangutans, Dr. Zira also expresses exasperation at the refusal of the entrenched scientific authorities to embrace evolution. That happens on our planet, too. The humans on the *Planet of the Apes* could never appreciate the evolution of their memory systems. On our planet, we can.

References

1. **Fleming, V.** (director) (1939) Metro-Goldwyn-Mayer.

2. **Corkin, S.** (2013) *Permanent Present Tense* (Basic Books, New York).

3. **Passingham, R.E.** and **Wise, S.P.** (2012) *The Neurobiology of the Prefrontal Cortex* (Oxford University Press, Oxford).

4. **Genovesio, A., Wise, S.P.,** and **Passingham, R.E.** (2014) *Trends Cogn. Sci.* **18**, 72–81.

5. **Ritchey, M., Libby, L.A.,** and **Ranganath, C.** (2015) *Prog. Brain Res.* **219**, 45–64.

6. **Darwin, C.** (1859, 2004) *The Origin of Species* (Castle Books, Hoboken, NJ).

7. **Hodgetts, C.J., Postans, M., Shine, J.P., Jones, D.K.** et al. (2015) *eLife.* **4**, 07902.

8. **Nadel, L.** and **Moscovitch, M.** (1997) *Curr. Opin. Neurobiol.* **7**, 217–227.

9. **Moscovitch, M., Nadel, L., Winocur, G., Gilboa, A.** et al. (2006) *Curr. Opin. Neurobiol.* **16**, 179–190.

10. **Squire, L.R.** and **Bayley, P.J.** (2007) *Curr. Opin. Neurobiol.* **17**, 185–196.

11. **Shaw, P., Kabani, N.J., Lerch, J.P., Eckstrand, K.** et al. (2008) *J. Neurosci.* **28**, 3586–3594.

12. **Gogtay, N., Nugent, T.F., Herman, D.H., Ordonez, A.** et al. (2006) *Hippocampus* **16**, 664–672.

13. **Gabrieli, J.D.E., Cohen, N.J.,** and **Corkin, S.** (1988) *Brain Cogn.* **7**, 157–177.

14. **Gardiner, J.M., Brandt, K.R., Baddeley, A.D., Vargha-Khadem, F.** et al. (2008) *Neuropsychologia* **46**, 2865–2868.

15. **Holdstock, J.S., Mayes, A.R., Isaac, C.L., Gong, Q.** et al. (2002) *Neuropsychologia* **40**, 748–768.

16. **Hartley, T., Bird, C.M., Chan, D., Cipolotti, L.** et al. (2007) *Hippocampus* **17**, 34–48.

17. **Mundy, M.E., Downing, P.E., Dwyer, D.M., Honey, R.C.** et al. (2013) *J. Neurosci.* **33**, 10490–10502.

18. **Pepperberg, I.M.** (2010) *Brain Lang.* **115**, 81–91.

19. **Poremba, A., Malloy, M., Saunders, R.C., Carson, R.E.** et al. (2004) *Nature* **427**, 448–451.

20. **Savage-Rumbaugh, E.S.** (1988) In: *Comparative Perspectives in Modern Psychology* (ed. Leger, D.W.), pp. 201–255 (University of Nebraska Press, Lincoln, NE).

21. **Shumaker, R.W., Walkup, K.R.,** and **Beck, B.B.** (2011) *Animal Tool Behavior: The Use and Manufacture of Tools by Animals* (The Johns Hopkins University Press, Baltimore, MD).

22. **Lameira, A.R., Hardus, M.E., Bartlett, A.M., Shumaker, R.W.** et al. (2015) *PLoS One* **10**, e116136.

23. **Boulle, P.** (1963) *Planet of the Apes* (Ballentine, New York).

Epilogue

Our part titles made use of construction metaphors, such as foundations and architecture. So, too, could our principal proposal: Human memory emerged though piecemeal additions—metaphorical bump-outs, sun rooms, conservatories, and the like—which occurred at various times in the distant past for reasons best understood in the context of those times.

Metaphors are especially apt because the evolution of memory systems empowered them, as both the Lion Man of Hohlenstein and the Cowardly Lion attest (see Fig. 11.1A). In a double metaphor, *The Lion in Winter*, King Henry II, faces his demise. "I will die sometime soon," he says, "One day I'll duck too slow, and at Westminster, they'll sing out 'long live the king' for someone else." The ability to face death in this way results from navigating representations of one's self through imaginary events. Paradoxically, this mental activity can create a peculiar kind of immortality: scenarios of afterlife, fantasies in which one's self survives death. As Hamlet (*III, i,* 67) wondered in a particularly memorable metaphor: "In that sleep of death what dreams may come?"

Through memory and metaphor we can even imagine the language parrot, Alex, flying off to that Great Cage in the Sky to spend his afterlife reading Shakespeare. With due respect to the never-ending squawking about uniquely human cognitive capacities, only people generate scenarios that reflect empathy for the postmortem intellectual life of another species, ascribe intentions to its members by analogy with our own, and engage in constructive episodic simulations on their behalf. Despite his impressive abilities, we doubt that Alex could ever have imagined a lion acting like a person—or a parrot—as people do so effortlessly.

The epigraph to Chapter 11 quoted a lion acting like a person. The Cowardly Lion asked "What makes the Hottentot so hot?" and "What have they got that I ain't got?" The proper name for Hottentots, Khoikhoi, means "people people," which is entirely appropriate to the Lion's query. He wanted to know what makes people people. The Cowardly Lion provides an answer all by himself. A metaphor for fearful valor, this creation emerged when a human brain navigated its social–subjective representations through scenarios embracing a broad scope of knowledge. The emergent trait that enabled this mental activity came to be called explicit or declarative memory by the only animals who can call it anything, and it's what we've got that they ain't got.

In this book, we have used memory and metaphor to advance a scenario about memory's past. Using our theory of mind, and with ample empathy, we encourage others to pursue our project and to mend our mistakes. It is inevitable, in any event, that others will take up the topic again some day. Because memory is born of biology, a powerful current runs relentlessly to its roots. Struggle as we might upstream, toward understanding memory in modern times, the surge will someday send us to the sea, where the vertebrate brain arose and the evolution of its memory systems began. Although much about memory eludes us:

> that's no matter—to-morrow we will run faster, stretch out our arms farther.... And then one fine morning—
> So we beat on, boats against the current, borne back ceaselessly into the past.

F. Scott Fitzgerald, *The Great Gatsby* (Scribner, New York, 1925, p. 180)

Index

Tables, figures, and boxes are indicated by an italic *t*, *f*, and *b* following the page number.

abstract rules 272, 278–9, 290, 358–9, 433–4
abstract strategies 279, 285, 287–90
abstractions 391–2
accumbens *see* nucleus accumbens; striatum; ventral
    basal ganglia; ventral striatum
action–effect associations 391, 418
action modules 194*f*, 209–11, 210*f*
action–outcome associations 94–5, 97, 104, 181–3
Aegyptopithecus xv, 62*f*, 69–71, 70*f*
affordance-competition model 212–14, 213*f*, 220
affordances 183, 211–12
agency 353, 359, 390, 418
agnathans xv, 45*f*, 46
agranular insular cortex 23, 24*t*, 40*f*, 54*f*, 56, 59, 65*f*,
    154–61, 171*t*, 179, 183, 269*f*, 271, 307, 314,
    366, 399, 415*f*
agranular orbital–insular cortex *see* agranular insular
    cortex; agranular orbitofrontal cortex; lateral
    agranular prefrontal cortex
agranular orbitofrontal cortex 166*f*, 171*t*, 179–83
agranular prefrontal cortex 64–6, 154, 156–84
    connections 157–60, 158*f*
    lateral 157–9, 171*t*, 179–83
        see also agranular insular cortex; agranular
        orbitofrontal cortex
    medial 158*f*, 159, 160–72
        see also anterior cingulate cortex; infralimbic
        cortex; prelimbic cortex
agreeableness 370
Alex the gray parrot 34, 476, 479
allocentric (extrinsic) reference frames 165–7, 180–1,
    452–4, 453*f*
allocortex xv, 20, 40*f*
    allocortical ring around neocortex 57–61
    amygdala transition area 161*f*
    amygdalohippocampal transition area 40*f*, 57
    amygdalopiriform transition area 40*f*, 57
    anterior olfactory nucleus 19*f*, 40*f*, 52*f*, 65*f*, 155*f*
    connections 159–60, 161*f*
    cortex–basal ganglia loops 41*f*, 42*f*, 59–61, 77,
        103, 159, 161*f*, 427, 459, 476, Plates 1–2
    dorsal cortex 40*f*, 51*f*, 52*f*, 53
    early amniotes 40*f*, 48–52
    early mammals 51*f*, 52*f*, 154, 155*f*
    hippocampus *see* hippocampus
    induseum griseum 18, 57
    lateral cortex 40*f*, 51, 55, 58
    olfactory bulb 45*f*, 46
    olfactory cortex *see* piriform cortex
    piriform cortex 19*f*, 40*f*, 46, 50–60, 76, 155–6*f*,
        158*f*, 198*f*, 415*f*, 466*f*

tenia tecta 18, 40*f*, 57
transition cortex 57–8
allometry 306, 347–9
Alouatta see howler monkeys
Alzheimer's disease 251–2, 317, 319
amalgam theory of cortical evolution 66
amnesia 319, 427–59
    amygdala plus hippocampus model 435*f*, 436–40, 455
    anterograde 3–4, 432, 473–4
    global 3–4, 397
    H.M.'s 3–5, 428–31, 473–5
    language impairments 373–5
    lesions 5, 397–400, 428–31
    monkey models 5, 429*b*, 432–41, 458
    neonatal 474
    receiver operating characteristic
        analysis 411–12, 412*f*
    retrograde 4, 474
amniotes (early) xv, 28*f*, 48–55, 76
    cerebral cortex 40*f*, 48–50
    navigation memory 147
amphibians xv, 48, 51*f*, 100
Amphioxus 43*f*, 44, 46, 477*f*
amygdala
    basolateral nuclei 97, 110
    central nucleus 90, 97, 109, 110
    extended 60
    lateral nucleus *see* basolateral nuclei
    lesions 398–9
    medial nucleus 90
    orbitofrontal interactions 214–16, 215*f*
    Pavlovian conditioning 88–90
    plus hippocampus lesions 435*f*, 436–40, 455
    reinforcer devaluation effects 96–7, 214–16, 215*f*
    striatal 41*f*, 42*f*, 54*f*, 59–60, Plates 1–2
amygdalohippocampal transition area 40*f*, 57
amygdaloid (temporal) hippocampus 17, 135, 147
    prefrontal cortex interactions 158*f*, 178
    semantic memory 317
    social–subjective memory system 362*f*, 369–70
amygdalopiriform transition area 40*f*, 57
analogical reasoning 311–13, 311*f*, 312*f*, 390–1, 418
analogy (vs. homology) 30, 35
anatomy *see* neuroanatomy
anemones *see* sea anemones
angiosperm trees 68–9, 268–9
animal learning theory 95, 98, 110–11, 113–14
    navigation 122, 125–6
    see also reinforcement memory system
animal models 136, 427–9, 432–41, 445, 458–9, 472
animal rights 361

animals, evolution of 86–7
animate items in semantic dementia 327–9, 367–8
annelids *see* protostomes
anomia 328, 330
anterior cingulate cortex 17, 21*f*, 169–70, 171*t*,
   182–3, 351
   on gyrus 351, 356–7
   in sulcus 357
anterior hippocampus *see* amygdaloid (temporal)
   hippocampus
anterior intraparietal area 21*f*, 201
anterior pituitary gland 47
anterior temporal lobe 246, 307, 390, Plates 2–4
   Herpes simplex virus encephalitis 327–8
   semantic dementia 318, 322, 323
   semantic hub *see* semantic hub
   semantic memory 10, 323–4, 330–1, 333,
      Plates 3–4
   social–subjective system 366–8
   surgical removal in epilepsy 329–30
anterior thalamic nuclei 407
anterograde amnesia 3–4, 432, 473–4
anthropoids xv, 61, 62*f*, 67–72, 468
   behavioral adaptations 67–9
   brain size 69–71, 70*f*, 345–6, 348*f*
   catarrhines *see* catarrhines
   cortical connections 196*f*, 197, 198*f*
   evolution 67–72, 230–1, 268–9, 471
   feature memory system 231–63
   goal memory system 267–97
   navigation memory 136–44, 147
   new cortical areas 40*f*, 64, 65*f*, 66, 71–2, 76,
      193*f*, 196*f*
   orbitofrontal–premotor interactions 219
   platyrrhine–catarrhine divergence 61, 68, 70–1
   platyrrhines *see* platyrrhines
   prefrontal cortex volume 73, 74*f*
   social cognition 345
   vision 67–8, 230–1, 260
   see also apes; hominins; humans; monkeys
anthropomorphism 361
anticipatory contrast effect 179
anxiety 135, 175
ape–human (hominoid) lineage 72, 74*f*, 306, 384*f*
apes 230*f*, 384*f*, 387, 403, 466*f*, 476–7
   brain size 347, 348*f*
   new cortical areas 74–6
   regional brain expansion 347–9
   see also chimpanzees; hominins
Aplysia 99
Appendicularians xv, 9, 44, 45*f*
arbitrary categorization 278
arbitrary mapping 259, 276–7
arboreal quadrupeds 68, 268
architectonics 24, 63–4, 74–5
arcuate fascicle 318, 430*f*
Ardipithecus 384*f*
area 5 205, 256–7, 256*f*
area 7 205
area TA 325, 367
area TE 21*f*, 24, 399

area TEO 21*f*, 24
ascidians xv, 9, 44, 45*f*
association cortex 307–8, 308*b*
attention
   goal memory system 292–5
   learning theory 99, 108, 110–11
   manual-foraging system 221
   representations of self and others 352–4, 355–6
   top-down biased competition 99, 185, 220–1,
      268–74, 291–6, 305, 307, 334–5, 352–4
attributes (attribute features) xv,
   232–5, 275–9, 468
audition 154, 262
auditory cortex, primary (A1) 55–6, 56*f*, 58
auditory stimuli 91, 105, 331, 407
Aurignacian culture 384*f*, 385, Plate 1
Australopithecus see australopiths; hominins
australopiths xv, 57, 348*f*, 384*f*
autism 403
autobiographical memory 355, 363, 418
autobiographical simulation 363–4, 418
automatic behavior 292, 294*f*
autonomic nervous system 160, 161*f*
autonomic responses 88, 169, 359
autopilot control 207–8
avoidance behavior 88, 100–1
awareness 222, 375, 413, 456
   see also self-awareness

baboons 259
basal forebrain xv, 60, 138
basal ganglia 17, 19–20, 19*f*, 42*f*, 76
   autopilot control 208
   dorsal 456–7
   extended 17, 59
   forward model 457–8
   habit–memory dichotomy 449–57
   habits vs. outcome-directed behavior 163–5,
      164*f*, 450–2
   homologues 46
   prevailing view 60–1, 77, 449, 470
   reinforcement learning 88, 89–90, 109, 111–12
   ventral 109, 111–12
   see also cortex–basal ganglia loops; pallidum;
      striatum
baseball 10, 305
basilar pontine nuclei 105, 106*f*
basolateral nuclei of amygdala 97, 110
bats 31, 32–3*b*, 33, 35
bed nucleus of the stria terminalis 19*f*, 41*f*, 60,
   Plate 1
behavioral inhibition 175–6
behaviorism 85–6, 113, 122, 126
biased-competition memory system 12–13,
   153–85, 467
   agranular prefrontal cortex, role in 156–83
   augmentation by goal memory system 291–5
   authors' proposal 157
   sensory neocortex 183–4
biconditional task 238
bipedalism 72–3, 387, 403

birds 32–3*b*, 35, 49*b*, 50, 51*f*, 53, 60, 98, 267
   explicit memory 408
   instrumental learning 101
blattopterans *see* cockroaches
blindness, congenital 206
blocking (Kamin blocking effect) 89*b*, 91–2, 107
bonobos *see* apes
boundary cells 127
brain
   anatomy 17–24, 18*f*, 19*f*
   evolution 9, 39–78, 465, 466*f*
   lesion effects 25–6
   regional expansion in hominins 73, 74*f*, 306–7,
      306*f*, 347–9
   social factors in evolution of 344–7
brain expansion *see* brain size
brain imaging 25–7
   attentional control of behavior 292
   general problem solving 311*f*, 312–13, 314*f*
   goal memory system 273–4
   metric coding 310
   navigation memory 144–5, 145*f*
   perception and memory 259
   perceptual learning 251–2
   semantic memory 324, 330–3, Plates 3–4
   social–subjective system 355–9, 355*f*, 361,
      367, 371
brain size
   anthropoids 69–71, 70*f*, 345–6, 346*f*, 348*f*
   early mammals 153, 184–5
   hominins 73, 345–7, 348*f*, 387–8
brainless conditioning 94*b*
brainstem 105, 108, 210
Broca's area 75
burial 385, 420
bushbabies 63–4, 193*f*, 194*f*, 195, 230*f*

callitrichids *see* marmosets; tamarins
Cambrian explosion 86
canine teeth, hominin 387–8
capuchin monkeys 259
Carpolestes xv, 62–3, 192, 193*f*
catarrhines xv, 61, 68, 71
categorical knowledge 318–19, 324
caudal prefrontal cortex (PFc) 21*f*, 22, 64, 197, 198*f*,
   200, 220–1
caudal primary motor cortex 72
caudate nucleus 19*f*, 20, 41*f*, 42*f*, 64, 164–5, 164*f*,
   294*f*, 450, 454–5
   see also striatum
cause-and-effect knowledge 390, 418–20
cave art 384*f*, 385, 389
Cebus monkeys *see* capuchin monkeys
central nucleus of the amygdala 90, 97, 109, 110
cephalochordates 44, 46
cerebellar cortex 105, 106*f*, 108
cerebellar flocculus 33*b*
cerebellum 90, 105–8
cerebral cortex 20–4
   basal ganglia loops *see* cortex–basal ganglia loops
   early mammals 55–61, 154–7, 155–6*f*

early primates 63–6, 192–5, 196*f*
   evolution 40*f*, 48–50, 51*f*, 76
   hominins 74–6, 306–7, 306*f*
   homologies 46, 50–5
   ring structure 40*f*, 57–61
   see also allocortex; neocortex
change–shift strategy 285, 290
Chauvet cave drawings 384*f*, 385, Plate 1
chicks/chickens 53, 54*f*, 60, 98
   see also hen
Chilecebus xv, 62*f*, 70*f*, 71
chimpanzees (and bonobos) 306, 384*f*
   brain size 345, 347, 348*f*
   metric abilities 308–10
   new cortical areas 75
   regional brain expansion 73, 74*f*, 306–7, 306*f*,
      Plate 2
   see also apes, panins
cholinergic neurons 109, 138
chordates xv, 43*f*, 44–6, 466*f*
cingulate cortex *see* anterior cingulate cortex;
      posterior cingulate cortex
cingulate motor areas 21*f*, 24, 270
cingulum bundle 361
clade xv, 28–30
cladistics xv, 28–30
claustrum 46–7
climatic cooling, global 71, 292
climbing fibers 105–8, 106*f*
clique size, social 345–6, 346*f*, 350–1
Cnidaria 93
cockroaches 94*b*
cognitive domains 307, 402
   models of semantic memory 324, 326
   semantic dementia 318–20, 323
cognitive maps 122–34, 147, 207, 255*b*, 365
cognitive modules 222, 309*b*, 402
cognitive psychology 95, 110, 125–6, 309*b*
cold-blooded animals 32*b*, 170
color 229, 231, 233–4, 277–9
color–place cues, conjunctive 142, 144
color vision, full (trichromatic) 68, 71, 138,
   260, 429*b*
common ground 373–5, 374*f*
communication 36, 372–5, 429*b*
comparative neuroanatomy 46, 56–8, 77,
   165, 450–2
comparator functions 103–8
compound discrimination learning 181
compound stimuli 89*b*, 238–40, 239*f*, 433
compulsivity 175–7
computational bottlenecks 293, 296
computational costs 98, 112, 292
computational models
   nonlinear scaling 306
   perception–memory dichotomy 252–4
   semantic memory 324–30
conceptual knowledge 318–20, 323–4
   see also semantic memory
concurrent discrimination learning *see*
      multiple-pair task

conditional motor learning 284–5, 285*f*, 290, 409–10, 410*f*, 433
conditioned inhibition 167–8
conditioned place preferences/aversions 406–7
conditioned responses/reflexes 87, 89–90, 410–11
conjunctive representations
 abstract dimensions 391–2
 false recognition 243, 244
 feature ambiguity 237–41, 246–9, 373–5
 feature memory system 234, 241, 253–5, 260
 feature overlap *see* feature ambiguity
 goal memory system 269, 271, 274–5, 296
 levels 233
 manual-foraging system 216
 mid-level 233–4, 260, 335, 390
 object representations 243, 391
 self-representations, included in 391–6, 400, 418, 469, 474
connectionist models 252–3, 326–8
constructive episodic simulation 363–4, 418
context pathway, goal memory system 269*f*, 270
contexts
 current vs. obsolete 177–8
 goal memory system 270–9
 hippocampal function 174–5, 364–5
control policies xv, 206–7
cooperation, social 358–9, 403–4
coordinate frames *see* reference frames
core neocortex 40*f*, 57–8, 154, 155*f*
 connections 160, 161*f*
 medial and lateral networks 361, 362*f*
corpus callosum 28–31, 33–4, 277
cortex–basal ganglia loops 41*f*, 59–60, 76–7, 476
 agranular prefrontal cortex 159–60
 cortical rings and 41*f*, 60
 early primates 192, 194*f*
 granular orbitofrontal cortex 217–18
 habit–memory dichotomy 455, 457–8
 memory systems and 42*f*, 60–1, Plate 1
 reinforcement learning 112
corticospinal projections 72, 209–10
cost–benefit analysis 111–12, 169–70, 177
Cowardly Lion, The 383–5, 384*f*, 389, 391*f*, 420, 465, 479
crabs 100
craniates 45*f*, 46
creative explosion 386, 388, 402, 404
credit assignment 280–2, 281*f*
crossed-disconnection lesions 25–6
 biased-competition system 172–7
 goal memory system 279, 283*f*, 284, 286*f*, 287–9
 navigation memory 138
crown group 28
cultural innovation 385–8, 402, 418–20
cultural knowledge 315–16, 396

Darwin, C. 119, 472
decapods *see* crabs
decision variables 213, 275
declarative memory *see* explicit memory

decontextualization 391–3
deep cerebellar nuclei 105–8, 106*f*
 see also cerebellum
default-mode network *see* medial network
defensive responses, conditioned 88–91
delay intolerance 179–80
delay tolerance 179–80
delayed alternation task 273
delayed copy-drawing test 322
delayed matching-to-sample task 25, 436
 see also matching tasks
delayed nonmatching-to-sample task 25, 436
 see also matching tasks
delayed response task 272–3
dentate gyrus 17, 50, 51*f*
depth perception 63, 138, 202
derived traits xv, 30
detour task 455
deuterostomes xv, 43–4, 43*f*, 46
 see also cephalochordates; chordates; tunicates
devaluation effects 96–7, 162*f*, 163, 214–16, 215*f*, 450
devaluation task 214–15
 see also devaluation effects; reinforcers, devaluation
D.F. (patient) 211–12
diencephalon 46, 112
difference vector 202*f*, 204*f*, 205–8
diffusion tractography xv, 75, 313–15, 318, 398, 400, 431*b*
discrimination reversal tasks 288–9
discrimination tasks
 learning set 287–9
 monkey models of amnesia 433–4, 439–40
 perception–memory dichotomy 235–41, 245–9
distance 192, 200, 229, 257, 259, 275, 308–9, 468
diversity denial 49*b*, 113, 441
dopaminergic neurons *see* dopaminergic system
dopaminergic system 64, 88, 89*b*, 217
 comparator functions 103, 105, 108
 cost–benefit analysis 111–12
 evolution 99, 112
dorsal basal ganglia 456–7
 see also pallidum; striatum
dorsal cortex 40*f*, 51*f*, 52*f*, 53
dorsal hippocampus *see* septal hippocampus
dorsal pallium 19*f*, 54*f*, Plate 2
dorsal prefrontal cortex (PFd) 21*f*, 22, 272
dorsal (visual) stream 195–7, 232
 see also vision, processing streams
dorsal striatum 64, 401, 456–7
 see also striatum
dorsolateral prefrontal cortex (PFdl) 21*f*, 23, 75, 170, 366
 goal memory system 270, 272–3, 274–5, 277, 294
 manual-foraging system 219
 relational reasoning 311*f*, 312
dorsolateral striatum 163–4, 164*f*, 450–4, 451*f*
dorsomedial prefrontal cortex (PFdm) 21*f*, 23
 goal and action pathway 270
 social–subjective system 355–6, 359, 364, 370–1

dorsomedial striatum 163–5, 164*f*, 449–51, 451*f*
Duncker illusion 396*b*
duration 200, 229, 257, 274–5

Ebbinghaus illusion 227–8, 228*f*
ectothermic animals 32*b*, 170
effort tolerance 170
egocentric (intrinsic) reference frames 165–7,
    180–1, 452–4, 453*f*
elemental features 233, 243–4
emotional conditioning 7
empathy 357, 359
encephalization quotient 346–7, 348*f*, 387
    hominin 384*f*, Plate 6
end-effector vector 202*f*, 203–5
end effectors 202–3
endothermic animals 32*b*, 154, 170, 183–4
energy conservation 68, 160, 170, 184
energy expenditure 160, 170, 183–4
entorhinal cortex 21*f*, 57, 184, 446
    equipotentiality principle 442, 443*f*
    explicit memory 414–16, 415*f*
    monkey models of amnesia 437–9, 440*b*
    navigation memory 127, 138
    one-trial learning 409, 410*f*
epilepsy 3, 329–30, 400
episodic-like memory 408–9
episodic memory xv, 395–6, 407–8
    autobiographical memory 355, 363, 418
    autobiographical simulation 363–4, 418
    constructive episodic simulation 363–4
    goal memory vs. 296–7
    H.M.'s 473–4
    semantic dementia 317, 322
    semantic memory vs. 368–9, 396
    summation principle 446
episodic retrieval 322
epithelium 93
equipotentiality principle 441–6, 459
euprimates xv, 62*f*, 63
eutherians *see* placental mammals
event memories, for goals 279–87, 291, 295
evolutionary accretion model 14–16, 14*t*, 15*t*, 476,
    Plate 1
    tests of 470–3
evolutionary psychology 307–8, 309*b*
exaptations xvi, 31, 305, 335, 394–5
experience-distant knowledge 368–9
experience-near knowledge 368–9
explicit memory 383–420, 469, 469*f*
    in animals 404–14, 452, 472
    authors' proposal 392–5
    definitions xvi, 389
    exaptations 394–5
    exclusivity to humans 395, 417, 472
    H.M.'s 4, 399–400, 432
    impaired *see* amnesia
    origin 395–404, 417–18
    prefrontal cortex–hippocampus
        interactions 414–17, 472
    prevailing view 7, 396–7, 427–8, 458

representational systems underlying 393–4
summation principle 446–8
tests, for monkeys 432–3, 439–40
see also episodic memory; semantic memory
explicit recollection 411–12, 434
explosive generalization 402–3, 418–20
extinction (of conditioning) 91–2, 101–2, 107–8,
    167, 179
    reinstatement 167–8, 168*f*
    spontaneous recovery 167–8, 168*f*
extrastriate visual areas 21*f*, 220–1, 234
extrinsic reference frames 165–7, 180–1,
    452–4, 453*f*
eye coordinates *see* reference frames
eye movements 47, 64
eyeblink conditioning 105–8, 106*f*
eyes 47, 63, 67–8

face perception 250–2
face recognition 34, 369
facial nucleus 105, 210
false recognition 242–3, 248
familiarity memory 251, 411–12, 412*f*, 444
Far Side, The 153, 184, 305
fast learning 286–7, 291, 296–7
fear conditioning 89, 135, 410–11
feature ambiguity 237–41, 246–9,
    369, 373–5
feature memory system 12, 13, 227–63, 468
    authors' proposal 231–2
    explicit memory 393
    goal memory system interactions 271–2,
        275, 276*f*
    hominins 307–37
    perception–memory dichotomy 235–55
    social–subjective system interactions 362*f*,
        372, 377
feature
    ambiguity 237–41, 246–9,
        369, 373–5
    conjunctions 233–4, 237–8, 241
    elemental 233, 243–4
    overlap *see* feature ambiguity
    see also attributes; metrics
feedback-based learning 456
feedback, forward models 208, 209*f*, 457
feeding movements 63, 99, 209–11, 210*f*
ferungulate *see* ungulate-carnivore clade
fiber tracts 103
    damage to 397–8, 400, 430*f*, 431, 431*b*,
        437–8, 473–4
    see also white matter tracts
fictional memories 363
fimbria 398
fine-branch niche 62–3, 197–9, 222
fins, paired 31, 48
fire, controlled 387
fish, teleost 100–1
    see also goldfish
Fitzgerald, F.S. 480
flexibility, behavioral 103, 134, 157

foraging
 anthropoids 67–9, 71–2, 233–4, 268–9
 auditory signs 262
 biased-competition memory 163, 169–70
 cognitive maps 122–5
 distance 233–4
 early animals 86–7
 early primates 62–3
 errors, reducing 269, 271, 284, 287–9, 290, 295–6
 goal memory system 268–9, 271–9, 282, 284
 hominins 72, 308–10
 instrumental learning 103
 journeys 126–8, 128f, 132
 metrics 257–9, 308–10
 open field 139t, 140–4
 patient 180
 scene memory 136, 138
 urgent 180
forelimbs 31, 35, 63, 305
foresight 394, 418
fornix
 lesions in human amnesia 398
 monkey models of amnesia 5, 434, 435f, 444
 navigation memory 124f, 125, 127–8, 128f, 137–8,
  137f, 142, 143f
 object-in-place scene learning 407–8, 408f
 object–place–context memories 174
 odd-stimulus-out task 400
 one-trial learning 409, 410f
forward models 207–8, 209f, 457–8
fovea 33, 67–8, 70–1, 260
FOXP2 gene 401
frontal eye fields 27, 64
 see also caudal prefrontal cortex
frontal-pole cortex *see* polar prefrontal cortex
frontotemporal dementia *see* semantic dementia
fruit eating 68–9, 72, 268–9
fusiform face area 324
fusiform gyrus 23f, 331
future-thinking 364, 394, 418

g (general intelligence) 307–13, 309b
 see also multiple demand cognition
Galago see bushbabies
gateway doctrine 414–16, 415f
genes, developmental regulatory 53, 54f, 60
gibbons 74–5
globus pallidus 111
glossiness 12, 200, 215–21, 229, 234, 262, 272, 275,
  276f, 294, 391
gnathostomes xvi, 29f, 48
goal and action pathway 269f, 270
goal-directed behavior *see* outcome-directed
  behavior
goal memory system 12–13, 267–97, 468
 abstract strategies 287–90
 augmenting older representational systems 290–5
 authors' proposal 271
 brain anatomy 230f
 event memories 279–87, 291, 295
 explicit memory 393

hominins 307–37
 new contexts 271–9
 processing pathways 269–71, 269f
 social–subjective system interactions 362f,
  372, 377
goal-related events, single 291, 295
goal tracking 87–8
goal vector 202f, 203
Godzilla 33
goldfish 100–1, 120, 121f, 147
goods models 212–14, 213f, 220–1
granular cortex, defined 20
granular orbitofrontal cortex (PFo) 21f, 23–4,
  64, 214–20
 amygdala interactions 214–16, 215f
 connections 197, 198f, 217, 270
 credit assignment 280–2
 goal memory system 270–1, 284–5
 influence on premotor areas 218–20
 lateral network, part of 367
 manual-foraging memory system 200
 properties 217–18, 218f
 social–subjective memory system 351, 367
granular prefrontal cortex 194f, 390
 attentive control 292–5
 connections 197, 198f, 415f, 416–17, 416f
 event memories 279–80
 evolution 63–6, 76, 471
 expansion in hominins 73, 74f, 348f, 349
 goal memory system 268, 270–1, 283–7,
  289–90, 296–7
 higher representational levels 335–6, 336f
 multiple demand cognition 313, 314f
 new areas in anthropoids 71–2, 76
 semantic memory 332–3
granule cells, cerebellar 105
grasping 63, 192, 201, 319–20
grasping–leaping locomotion 62–3, 192, 222, 268
Great Gatsby, The 480
grid cells 127
grivets 231
gustatory inputs 158f, 159
gustatory stimuli 91

H.M. (patient) vii, 3–6, 473–5
 explicit memory 4, 399–400, 432
 habit–memory dichotomy 455–6
 implicit/skill memory 4, 191–2, 475
 language impairments 373
 lesion 397–400, 428–31, 430f, 431b
 monkey models 5, 433–4, 436–7
 navigation memory 146
 perceptual function 235, 237, 250, 448, 475
 other mentions 8, 11, 16, 200, 222, 319, 409,
  417, 465
habit–memory dichotomy 405, 449–59
habits 7, 60, 95, 433, 449
 behavioral dichotomies 405
 medial agranular prefrontal cortex 161–5, 168–9
 outcome-directed behavior vs. 96, 98, 163–5,
  164f, 450–2, 451f

resource volatility and 98, 292
see also stimulus-response associations
hagfish 45*f*, 46
Haikouella 45
Haikouichthys 45
hand coordinates 202–3
haplorhines xvi, 61–2, 67–8
head-direction cells 127
Heart of Darkness, The 343–4, 377
Heidelberg people *see Homo heidelbergensis*
hen 267
Herpes simplex virus encephalitis (HSVE) 327–9, 335
hidden layer/units, connectionist models 326–9
hierarchies, cortical processing 326–7, 352–4, 366, 376, 403
high-level conjunctive representations 233, 260, 335–6, 336*f*
hindlimb-dominated locomotion 63
hippocampal complex xvi, 17
hippocampal–navigation system, extended
  explicit memory 393, 395, 397, 399, 414, 416–18
  social–subjective system 365, 377
hippocampus 17
  amygdaloid *see* amygdaloid hippocampus
  cognitive maps 122–5
  computational modeling 254
  context information provided by 174–5, 364–5
  equipotentiality principle 442–5, 443*f*
  evolution 50–3, 58, 66, 67*f*, 76
  explicit memory 394, 409–17, 428
  feature-ambiguity experiments 239–41, 240*f*, 246–7
  functions 134–5, 148, 470–1
  goal memory system and 296–7
  habit–memory dichotomy 452–5
  higher representational levels 335–6, 336*f*
  homologues 49*b*, 50–3
  instrumental learning 103, 104*f*
  lesions causing amnesia 398–9, 428–32
  linguistic function 373, 375
  London taxi drivers 145, 145*f*, 370
  medial prefrontal cortex interactions 172–8
  monkey models of amnesia 5, 434–9
  navigation function 120–1, 125, 127–48, 470
  object memory 242
  perception–memory dichotomy 248–52, 254–5
  prefrontal cortex connections 158*f*, 159, 414–17, 472
  scene memory 136–8, 146–7
  semantic memory 317, 446–8
  septal *see* septal hippocampus
  social–subjective system 361–4, 369–70
homeostasis 47
hominids xvi, 384*f*
hominins xvi, 72–6, 384*f*, Plate 1
  Ardipithecus 384*f*
  artifacts 385–8
  brain size 73, 345–7, 348*f*, 387–8
  evolution 306–7, 344–9, 384*f*, 385–9
  explicit memory 383–420, 469
  goal and feature memory systems 305–37

new cortical areas 74–6
parietal–prefrontal networks 308–15
regional brain expansion 73, 74*f*, 306–7, 306*f*, 347–9
Sahelanthropus 384*f*
social–subjective memory system 343–77
temporal–prefrontal networks 315–35
see also australopiths; humans
hominoids xvi, 384*f*
Homo erectus 384*f*, 387, Plate 1
Homo ergaster 348*f*, 384*f*, 387, Plate 1
Homo habilis 348*f*, 384*f*, 387, Plate 1
Homo heidelbergensis (Heidelberg people) 348*f*, 384*f*, 387, Plate 1
Homo neanderthalensis see Neanderthals
Homo sapiens see humans
homologies xvi, 29*f*, 30–1, 35
Homunculus 71
honeybees 93, 100–1, 112
howler monkeys 68
hub-and-spoke model 324–7, 325*f*, 329–30, 331, 333–4
see also semantic hub
humans
  brain map 23*f*
  brain size 347, 348*f*
  cortical homologues 54*f*, 64, 65*f*
  cultural innovation 385–8, 402, 418–20
  evolution 384*f*, 385–9, 420, 476–7
  explicit memory *see* explicit memory
  navigation memory 144–8
  new cortical areas 74–5, 193*f*
  perception–memory dichotomy 246–55
  regional brain expansion 73, 74*f*, 307, 347–9
  scene memory 138, 362*f*, 369, 371–5
  species-specific self-representation 15, 343, 349, 352, 366, 377, 390–5, 400, 416–18, 468–9, 472–3, 476
  unique features 383–5, 389, 390, 420
  visually guided movements 191–2, 207–8, 222
  see also hominins
hunter-gatherers 386, 403–4
hunting 191, 403–4
Huntington's disease 208, 456
hypothalamus 47, 55, 60, 159

ideational apraxia 211
illusions
  Duncker 396*b*
  of otherness 361, 371
  out-of-body experience 353
  visual 227–8, 228*f*, 260, 262, 396*b*
imagined events 363–4
imitation 388*b*
impatience 179–80
implicit memory 395–6, 396*b*, 409
  H.M.'s 4, 191–2, 475
  nonhuman animals 404
imprinting 291
impulsivity 175–7, 180
  see also delay intolerance

inadvertent fiber-tract damage 26, 49*b*, 139, 399,
    437–42, 458
inanimate items in semantic dementia 327–9,
    361, 367–8
independent evolution 31–4
individual identity 371
induced-motion illusion 396*b*
induseum griseum *see* allocortex
inferior longitudinal fascicle 318, 400, 430*f*
inferior olivary nuclei 105–8, 106*f*
inferior temporal cortex 17, 21*f*, 22*f*, 23, 390
    evolution 34, 76
    feature memory system 232–5
    goal memory system 270–1, 277, 284–9
    manual-foraging system 200
    network modeling 253–4
    orbitofrontal cortex interactions 158*f*, 215–17
    perception–memory dichotomy 235, 236*b*, 448
    perceptual learning 71
    social–subjective system 367–8, 370
information overload 99, 111
infralimbic cortex 21*f*, 161–5, 162*f*, 167–9, 170, 171*t*
innate behavior 88, 169
insects
    reinforcement learning 93–4, 100
    wings 32–3*b*
    see also protostomes
instrumental conditioning 95–103, 467
    evolution 99–103
    explaining human behavior 405–7
    interactions with Pavlovian conditioning 97–8,
        165, 176–7
    mechanisms 103–12
    new vs. old memories 167–8
    possible selective factors 98–9
intelligence, general *see* multiple demand cognition
interference 171, 239–40, 243, 248
    proactive 167, 169, 181
internal models 207
internal states
    one's own 353, 355, 359
    other people's 359–60
intraparietal sulcus 22*f*, 23, 211
intrinsic reference frames 165–7, 180–1, 452–4, 453*f*
inverse models 207
invertebrates 43, 91, 94
    see also protostomes
isocortex *see* neocortex
item-in-context task 177–8

jaw, vertebrate 30–1
journeys 126–8, 128*f*, 132, 147
Jurassic Park 58
juxtallocortex 20, 58
    see also ring neocortex

Kamin blocking effect 89*b*, 91–2, 107
Knowledge, The (London taxi drivers) 145, 145*f*, 370

lampreys 45*f*, 46, 112
lancelet *see* Amphioxus

landmark-vector cells 129
language 371–5
    evolution 401–2
    impairments in amnesia 373–5
    "precursors" 34–6, 429*b*
    stroke-induced impairments 331–3
    topic–comment grammar 372, 401
    see also speech; vocalizations
large-scale networks 361–77, 468
    default-mode network *see* medial network
    disconnections in amnesia 397, 400
    interactions between 370–5
    lateral network *see* lateral network
    medial network *see* medial network
    specializations 368–70
latent inhibition 93, 101
lateral agranular prefrontal cortex 157–9,
        171*t*, 179–83
    see also agranular insular cortex; agranular
        orbitofrontal cortex
lateral cortex 40*f*, 51*f*, 55, 58
    see also allocortex
lateral frontal-pole cortex 75
lateral intraparietal area 21*f*, 201, 205, 221
lateral network, large-scale 362*f*, 366–8, 377, 468
    disconnections in amnesia 397, 400
    medial network interactions 370–5
    specializations 368–70
lateral pallium 50, 51*f*, 53–5, 54*f*
lateral septal nucleus 59–60
leaf discrimination 71
leaf eating 62, 71
leaping–grasping locomotion 62–3, 192, 222, 268
learning set 287–9, 288*f*
learning theory *see* animal learning theory
length, relative 257, 258*f*
lexical decisions 375
limbic system 55, 76, 449
linguistic ambiguity 375
linguistic common ground 375
Linnaeus 337
Lion Man of Hohlenstein 384*f*, 385, 389, Plate 1
lions 383–5, 389, 391*f*, 420, 465, 479, Plate 1
lizards 28*f*, 29*f*, 33, 48, 50–3, 51*f*, 52*f*, 120, 121*f*, 147,
        185, 477*f*
locomotion 31, 35, 49*b*, 62–3, 68, 72, 192, 200, 209,
        222, 268, 284, 387, 404, 467
locusts 94*b*
London taxi drivers 145, 145*f*, 370
long-term depression 107–8
long-term potentiation 107–8
lose–shift strategy 289, 434
low-level representations 233, 260, 335
lunar landing 39, 77–8

macaque monkeys
    brain size 70*f*, 184–5
    cerebral cortex 20–4, 21*f*, 22*f*, 193*f*, 307
    feature memory system 230*f*, 233*f*
    goal memory system 272, 287
    neocortex 74

prefrontal cortex 64, 65f, 75
see also monkeys
MacLean, P.D. 55, 449
magnitude of reinforcement extinction (MRE)
 effect 102–3
mammals (early) 29–30, 29f, 467
 biased-competition memory 153–85
 derived traits 57, 154
 instrumental learning 101–3
 neocortex 55–61, 76, 154–7, 155–6f
 see also placental mammals
mammillary bodies 138, 398, 407
manipulating objects 63, 72, 201, 319–20
manual-foraging memory system 12–13, 197–223, 467
 augmentation by goal memory system 290–1
 authors' proposal 200
 caudal prefrontal cortex 220–1
 challenges in fine-branch niche 199–200
 connections 197, 198f
 parietal–premotor networks 201–13
 temporal–orbitofrontal networks 213–20
marmosets 180, 272
marsupials 28f, 29f, 30, 52f
matching tasks
 goal memory system 277–9, 286
 short interval *see* short-interval matching task
 spatial 139–43, 261–2b
 terminology 25, 434
matching-to-position task 169, 174
maze learning 121f, 126b
maze tasks 102–3, 145–6
 see also Morris water maze; plus-maze task; radial-
 arm maze task; T-maze task
medial cortex 40f, 50–3, 51f, 55, 58
 distortions in primates 66, 67f
 lesions in reptiles 53, 147
 navigation function 52f, 53, 120, 147
 see also allocortex; hippocampus
medial frontal-pole cortex 75, 355–6, 355f, 357
medial intraparietal area 21f, 201, 205
medial network, large-scale 361–6, 377, 468
 disconnections in amnesia 397, 400
 lateral network interactions 370–5
 specializations 368–70
medial nucleus of amygdala 90
medial pallium 50, 51f, 53, 54f, 120, 121f
 see also hippocampus; medial cortex
medial prefrontal cortex 24, 24t, 75
 agranular 158–72
 hierarchical organization 352–4
 hippocampus interactions 172–8
 social–subjective system 350–1, 355–60,
 364–6, 368
medial septal nucleus 60
medial temporal lobe memory system 7, 10, 427–8,
 441–59, 470
 alternative view 7–9, 14–16, 458–9, 475–6
 equipotentiality principle 441–6, 459
 evolutionary context 60–1, 77
 habit–memory dichotomy 449–58, 459
 monkey models of amnesia 437–8, 440–1

perception–memory dichotomy 235, 246, 248,
 448–9, 459
summation principle 446–8, 459
mediodorsal nucleus of thalamus 64, 399
Meissner corpuscles 72
memory awareness 413
memory tests
 artificiality 99, 245
 perception tasks vs. 235–7
 task naming 25
mental states
 one's own 356
 of others *see* theory of mind
mental time travel 343, 363–4, 384f, 389, 394, 418,
 419f, 467–8
mental trial and error 113, 350, 363–4, 384f, 388b,
 418, 419f, 467–8
mentalizing *see* constructive episodic simulation
meta-analysis 454b
metamemory 413
metaphor 113, 315, 333, 336f, 377, 384f, 385, 391f,
 392, 402, 418, 467, 479
metaphorical reasoning 384f, 418
metric contexts 274–5, 276f, 366
metrically abstract goals 213, 221
metrically concrete goals 214, 221
metrics xvi, 256–9, 310, 468
 cortical encoding 256–7, 256f, 258f, 274–5, 310
 foraging-related 257–9, 308–10
 goal memory system 272–5
 relational 257–9, 308–10, 366
 visuomotor 192, 201–7, 211–12, 275
mid-level conjunctive representations 233–4, 260,
 335, 390
midbrain 88–90, 103, 108
middle temporal gyrus 23f, 66, 333, 368
misbehavior 97, 165, 177
mobility, animal 86–7
model-free reinforcement learning 126b, 292
Molaison, Henry *see* H.M.
molar teeth 57
mollusks 91, 99–100
monkeys 5–7, 9
 conditioned responses 89b, 91
 episodic memory 407–8
 equipotentiality principle 442, 443f
 explicit memory 409–10, 412–14
 explicit memory testing 432–3, 439–40
 goal memory system 272–4, 277–9, 280–90, 294
 granular orbitofrontal cortex 214–20
 habit–memory dichotomy 454b
 manual-foraging system 203, 205, 209–11, 210f
 metrics 256–9
 models of human amnesia 5, 429b, 432–41
 navigation memory 136–44, 147
 perception–memory dichotomy 235–42
 reinforcer devaluation 96–7
 social cognition 350–1
 stimulus–action dichotomy 182–3
 see also anthropoids; catarrhines; macaque
 monkeys; platyrrhines

monophyletic group 29*f*
monotremes 29*f*, 30
morphed stimuli 238–41, 239*f*, 244
Morris water maze 52*f*, 53, 125, 127, 145–6
mossy fibers 105, 106*f*
motor cortex 21*f*, 24, 72
motor plans
   affordance competition 212–13
   caudal prefrontal cortex 221
   control policies 206–7
   difference vector 204*f*, 205–6
   parietal–premotor networks 218–19
motor skill learning, H.M.'s 4, 191–2, 475
MPTP 112, 455
MRE *see* magnitude of reinforcement
     extinction effect
multiple demand cognition 309*b*, 313–15, 314*f*, 471
multiple-pair task 235–7, 246–8, 249, 287–9, 454–5
muscle memory 222
muscles
   segmented 45
   vertebrate 32*b*, 47
music 406
myelination in cortical areas 63–4, 73

n-back task 273
navigation memory system 12–13, 119–48, 467
   augmentation by goal memory system 290–1
   authors' proposal 121
   evolution 120–1, 147–8
   explicit memory 393
   extrinsic vs. intrinsic coordinates 165–7,
     452–4, 453*f*
   humans 144–8
   monkeys 136–44, 147
   nonspatial representations 128–34
   reptiles 52*f*, 53
   rodents 121–36, 147
   social–subjective system interactions 362*f*,
     365, 377
Neanderthals (*Homo neanderthalensis*) 348*f*, 384*f*,
    386, 401
nematodes 92*f*
neocortex 17, 20, 154–7, 155–6*f*
   advantages of 156–7
   allocortex vs. 48, 50
   core *see* core neocortex
   early 155–6*f*, 156
   early primates 63
   evolution 40*f*, 55–61, 76, 185
   hominins 74–5, 307
   ring *see* ring neocortex
   sensory 183–4
   size and social complexity 345–7
   transition cortex 57–8, 154
neonatal amnesia 474
neural crest 47
neuroanatomy 17–24
neuroendocrine systems 18, 47, 60
neuropsychology 24–7
   conventions 24–5

lesion effects 25–6
   task names 25
neurosecretory systems 18, 47, 60
New World monkeys *see* platyrrhines
newts 100
nictitating membrane response 88
nondeclarative memory *see* implicit memory
nonmatching-to-position task 169, 174
nonspatial representations 128–34
nonspatial visual stimuli 128–9
notochord 44
nucleus accumbens 19*f*, 41*f*, 42*f*, 88, 97, 164*f*,
    294*f*, 357
number 229, 256–9, 275, 308–9
numeracy skills 319

object-in-place scenes task 136–8, 137*f*, 146, 282–4,
    283*f*, 407–8, 408*f*
object–order conjunctions 172–4
object–place conjunctions 139, 139*b*, 172–5
object–place–context conjunctions 174
object recognition 233–4
   false 242–3, 248
   spontaneous 243, 244*f*
   tasks *see* matching tasks
object reversal learning 182–3, 216
object
   analysis 233–4
   features *see* features
   identification 234, 237
   manipulation 63, 72, 201, 319–20
   perception of moving 396*b*
obsolete contexts 177–8
occipital cortex 22*f*
   feature memory system 232–3, 233*f*
   see also visual cortex
oculomotor system 47
odd-stimulus-out task 242, 245, 248–51,
    250*f*, 400
odors 129–32, 130*f*, 131*f*, 133–5, 133*f*, 177–8
Old World monkeys 68, 75, 231, 429*b*
   see also catarrhines
olfactory bulb 45*f*, 46
olfactory stimuli *see* odors
olfactory tubercle 19*f*, 41*f*, 155–6*f*
   see also striatum; ventral basal ganglia; ventral
     striatum
one-trial learning 282, 284, 291, 407, 409–10
open-field foraging 139*t*, 140–4
operant conditioning *see* instrumental conditioning
optic ataxia 211
optogenetics 174, 472–3
orangutans xix, 74*f*, 230*f*, 384*f*, 476–7
   fictional, as scientific authorities xix, 476–7
   see also apes
orbitofrontal cortex 23–4, 24*t*, 75
   agranular 166*f*, 171*t*, 179–83
   connections 157–9, 158*f*
   goal memory system 270
   granular *see* granular orbitofrontal cortex
   lateral network, part of 366–7

order/ordered sequences 131–2, 200, 256,
    275, 308–10
orienting, conditioned 88
otherness, illusions of 361, 371
others (other people)
    goals appropriate to social categories 360
    representations 344–5, 352–7, 365
    representing mental states 358–60
    see also social cognition; theory of mind
out-of-body experience 353
outcome-directed behavior 95–6, 98, 450–2, 451*f*
    explicit and implicit, in humans 405–6
    medial prefrontal cortex, role in 161–5
outcome pathway, goal memory system 269*f*, 270–1
over-training 161–3, 162*f*, 452, 454

pain responses, conditioned 90
pair coding 277
paired-associate task 259, 276–7
pallidum 17, 19–20, 19*f*, 42*f*, 60
    amygdala 54*f*, Plates 1–2
    bed nucleus of the stria terminalis xii, 19*f*, 41*f*,
        60, 111
    cortex–basal ganglia loops 15, 41*f*, 42*f*, 54*f*, 60–1,
        103, 112, 159, 165, 194*f*, 201, 218, 270, 292,
        427, 451, 455, 457, 459, 476, Plates 1–2
    dorsal *see* globus pallidus
    globus pallidus xiii, 18–20, 41*f*, 59
    medial septal nucleus 19*f*, 41*f*, 42*f*, 60, Plates 1–2
    substantia innominata 18, 41*f*, 109, Plate 1
pallium 19*f*, 46, 48
    homologies 50, 51*f*, 53, 54f
    see also lateral pallium; medial pallium
panins xvi, 72, 384*f*
parahippocampal cortex 21*f*, 57
    connections 158*f*, 217
    equipotentiality principle 445
    function 446
    gateway doctrine 414
    spatial memory 139, 146, 184
parahippocampal place area 324
parallel evolution 32–3*b*
parallel fibers 105–8, 106*f*
paraphyletic group xvi, 30
Parapithecus xvi, 70*f*, 71
parasubiculum 57
parietal cortex 193*f*, 195, 196*f*
    hominins 306–7, 306*f*
    parietal–prefrontal networks 308–15, 389–90
    parietal–premotor networks 201–13
    see also posterior parietal cortex
parietal reach region *see* medial intraparietal area
Parkinson's disease 111, 456
parrots 34, 476, 479
parsimony 14–15, 126
partial reinforcement extinction (PRE)
    effect 101–3, 102*f*
patience 180
Pavlov, I.P. 85–6, 113–14
Pavlovian approach behavior 87–8, 97
Pavlovian conditioning 87–94, 466–7

evolution 91–4
humans 406–7, 433
instrumental learning interactions 97–8,
    165, 176–7
mechanisms 103–14
neural substrates 88–90, 94
new vs. old memories 167–8, 169
Pavlovian-to-instrumental transfer 97
perception 227–9, 259–60
    H.M.'s abilities 235, 237, 250, 448, 475
    perception–action dichotomy 228–9, 228*f*, 285
    perception–memory dichotomy 228–9, 228*f*, 235–
        55, 259, 448–9, 459
    computational models 252–4
    humans 246–55
    monkeys 235–42
    prevailing doctrine 235–7
    rodents 242–5
perception tasks 235–7
perceptual learning, visual 70–1, 251–2, 253*f*
periallocortex 20, 58
perirhinal cortex 21*f*, 55, 184, 400, 446
    equipotentiality principle 442, 443*f*
    feature-ambiguity experiments 237–8, 240–2,
        240*f*, 246–7
    feature memory system 233–4, 253–4
    gateway doctrine 414
    goal memory system, and 270–1, 277
    manual-foraging memory system 200, 215–17
    monkey models of amnesia 437–9, 440*b*
    perception and memory functions 243–5,
        248–52, 254–5
    perception–memory dichotomy 235, 236*b*, 448
    semantic memory 317
personality traits 356, 370–1
perspective-taking 365–6, 375, 471
physiological responses, conditioned 88
picture-naming task 321*f*, 322
pigeons 85, 101, 104*f*, 121*f*, 414
pigs vii, 29*f*, 85, 97, 254, 316, 328, 331, 335, 391*f*, 392
piriform cortex 40*f*, 54*f*, 76
    early mammals 57
    homologies 50, 51*f*, 53–5, 58
    see also allocortex; lateral cortex; lateral pallium
pituitary gland, anterior 47
place cells, hippocampal 122–4, 127–9, 135
placental mammals 29–34, 29*f*, 466*f*
    cerebral cortex 40*f*, 57
    cortical connections 195, 196*f*
placodes, embryonic 47
Planaria 91
Planet of the Apes viii, xix, 476–7
platyrrhines xvi, 56*f*, 61, 68, 71, 180,
    259, 272, 348*f*
plesiadapiforms xvi, 61–3, 193*f*
plus-maze task 122, 124–5, 147, 165, 175,
    452–3, 453*f*
polar prefrontal cortex (PFp) 21*f*, 24, 74–5, 283*f*,
    284, 471
pop out 221
posterior cingulate cortex 21*f*, 361, 368

posterior granular cortex in bushbabies 64
posterior hippocampus *see* septal hippocampus
posterior parietal cortex 73, 76, 193*f*, 195
  action modules 209–10
  affordances 211
  anthropoids 230–1
  connections 197, 198*f*
  feature memory system 231–2
  general problem solving 311*f*, 312–13, 314*f*
  goal memory system 275
  metric representations 256–7, 256*f*, 258*f*, 275, 310
  semantic memory 333
  social–subjective system 357–8, 371
  visually-guided movements 200, 202–5, 208
postrhinal cortex 242
PRE *see* partial reinforcement extinction effect
precuneus cortex 23*f*, 361
precursors 35–6
predation 13, 15–16, 39, 43, 46, 63, 67–71, 76, 87–90,
    120, 147, 262, 267–8, 292, 295, 345, 387,
    393, 467–8
  risk, behavioral responses 68–9, 175
  social complexity and 345–6
prediction-error signals 105–10
prediction signals 105–8, 110–11
preferential viewing 236*b*
prefrontal cortex 21*f*, 22–4
  agranular *see* agranular prefrontal cortex
  anthropoid elaborations 71–2, 76, 275, 276*f*
  caudal (PFc) 21*f*, 22, 64, 198*f*, 200, 220–1
  disconnections in amnesia 397–400
  dorsal (PFd) 21*f*, 22, 272
  dorsolateral *see* dorsolateral prefrontal cortex
  dorsomedial *see* dorsomedial prefrontal cortex
  early primate innovations 63–6, 76, 275, 276*f*
  general problem solving 311*f*, 312–13, 314*f*
  goal memory system 267–71, 277–89, 294–7
  granular *see* granular prefrontal cortex
  hierarchy 352–4, 403
  hippocampus connections 158*f*, 159, 414–17, 472
  hominins 73–6, 74*f*, 306–7, 347–9
  medial *see* medial prefrontal cortex
  metric representations 257, 258*f*, 274–5, 310
  parietal–prefrontal networks 308–15, 389–90
  polar (PFp, frontal-pole cortex) 21*f*, 24, 74–5,
      283*f*, 284, 471
  semantic memory 332–5
  temporal–prefrontal networks 315–35
  ventrolateral *see* ventrolateral prefrontal cortex
  ventromedial 24, 356–7, 359–60
  working memory theory 273
prelimbic cortex 21*f*, 161–5, 162*f*, 167, 169, 170,
    171*t*, 180–1
premotor cortex 24, 195
  action modules 209–11
  connections 197
  goal memory system, and 270
  granular orbitofrontal cortex influences 218–20
  manual-foraging system 200
  parietal–premotor networks 201–13
  vision-for-action 261–2*b*

presubiculum 57
presupplementary motor area 356
primary auditory cortex (A1) 55–6, 56*f*, 58
primary motor cortex (M1) 21*f*, 24, 72
primary somatosensory cortex (S1) 55–6, 56*f*, 58
primary visual cortex (V1) 21*f*, 55–6, 56*f*, 58, 184
  feature memory system 233–4, 260
primates (early) 191–223, 467
  cladogram 230*f*
  evolution 61–7, 62*f*, 192–7, 471
  fine-branch niche 62–3, 197–9, 222
  frontal cortex connections 197, 198*f*
  manual-foraging memory system 197–223
  medial cortex distortion 66, 67*f*
  new cortical areas 63–6, 76, 192–5, 196*f*
  social cognition 345
  stimulus–action dichotomy 182–3
  visual and behavioral adaptations 63
  see also anthropoids; hominins; monkeys
priming 7
principal sulcus 17, 22*f*
prisoner's dilemma 351
proactive interference 167, 169, 181
probabilistic classification tasks 456
probe tests 133–4, 214, 241
problem solving, general 309*b*, 310–13, 314*f*
  see also g; multiple demand cognition
procedural memory *see* implicit memory
process and knowledge distinction 171–2, 268, 271,
    334, 353
proisocortex 20, 58
  see also ring neocortex
proprioception 203–5
prosimians xvi, 61–4
prosopagnosia 329
prospection/prospective coding 287–9, 363–4,
    394, 418
prosubiculum 57
protolanguage 401–2
protostome–deuterostome ancestor (PDA) 43–4
protostomes xvi, 43–4, 43*f*, 46
  reinforcement learning 91–4, 92*f*, 99–100, 112
proxy terms 404, 409, 414
pterosaurs 31, 32–3*b*, 305
Purkinje cells 105, 107–8
putamen 450–1, 455
  see also striatum
pyramids and palm trees test 316, 330

quadrupedal locomotion 68, 72, 76, 268, 322

raccoons 192
radial-arm maze task 125, 145–6, 454
rats *see* rodents
Raven's matrices 311, 311*f*
re-representations 351–4, 365, 372, 376, 395–6
reaching movements 192, 193*f*, 200
  parietal–premotor networks 201–8, 211
  spatial memory 138–40
  see also visually guided movements
reality monitoring 364

receiver operating characteristic (ROC)
    curves 411–13, 412*f*
recency memory 132, 413, 436, 444
recognition memory tasks *see* matching tasks
reference frames
    extrinsic vs. intrinsic 165–7, 180–1, 452–4, 453*f*
    visual 201–7
reflected self-knowledge 356
reinforcement memory system 12, 85–114,
    292, 466–7
    augmentation by goal memory system 291
    authors' proposal 114
    evolution 86–7
    instrumental conditioning 95–103
    mechanisms 103–12
    model-based 126*b*, 292
    model-free 126*b*, 292
    Pavlovian conditioning 87–94
reinforcer
    devaluation 96–7
    primary and secondary 95
relational memory 132
relational reasoning 310–13, 311*f*, 468
repeat–stay strategy 285, 290
representational systems 6, 465
    evolution 11–13
    evolutionary accretion model 14–15, 14*t*, 15*t*,
        470, 476
    reptiles xvi, 29*f*, 32–3*b*, 48, 50–3, 51*f*, 52*f*, 121*f*, 153,
        184, 477*f*
"reptilian brain" 15–16, 55, 185, 449
resource volatility 71, 98, 292–3
response–outcome (R–O) associations *see* action–
    outcome associations
retina
    coordinate frames 201–2, 205–6
    image stabilization 33
    see also fovea; vision
retrograde amnesia 4, 474
retrosplenial cortex 23*f*, 146, 184
reversal learning 166*f*, 168*f*, 180–3, 216
reversal set 289
reversal tasks 139*t*, 165–6, 168*f*, 180–3, 216
ring neocortex 40*f*, 57–8, 61, 154, 155*f*
    caudal 183–4
    connections 159–60, 161*f*
    medial and lateral networks 361, 362*f*
    rostral *see* agranular prefrontal cortex
    transition areas 57–8
    see also juxtallocortex; periallocortex; proisocortex
Road Not Taken, The 8, 427–8, 439, 441, 458–9
rodents (including rats)
    biased-competition memory 157, 161–83
    explicit memory 411–12, 452
    frontal cortex 64–6, 65*f*
    habit–memory dichotomy 449–54
    instrumental learning 96–7, 102–3, 104*f*
    navigation memory 121–36, 147
    parietal cortex 193*f*, 195
    Pavlovian conditioning 88–9
    perception–memory dichotomy 242–5

role-based categories 390–2
routine trichromatic vision *see* trichromatic vision
rule-switching tasks 279

saccadic eye movements 206–8, 374*f*, 375
Sahelanthropus 384*f*
salience 201, 221
satiety/satiation 96–7, 142, 162*f*, 214–16
scenario construction 146–7, 363–4, 418
    see also constructive episodic simulation
scene memory 121, 128–9, 132, 135–40, 146–7, 369
schizophrenia 403
sea anemones 43*f*, 87, 91, 92*f*, 93–4, 113, 466,
    476, 477*f*
sea hare/slug *see* Aplysia
secondary visual cortex (V2) 21*f*, 34, 40*f*, 55, 155–6*f*,
    194*f*, 198*f*, 259–60
selective satiation procedure 96–7, 142, 162*f*, 214–16
    see also devaluation effects; reinforcer devaluation
selective-value effect 310
self, representations of 344–5, 355–6, 359
    decontextualization 392–3
    species-specific hominin 15, 343, 349, 352–4,
        365–6, 377, 390–6, 400, 416–18, 468–9,
        472–3, 476
self-awareness 113, 359, 367, 383, 389, 394
self-knowledge, reflected 356
self-reference effect 357–8
semantic aphasia 331–3, 335
semantic association tasks 325*f*, 330–1
semantic categories 326–7, 390–1
semantic concepts 326–7, 390–1
semantic control 331–4
semantic dementia 316–23, 335, 447
    anatomy 316–18
    computational models of 326–7
    Herpes encephalitis vs. 328
    learning integrative concepts 323
    perception–memory dichotomy 246–9, 251–2
    social knowledge 367
    specific impairments 318–20, 330, 332–3
    typicality and frequency effects 320–2, 321*f*, 326
semantic generalizations 316, 327, 420
semantic hub 323–7, 325*f*, 329–30, 331, 333–4, 471,
        Plates 3–4
    disconnection in amnesia 397, 399
    human cultural innovation 402, 418–20
    social–subjective system 367–8, 377
semantic judgment test 332–3
semantic knowledge 319, 320–3, 326–7, 371
semantic memory xvi, 315–35, 390
    animate vs. inanimate items 327–9
    anterior temporal lobe hub *see* semantic hub
    basic-level concepts 326–7, 376
    brain imaging 324, 330–1
    computational models 324–7, 329–30
    decontextualization 391–3
    dimming vs. distortion 328–9
    episodic memory vs. 368–9, 396
    exaptations 335
    general-level concepts 326–7, 376

semantic memory (*Cont.*)
  Herpes simplex virus encephalitis 327–9
  H.M.'s 474–5
  hub-and-spoke model 324–7, 325*f*, 329–31, 333–4
  impairments 318–22, 327–33
  social concepts and categories 344, 367–8
  specific-level concepts 326–7, 376
  summation principle 446–8
  temporal–prefrontal interactions 334–5
semantic representations 322, 328, 332
  see also semantic memory
sensory modalities 307
  in agranular prefrontal cortex 158*f*, 159
  in posterior parietal cortex 202–4
septal hippocampus 17, 67*f*, 134–5, 159, 246, 317,
     319, 362*f*, 431*b*
  London taxi drivers 145, 145*f*, 370
  perceptual learning 251–2
  prefrontal cortex interactions 158*f*, 178
  social–subjective system 362*f*, 369–70
septal nuclei 59–60, 103
  see also lateral septal nucleus; striatum
sequences *see* order/ordered sequences
serial discrimination learning *see* single-pair task
sexual dimorphism 387–8
shape 229, 231, 233–4, 248
shared knowledge 373–5
short-interval matching task 25, 113, 130, 139–40,
     142–4, 169, 174, 236*b*, 242, 251, 257–62,
     411, 413–14
  equipotentiality principle 442–5, 443*f*
  feature memory system 257, 258*f*
  goal memory system 274, 277–9, 286
  habit–memory dichotomy 455
  monkey models of amnesia 434–58
  see also matching tasks
short-term memory 4, 311, 409, 475
  see also working memory
sign tracking 87–8, 433
single events, memories of 273, 282, 291, 296
  goal related 291, 379–87, 468
  see also one-trial learning
single-pair task 235, 236*b*, 238, 287–9
sister group xvi, 30
situational contexts 364–6
situational models *see* situational contexts
skill memory *see* implicit memory
small-branch niche *see* fine-branch niche
Smith, H.W. 11, 15
snails 91, 99–100
snakes 28*f*, 29*f*, 34, 48, 67*f*, 91, 254, 313, 351,
     466*f*, 477*f*
snapshot memory 53, 136, 255*b*
SNc *see* substantia nigra pars compacta
SNC *see* successive negative contrast effect
social categories 360, 367–8
social classifications 368
social cognition 344–7
  ancestral mechanisms 350–1
  interactions of self and others 356–7
  representations of others 344–5, 356–7

representations of self 344–5, 355–6
somatic marker hypothesis 359
theory of mind 353, 358–60, Plate 5
social communication 429*b*
  see also language; speech; vocalizations
social concepts 367–8
social groups
  competition and cooperation 358
  size 345–6, 346*f*, 350–1
social modeling 363–4
social rules/norms 359–60, 367
social–subjective memory system 12–13,
     343–77, 468
  authors' proposal 349–50
  emergent properties 358–61
  evolution 344–9
  explicit memory 393
  large-scale cortical networks 361–75, 376–7
  medial prefrontal cortex 355–8, 355*f*
social–subjective representations 351–8, 376
  see also others; self
social threats 90
social transmission of food preferences 134–5
somatic marker hypothesis 359
somatosensory cortex, primary (S1) 55–6, 56*f*, 58
source memory 319, 391–3
spatial delayed response task 272–3
spatial goals 122, 147, 212–13, 273
spatial layouts 122, 145, 184
spatial matching tasks 139–143, 261–2*b*
spatial memory 139–44
spatial perception 195–7
spatial reversal task 139*t*, 273
species-specific re-representations of self 15, 343,
     349, 352–4, 365–6, 377, 390–6, 400, 416–18,
     468–9, 472–3, 476
speech
  origin of 35–6, 372, 401–2
  related pathway 313–15
  see also language; vocalizations
spinal cord 18*f*, 19*f*, 72, 210
spontaneous alternation (or exploration) 169, 172–4,
     173*f*, 242–3, 291
spontaneous recognition 236*b*, 243, 244*f*
spontaneous recovery 167–8, 168*f*
squirrels 193*f*, 195
stage models 212–14, 213*f*, 221
stegosaurus 153, 184–5
stem group 28
stereopsis 63, 68, 202
stimulus–action dichotomy 182–3
stimulus associability 99, 108–10
stimulus generalization 98, 278
stimulus–outcome (S–O) associations 87, 93, 97,
     104, 181–3, 405–6, 433
stimulus–response (S–R) associations 95–6,
     163, 450
  see also habits
stimulus–response–outcome (S–R–O)
     associations 95–6, 126, 433
strategy task 279, 280*f*

strepsirrhines xvi, 28*f*, 61–4, 67–8, 70*f*, 71, 193*f*,
    194*f*, 195–7, 209–10, 220, 230*f*, 345–6, 348*f*,
    349–50, 466*f*, 477*f*
striate cortex *see* primary visual cortex
striatum 17, 19–20, 19*f*, 59–60, 64
    amygdala 54*f*, Plates 1–2
    caudate nucleus 19*f*, 20, 41*f*, 42*f*, 64, 164–5, 164*f*,
        294*f*, 450, 454–5
    central nucleus of the amygdala 90, 97, 109, 110
    cortex–basal ganglia loops 15, 41*f*, 42*f*, 54*f*, 60–1,
        103, 112, 159, 165, 194*f*, 201, 218, 270, 292,
        427, 451, 455, 457, 459, 476, Plates 1–2
    dorsal 64, 401, 456
    dorsolateral 163–4, 164*f*, 450–4, 451*f*
    dorsomedial 163–5, 164*f*, 449–51, 451*f*
    habit–memory dichotomy 449–57
    lateral septal nucleus 19*f*, 41*f*, 42*f*, 54*f*, 59–60,
        161*f*, Plates 1–2
    nucleus accumbens 19*f*, 41*f*, 42*f*, 88, 97, 164*f*,
        294*f*
    olfactory tubercle 19*f*, 41*f*, 155–6*f*
    putamen 19*f*, 20, 41*f*, 42*f*, 164*f*, 294*f*, 450, 455
    septal nuclei *see* lateral septal nucleus
stroke 331–3
subiculum 57, 414, 416*f*
subjective memory xvii, 344
    see also social–subjective memory system
subjective value 90, 96, 212, 215–16
substantia innominata 18, 41*f*, 109, Plate 1
substantia nigra pars compacta (SNc) 18, 105, 109
subthalamic nucleus 59
successive negative contrast (SNC) effect 102–3,
    104*f*, 179
summation principle 446–8, 459
superior frontal cortex 23*f*
superior longitudinal fascicle 75, 430*f*
superior parietal cortex 21*f*, 22*f*, 23
superior temporal cortex 21*f*, 22*f*, 23, 75, 192, 194*f*,
    197, 198*f*, 230*f*, 234, 262, 269*f*, 270, 277, 324,
    331, 350, 353, 366, 371, 399, 415*f*, 468, 473
superior temporal gyrus 331
superior temporal sulcus 22*f*, 234, 371
supplementary motor area 21*f*, 24
supramarginal gyrus 23*f*, 313–15
surprise 109–11, 110*f*

T-maze tasks 122, 123*f*, 142, 143*f*, 179–80
tamarins 180
tarsiers xvi, 61, 67–8, 70*f*, 71, 230*f*, 466*f*, 477*f*
task names 25
task rules 257, 278–9
taste aversion learning 91, 96, 291, 450
tastes, recalling 179
taxi drivers, London 145, 145*f*, 370
teaching signal 89*b*, 105–7, 110–12
teeth 57, 387–8
telencephalon xvii, 19–20, 19*f*
    evolution 46–7
    homologies 50, 51*f*
    motor outputs 159, 160*f*
temperature regulation 53, 100, 147

temporal cortex 66, 232
    anthropoids 230–1
    elaboration 75–6
    feature memory system 231–4, 233*f*
    hominins 306–7, 306*f*
    semantic memory 318, 330–1
    social–subjective memory system 367–8
    temporal–orbitofrontal networks 213–20
    temporal–prefrontal networks 315–35
    see also anterior temporal lobe, inferior temporal
        cortex; medial temporal lobe memory
        system; perirhinal cortex; semantic hub;
        superior temporal cortex
temporal hippocampus *see* amygdaloid (temporal)
        hippocampus
temporal-order task 172–4, 173*f*
temporal–parietal junction 331, 353, 367, 368
temporal-pole cortex 318, 325*f*, 366
temporal stem 137–8, 137*f*, 397–9, 430*f*, 437
    see also white matter tracts, lesions/damage
temporally extended events 132, 147, 285–7, 286*f*
tenia tecta 18, 40*f*, 57
    see also allocortex
tenrecs 28*f*, 155–6*f*, 466*f*
tetrapods xvii, 16, 29*f*, 34–5, 48, 51*f*, 121*f*, 305,
    466*f*, 477*f*
thalamus 18–19, 41*f*, 42*f*, 50, 51*f*, 53, 55, 59–60, 64,
    68, 106*f*, 138, 158*f*, 159–60, 194*f*, 294, 317,
    369, 397–9, 431*b*, 438
    anterior nuclei 138, 407
    mediodorsal nucleus 42*f*, 64, 317, 369, 399
theory of mind 353, 358–60, Plate 5
three-arm bandit task 280–2
    see also credit assignment
time cells 132
Tolman, E.C. 122–3, 125–6, 163
tools 39, 200, 203, 211, 315, 384*f*, 387–90, 392, 402,
    404, 420
    Acheulean 384*f*, 387–8
    Oldowan 384*f*, 387–8
top-down attention *see* attention
topic–comment grammar 372, 401
topographic maps 146
topographical memory 319
trace conditioning, Pavlovian 169
tractography *see* diffusion tractography
transcranial magnetic stimulation, repetitive
    (rTMS) 208, 310, 325*f*, 330, 472
transition cortex 57–8, 154
    see also ring neocortex
transitive inference task 310
transverse patterning task 238–40
trash-can categories 94, 292, 405
    see also paraphyletic group; two-factor theories of
        behavior
tree shrews 28*f*, 62*f*, 192, 195, 211, 466*f*, 477*f*
trichromatic (full color) vision 68, 71, 138,
    260, 429*b*
tubes test 413–14
tunicates xvii, 4–5
    see also appendicularians; ascidians

turtles 28*f*, 29*f*, 35, 48, 52*f*, 53, 120, 121*f*, 147, 153, 466*f*, 477*f*
two-factor theories of behavior 291–2, 293*t*, 405
typicality effects 320–2, 321*f*, 326

uncinate fascicle 277, 318, 398–9, 431*b*
ungulate–carnivore (ferungulate) clade 34
upward grade shift, brain size 69–71, 70*f*, 345, 471
urgent foraging 180
    see also delay intolerance

valuation 214–20, 222, 282
ventral basal ganglia 64, 97, 109, 111–12
    see also nucleus accumbens; striatum
ventral hippocampus *see* amygdaloid (temporal) hippocampus
ventral premotor cortex 21*f*, 209–11
ventral stream
    auditory 262
    visual 232–4, 237–8
    see also vision, processing streams
ventral striatum 64, 97
    see also nucleus accumbens; olfactory tubercle; ventral basal ganglia
ventral tegmental area 105
ventrolateral prefrontal cortex (PFvl) 21*f*, 24, 75, 216
    event memories 280–2
    goal memory system 270, 275, 277–9, 284–5, 294
    lateral network 366
    semantic memory 332–5
    social–subjective system 371
ventromedial prefrontal cortex 24, 356–7, 359–60
verbal instructions 371–2
verbal tests 320–2, 321*f*, 330–2
vertebrates (early) 41–8, 76, 466*f*, 467, 477*f*
    brain evolution 45–8, 465, 466*f*
    navigation memory 119–48
    origin 43–5
vicarious reinforcement task 351
virtual reality 129, 145–6, 406
visceral stimuli 158*f*, 159
vision
    anthropoids 67–9, 230–1, 260
    depth perception 63, 138, 202

processing streams 195, 227, 232–4, 237–8, 257, 260–2, 270–2
trichromatic (full color) 68, 71, 138, 260, 429*b*
    see also fovea; retina
vision-for-action 260–2
vision-for-perception 261–2*b*
visual agnosia 211–12
visual cortex
    anthropoids 69–71, 230–1
    extrastriate 21*f*, 220–1, 234
    perception and memory 259–60
    primary (striate) *see* primary visual cortex
    secondary (V2) 21*f*, 34, 40*f*, 55, 155–6*f*, 194*f*, 198*f*, 259–60
visual recognition tasks *see* matching tasks
visual reference (coordinate) frames 201–7
visual scene memory *see* scene memory
visual texture (glossiness, translucence) 12, 200, 215–21, 229, 234, 262, 272, 275, 276*f*, 294, 391
visually guided movements 63, 140, 148, 199–209, 222–3
    autopilot control 207–8
    coordinate frames and transforms 201–7
    object affordances 211–12
    parietal–premotor networks 201–13
vocalizations 34–6, 401–2, 429*b*, 476, 479
    see also language; speech
volatile resources *see* resource volatility

walnut-size brains 153, 185
warm-blooded animals *see* endothermic animals
weather prediction task 456
white matter tracts 75, 361, 430–1
    lesions/damage 137–8, 277, 318, 397–9, 430*f*, 431, 431*b*, 437, 474
    specializations 400
    see also fiber tracts
win–stay strategy 181, 289, 434, 454
wings 6, 31–3, 32–3*b*, 35, 49*b*, 305, 394
Wisconsin card sorting task 278
Wizard of Oz 49*b*, 334, 383–5, 389, 391, 420, 465, 476, 479, Plate 1
word deafness 329
working memory 4, 169, 268, 272–4, 277, 287, 309*b*, 311, 409, 413–14, 434, 475

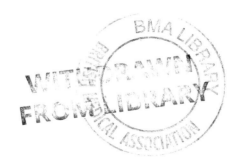